CEREBRAL CORTEX

Volume 1
Cellular Components of
the Cerebral Cortex

CEREBRAL CORTEX

Volume 1
Cellular Components of the Cerebral Cortex

Edited by
ALAN PETERS
Boston University School of Medicine
Boston, Massachusetts

and

EDWARD G. JONES
Washington University School of Medicine
Saint Louis, Missouri

Plenum Press • New York and London

Library of Congress Cataloging in Publication Data

Main entry under title:

Cerebral cortex.

Includes bibliographical references and index.
Contents: v. 1. Cellular components of the cerebral cortex.
1. Cerebral cortex—Collected works. I. Peters, Alan, 1929–   . II. Jones,
Edward G., 1939–   . [DNLM: 1. Cerebral cortex—Anatomy and histolo-
gy. 2. Cerebral cortex—Physiology. WL 307 C4136]
QP383.C45   1984   612′.825   84-1982
ISBN 0-306-41544-5 (v. 1)

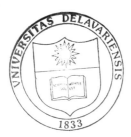

© 1984 Plenum Press, New York
A Division of Plenum Publishing Corporation
233 Spring Street, New York, N.Y. 10013

Printed in the United States of America

Contributors

Heiko Braak — Anatomical Institute, 6000 Frankfurt/Main 70, Federal Republic of Germany

Alan Cowey — Department of Experimental Psychology, University of Oxford, Oxford OX1 3UD, England

Javier DeFelipe — Unidad de Neuroanatomia, Instituto Cajal, CSIC, Madrid 6, Spain. *Present address:* James L. O'Leary Division of Experimental Neurology and Neurological Surgery, Washington University School of Medicine, St. Louis, Missouri 63110

Alfonso Fairén — Unidad de Neuroanatomia, Instituto Cajal, CSIC, Madrid 6, Spain

Martin L. Feldman — Department of Anatomy, Boston University School of Medicine, Boston, Massachusetts 02118

Albert M. Galaburda — Neurology Unit, Beth Israel Hospital, Boston, Massachusetts 02215

Stewart H. C. Hendry — James L. O'Leary Division of Experimental Neurology and Neurological Surgery and McDonnell Center for Studies of Higher Brain Function, Washington University School of Medicine, Saint Louis, Missouri 63110

Edward G. Jones — James L. O'Leary Division of Experimental Neurology and Neurological Surgery and McDonnell Center for Studies of Higher Brain Function, Washington University School of Medicine, Saint Louis, Missouri 63110

Thomas Le Brun Kemper — Department of Neurology, Boston City Hospital, Boston, Massachusetts 02118

Jennifer S. Lund   Departments of Psychiatry, Neurology, and Ophthalmology, University of Pittsburgh School of
Medicine, Pittsburgh, Pennsylvania 15261

Miguel Marin-Padilla   Department of Pathology, Dartmouth Medical
School, Hanover, New Hampshire 03756

Alan Peters   Department of Anatomy, Boston University School
of Medicine, Boston, Massachusetts 02118

José Regidor   Departamento de Biología, Colegio Universitario
de Las Palmas, División de Medicina, Las Palmas
de Gran Canaria, Spain

Richard L. Saint Marie   Department of Anatomy, Boston University School
of Medicine, Boston, Massachusetts 02118

Peter Somogyi   First Department of Anatomy, Semmelweis University Medical School, Budapest 1450, Hungary.
Present address: Department of Human Physiology, The Flinders Medical Centre, Bedford Park,
Australia 5042

Teréz Tömböl   First Department of Anatomy, Histology, and
Embryology, Semmelweis University Medical
School, Budapest 1450, Hungary

Preface

The process of compiling this treatise on the cerebral cortex has been long and has not been easy. For a number of years we had both felt that a series of volumes reviewing the present state of knowledge of the structure and function of the cerebral cortex would be a useful addition to the literature, but we were daunted by fears. At first we felt that we were being too presumptuous in trying to undertake such a task. Then we wondered whether the time was right for producing such a treatise, given the fact that the field is moving so rapidly. Finally, we wondered how the work would be received by our fellow neuroscientists. Eventually we concluded that we had to be presumptuous and that if we waited until we understood everything about the organization and function of the cerebral cortex, the volumes would *never* be published. As to how the work will be received, we will only know after it has been completed and published. Then we shall be able to reflect on what we did wrong! At present, we only know that approaches to our colleagues to contribute chapters have been generally met by enthusiasm, and we have been fortunate in that most of them have readily agreed to make contributions. For their support we are particularly grateful.

The general plan we have formulated in putting together this treatise is as follows. The first volume, the present one, deals with morphological aspects of cortical neurons. It covers the history of studies of cortical neurons and includes sections devoted to cytoarchitectonics and the different types of neurons encountered within the cerebral cortex. Because of their unique and special features, the inner and outer cortical layers are the subjects of separate chapters.

Having thus dealt with the morphology of cortical neurons in this first volume, we will be concerned in the second with the general physiological properties of cortical neurons, with transmitters and receptors in the cortex, with what is presently known about the physiological properties of neurons that have subsequently been recovered morphologically, and with the cortical neuroglial cells.

Later volumes will describe the functional properties of the various known areas of the cerebral cortex and the afferent and efferent connections of the neurons that they contain. We hope to follow these with volumes devoted to the evolution and development of the cerebral cortex, and accounts of how the cortex may be affected by various perturbations.

Clearly, the treatise cannot hope to be totally comprehensive. In choosing what to include, we have been guided by advice from the members of our editorial board. However, if topics dear to the hearts of some scientists have had to be omitted, the responsibility for this rests with us.

In the present volume the authors were asked to write about rather broadly defined topics, and, as a consequence, there may be some overlap in the information contained in the various chapters. This is unavoidable, and we believe that it is an advantage, for in many instances it illuminates the fact that not all scientists agree about how cortical neurons should be categorized or about how the information we have about them should be interpreted. Efforts to eliminate any overlap would not be productive, because such streamlining could only be brought about by the imposition of our own views. Consequently, we have not attempted to change the opinions expressed by any of the authors, but have confined our editing, as far as possible, to inserting references in the text to indicate where the reader can find additional information or further discussion of various topics.

We would like to extend our sincere thanks to the members of the editorial board, and to Kirk Jensen of Plenum Press for encouraging us to develop this series. Without his frequent prompting we would probably still be thinking about this volume. We would also like to thank our secretaries, Ms. Janet Harry and Ms. Margo Gross, for their efforts.

Alan Peters
Edward G. Jones

Boston and Saint Louis

Contents

ix

II. Neurons

Chapter 4

Classification of Cortical Neurons

Alan Peters and Edward G. Jones

Chapter 5

Morphology of the Neocortical Pyramidal Neuron

Martin L. Feldman

Chapter 6

Nonpyramidal Neurons: General Account

Alfonso Fairén, Javier DeFelipe, and José Regidor

Chapter 7

Spiny Stellate Neurons

Jennifer S. Lund

Chapter 8

Basket Cells

Edward G. Jones and Stewart H. C. Hendry

Chapter 9

Double Bouquet Cells

Peter Somogyi and Alan Cowey

Chapter 10

Chandelier Cells

Alan Peters

Chapter 11

Bipolar Cells

Alan Peters

Chapter 12

Neurogliaform or Spiderweb Cells

Edward G. Jones

Chapter 13

Smooth and Sparsely Spinous Nonpyramidal Cells Forming Local Axonal Plexuses

Alan Peters and Richard L. Saint Marie

Chapter 14

Neurons of Layer I: A Developmental Analysis

Miguel Marin-Padilla

History of Cortical Cytology

EDWARD G. JONES

1. The Discovery of Cortical Neurons

It is difficult to ascertain who first *saw* a neuron in the cerebral cortex. It seems evident from modern studies which have attempted to duplicate the conditions of Malpighi's (1666) experiments that the "glands" he described in the human cerebral cortex cannot have been cells (Clarke and Bearn, 1968). Similarly, the often-reproduced figures of Gennari (1782) and Baillarger (1840) that accompanied their descriptions of the laminar structure of the cortex are based upon alternating patterns of gray and white matter as detected with the naked eye or with a hand lens. Cells were obviously not visualized.

Ehrenberg (1833, 1836), an early microscopist, appears to have been aware of neurons in the cerebral cortex of man and animals, referring to them as "granules" or "globules," but he did not illustrate them. Clearer descriptions of nucleated "ganglion bodies" in the cortex are given by Valentin (1836) and Remak (1841). Remak also detected bundles of axons ascending from the white matter and deflecting horizontally especially near the surface of the brain. Remak makes it clear that he felt he could see myelinated fibers in continuity with the processes emanating from the ganglion cells in the cortex, as he had in the spinal and sympathetic ganglia.

EDWARD G. JONES • James L. O'Leary Division of Experimental Neurology and Neurological Surgery and McDonnell Center for Studies of Higher Brain Function, Washington University School of Medicine, Saint Louis, Missouri 63110.

The early observations on the cortex were made on tissue that was unfixed, or, at best, poorly fixed in alcohol; usually it was compressed in water under a cover glass, rather than sectioned, and it was unstained. Fixation in chromic acid was introduced by Hannover in 1840 and the use of carmine as a stain for nerve cells not until 1858 (Von Gerlach, 1872). Between the discovery of the "ganglion cells" in the cortex and the introduction of carmine, von Kölliker (1849) was able to make some crude sketches of cells some of which he called "pyramidal" (Fig. 1). The idea was also gaining acceptance that the myelinated fibers of the white matter were probably continuations of nerve cell processes (reviewed e.g. in Liddell, 1960). But in 1860 von Kölliker still felt obliged to say: "although the conection of the fibres entering into the cortical substance with nerve cells has not, as yet, been actually demonstrated, still I do not hesitate in affirming it; and I regard the cortical substance as the place of origin of all the nerve fibres of the hemispheres and *corpus callosum*." Final confirmation of the original statement by Remak in the cerebral cortex and elsewhere had to await the work of Dieters in 1865. Even by 1905, however, Campbell could still believe that some fibers in the cortex might be "autochthonous."

Von Gerlach in 1858 stained sections cut from material fixed in potassium dichromate with ammoniacal carmine. In the same year, Berlin (1858) applied

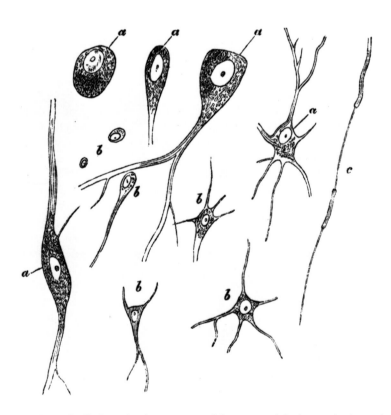

Figure 1. Drawings of cells from the deeper parts of the cortex of the human brain; probably from chromic acid-fixed but unstained material. Cell a at top center is a "pyramidal cell." Reproduced from von Kölliker (1860); drawn in 1852 or earlier for the second edition of his textbook.

the new method to the cerebral cortex for the first time and was able to distinguish not only its arrangement in layers but also several forms of cells that he called pyramidal, granular and spindle-shaped or fusiform (Fig. 2). The originality of these names is, perhaps, questionable since von Kölliker (1852) had already referred to triangular, round, and spindle cells in addition to pyramidal cells in the cortex.

2. Laminar Patterns in the Cortex

Making his first studies on the brains of bats, but later extending them to man and other animals, Meynert (1867–1868, 1869–1872) provided the first systematic descriptions of cortical layering (Fig. 3). His preparations were sections of material fixed in potassium dichromate, stained with carmine, dehydrated in alcohol, and cleared in oil of cloves. To him, the commonest type of cortical stratification, covering the surface of much of the human brain, was a five-layered one (Fig. 3A), consisting of an outer "neuroglia layer" containing a few angular nerve cells, a second layer of small pyramidal cells, a third layer of large pyramidal cells, a fourth layer of multiform or granular cells, and a fifth layer composed of large short pyramids and deeper spindle-shaped cells. His fifth layer, obviously, includes both our layers V and VI. Meynert was also able to detect what he called projection fibers and association fibers entering and leaving the cortex and to trace some of them in continuity with the axons arising from pyramidal cells. The radial fasciculi of the cortex were also his discovery.

Meynert noted three additional layers in the cortex of the calcarine sulcus (Fig. 3B). Examining his drawings, one can see that he merged layers II and III of the five-layered cortex, recognized the three divisions of what many workers now call layer IV in the primate visual area, noted a distinct layer V containing the large solitary pyramidal cells that now bear his name, and divided our layer VI into superficial and deep parts.

The next significant series of studies on cortical lamination were made by Lewis (1878a) and his collaborator, Clarke (Lewis and Clarke, 1878). In the intervening years, Betz (1874) had discovered in the motor cortex of man, dog, and monkey the large pyramidal cells that have come to bear his name.

Lewis gives an account of his methods in the same volume of *Brain* (Vol. 1) that carries his paper on the comparative structure of the cortex in man, sheep, and cat (Lewis, 1878b). He cut unfixed brain tissue on a small freezing microtome, freezing thin blocks in less than 20 sec by the use of an ether spray. They were then cut (at an unspecified thickness) into water. From there, they were mounted on glass slides, fixed in 0.1–0.2% osmium tetroxide and stained with 0.25% aniline black. Before mounting in Canada Balsam, they were dehydrated in sulfuric acid vapor to avoid leaching of the stain by alcohol. Apart from superior staining, Lewis rightly considered that his method of preparation resulted in far less shrinkage of the cortex than occurred after prior dichromate fixation.

The paper by Lewis and Clarke (1878) is devoted to the human motor cortex, as delimited from a comparison with Ferrier's (1874) stimulation maps in mon-

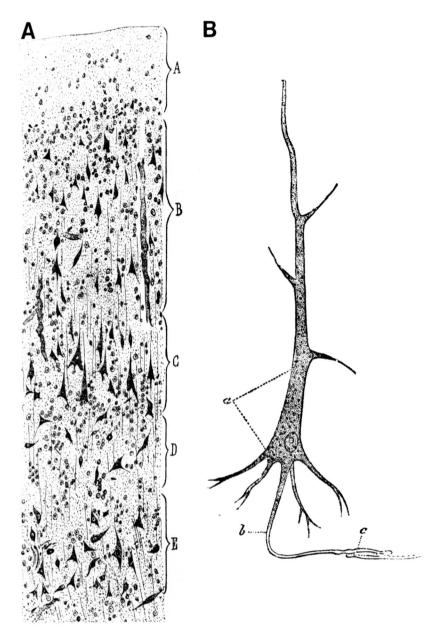

Figure 2. (A) Drawing of part of a section of the cerebral cortex from the brain of a "simpleton," stained with carmine probably after fixation in chromic acid, showing the five layers (A–E) of Meynert with pyramidal, small angular, and fusiform cells. From Dejerine (1895); said to be from an earlier work of Vignal. (B) Pyramidal cell, probably from fixed but unstained material. From Bastian (1880); said to be from an earlier work by Charcot.

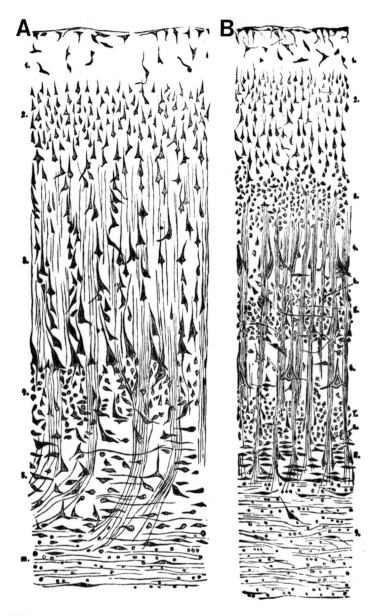

Figure 3. (A) Meynert's drawing of his typical five-layered cortex, from the frontal lobe. (B) Meynert's drawing of "the cortex of the calcarine fissure," showing four additional layers but fusion of layers 2 and 3. From Meynert (1884).

keys. In this, they illustrated the human Betz cells for the first time* and noted that the motor cortex was five-layered. But in his subsequent paper on the comparative anatomy of the cortex, Lewis (1878a) took issue with Meynert and concluded that, apart from the motor area, the cortex was fundamentally six-

* Betz did not illustrate them in 1874, nor in his more comprehensive account of 1881.

layered (Fig. 4). Layer I was regarded as containing no nerve cells. Layers II and III formed a continuum of pyramidal cells of increasing size. Layer IV he regarded as a further layer of small pyramidal cells, exactly similar to those of layer II. This layer he regarded as absent from the motor area. Layer V was the ganglionic layer and layer VI the spindle cell layer. In his later work, seemingly published only as part of the enlarged second edition of Ferrier's work *The Functions of the Brain* (1886), Lewis more clearly identified the granule cells of layer IV in the monkey brain (Fig. 5) and noted seven layers in the visual cortex, the additional layer being formed by a splitting of layer IV.

The subsequent history of cortical lamination has been often told (see Chapter 2). During his brief career, the Swedish worker Hammarberg (1895) sampled a number of cortical regions in man and described laminar variations among

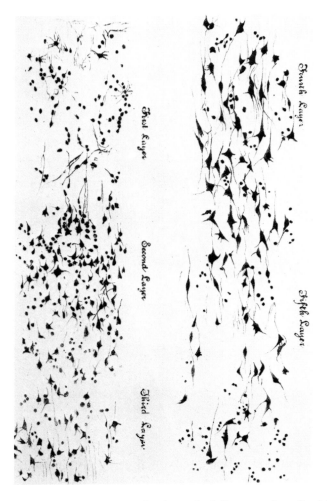

Figure 4. Lamination of the motor cortex of a sheep; fresh frozen sections, fixed in osmium and stained with aniline black. From Lewis (1878a).

them, mainly in terms of a five-layered plan, the internal granular layer being termed layer 4 and described as a layer of small irregular cells.

The first complete description based upon cytoarchitectonic criteria of the extent of a single cortical area was that of Bolton (1900) who delimited the human visual cortex with remarkable accuracy. He numbered the layers only 1 through 5 and though fusing our layers II and III, he clearly identified the three components of layer IV, naming them the outer granular layer, the stria of Gennari, and the inner granular layer (Fig. 6).

Campbell (1905), in the first comprehensive architectonic work on the cortex of man and animals, adopted a seven-layered scheme derived from that of Ramón y Cajal (1904) and seemingly obtained from German translations of Ramón y Cajal's earlier Spanish works (1900–1906). The scheme is not fundamentally different from the six-layered plan of Lewis, the seventh layer being obtained simply by a division of Lewis's (and our) layer III into an outer layer of medium-sized pyramids and an inner layer of large pyramids. Campbell relied upon thionin-stained,* celloidin sections from brains fixed in Müller's fluid, and in addition to pyramidal cells, he observed what he called stellate cells in layer 5 (our layer IV) and spindle-shaped or fusiform cells in layer 7 (our layer VI) (Fig. 7). In the visual area he described two layers of stellate cells in the equivalent of our layer IV.

The idea of six layers as the fundamental cortical pattern became rooted in the literature as the result of its adoption by Brodmann (1903, 1909, 1912) and his teachers, C. and O. Vogt (1919; O. Vogt, 1903). Brodmann's principal reason for adopting this plan stemmed from his belief that it represented the fundamental embryological and evolutionary scheme of cortical organizaiton. The cell types that Brodmann and the Vogt school identified on the basis of Nissl staining were: granular, pyramidal and triangular or fusiform but they made little point of these, their principal emphasis being on the laminar structure as a means of cytoarchitectonic parcellation. By adhering rigidly to a six-layered scheme, they found it necessary in areas like the visual cortex to divide certain layers such as layers IV and VI into sublayers (Fig. 8). These are with us to this day and have often led to endless confusion, especially when cross-species homologies are involved.

As the years passed, the architectonicists of the German school came to place more and more emphasis on myelin stains as a means of delineating cortical areas (Mauss, 1908; Vogt and Vogt, 1919). The Weigert method based on hematoxylin staining, had been introduced in 1882 and the modification of Wolters was used to survey cortical lamination in the human brain by Kaes (1893) who was warmly praised for his observations by Campbell (1905). From Kaes's studies and from the later ones of Edinger (1896), Bechterew (1894), Flechsig (1898), Ramón y Cajal (1909–1911), Campbell (1905), and Brodmann (1909) some of whom used the Pal variant of the stain, a nomenclature relating to the fiber lamination of the cortex emerged (Fig. 8). At the surface is the zonal or plexiform

---

* Nissl had introduced his aniline dye stain in about 1885 but it was not perfected for several years (Nissl, 1903).

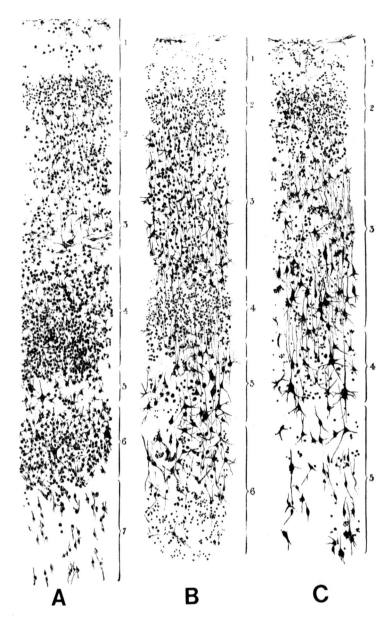

Figure 5. Later drawings by Lewis showing cortical lamination in the monkey. From Ferrier (1886). (A) Occipital lobe; (B) temporal lobe; (C) frontal lobe (probably area 6); (D) motor area; (E) hippocampus; (F) entorhinal area.

layer, consisting of a rather dense plexus of horizontal myelinated axons usually thought by the early workers to arise mostly from Martinotti cells. A thick but lightly myelinated supraradiary plexus corresponds to layers II and III of Nissl stains. In some areas, a thin stria of Kaes–Bechterew may occupy the upper part of layer II. The external band of Baillarger (sometimes called the stria of Gennari

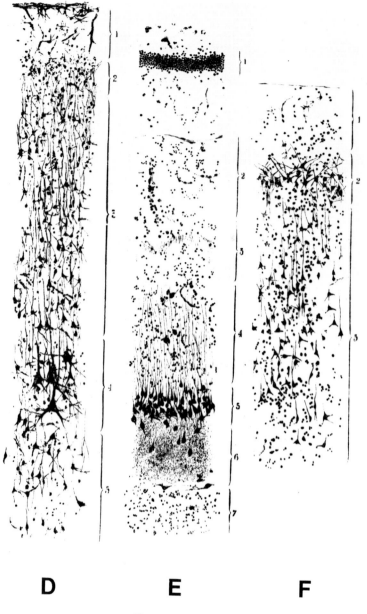

D   **E**   **F**

Figure 5. *(continued)*

even outside the striate area, e.g., by Campbell) corresponds to layer IV and is composed of a dense horizontal plexus. The internal band of Baillarger, another dense horizontal plexus, lies deep in layer V separated from the external band by a lightly myelinated, intrastriate layer. Layer VI often has several strata of horizontal fibers, the most obvious being at the border of the white matter.

TABLE SHOWING THE RELATION TO ONE ANOTHER OF THE VARIOUS PUBLISHED CLASSIFICATIONS OF "OCCIPITAL" LAMINATION.

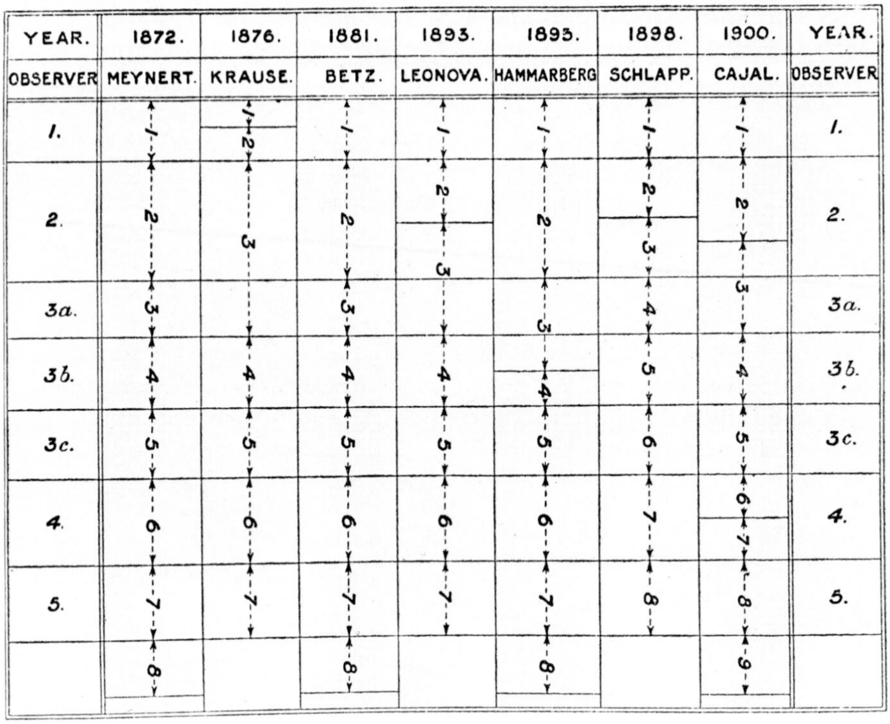

YEAR.	1872.	1876.	1881.	1893.	1895.	1898.	1900.	YEAR.
OBSERVER	MEYNERT.	KRAUSE.	BETZ.	LEONOVA.	HAMMARBERG	SCHLAPP.	CAJAL.	OBSERVER
1.	1	1 / 2	1	1	1	1	1	1.
2.	2	3	2	2	2	2 / 3	2	2.
3a.	3		3	3	3	4	3	3a.
3b.	4	4	4	4	4	5	4	3b.
3c.	5	5	5	5	5	6	5	3c.
4.	6	6	6	6	6	7	6 / 7	4.
5.	7	7	7	7	7	8	8	5.
	8		8		8		9	

Figure 6. Bolton's (1900) comparative table of schemes of lamination for the human visual cortex. His own layers are placed at left and right.

Traversing the horizontal layers of myelinated fibers are the vertical radiations of Meynert, with the intervening, delicate, interradiary plexus of Edinger.

The myelin stains naturally, however, added no information in the area of cellular morphology. Relatively little was contributed by the reduced silver or neurofibrillar stains either. The first of these was introduced by Bielschowsky in 1902 and perfected in 1904. In 1905, he and Brodmann published a joint paper on the application of silver staining to the human cerebral cortex (Fig. 9). Ramón y Cajal used the method to complement some of his observations made with the Golgi technique, particularly on the nature of the axonal endings around pyramidal cells. However, in requiring the use of relatively thin sections and in staining, unlike the Golgi or methylene blue method, every soma and every process present, the reduced silver methods made it very difficult to build up a satisfactory three-dimensional picture of individual cells. Ramón y Cajal (1954), who stated that he first used neurofibrillar stains in 1903, remarked that the method was also unsatisfactory for staining short-axon cells.

Some of the early studies of connectivity on the cortex were also made during the heyday of architectonics. Many of these are referred to in Chapter 16. Several workers had by about 1910 clearly recognized that retrograde degeneration of Betz cells ensued after spinal cord lesions or long-standing amputations (e.g., Campbell, 1905; Holmes and Page May, 1909), thus leading to the belief that the infragranular layers of all cortical areas were efferent and the supragranular layers receptive or associative (e.g., Bolton, 1910). It was to be many years, however, before the details or even an outline of efferent and afferent connections of the cortex was established. Retrograde degeneration (e.g., Nissl, 1913;

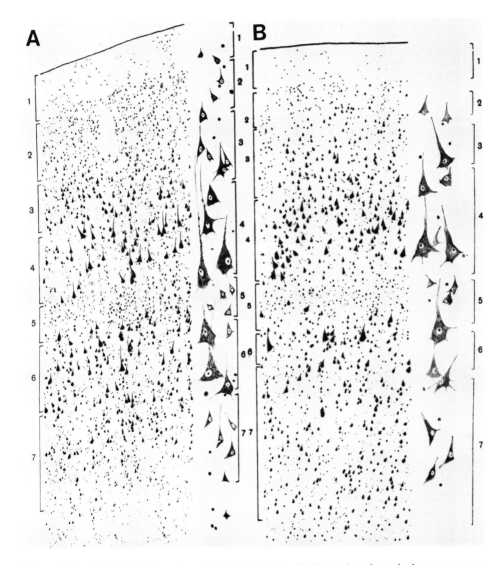

Figure 7. Campbell's (1905) drawings of thionin-stained, celloidin sections from the human postcentral gyrus (A) and superior parietal lobule (B). The layering scheme is that of Ramón y Cajal and the cells are all drawn as small pyramids.

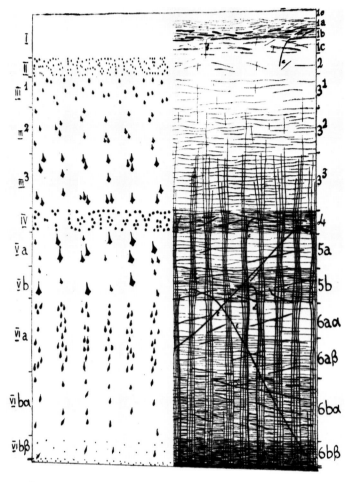

Figure 8. Vogt's scheme of the fundamental plans of cellular (left) and fiber (right) layering in the cerebral cortex. Fiber layers 4 and 5b are the bands of Baillarger; the stria of Kaes–Bechterew when present is layer lc. From Vogt and Vogt (1919).

von Monakow, 1914; Walker, 1938), the Marchi method (e.g., Polyak, 1932), the Nauta methods (e.g., Brodal, 1969), and electrophysiology (e.g., Fulton, 1949) eventually gave us a fairly thorough understanding of the broad organizational plan of efferent and afferent connections in the cortex but the exact origins and terminations of efferent and afferent fibers in cellular terms had to await studies carried out in the last 7 or 8 years.

3. Staining of Individual Cell Types

Although the broad distinction between pyramidal and nonpyramidal cell types was evident in the earliest studies utilizing carmine as a stain, full recognition of the variety of cell types and the extent of the ramifications of individual

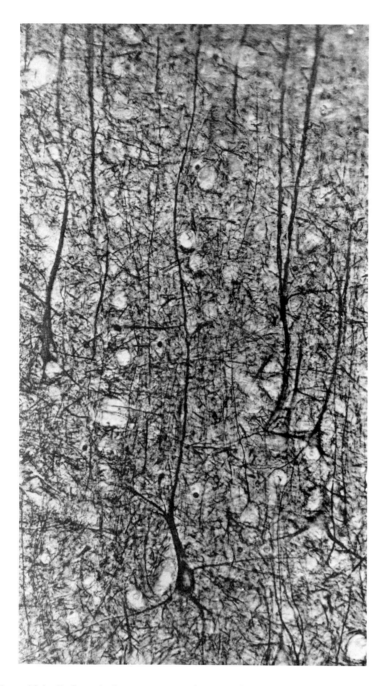

Figure 9. Pyramidal cells from the human precentral gyrus stained with Bielschowsky's neurofibrillar stain. From Bielschowsky and Brodmann (1905).

cells only emerged with the application of the Golgi and methylene blue stains. Golgi discovered the silver stain that bears his name in 1873 and by 1874 had applied it to the cerebellar cortex. When he first used it to examine the cerebral cortex is difficult to ascertain but by 1883, he had described both pyramidal cells and large star-shaped cells in some detail (see Chapter 5). According to Ramón

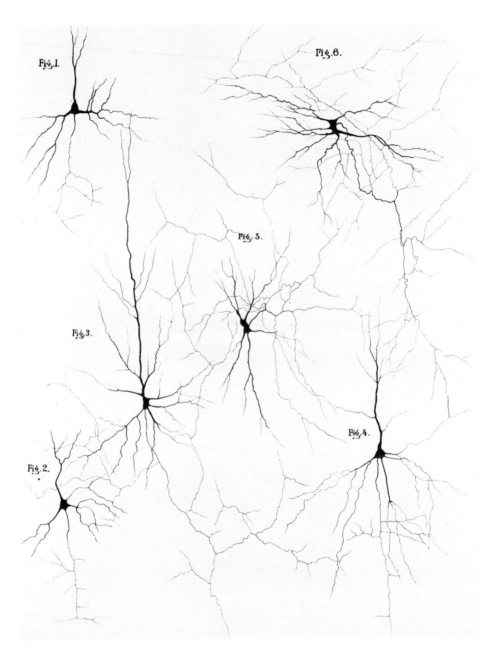

Figure 10. Drawings by Golgi of pyramidal and nonpyramidal cells from the human cerebral cortex. The original drawing showed axons in red. From Golgi (1883b).

y Cajal (1954), one of Golgi's chief contributions at this stage was to indicate that the dendrites ended freely, not by anastomosing with one another. Probably Golgi should also be credited with the first clear distinctions between axons and dendrites in the cortex, though Deiters had indicated this much earlier in other regions. Golgi was able to stain the axons of many of the cortical cells and observed collateral branches, probably for the first time (Fig. 10). He did not draw spines on the dendrites of any cells though Ramón y Cajal, who first described them on pyramidal cells in 1891, stated (1954) that Golgi must have seen them.

Between 1883 and publication of Volume 2, Part 2 of the original Spanish version of Ramón y Cajal's *Histologie du Système Nerveux,* in 1904, there were several excellent studies of the cerebral cortex made by using the Golgi method particularly by Golgi himself (1884, 1885, 1886, 1894), by Ramón y Cajal (1891, 1894, and other references in his books of 1904, 1911, and 1954), and by Retzius (1893, 1896). Many others dabbled with the staining of cortical cells (Fig. 11), but by far the most comprehensive surveys of cortical cell types are those of Ramón y Cajal and of Retzius (Fig. 12), who in general concurred with most of Ramón y Cajal's descriptions. A further readable and well-illustrated account, also in line with that of Ramón y Cajal, is the one published by von Kölliker

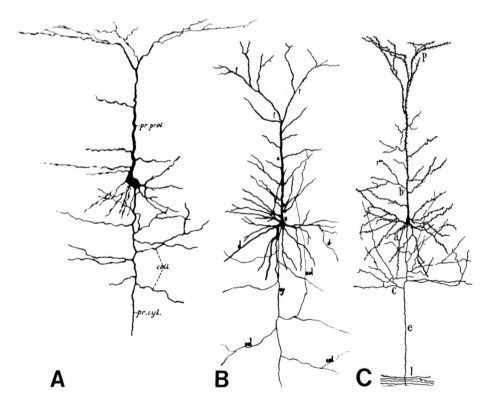

A　　　　**B**　　　**C**

Figure 11. Drawings of Golgi-impregnated pyramidal cells from the cortex of a 9-day-old mouse (A), adult man (B), and a mouse of unspecified age (C). By Van Gehuchten (1897, A), by Ramón y Cajal's translator, Azoulay (from Dejerine, 1895, B) and by Ramón y Cajal himself (1909–1911, C). All indicate the axon and its collaterals. (B) and (C) show dendritic spines.

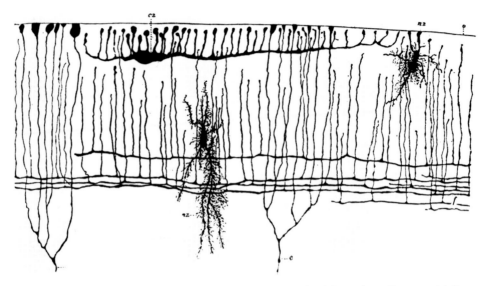

Figure 12. Drawing by Retzius (1893) of a Golgi-impregnated Cajal–Retzius cell, tangential fibers, astrocytes, and radial glial processes from layer I of the temporal cortex of a human fetus.

(1896) in the sixth edition of his *Handbuch der Gewebelehre des Menschen* (Fig. 13). This was based on a series of studies carried out as the result of his "discovery" of Ramón y Cajal and Ramón y Cajal's preparations at the meeting of the German Anatomical Society in Berlin in 1889 (Ramón y Cajal, 1937).

Ramón y Cajal based his studies not only on Golgi preparations but also on those stained with methylene blue (Figs. 14, 15) introduced by Ehrlich in 1868, and like the Golgi method staining only a small proportion of the neurons present but in their entirety. He stated (Ramón y Cajal, 1954), however, that he found methylene blue less satisfactory than the Golgi method, except for demonstrating the large fusiform cells.

Ramón y Cajal described the cells of the cortex systematically, layer by layer, both in general terms and in selected specific areas such as the visual and auditory. His emphasis was on the human brain and he made extensive use of preparations from human infants, supplemented by some material from cats, dogs, and rodents. Later in life he was to make a detailed study of the visual cortex of the cat alone (Ramón y Cajal, 1922). His basic classification is into pyramidal cells and cells with short axons (Fig. 14; and see Chapter 6). He thought that the number of short-axon cells increased greatly in the human brain and he saw this feature as one of the keys to understanding the functional complexity of the brain of man. He recognized the similarity between pyramidal cells of all layers, despite considerable variations in size. But he also detected subtle differences in their dendrite branching patterns and in the patterns of collateral branching of their axons. Among the cells with short axons, he detected a number of different varieties based on dendritic and/or axonal arborizations. Unfortunately, he was not always consistent in his naming of these, sometimes using several synonyms for the same cell type and sometimes giving the same name to clearly different kinds of cells. His use of the term *double bouquet cell,*

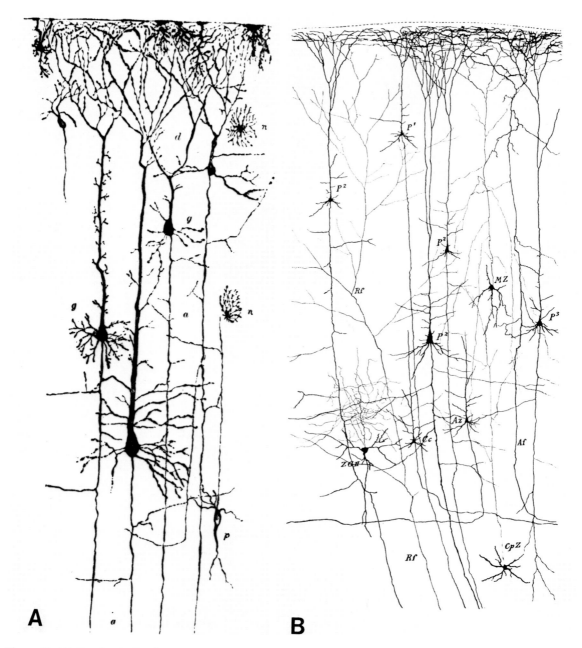

A

B

Figure 13. (A) Drawing by Retzius (1896) of Golgi-impregnated neurons and glial cells in the cerebral cortex of a young rabbit. (B) Drawing by von Kölliker (1896) summarizing his view of cortical organization, as based on Golgi preparations of mice and rabbits: Af: ending of a callosal or association fiber; Az: association cell; Cc: cell of corpus callosum; CpZ: cell of corpus striatum; MZ: Martinotti cell; P: pyramidal cells; Rf: "Ramon's centripetal sensory fiber"; ZGII: Golgi type II cell. The original drawing showed axons in blue or red.

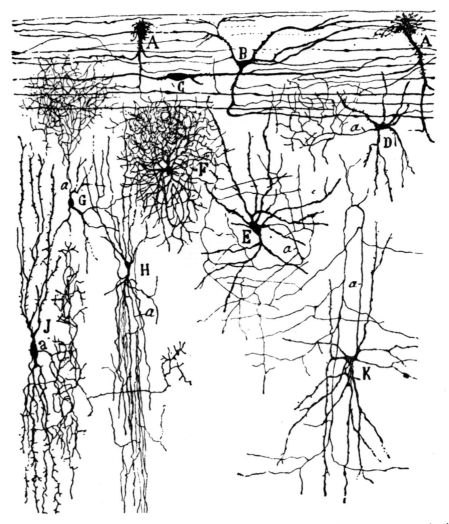

Figure 14. Drawings by Ramón y Cajal (1911) of Golgi-impregnated short-axon neurons in the superficial layers of the motor cortex of a human infant. A–C: "horizontal cells"; D–F: "short-axon cells"; G: "cell with ascending axon"; H, J: "double bouquet cells"; K: "large short-axon cell."

for example, is notoriously inconsistent, sometimes being based on dendritic characteristics, sometimes on one kind of axonal characteristic, and sometimes on another (see Chapter 6). This may be one reason why until recent times Ramón y Cajal's terms did not come into common usage, his followers such as Lorente de Nó (1922, 1949) preferring to use the term *short-axon cell* to cover all forms.

Generally speaking, Ramón y Cajal described short-axon cells in all layers and in all areas, dividing them into forms with local axons, vertical axons, or horizontal axons. Most have been recognized in recent studies (e.g., Jones, 1975). The relatively large numbers of spines shown by Ramón y Cajal on many of them, however, has on the whole not been reproducible, possibly because he

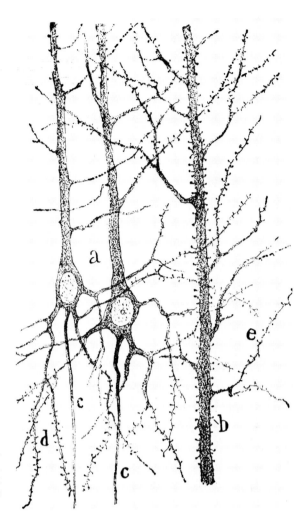

Figure 15. Drawings by Ramón y Cajal (1954) of methylene blue-stained pyramidal cells in the cerebral cortex of a cat, used by him to reinforce his belief in dendritic spines.

mostly used material from immature brains. Unique forms of neurons found in layer I particularly of infant animals were the Cajal–Retzius cells (Fig. 12; and see Chapter 14), and the short-axon and pyramidal cells of layer VI adopted a variety of forms different from those of other layers. Unique, he thought, to the auditory area was a special form of giant cell and unique to layer IVb of the visual cortex a type of large spiny nonpyramidal cell with an axon that, unlike those of other nonpyramidal cells, entered the white matter (Ramón y Cajal, 1922). Various forms of afferent fibers were also described and he was probably the first to clearly identify the terminal territories of thalamic afferents in layer IV. In his final work (1954) he concluded the section on the cerebral cortex thus: "One thing is certain: classification of the manner of connection between the innumerable centrifugal and centripetal, terminal and collateral branches emanating from thalamic, callosal and association fibers constitutes at present an overwhelming problem. In it many generations of future neurologists will put their sagacity and their patience to the test."

4. Golgi Studies after Ramón y Cajal

The chief aficionado of the Golgi technique in the years that followed Ramón y Cajal's death in 1934 was undoubtedly Lorente de Nó, who had completed his first study of what he took to be the auditory cortex of the mouse under Ramón y Cajal's direction in 1922. The area he was studying was probably the first somatic sensory area. In it he was able to detect many of the cell forms described earlier by Ramón y Cajal and made pertinent observations on the relationships of certain short-axon cells and of the dendritic fields of certain pyramidal cells to the terminal ramifications of thalamocortical axons. Lorente de Nó's subsequent published work on the cortex was mostly devoted to the hippocampal formation and adjoining areas. However, for Fulton's *Physiology of the Nervous System*, the last edition of which was published in 1949, he provided a general account of neuronal organization in the neocortex that stands as a frequently quoted classic (Fig. 16). In it he proposed a model of cortical circuitry based on thalamocortical axons terminating in layer IV on the dendrites of both pyramidal

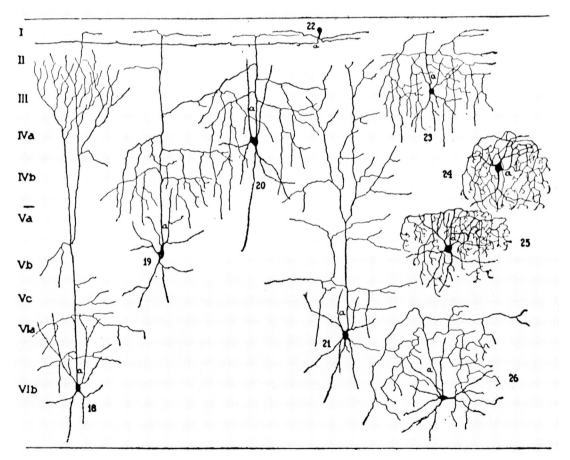

Figure 16. Drawings by Lorente de Nó (1949) showing his three types of neurons with intracortical axons. 18–21: cells with ascending axons; 22: cell with horizontal axon; 23–26: cells with short axons.

and short-axon cells. From these, activity was conducted upwards and downwards in the cortex by pyramidal cell axons and by short-axon cells with vertical axons. At all levels there were reentrant loops formed by the collateral axon branches of pyramidal cells and by short-axon cells with local axon plexuses. Hence, a vertically oriented, reverberating circuit of activity would be set up. In this scheme we can detect the first glimmerings of a concept of columnar organization in the cortex, a fact that was recognized by Mountcastle (1957) in his original paper on the cortical column.

Lorente de Nó is often taken to task for describing too many cortical cell types. He mentioned some 40 in his first paper, though he later reduced the number to about 5. It is doubtful, however, that he meant these to be more than but variants of a much more fundamental plan of organization in which some short-axon cells operated over relatively long intracortical distances, commonly in the vertical dimension, while others exerted extremely local effects.

There were a number of descriptive Golgi studies subsequent to Lorente de Nó's account but those published between 1940 and about 1970 seem remarkably superficial and it is doubtful that any truly lasting data emerged from them. A possible exception is the work of Sholl (1956) who made rather more use of the mercury-based Golgi–Cox method (Cox, 1891) than had previous investigators and directed his major efforts at the quantification of dendritic field architecture. His methods for graphic representation of the lengths of dendritic branches (Fig. 17) and for measuring dendritic field complexity in terms of numbers of dendritic profiles that intersect a series of circles of increasing radius centered on the cell soma (Fig. 17), are still widely used.

Sholl is now coming to be criticized for his classification of cortical neurons simply into pyramidal and stellate forms and for making little attempt to define different classes of stellate cells. One reason for this was undoubtedly that the Golgi–Cox method as used by him did not reliably stain the axons which are the major distinguishing feature of the different classes of nonpyramidal cells (Jones, 1975). Within his frame of experimental reference, however, this was unnecessary for Sholl.

The advent of electron microscopic studies of the central nervous system resulted in a new phase of descriptive morphology using Golgi preparations, since there was a need to correlate the profiles identified electron microscopically with components of particular cell classes of light microscopy (see Chapter 4 on neuronal classification). The first return to the cortex was in the work of Szentágothai (1969) and of Valverde (1971) who noted again some of the forms of short-axon cells described by Ramón y Cajal (Figs. 18, 19). A second significant contribution was that of Lund (1973) who defined two classes of nonpyramidal cells, spiny and nonspiny. In 1975 the author made a concerted effort to define nonpyramidal cells in terms of their axonal arborizations (Jones, 1975). From this emerged eight or nine distinctive cell classes, all of which seem to have stood the test of time and subsequent studies (e.g., Peters and Regidor, 1981; and other chapters of this book). In many respects the new Golgi studies have led to a rediscovery of the cortical cell types of Ramón y Cajal. However, the work has generally been carried out in a more systematic manner than in the past, and in the light of knowledge of cortical connectivity derived from experimental studies. There has also been an emphasis on classifying nonpyramidal cells according to their axonal ramifications which can be remarkably stereotyped and more useful than classification in terms of dendritic field shapes (Jones, 1975; see Chapter 13). From these types of studies a number of hypothetical schemes have been put forward, particularly by Szentágothai (1969, 1970, 1973, 1975, 1978) in an effort to provide a circuit diagram that underlies the functional columnarity of the cortex (Fig. 19).

Two major contributions have been technical. The first was that of Colonnier (1964a) who showed that by slightly modifying a variant of the Golgi stain originally introduced by Kopsch (1896), tissue from the same animal fixed by

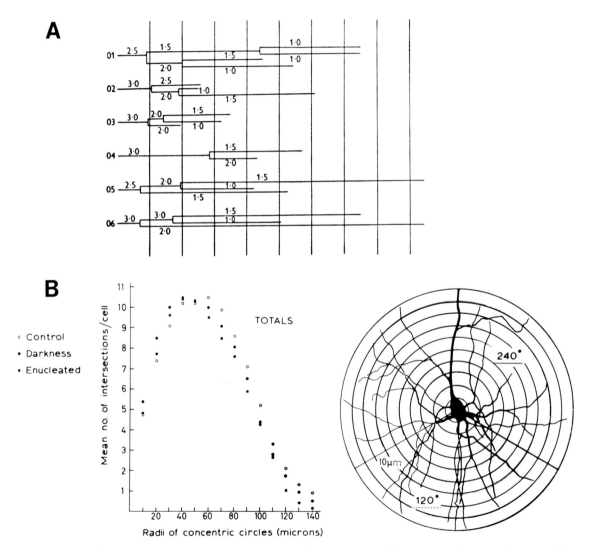

Figure 17. (A) Sholl's (1956) method of "graphical representation of the lengths of dendritic branches for a single neuron." (B) Sholl-type analysis for complexity of dendritic branching based on number of intersections made by dendrites with circles of increasing radii centered on soma. For basal dendrites of layer III pyramids in the visual cortices of normal mice (control), mice reared in darkness, and mice enucleated at birth. From Valverde (1971).

perfusion with mixed aldehydes could be used both for Golgi impregnation and for electron microscopy. This method has become one of the most widely used of all the Golgi methods. Derivative of it is the method of perfusing with the initial Golgi reagent, potassium dichromate, mixed in with the aldehydes (Rethélyi, 1972). A second major innovation was that of Fairén *et al.* (1977) who showed that the silver chromate precipitate filling a well-impregnated neuron could be replaced with finer gold particles that were not only more amenable to electron microscopic study but left the ultrastructure remarkably well preserved (see Chapters 9–13). In this way a cell identified light microscopically can be examined electron microscopically, often in conjunction with another marker (e.g., axon terminal degeneration) and the afferent and efferent connectivity of the cell defined. In the future it seems inevitable that the Golgi method will also be made compatible with other techniques, particularly those involving immunocytochemistry, autoradiography, and labeling by axoplasmic transport.

Scheibel and Scheibel posed the question in 1971: "The rapid Golgi method: Indian summer or renaissance?" There can be no question that there has been a definite renaissance in this time-honored method and despite advances in other forms of cell labeling it seems likely that it will hold its place as a major method on which we base our classifications of cortical cells for many years.

5. Recent Innovations

Most of the methods that have been introduced for the study of cortical neurons in recent years are outlined in Chapter 4. The first of these was undoubtedly electron microscopy. Probably the first significant contributions with the new technique were made by Gray (1959) whose method of fixation involved dripping osmium tetroxide onto the cortex or dicing it into small pieces prior to immersion in osmium. Gray was also one of the first to embed neural tissue in Araldite prior to sectioning. Among his fundamental observations were the identification of asymmetrical and symmetrical synapses (which he called types I and II) and the clear delineation of dendritic spines as biological entities rather than, as some had supposed, artifacts of the Golgi stain or impregnated synaptic terminals. He showed that most synapses were on spines rather than on the dendritic shafts of pyramidal cells. Soon after the introduction of perfusion with mixed aldehydes as the primary fixative of choice in electron microscopy of the nervous system (Karnovsky, 1965; Vaughn and Peters, 1966), two further observations of fundamental significance were made by Colonnier (1968). He showed (in a classic plate illustrating 100 synapses with parallel sectioned membranes) that axon terminals making Gray's asymmetrical synapses invariably contained synaptic vesicles that were spherical in shape, while those making symmetrical synapses invariably contained vesicles that were flattened or pleomorphic when fixed in aldehyde mixtures of relatively high osmolarity. An association of symmetric, flattened vesicle-containing synapses with inhibitory synapses had already been made in the cerebellar cortex by Uchizono (1965). Colonnier also pointed out that pyramidal and nonpyramidal cells could be distinguished by differences

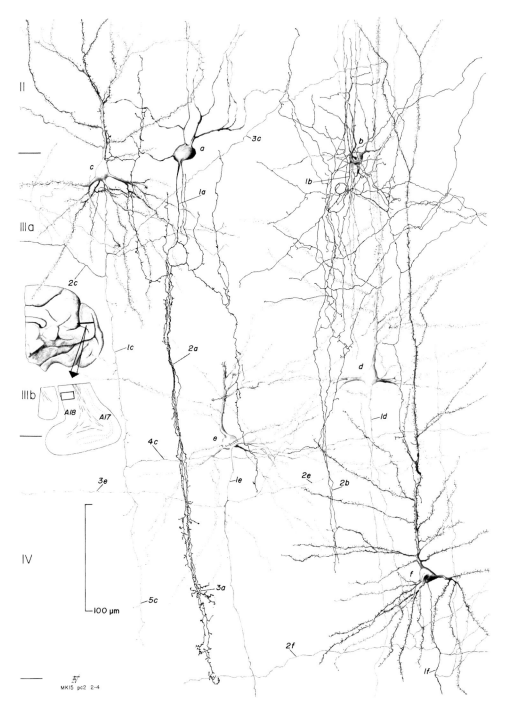

II

IIIa

IIIb

IV

100 μm

MKI5 pc2 2-4

Figure 18. A modern master of the Golgi technique. Drawings of impregnated cells by Valverde (1978) to illustrate his paper on area 18 of the monkey cortex.

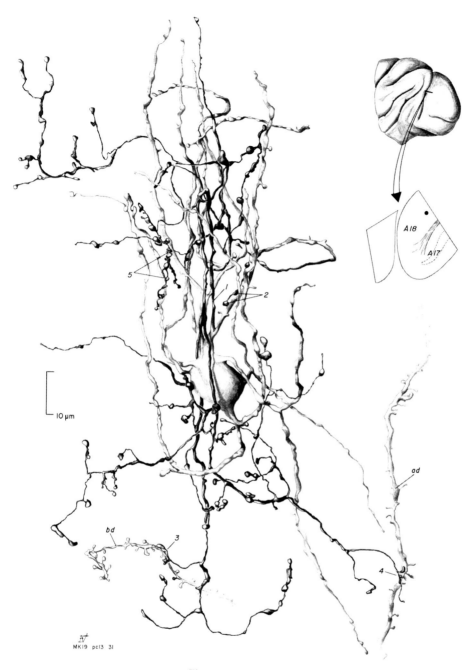

Figure 18. *(continued)*

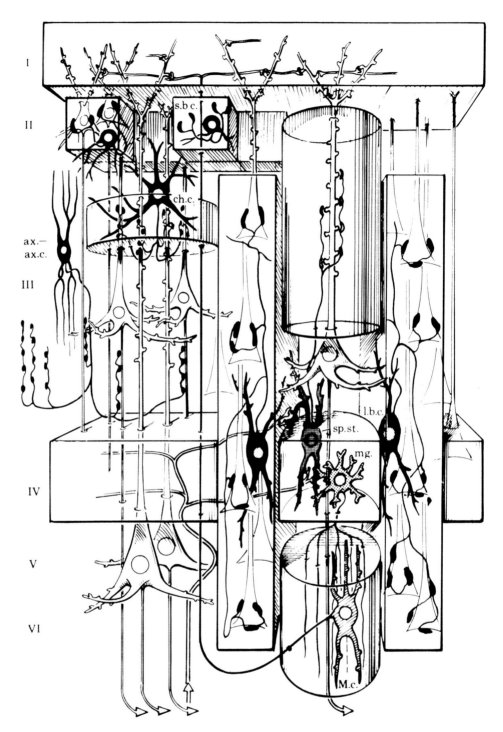

Figure 19. Another modern master. Szentágothai's (1978) "Synthetic stereoscopic view of the modular arrangement of local neuronal connections" in the cortex, based on Golgi and experimental studies. Here, he attempts to relate the different classes of intrinsic neurons (inhibitory in black, excitatory shaded), to the chain of synaptic events that should ensue following the arival of an afferent volley and which must underlie the functional columnarity of the cortex.

in their complements of organelles and in the numbers and proportions of different types of synapse that they received. For example, pyramidal cell somata received relatively few synapses, all of the symmetric type, while most nonpyramidal cells received many synapses of both types on their somata and dendrites. Colonnier's two observations have formed the basis for many subsequent fine structural studies of the cerebral cortex. He was also able to demonstrate the morphological characteristics of axon terminal degeneration that ensued in the cortex following undercutting (Colonnier, 1964b). The use of Wallerian degeneration to promote identifiable labeling of the terminals of specific afferent pathways entering the cortex was first applied by Jones (1968; Jones and Powell, 1970).

More recent technical innovations include the labeling of cortical cells by retrograde axoplasmic tracers, which between 1974 and 1977 enabled us to say conclusively not only that pyramidal cells are the major output cells of the cortex, and nonpyramidal cells intrinsic (Chapter 16), but also that the layers of the cortex have different output connections (see list of all early references in Wise and Jones, 1977). Their input connections have, similarly, been more thoroughly characterized than ever before by studies using anterograde axoplasmically transported markers (see Jones and Hartman, 1978).

Through the use of both techniques, coupled with [^{3}H]thymidine autoradiography, the developmental history of the cortex has been elucidated (Angevine and Sidman, 1961; Rakic, 1974, 1976; Jones, 1981). Labeling of individual cell classes by immunocytochemistry or by autoradiography following uptake of their radiolabeled transmitter has given us the information that a large population and several varieties of the intrinsic neurons are GABAergic and that GABA is associated with symmetric synapses (Ribak, 1978; Hendry and Jones, 1981; Hendry *et al.*, 1983; Houser *et al.*, 1983; Peters *et al.*, 1982; see also chapter by Houser *et al.* in Volume 2). A number of forms of intrinsic neurons also contain various brain–gut peptides (Emson and Hunt, 1981). Receptor localization (Palacios *et al.*, 1981; Wise and Herkenham, 1982; see also chapter by Wamsley in Volume 2) is only just beginning in the cortex, one of the methods being used representing a return to that of Lewis (1878b).

The definition of individual cell classes in terms of their receptive field properties by intracellular recording followed by intracellular injection was commenced by Kelly and Van Essen in 1974 when they injected a small population of pyramidal and nonpyramidal cells in the cat visual cortex with procion yellow. This exhausting but rewarding work has been continued using horseradish peroxidase as the intracellular marker in the hands of Deschênes *et al.* (1979), Gilbert and Wiesel (1979), and Lin *et al.* (1979). The yield of cells to date is rather too small to make any generalizing statements about the relationship of cell type to receptive field type but already better information has been derived about the distribution of collateral branches of different types of pyramidal cells than had ever appeared in any previous Golgi studies.

Other types of study that are just commencing on the cortex include those on regional blood flow and metabolism (Sokoloff *et al.*, 1977) and the histochemical detection of oxidative enzymes (Wong-Riley, 1979). All of these methods, though not yet having reached the level of resolution of the single cell, lend themselves to experimental manipulation. It seem inevitable that further advances, perhaps using these in combination with other methods, will eventuate.

With so many new techniques appearing, the future of cortical studies is likely to be an active one. Among new technical innovations that may be envisaged are the recording of the activities of groupings of neurons working as functional units by the use of multiple, closely spaced microelectrodes and the specification of individual cell classes through a knowledge of their individual antigenic characteristics and, ultimately, through a knowledge of their genome. Perhaps in the not too distant future we shall understand not only why cortical cells express certain transmitters but also why they adopt individual morphologies and connectivities.

6. References

Angevine, J. B., Jr., and Sidman, R. L., 1961, Autoradiographic study of cell migration during histogenesis of cerebral cortex in mouse, *Nature (London)* **192**:766–768.

Baillarger, J.-G.-F., 1840, Recherches sur la structure de la couche corticale des circonvolutions du cerveau, *Mém. Acad. R. Med.* **8**:149–183.

Bastian, H. C., 1880, *The Brain as an Organ of Mind,* Kegan Paul, London.

Bechterew, W., 1894, *Die Leitungsbahnen in Gehirn und Ruckenmark: Ein Hanbuch für das Studium des Nervensystems* (translated by V. Weinberg), Besold, Leipzig.

Berlin, R., 1858, *Beiträge zur Strukturlehre der Grosshirnwindungen,* Junge, Erlangen.

Betz, W., 1874, Anatomischer Nachweis zweier Gehirnzentra, *Zentralbl. Med. Wiss.* **12**:578–580, 595–599.

Betz, W., 1881, Über die feinere Struktur der Grosshirnrinde des Menschen, *Zentralbl. Med. Wiss.* **19**:193–195, 209–213, 231–234.

Bielschowsky, M., 1902, Die Silberimprägnation der Achsenzylinder, *Neurol. Zbl.* **21**:579–584.

Bielschowsky, M., 1904, Die Silberimprägnation der Neurofibrillen, *J. Psychol. Neurol.* **3**:169–188.

Bielschowsky, M., and Brodmann, K., 1905, Zur feineren Histologie und Histopathologie der Grosshirnrinde mit besonderer Berücksichtigung der Dementia paralytica, Dementia senilis und Idiotie, *J. Psychol. Neurol.* **5**:173–199.

Bolton, J. S., 1900, The exact histological localisation of the visual area of the human cerebral cortex, *Philos. Trans. R. Soc. London* **193**:165–122.

Bolton, J. S., 1910, A contribution to the localization of cerebral function, based on the clinico-pathological study of mental disease, *Brain* **33**:26–147.

Brodal, A., 1969, *Neurological Anatomy in Relation to Clinical Medicine,* 2nd ed., Oxford University Press, London.

Brodmann, K., 1903, Beiträge zur histologischen Lokalisation der Grosshirnrinde. Erste Mitteilung. Die Regio Rolandica, *J. Psychol. Neurol.* **2**:79–132.

Brodmann, K., 1909, *Vergleichende Lokalisationslehre der Grosshirnrinde in Ihren Prinzipien dargestellt auf Grund des Zellenbaues,* Barth, Leipzig.

Brodmann, K., 1912, Neue Ergebnisse über die vergleichende histologische Lokalisation der Grosshirnrinde mit besonderer Berücksichtigung des Stirnhirns, *Anat. Anz.* **41**(Suppl.): 157–216.

Campbell, A. W., 1905, *Histological Studies on the Localisation of Cerebral Function,* Cambridge University Press, London.

Clarke, E. C., and Bearn, J. G., 1968, The brain "glands" of Malpighi elucidated by practical history, *J. Hist. Med.* **23**:309–330.

Colonnier, M., 1964a, The tangential organization of the visual cortex, *J. Anat.* **98**:327–344.

Colonnier, M., 1964b, Experimental degeneration in the cerebral cortex, *J. Anat.* **98**:47–53.

Colonnier, M., 1968, Synaptic patterns on different cell types in the different laminae of the cat visual cortex: An electron microscopic study, *Brain Res.* **9**:268–287.

Cox, W., 1891, Imprägnation des centralen Nervensystems mit Quecksilbersalzen, *Arch. Mikrosk. Anat. Entwicklungsmech.* **37**:16–21.

Dejerine, J. (with collaboration of Mme. Dejerine-Klumpke), 1895, *Anatomie des Centres Nerveux*, Vol. 1, Rueff, Paris.

Deschênes, M., LaBelle, A., and Landry, P., 1979, Morphological characterizations of slow and fast pyramidal tract cells in the cat, *Brain Res.* **178:**251–274.

Dieters, O. F. K., 1865, *Untersuchungen über Gehirn und Ruckenmark des Menschen und der Säugethiere* (M. Schultze, ed.), Vieweg, Braunschweig.

Edinger, L., 1896, *Vorlesungen über Bau der nervosen Centralorgane des Menschen und der Thiere*, 5th ed., Vögel, Leipzig.

Ehrenberg, C. G., 1833, Notwendigkeit einer feineren mechanischen Zerlegung des Gehirns und der Nerven, *Poggendorff's Ann. Phys. Chem.* **28:**449–465.

Ehrenberg, C. G., 1836, Beobachtung einer bisher unbekannten auffallenden Struktur des Seelen-organs bei Menschen und Tieren, *Abh. Akad. Wiss. Berlin (Phys. Math. Kl.)* **1836:**665–723.

Ehrlich, P., 1868, Über die Methyleneblaureaction der lebenden Nervensubstanz, *Dtsch. Med. Wochenschr.* **12:**49–52.

Emson, P. C., and Hunt, S. P., 1981, Anatomical chemistry of the cerebral cortex, in: *The Organization of the Cerebral Cortex* (F. O. Schmitt, F. G. Worden, G. Adelman, and S. G. Dennis, eds.), pp. 345–346, MIT Press, Cambridge, Mass.

Fairén, A., Peters, A., and Saldanha, J., 1977, A new procedure for examining Golgi impregnated neurons by light and electron microscopy, *J. Neurocytol.* **6:**311–337.

Ferrier, D., 1874, *Experimental Researches in Cerebral Physiology and Pathology, West Riding Lunatic Asylum Medical Reports* (1873) **3:**1–50.

Ferrier, D., 1886, *The Functions of the Brain*, 2nd ed., Smith Elder, London, and Putnam, New York.

Flechsig, P., 1898, Neue Untersuchungen über die Markbildung in den menschlichen Grosshirn-lappen, *Neurol. Zbl.* **17:**977–996.

Fulton, J. F. (ed.), 1949, *Physiology of the Nervous System*, 3rd ed., Oxford University Press, London.

Gennari, F., 1782, *De Peculiari Structura Cerebri Nonnullisque Ejus Morbis. Paucae aliae. Anatom. Observat. Accedunt*, Regio Typographeo, Parma.

Gilbert, C. D., and Wiesel, T. N., 1979, Morphology and intracortical projections of functionally characterised neurones in the cat visual cortex, *Nature (London)* **280:**120–125.

Golgi, C., 1873, Sulla sostanza grigia del cervello, *Gaz. Med. Ital. Lombardia* **6:**244–246. (Quoted from *Opera Omnia*, 1903, Vol 1, pp. 91–98, Hoepli, Milan.)

Golgi, C., 1874, Sulla fina anatomia del cervelleto umano, *Reale Instituto Lombardia Rep. II* **7:**1–69. (Quoted from *Opera Omnia*, 1903, Vol. 1, pp. 99–111, Hoepli, Milan.)

Golgi, C., 1883a, Recherches sur l'histologie des centres nerveux, *Arch. Ital. Biol.* **3:**285–317.

Golgi, C., 1883b, Sulla fina anatomia degli organi centrali del sistema nervoso, *Riv. Sper. Freniatr. Med. Leg. Alienazioni Ment.* **9:**1–17, 161–192, 385–402. (Quoted from *Opera Omnia*, 1903, Vol. 1, pp. 295–375, Hoepli, Milan.)

Golgi, C., 1884, Recherches sur l'histologie des centres nerveux, *Arch. Ital. Biol.* **4:**92–123.

Golgi, C., 1885, Sulla fina anatomia degli organi centrali del sistema nervoso, *Riv. Sper. Freniatr. Med. Leg. Alienazioni Ment.* **11:**72–123, 193–220.

Golgi, C., 1886, Sur l'anatomie microscopique des organes centraux du système nerveux, *Arch. Ital. Biol.* **7:**15–47.

Golgi, C., 1894, *Untersuchungen über den feineren Bau des centralen und peripherischen Nervensystems* (translated by R. Teuscher), Fischer, Jena.

Gray, E. G., 1959, Axo-somatic and axo-dendritic synapses in the cerebral cortex: An electron microscopic study, *J. Anat.* **93:**420–433.

Hammarberg, C., 1895, *Studien über Klinik und Pathologie der Idiotie, nebst Untersuchungen über die normale Anatomie der Hirnrinde* (translated by W. Berger), Druck der Akad. Buchdruckerei, Upsala.

Hannover, A., 1840, Die Chromsäure, ein vorzügliches Mittel bei mikrokopischen Untersuchungen, *Arch. Anat. Physiol. Physiol. Abt.* 549–558.

Hendry, S. H. C., and Jones, E. G., 1981, Sizes and distributions of intrinsic neurons incorporating tritiated GABA in monkey sensory-motor cortex, *J. Neurosci.* **1:**390–408.

Hendry, S. H. C., Houser, C. R., Jones, E. G., and Vaughn, J. E., 1983, Synaptic organizaiton of immunocytochemically identified GABAergic neurons in the monkey sensory-motor cortex, *J. Neurocytol.* **12:**639–660.

Holmes, G., and Page May, W., 1909, On the exact origin of the pyramidal tracts in man and other mammals, *Brain* **32:**1–43.

Houser, C. R., Hendry, S. H. C., Jones, E. G., and Vaughn, J. E., 1983, Morphological diversity of GABA neurons demonstrated immunocytochemically in monkey sensory-motor cortex, *J. Neurocytol.* **12**:617–638.

Jones, E. G., 1968, An electron microscopic study of the terminations of afferent fibre systems within the somatic sensory cortex of the cat, *J. Anat.* **103**:595–597.

Jones, E. G., 1975, Varieties and distribution of non-pyramidal cells in the somatic sensory cortex of the squirrel monkey, *J. Comp. Neurol.* **160**:205–268.

Jones, E. G., 1981, Development of connectivity in the cerebral cortex, in: *Studies in Developmental Neurobiology in Honor of Victor Hamburger* (W. M. Cowan, ed.), Oxford University Press, London.

Jones, E. G., and Hartman, B. K., 1978, Recent advances in neuroanatomical methodology, *Annu. Rev. Neurosci.* **1**:215–296.

Jones, E. G., and Powell, T. P. S., 1970, An electron microscopic study of the laminar pattern and mode of termination of the afferent fibre pathways to the somatic sensory cortex, *Philos. Trans. R. Soc. London Ser. B* **257**:45–62.

Kaes, T., 1893, Beiträge zur Kenntniss des Reichtums der Grosshirnrinde des Menschen an markhaltigen Nervenfasern, *Arch. Psychiatr. Nervenkr.* **25**:695–758.

Karnovsky, M. J., 1965, A formaldehyde–glutaraldehyde fixative of high osmolality for use in electron microscopy, *J. Cell Biol.* **27**:137a.

Kelly, J. P., and Van Essen, D. C., 1974, Cell structure and function in the visual cortex of the cat, *J. Physiol. (London)* **238**:515–547.

Kopsch, F., 1896, Erfahrungen über die Verwendung des Formaldehyds bei der Chromsilber Impragnation, *Anat. Anz.* **11**:727–729.

Lewis, W. B., 1878a, On the comparative structure of the cortex cerebri, *Brain* **1**:79–86.

Lewis, W. B., 1878b, Application of freezing methods to the microscopic examination of the brain, *Brain* **1**:348–359.

Lewis, W. B., and Clarke, H., 1878, The cortical lamination of the motor area of the brain, *Proc. R. Soc. (London)* **27**:38–49.

Liddell, E. G. T., 1960, *The Discovery of Reflexes*, Clarendon Press, Oxford.

Lin, C.-S., Friedlander, M. J., and Sherman, S. M., 1979, Morphology of physiologically identified neurons in the visual cortex of the cat, *Brain Res.* **172**:344–348.

Lorente de Nó, R., 1922, La corteza cerebral del ratón (Primera contribución-La corteza acústica), *Trab. Lab. Invest. Biol. Madrid* **20**:41–78.

Lorente de Nó, R., 1949, Cerebral cortex: Architecture, intracortical connections, motor projections, in: *Physiology of the Nervous System* (J. F. Fulton, ed.), 3rd ed., pp. 288–313, Oxford University Press, London.

Lund, J. S., 1973, Organization of neurons in the visual cortex, area 17, of the monkey *Macaca mulatta*, *J. Comp. Neurol.* **147**:455–496.

Malpighi, M., 1666, De cerebre cortice, in: *Viscerum Structura Excercitatio Anatomica*, pp. 50–70, Montius, Bologna.

Mauss, T., 1908, Die faserachitektonische Gliederung der Groshirnrinde bei den niederen Affen, *J. Psychol. Neurol.* **13**:263–325.

Meynert, T., 1867–1868, Der Bau der Grosshirnrinde und seine örtichen Verschiedenheiten, nebst einen pathologisch–anatomischen Corollarium, *Vierteljahrsschr. Psychiatr.* 1867, **1**:77–93, 125–217; 1868, **1**:381–403, **2**:88, 113.

Meynert, T., 1869–1872, *Von Gehirne der Saugethiere*, in: *Handbuch der Lehre von der Geweben des Menschen und der Thiere* (Stricker, ed.), **2**:694–808.

Meynert, T., 1884, *Psychiatrie: Klinik der Erkrankungen des Vordeshirns* (Erste Halfe), Braumüller, Vienna.

Mountcastle, V. B., 1957, Modality and topographic properties of single neurons of cat's somatic sensory cortex, *J. Neurophysiol.* **20**:408–434.

Nissl, F., 1903, *Die Neuronlehre und ihre Anhanger*, Fischer, Jena.

Nissl, F., 1913, Die Grosshirnanteile des Kaninchens, *Arch. Psychiatr. Nervenkr.* **52**:867–953.

Palacios, J. M., Wamsley, J. K., and Kuhar, M. J., 1981, High affinity GABA receptors—Autoradiographic localizaiton, *Brain Res.* **222**:285–308.

Peters, A., and Regidor, J., 1981, A reassessment of the forms of nonpyramidal neurons in area 17 of cat visual cortex, *J. Comp. Neurol.* **203**:685–716.

Peters, A., Proskauer, C., and Ribak, C. E., 1982, Chandelier cells in rat visual cortex, *J. Comp. Neurol.* **206**:397–416.

Polyak, S., 1932, *The Main Afferent Systems of the Cerebral Cortex in Primates,* University of California Press, Berkeley.

Rakic, P., 1974, Neurons in rhesus monkey visual cortex: Systematic relation between time of origin and eventual disposition, *Science* **183**:425–426.

Rakic, P., 1976, Prenatal genesis of connections subserving ocular dominance in the rhesus monkey, *Nature (London)* **261**:467–471.

Ramón y Cajal, S., 1891, Sur la structure de l'écorce cérébrale de quelques mammifères, *La Cellule* **7**:125–176.

Ramón y Cajal, S., 1894, La fine structure des centres nerveux, *Proc. R. Soc. London* **55**:444–468.

Ramón y Cajal, S., 1900–1906, *Studien über die Hirnrinde des Menschen,* Parts 1–5 (translated by J. Bresler), Barth, Leipzig.

Ramón y Cajal, S., 1904, *Textura de sistema nervioso de hombre y de los vertebrados: Estudios sobre el plan estructural y composición histológica de los centros nerviosos adicionados de consideraciones fisiológicas fundadas en los neuvos descubrimientos,* Vol. 2, Part 2, Moya, Madrid.

Ramón y Cajal, S., 1909–1911, *Histologie du système Nerveux de l'Homme et des Vertébrés* (translated by L. Azoulay), Maloine, Paris.

Ramón y Cajal, S., 1922, Studien über die Sehrinde der Katze, *J. Psychol. Neurol.* **29**:161–181.

Ramón y Cajal, S., 1937, *Recollections of My Life* (translated by E. H. Craigie with the assistance of J. Cano), The American Philosophical Society, Philadelphia.

Ramón y Cajal, S., 1954, *Neuron Theory or Reticular Theory? Objective Evidence of the Anatomical Unity of Nerve Cells* (translated by M. Ubeda Purkiss and C. A. Fox), Consejo Superior de Investigaciones Científicas, Madrid.

Remak, R., 1841, Anatomische Beobachtungen über das Gehirn, das Ruckenmark und die Nervenwurzeln, *Müller's Arch. Anat. Physiol. Wiss.* **1841**:506–522.

Rethélyi, M., 1972, Cell and neuropil architecture of the intermediolateral (sympathetic) nucleus of cat spinal cord, *Brain Res.* **46**:203–213.

Retzius, M. G., 1893, Die Cajalschen Zellen der Grosshirnrinde bein Menschen und bei Säugethieren, *Biol. Untersuch. N.F.* **4**:1–9.

Retzius, M. G., 1896, *Das Menschenhirn: Studien in der makroskopischen Morphologie,* Norstedt, Stockholm.

Ribak, C. E., 1978, Aspinous and sparsely-spinous stellate neurons in the visual cortex of rats contain glutamic acid decarboxylase, *J. Neurocytol.* **7**:461–478.

Scheibel, M. E., and Scheibel, A. B., 1971, The rapid Golgi method: Indian summer or renaissance? in: *Contemporary Research Methods in Neuroanatomy* (W. J. H. Nauta and S. O. E. Ebbesson, eds.), Springer, Berlin.

Sholl, D. A., 1956, *The Organization of the Cerebral Cortex,* Methuen, London.

Sokoloff, L., Reivich, M., Kennedy, C., Des Rosiers, M. H., Patlak, C. S., Pettigrew, K. D., Sakurada, O., and Shinohara, M., 1977, The [^{14}C]deoxyglucose method for the measurement of local cerebral glucose utilization: Theory, procedure and normal values in the conscious and anesthetized albino rat, *J. Neurochem.* **28**:897–916.

Szentágothai, J., 1969, Architecture of the cerebral cortex, in: *Basic Mechanisms of the Epilepsies* (H. H. Jasper, A. A. Ward, and A. Pope, eds.), pp. 13–28, Little, Brown, Boston.

Szentágothai, J., 1970, Les circuits neuronaux de l'écorce cérébrale, *Bull. Acad. R. Med. Belg.* **10**:475–492.

Szentágothai, J., 1973, Synaptology of the visual cortex, in: *Handbook of Sensory Physiology,* Vol. VII/3, *Central Processing of Visual Information,* Part B, *Visual Centers of the Brain* (R. Jung, ed.), pp. 269–324, Springer, Berlin.

Szentágothai, J., 1975, The "module-concept" in cerebral cortex architecture, *Brain Res.* **95**:475–496.

Szentágothai, J., 1978, The neuron network of the cerebral cortex: A functional interpretation, *Proc. R. Soc. London Ser. B* **201**:219–248.

Uchizono, K., 1965, Characteristics of excitatory and inhibitory synapses in the central nervous system of the cat, *Nature (London)* **207**:642–643.

Valentin, G. G., 1836, Über den Verlauf und die letzten Ende der Nerven, *Nova Acta Phys.-Med. Acad. Leopoldina, Breslau,* **18**:51–240.

Valverde, F., 1971, Short axon neuronal subsystems in the visual cortex of the monkey, *Int. J. Neurosci.* **1**:181–197.

Valverde, F., 1978, The organization of area 18 in the monkey: A Golgi study, *Anat. Embryol.* **154**:305–334.

Van Gehuchten, A., 1897, *Anatomie du Système Nerveux de l'Homme: Lecons professées à l'Université de Louvain,* 2nd ed., Uystpruyst-Dieudonné, Louvain.

Vaughn, J. E., and Peters, A., 1966, Aldehyde fixation of nerve fibers, *J. Anat.* **100:**687.

Vogt, C., and Vogt, O., 1919, Allgemeinere Ergebnisse unserer Hirnforschung, *J. Psychol. Neurol.* **25:**279–462.

Vogt, O., 1903, Zur anatomischen Gliederung des Cortex cerebri, *J. Psychol. Neurol.* **2:**160–180.

Von Gerlach, J., 1872, Über die Struktur der grauen Substanz des menschlichen Grosshirns, *Zentralbl. Med. Wiss.* **10:**273–275.

von Kölliker, A., 1849, Neurologische Bemerkungen, *Z. Wiss. Zool. Abt. A* **1:**135–163.

von Kölliker, A., 1852, *Handbuch der Gewebelehre des Menschen,* 2nd ed., Englemann, Leipzig.

von Kölliker, A., 1860, *A Manual of Human Microscopic Anatomy,* Parker, London.

von Kölliker, A., 1896, *Handbuch der Gewebelehre des Menschen,* 6th ed., Vol. 2, *Nervensystem des Menschen und der Thiere,* Engelmann, Leipzig.

von Monakow, C., 1914, *Die Lokalisation im Grosshirn und der Abbau der Funktion durch kortikale Herde,* Bergmann, Wiesbaden.

Walker, A. E., 1938, *The Primate Thalamus,* University of Chicago Press, Chicago.

Weigert, C., 1882, Über eine neue Untersuchungsmethode des Zentralnervensystems, *Zentralbl. Med. Wiss.* **20:**753–757, 772–774.

Wise, S. P., and Herkenham, M., 1982, Opiate receptor distribution in the cerebral cortex of the rhesus monkey, *Science* **218:**387–389.

Wise, S. P., and Jones, E. G., 1977, Cells of origin and terminal distribution of descending projections of the rat somatic sensory cortex, *J. Comp. Neurol.* **175:**129–158.

Wong-Riley, M., 1979, Changes in the visual system of monocularly sutured or enucleated cats demonstrable with cytochrome oxidase histochemistry, *Brain Res.* **171:**11–28.

Cytoarchitectonics

I

2

Principles of Cytoarchitectonics

THOMAS LE BRUN KEMPER and
ALBERT M. GALABURDA

1. Introduction

Before proceeding with the history and methods of cytoarchitecture and cytoarchitectonics it will be useful to define the terms used. The term *cortical architecture* refers to the arrangement of a particular cortical unit into layers and columns. Since this arrangement is not homogeneous throughout the cortical mantle, it forms the basis for subdividing the cortex into separate areas. The term *cortical architectonics* refers to the anatomical field of study dealing with the identification and characterization of these different areas. The particular method used is denoted as a prefix. Thus, cytoarchitectonics refers to the study of the arrangement of neurons which have been stained with Nissl stain and myeloarchitectonics to the study of myelin-stained sections. There are also angioarchitectonics, glioarchitectonics, pigmentoarchitectonics, chemoarchitectonics, and pathoarchitectonics.

THOMAS LE BRUN KEMPER • Department of Neurology, Boston City Hospital, Boston, Massachusetts 02118. ALBERT M. GALABURDA • Neurology Unit, Beth Israel Hospital, Boston, Massachusetts 02215.

2. Historical Background

Cytoarchitectonics had its roots in myeloarchitectonics. Its beginning can be dated to February 2, 1776, when an Italian medical student, Francesco Gennari (1782), stated in a footnote that he first saw a prominent little white line (lineola albidior) within the cerebral cortex of the internal part of the posterior lobe of the brain in frozen human cadaver. Its presence was later independently described and illustrated by Vicq d'Azyr (1786) and Soemmering (1788), and this band in the visual cortex is often referred to as the band of Gennari or of Vicq d'Azyr.

The next major advance in myeloarchitectonics of the cerebral cortex was made by Baillarger (1840), a Parisian alienist (psychiatrist). He commented that at that time there was a controversy regarding the existence of layering in the cerebral cortex and whether three layers might become evident in mental illness (mania). He placed thin sections of fresh brain tissue between glass and observed for the first time a six-layered pattern that showed regional differences. When viewed with transilluminated light the layers alternated between opaque and transparent and he numbered them from within out, with his layer VI corresponding to the molecular layer. His opaque layers II and IV corresponded respectively to what are now referred to as the inner and outer stripes of Baillarger, tangential bands of myelinated fibers that occur in layers Vb and IV of modern nomenclature. He also noted a system of radial fibers that extended from the cerebral white matter into the cerebral cortex that were most prominent in the crests of gyri. He attributed considerable importance to these fibers since they clearly showed that the cerebral cortex was intimately connected to the underlying white matter and was not therefore merely a "precipitate furnished by the inner surface of the pia matter," a view put forth by Reil (1759–1813) and apparently still popular at that time. He further noted that in lower mammals the cerebral cortex was less stratified and that in nonmammalian vertebrates it was absent. Using Baillarger's method Smith (1907) studied over 200 human cerebral hemispheres and produced a complete myeloarchitectonic map. In it he recognized approximately 50 different regions with "exact boundaries of each area."

Another significant myeloarchitectonic contribution was that of Flechsig (1920) who introduced the concept of association areas. He studied the sequence of myelination of the cerebral cortex and underlying white matter, eventually recognizing in a series of publications 45 different fields. Fields which showed stainable myelin at birth he called premature fields. These included allocortical formations, limbic cortices, and primary sensory and motor cortices. Surrounding the premature fields were concentric rings of postmature fields that myelinated next. These he called marginal zones. The fields that myelinated last he called association areas. These he felt had their major connectivity to the sensory spheres rather than subcortical formations and provided the substrate for specifically human "psychic function."

The first important contribution to cytoarchitectonics was that of Berlin (1858), who introduced cell staining to the study of the cerebral cortex. With the use of the carmine stain he recognized six layers and numbered them, like

Baillarger, from within out and coined the terms pyramidal, spindle, and granule cell (see Chapter 1).

Credit for the origins of cytoarchitectonics goes to Meynert (1867, 1869, 1872). He recognized two fundamentally different areas, a cortex with a white surface (weissen Rinde) and one with a gray surface (grauer Rinde) (Fig. 1) each of which was composed of pyramidal, granular, and spindle cells with local variations in their emphasis. The weissen Rinde, with a myelinated outer stratum, included the olfactory bulb, septum pellucidum, and uncus and Ammon's horn formation. According to Meynert these were respectively a granular formation, a defective cortex with pyramidal and spindle forms, and a defective cortex with pyramidal forms. In his grauer Rinde, which contained an outer stratum "characteristic of the gray matter of the brain," he also recognized three types. The most extensive was a five-layered common type in which pyramidal cells prevailed (Fig. 2B). It covered the convexity of the cerebral hemispheres and part of the cingulate gyrus. His layers I to IV corresponded to those of modern nomencla-

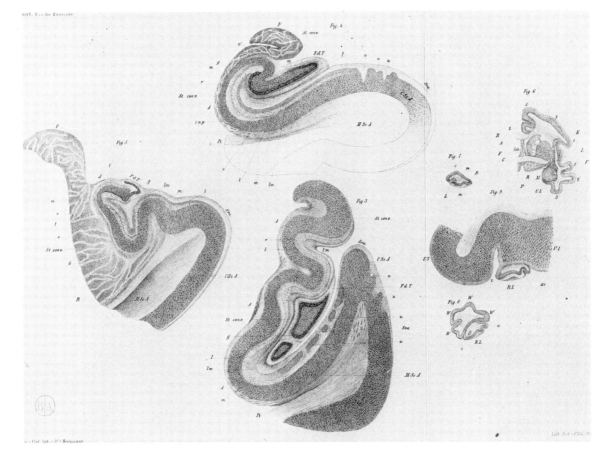

Figure 1. Meynert's illustration (1867) of his weissen Rinde and grauer Rinde. The three figures on the left are from the hippocampal formation with the white outer stratum of his weissen Rinde indicated by a "u." The point at which this stratum terminates in the parahippocampal gyrus is the transition to his grauer Rinde.

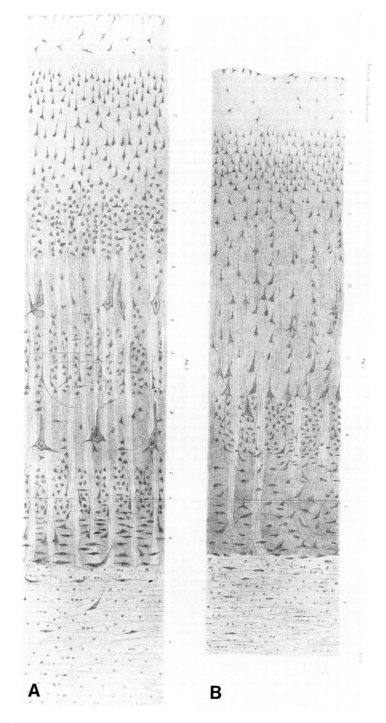

Figure 2. Meynert's illustration (1867) of his eight-layered cortex (A) and his five-layered cortex (B).

ture and his layer V to layers V and VI. The pyramidal cells of layer III he equated with those of Ammon's horn and the characteristic spindle cells in V to those of the claustrum. The second type was an eight-layered cortex (Fig. 2A) in which the prevailing neuron was the granule cell. It occurred in the under part of the cuneus and upper part of the lingula, i.e., in the primary visual cortex as defined in man by later studies. The only layer designated pyramidal in this cortex was his layer II. Layers III through VII contained three granule cell layers separated by two "barren" intermediate layers containing occasional large cells which he called pyramidal. These large cells in layers IV and VI are now often referred to respectively as the solitary stellate and pyramidal cells of Meynert and are characteristic of the primary visual cortex. Layer VIII contained spindle cells. The third type, a five-layered cortex found in the sylvian fossa, was characterized by the presence of the claustrum and therefore contained spindle cells as the dominant element. For Meynert the claustrum was "a layer of the innermost stratum of the cortex, cut off from the main body of the same."

Betz, in a series of five papers (1874b,c, 1881a,b,c) dedicated to Broca, made significant further contributions to cytoarchitectonics. In the first of these papers (1874b) he pointed out that the cerebral cortex was divided by the plane of the fissure of Rolando (central sulcus) into an anterior part in which pyramidal cells predominate and a posterior part where granule cells predominate. In the anterior part he described the giant pyramidal cells that bear his name, pointing out that no one had seen them before. These he felt were more numerous and larger in the right cerebral hemisphere. He provided measurements of their size and number of processes and noted their occurrence in groups of two or three or more. He further noted that they were in the same place in every human brain including the brains of idiots, and in the brains of chimpanzees, baboons, monkeys, and dogs. Betz considered them to have all the attributes of motor cells, noting that in the dog they occurred in the same area identified by Fritsch and Hitzig (1870) as the motor area in this animal. In the next paper (1874c) he described, among other things, the calcarine cortex along lines similar to Meynert, stating that he considered it a sensory center. By 1881 (a,b,c), he had accumulated over 5000 preparations from fetuses to adults, from right and left hemispheres, and from males and females. From these, he stated (1881a), without giving details, that the peculiarities of the structure of the cerebral cortex are present precisely in the same region in most brains, that some cortical regions show differences in size in the two cerebral hemispheres and between different brains, and that most cytoarchitectonic variations occurred in the third cortical layer. He then described (1881b), without illustrating them, regional differences in cytoarchitecture and provided a particularly detailed description of the inferior frontal convolution and of the cingulate gyrus. In that paper he noted that the cortex of the transverse temporal gyrus (primary auditory cortex) resembled that of the post central convolution (primary somesthetic cortex). In his final paper (1881c) he stated that the frontal lobe of the female brain, as compared to the male, has smaller and less frequent pyramidal cells in the third layer as well as smaller and less frequent giant cells. In contrast, the occipital and posterior parietal lobes of the female brain contained more and larger cells in the third layer. He concluded by promising an atlas that unfortunately never materialized.

Lewis and Clarke (1878) studied the motor cortex of man in greater detail, including serial sections, and provided the first illustration of it (Fig. 3A). In agreement with Betz they found that the motor area was distributed over a very definite area that included the posterior part of the superior and middle frontal convolutions and thus probably comprised areas 4 and 6 of Brodmann. Lewis (1879a) repeated these observations in the human and extended them to the cat and sheep. This cortex was described as five-layered, a cortex which he felt was "preeminently" characteristic of the motor area. Further, in agreement with Betz, he noted an abrupt shift in cytoarchitecture in the plane of the fissure of Rolando with the cortex behind it being six-layered. Lewis's description of this six-layered cortex (Fig. 3B), which was achieved by dividing Meynert's layer V into a ganglionic layer (layer V) and a spindle cell layer (layer VI), has been almost universally adopted. In 1880, Lewis mapped the topography of his five- and six-layered cortices in the Barbary ape, ocelot, cat, pig, and sheep, noting the similarity of their appearance and location in all animals studied.

The first atlas illustrating regional variation in the cerebral cortex is a mag-

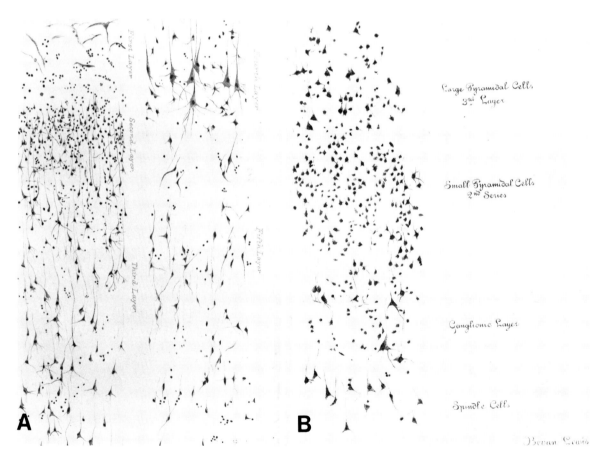

Figure 3. (A) Lewis and Clarke's illustration (1878) of the motor cortex. (B) Lewis's illustration (1879a) of the six- layered cortex behind the plane of the Rolandic fissure.

nificent one provided by Hammarberg in 1895. The goal of his study was to investigate the brains of nine individuals with mental retardation by comparing them to 12 normal controls aged five fetal months to 50 years of age. Detailed descriptions of approximately 20 different cortical regions in the control brains were given, 10 of which were in the frontal lobe, all other lobes having at most three different regions. Layer-by-layer descriptions included measurements of layer thickness, cell size, and cell packing density. Nine neocortical regions, the entorhinal cortex, and three different regions of the hippocampal complex were illustrated with exact scale drawings made at a linear magnification of 200 × (Fig. 4). Comparable drawings were made of the cerebral cortex of the patients with mental retardation. These latter Hammarberg thought showed various stages of curtailed maturation commensurate with the severity of their mental retardation.

The first attempt to provide a complete cytoarchitectonic map with exact borders between the various areas was that of Schlapp (1898). In the macaque cynomolgus monkey he recognized three basic cortical types (Figs. 5A, B, and C). A five-layered type occupied the frontal lobe and an eight-layered type the occipital lobe. Between these was a seven-layered type in which the third layer of modern nomenclature was divided into two separate layers. In all but the occipital cortex he described regional variation.

In 1900, Bolton, in a study on the exact localization of the visual area, introduced the use of human disease states to define cytoarchitectural areas. In his carefully blocked serial sections he recognized a visuo-sensory and a visuo-psychic area, the former corresponding to primary visual cortex and the latter to its surrounding association area. In cases of long-standing blindness and congenital absence of the eyes, he noted, when compared to controls, a decrease in the width of the visuo-sensory but not the visuo-psychic cortex. In a case with congenital absence of the eyes the extent of the visuo-sensory area was decreased as well.

In 1905 Campbell produced the first cytoarchitectonic (and myeloarchitectonic) map of the human brain with comparable maps for the orangutan, chimpanzee, dog, cat, and pig. Prior to 1905, only the motor cortex (Lewis and Clarke, 1878; Brodmann, 1903a) and visual cortex (Bolton, 1900; Brodmann, 1903c) had been accurately defined in man. The motor and primary sensory cortices were defined not only by cyto- and myeloarchitectonic criteria, but also by changes noted in diseases that specifically affected the motor and ascending sensory systems. In the motor system he cited cases of amyotrophic lateral sclerosis in which selective loss of Betz cells occurred and cases of limb amputation in which he found transneuronal reactive changes in these cells. This latter change he called a "reaction at a distance." For sensory disorders he used cases of tabes dorsalis, a disease discreetly affecting the posterior columns of the spinal cord. In this disease he also noted transneuronal changes that were confined to the postcentral sensory cortex. The remaining cortical areas were defined solely on the basis of cyto- and myeloarchitecture. Surrounding the primary sensory cortices were areas he referred to as psychic centers, and in front of the primary motor cortex he described an intermediate precentral area that he postulated was involved in skilled movements. Surrounding these were areas of more elab-

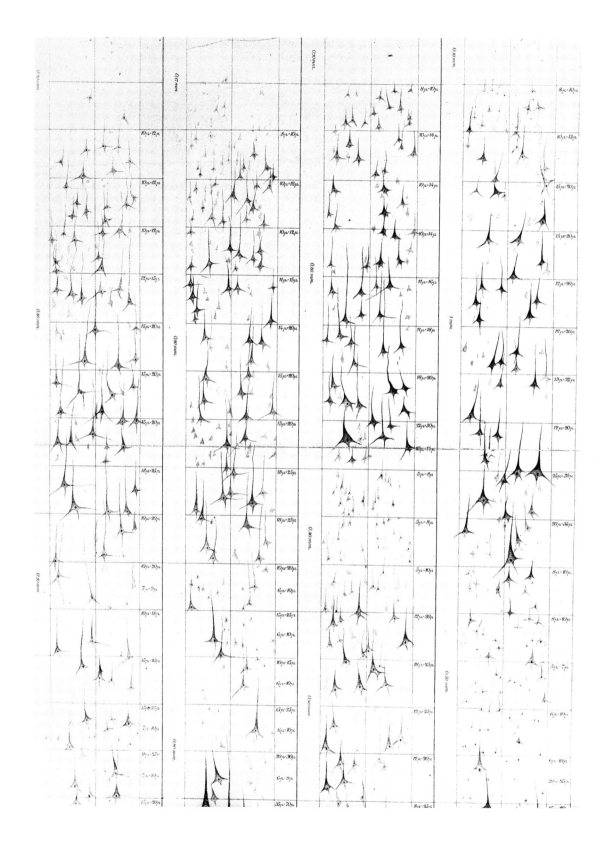

orate sensory and motor function, which from his comparative studies, he indicated were the primary locus of evolutionary elaboration and equated them with higher associative intellectual activity.

Brodmann began his classic studies in 1903 utilizing serial sections of blocks taken from three adult, two infant, and two fetal human brains. In his first study (1903a), he provided an exact localization of what he later called area 4, the primary motor cortex. Although this area had been considered by Betz and later workers as the motor cortex, Brodmann at that time was not convinced of this. In this paper the beginnings of his concept of a six-layered fundamental tectogenetic cortical type during fetal development can be seen. He noted that the motor cortex, which has five layers in the adult, had six layers during fetal development. Later that same year (1903b), using the same brains, Brodmann provided an exact topography for the primary visual cortex, and in agreement with Bolton (1900), showed variation in its position in different brains. In 1905 he published his first complete brain map (1905a) using what he called a *Cercopithecus* monkey, a monkey that von Bonin and Bailey (1947) later suggest was the *Lasyopyga campbelli*. The right cerebral hemisphere of a single monkey was cut in toto in the horizontal plane (Fig. 6A) and 28 cytoarchitectonic areas were defined (Fig. 6B) and illustrated with photomicrographs. It is here that his famous numbering system first appears, with those fields first encountered in the serial sections receiving the lowest numbers. In this paper he noted that some areas are more or less circumscribed while others show sharp borders. In agreement with the earlier findings of Betz (1874b) and Lewis (1879a) he also noted a fundamental difference in the cortices rostral and caudal to the sulcus of Rolando and extended this plane of separation to include the cingulate and insular cortices. In the former it was marked by the separation of his areas 23 and 24 and in the latter by the central sulcus of the insula. Anterior to this plane he identified agranular fields and posterior to it cortices with a well-developed fourth granule cell layer. Later that same year (1905b) he published maps of the giant pyramidal cell cortex in carnivores.

A major paper by Brodmann appeared in 1906 on the general plan of the cerebral cortex in mammals, citing as evidence the brains of primates, prosimians, bats, carnivores, seals, insectivores, rodents, ungulates, armadillos, sloths, and marsupials. He felt that the basic cortical layering was the same in all of these animals and that differences could be understood by the differentiation within a particular layer, the loss of a layer, the condensation of two or more layers, or the rearrangement of layers. He further noted, as he had in earlier papers, that with few exceptions the cytoarchitectonic fields showed no exact relationship to gyri. In 1908, he published his famous map of the human brain (1908a), with later modifications and additions in 1909, 1912, and 1914. In these he recognized 44 cortical areas and provided only a surface map of their locations, leaving the sulcal cortices largely unexplored. The descriptions of the areas were brief and no histological details or photomicrographs were provided. However, in his last major cytoarchitectonic study, on the brain of a lemur (1908b), all these details

---

← ——————————————————————————————————

Figure 4. Plate 2 from Hammarberg (1895). On the left is the cortex in the posterior part of the superior frontal gyrus, followed by motor cortex, the cortex of the postcentral gyrus, and the cortex of the posterior part of the inferior frontal convolution. The original plate measures 24 × 63 cm.

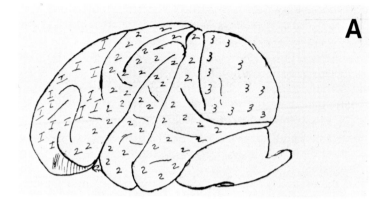

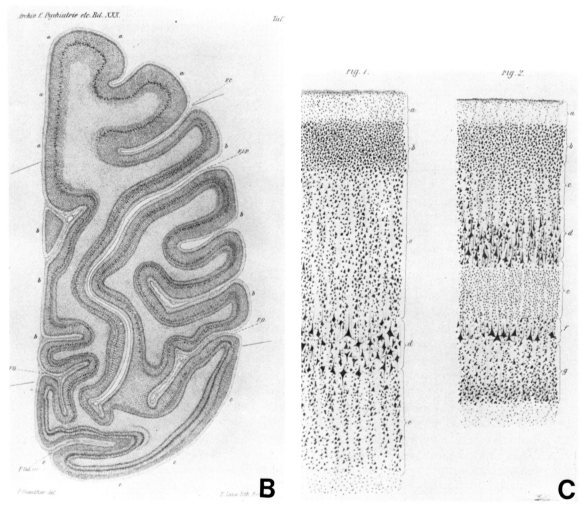

Figure 5. The first cytoarchitectonic map, made by Schlapp (1898). (A) The map; (B) the distribution of his three cortical types in a Nissl-stained horizontal section; (C) his first and second type shown at a higher magnification.

were provided. There was a complete surface map, diagrams of the location of the areas within the sulci, and photomicrographs.

In 1909 Brodmann expanded these works into a monograph on comparative localization in the cerebral cortex in which he provided complete surface maps for many of the animals that he had studied. He discussed in detail the problems of cytoarchitectonic parcellation, emphasizing the need for other types of investigation to supplement these studies, particularly physiological studies. Based on these comparative studies and his studies of ontogenetic development of the cerebral cortex, he felt that the original form of the cerebral cortex consisted of six layers, i.e., his six-layered tectogenetic basic type. In human development he noted the appearance of this fundamental type during the sixth to eight fetal month. Those cortical areas that retained this six-layered pattern he called homotypical homogenetic cortex and those in which the six layers were no longer evident in the adult brain heterotypical homogenetic cortex. The latter included, among others, the rostral and retrosplenial cingulate cortices, part of the insula, his areas 4 and 6, and the primary visual cortex. Cortical areas that failed to show a six-layered pattern during fetal development he called heterogenetic. Areas included in this group were the olfactory bulb, tuberculum olfactorium,

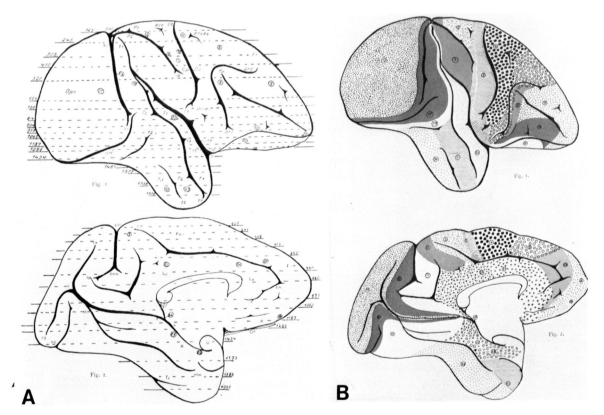

A　　　　　　　　　　　　　　　　　　**B**

Figure 6. Brodmann's map (1905a) of the *Cercopithecus* monkey. (A) The plane of section and cutting sequence. (B) The map. The first sections have the lowest number on the map. Although shown here in black and white, the original was in color.

anterior perforant space, amygdala, hippocampal formation, presubiculum, entorhinal cortex, septum, and prepyriform cortex. These two basic cortical types, homogenetic and heterogenetic, were later called isocortex and allocortex by Vogt and Vogt (1919) and correspond to Meynert's grauer Rinde and weissen Rinde. The first of these two types Smith (1901) called neopallium.

In 1925 a scholarly study of the cytoarchitecture of the human cerebral cortex was published by von Economo and Koskinas. It was the result of 15 years of work, with the initial plans drawn up by von Economo in the same house where Meynert had worked (van Bogaert and Théodoridès, 1979). Von Economo and Koskinas recognized 107 fields and illustrated them in an atlas containing 112 actual photographic enlargements. One hundred and two fields were magnified 100 times so that 1 mm equaled exactly 10 μm. Each area was described in detail with data on layer thickness, cell size, and cell packing density. They introduced the term *koniocortex* as a general term describing primary sensory cortices, calling attention to their dustlike appearance.

The most recent attempt at parcellation of the human brain is that of Sarkissov *et al.* (1955) at the Moscow Brain Institute. According to Braak (1980) this map was patterned after that of Brodmann. It, however, has the decided advantage over Brodmann's version in that the areas are systemically described and illustrated.

The seemingly unrelenting progress of architectonics toward greater refinement resulting in increasing numbers of areas did not go unchallenged, particularly Brodmann's concept that the cerebral cortex was a discrete mosaic of juxtaposed centers which, according to Vogt and Vogt, had hair-sharp borders raised many objections. Also under attack was Brodmann's concept of a six-layered tectogenetic basic cortical lamination during fetal development. This latter concept was challenged by Lorente de Nó (1933, 1938) as fundamentally wrong. He claimed that the six-layered pattern seen during the sixth fetal month in the human brain did not correspond to the six-layered pattern of the adult. According to Lorente de Nó the fetal six-layered pattern was the result of protoplasmic (dendritic) plexuses and not cell layering. Further he stated that in the fifth fetal month, in Golgi preparations, "every layer is recognizable with the same fundamental characteristic as in the adult cortex."

Lashley and Clark (1946) published a particularly sharp criticism of the cytoarchitectonic method. They independently parcellated the cerebral cortex of two spider monkeys (*Ateles geoffroyi*) and noted little agreement between the resultant maps. On the basis of these differences they raised a number of criticisms of cytoarchitectonic parcellations. They felt that most of the architectonic fields changed gradually at their borders, that there was individual variation in size and appearance of comparable areas from brain to brain, and that some areas could be seen in some brains and not others. Furthermore, they were unable to locate the majority of the isocortical areas recognized by other investigators in this monkey and in the macaque. They emphasized the need for developing objective criteria and uniform standards that would result in maps that better represent functional units and the need of other methods of confirmation, particularly studies of specific fiber connectivity. Additional difficulties with the cytoarchitectonic method were cited by von Bonin and Bailey (1947), Bailey *et al.* (1950), and Bailey and von Bonin (1951) in their cytoarchitectonic studies respectively of *Macaca mulatta*, chimpanzee, and man, particularly in their study of the human brain. They were struck by their perception of the homogeneity of vast areas of the cerebral cortex that had previously been subdivided and felt that knowledge of the functional significance of the subdivisions would be needed for proper parcellation. Bailey and von Bonin (1951) stated that "after long and careful study of the human isocortex the main impression we have retained is that vast areas are so closely similar in structure as to make any attempt at subdivision unprofitable, if not impossible."

All these criticisms pointed to the need to correlate architectonic subdivisions to physiological and connectional observations. Such studies, which have helped in the renaissance of architectonics, were first carefully explored by Walker (1938) and Rose and Woolsey (1948, 1949). There then followed numerous studies showing a close correlation between architectonics and specific connectivity as illustrated by the work of Leonard (1969), Jones and Powell (1970), Jones and Burton (1976), Allman and Kaas (1971), Pandya and Sanides (1973), Seltzer and Pandya (1978), and Mesulam and Mufson (1982) to name but a few. Similar support for architectonic parcellation has been provided by recent physiological analysis showing changes across borders (Merzenich and Brugge, 1973; Powell and Mountcastle, 1959; Hubel and Wiesel, 1965). In some cases this agreement has not been forthcoming (Zeki, 1978).

During recent times few architectonic studies have been published that claim to stand on their own. Complete maps have been generally provided in the framework of stereotaxic atlases or as an aid to research in physiology and connectivity,* and have relied heavily on old parcellations. In human studies, where interventional anatomical techniques are not possible, purely architectonic studies still maintain a strong foothold for advances in the understanding of specific issues. Among these are studies of cerebral asymmetries and architectonic analysis of lesions. Such studies are necessary for structure–function relationships in normative cerebra as well as in acquired and congenital neurological disorders.

A modern exponent of the architectonic method for the purpose of advancing theories in brain evolution is Sanides (1972). He has stressed less issues of cortical parcellation than concepts of trends of cortical evolution capable of illustrating similarities and differences along the phylogenetic scale and of providing predictive capabilities on questions of homology (cf. Galaburda and Pandya, 1982).

3. Methods of Processing

The methods of processing have varied throughout the history of architectonics (see Chapter 1). The early workers, Berlin, Meynert, and Betz, used Gerlach's carmine stain, a deep red dye extracted from the dried bodies of female

---

* Such parcellations are available for the snake (Ulinski, 1974), opposum (Oswaldo-Cruz and Rocha-Miranda, 1968), rat (Krieg, 1946; Zilles *et al.*, 1980), mouse (Caviness, 1975), cat (Gurewitsch and Chatschaturian, 1928), *Tupaia* (Zilles *et al.*, 1978), *Galago* (Zilles *et al.*, 1979), and man (Braak, 1980).

cochineal insects (Mallory, 1938). A detailed description of the carmine stain is provided by Betz (1874a). In his method, nervous tissue is initially fixed in 70–80% alcohol stained light brown with iodine and, as also did Berlin and Meynert, hardened in a chromate solution. Unembedded sections are cut on a microtome, stained, dehydrated in graded alcohols, cleared with terpentine, and mounted in damarlack.

Lewis and Clarke (1878) and Lewis (1877) introduced frozen sectioning and serial sectioning to cytoarchitectonic studies. Lewis has provided a complete description of his methods together with a woodcut illustration of a freezing microtome of his own design (Lewis, 1877, 1879b). Frozen sections of fresh brain tissue cut on his microtome were fixed with a 0.1 to 0.2% solution of osmic acid and stained with aniline black. According to Lewis (1879b), "such preparations exhibit the structure of the cortex cerebri with a distinctness and beauty unrivaled by any other process which I have seen adopted." The "nerve cells [are] far more crowded and their processes more numerous, more distinct, and more complicated than seen in corresponding sections prepared by the chrome method." Added advantages were that shrinkage during processing was greatly reduced, myelin was not stained, and the process was rapid and reliable. Some of these advantages can be readily seen by comparing the illustrations of Meynert with Lewis and Clarke and Lewis (cf. Fig. 2 with Fig. 3).

The Nissl method for staining nervous tissue was introduced by 1894. Nissl (1894) stated that his method gave best results after fixation in 96% alcohol and sections cut from unembedded blocks stained with methylene blue to which Venetian soap had been added. Hammarberg (1895), although not acknowledging Nissl, used both alcohol fixation and methylene blue staining. However, he embedded his blocks in paraffin wax. Since his purpose was to compare control brains of different ages with those of the mentally retarded, it was essential that shrinkage and/or swelling of the tissue during processing be held to a minimum. After extensive trials on the effects of different methods of fixation and embedding, in which he monitored the blocks for changes in volume and linear dimensions during processing, he settled on his final method. It showed the least change in the width of the cortex and the least variation in shrinkage from brain to brain. On the material thus prepared, he developed a method for cell counting in serial sections using an ocular reticle and counting either nucleoli or pyramidal cells with at least a 10-μm apical dendrite, thus avoiding counting the same cell twice in adjacent sections. He expressed his results as the number of neurons per 0.1 mm^3, a unit of measure that has become the standard in quantitative cytoarchitectonics.

Schlapp (1898) introduced whole brain serial sectioning to architectonics. He used alcohol fixation, celloidin embedding, and the Nissl stain. Bolton (1900) carefully blocked formalin-fixed tissue "in such a manner and of such size as to enable sections to be made from them at right angles to the course of the gyri without more waste of tissue than was absolutely unavoidable." For his studies of the visual cortices this required 20 to 69 blocks per brain with frozen sections stained with Nissl stain. This complex method was essential for his studies since he was measuring the width of the cortex and its various layers as well as the cortical extent.

Brodmann used paraffin embedding and thionin Nissl staining using a microtome of his own design (1903c) (Fig. 7). Of paramount importance to him

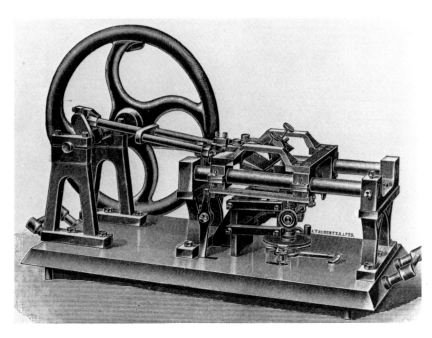

Figure 7. Brodmann's Doppelschlittenmikrotom (1903c). Brodmann designed this microtome with a double slide to provide greater stability for the knife carrier.

were uniformly cut paraffin sections of thickness 10 to 20 μm which he felt was the best thickness for photography. Noting that available microtomes were unable to produce sections of adequate size and uniform thickness, he designed and built one with a double slide to provide greater stability for the knife carrier. This microtome could only accommodate a block size of 70 × 80 mm. He therefore was limited in his human studies to blocking the brains, generally cutting the blocks in serial sections that were oriented as much as possible at right angles to the gyri. For smaller brains he used whole brain serial sectioning.

Campbell (1905), in order to cut as much of the brain as possible at right angles to the gyri, took approximately 50 blocks per human brain. He recorded their positions on orthogonal drawings and on photographs. The blocks were embedded in celloidin and cut in serial sections at a thickness of 15 or 25 μm. Staining of nerve cells was accomplished with thionin and myelin staining with Wolters–Kulschitzky stain. For some of his pathological brains, serial frozen sections were used. Animal brains were cut whole in the coronal plane and stained by the same methods.

The most elaborate method was that of von Economo and Koskinas (1925). Using a modification of the method devised by Bolton (1900), they hand cut the brain into several hundred blocks, always cutting at right angles to gyri (Fig. 8). Each block was flattened between filter paper, embedded in paraffin, and serially cut at 25 μm, a thickness selected in order to clearly show both cortical layers and the details of individual neurons. The sections were deparaffinated and stained unmounted with toluidine blue. They felt that the shrinkage during this process was negligible, amounting to about 10%.

No new approaches were used in the studies of von Bonin and Bailey.

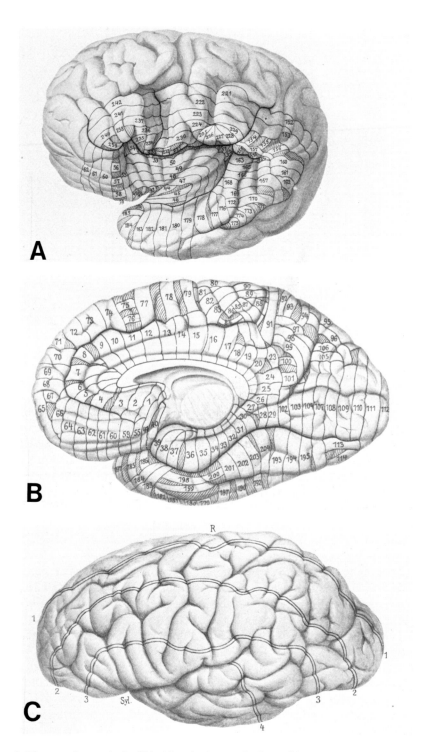

Figure 8. The complex method of blocking the human brain used by von Economo and Koskinas (1925) is shown in (A) and (B). Their method of sampling a large area of the human brain in single sections is shown in (C).

Cytoarchitectonics is the most widely used approach to the parcellation of the cerebral cortex. The only other commonly used technique is myeloarchitectonics. The latter is technically more difficult and its relationship to cytoarchitectonic parcellations not universally agreed upon. It requires careful differentiation during staining, during which the density of myelin staining, the extent and number of myelinated fibers, and the background staining will vary. Another possible source of concern in man is that myelination within the cerebral cortex continues well into adult life with prominent changes also noted with aging (Kaes, 1907). Early workers with experience in both techniques found a good correspondence between cyto- and myeloarchitecture (Campbell, 1905; Brodmann, 1909; Vogt, 1910, 1911, 1927; Vogt and Vogt, 1919). Brodmann (1909) felt that this was particularly the case in animals. In man he felt myeloarchitecture provided a finer differentiation within the cerebral cortex, leading to the recognition of more areas. In support of this notion Vogt and Vogt (1910–1927) recognized some 200 myeloarchitectonic areas in the human brain which they felt showed good correspondence with cytoarchitecture. In contrast, von Economo and Koskinas (1925), von Bonin and Bailey (1947), Bailey *et al.* (1950), and Bailey and von Bonin (1951), who used only cytoarchitectonic criteria in their studies, doubted the usefulness and validity of myeloarchitectonics. Von Economo and Koskinas, after reviewing the myeloarchitectonic maps of Vogt and Vogt, felt there was little agreement between these maps and cytoarchitectonic maps of the human brain including their own. Bailey and von Bonin (1951) went further in their criticism of the myeloarchitectonic technique stating that "slight, almost unavoidable, local variations in the degree of differentiation suggest areal differences which, on closer scrutiny, could not be upheld." Modern workers apparently are on the side of those who feel that there is a good correspondence between these two techniques (Braak, 1980; also see Chapter 3).

The recently introduced pigmentoarchitectonics technique (Braak, 1980) is reviewed elsewhere in this book (Chapter 3). It is of note that this technique, which uses sections stained only for lipofuscin pigment, has the decided advantage of showing borders between adjacent fields with great clarity in many fields. Unlike cytoarchitectonics, the lipofuscin method does not stain every neuron and therefore represents a chemoarchitectonic variant which cannot at this time be clearly related to the Nissl patterns outlined by cytoarchitectonics.

5. Techniques of Parcellation

A major aid in architectonic parcellation is the identification of gross anatomical landmarks, because they often correspond to architectonic borders. Thus, gyri often contain separate architectonic areas, while sulci, fissurets, and often even small cortical dimples commonly outline a border between two architectonic areas (Sanides, 1972; Galaburda, personal observations). For example, in the human brain the precentral gyrus contains the gigantopyramidal motor area, the central sulcus delimits its posterior margin, and the precentral sulcus (at least dorsally) delimits its anterior border. The human frontal operculum contains architectonic areas of distinctive granular appearance which are separated from other areas on the frontal convexity by portions of the inferior frontal sulcus. Various opercular areas are themselves separated by sulci such as the anterior horizontal and vertical limbs of the sylvian fissure. In the rhesus monkey similar gross landmarks on the surface aid in parcellating that cortex. The superior temporal region of the macaque is organized in an orderly fashion such that primitive root fields are located in the circular sulcus, granular core fields on the superior temporal plane, and surrounding belt fields having well-developed layer III pyramidal neurons on the superior temporal gyrus (Galaburda and Pandya, 1982) all remarkably faithful to their topographical locations. Lissencephalic brains of lower mammals do not offer the same degree of assistance, but even in those brains small cortical dimples often herald the border between adjacent fields.

Parcellation of architectonic fields is best carried out under low-power microscopy. In larger brains a stereomicroscope is most useful, but in smaller specimens low-power compound microscopy may be needed. An "impressionistic" view of the cortex is required, rather than attention to special histological features. Therefore, relative tinctorial patterns rather than size and shape of individual neurons, provide the best approach to parcellation. Assuming an evenly stained section, different architectonic areas will appear to take up different amounts of stain. Further analysis will show that this is the result of different staining properties of the layers. Thus, one field may be noted to stain more heavily in layers II and III whereas its neighboring area will stain more darkly in the deeper layers. It is probably a safe general principle that at a reliable and reproducible architectonic border, a tinctorial change will be evident in each layer. These differences in staining properties will reflect differences in average cell size and cell packing density, as well as differences in the relative widths of the layers. In addition, in certain areas, differences in staining pattern will also reflect the presence or absence of a columnar arrangement perpendicular to the pial surface. The manner in which cell layers border each other, whether sharply or indistinctly, will affect the "impressionistic" view of a field, and may provide an additional distinguishing feature for parcellation. This also applies to the way in which layer VI meets the subcortical alba. In granular koniocortices, for instance, the cortical–subcortical border is often razor sharp, whereas in adjacent fields this border is tapered.

Although impressions of general degree of staining are useful in telling architectonic borders, experience shows that architectonic changes occur most commonly in ways which relate to specific laminar features. Thus, it is often very useful to note differences in depth of staining between the superficial and deep strata, i.e., the layers lying superficial to layer IV and deep to it. Cortical areas, then, may be externodense, i.e., the superficial stratum is darker than the deeper one; they may be internodense, i.e., the deeper stratum is more heavily stained; or an area may be eudense, a situation in which both inner and outer strata are roughly equally dark. In general more primitive cortices, e.g., the proisocortices of the anterior cingulate gyrus and insula, are strongly internodense, whereas the evolutionarily newer cortices are eudense, e.g., homotypical areas of the frontal and parietal lobe, or externodense, e.g., the somesthetic, visual, and auditory koniocortices. One exception to this rule is the picture provided by the primary motor field and immediately adjacent belt areas which, although highly evolved, are internodense, due in great part to the specialized nature of layer V.

Another laminar characteristic which proves useful in parcellation of areas is the appearance of layer IV. This layer often shows sharp changes in thickness and density across architectonic borders when other clues are more difficult to visualize. The rostro-caudal borders of fields lying along the circular sulcus of the monkey and human brain, for instance, are best resolved by the change in the appearance of layer IV. Similarly, areas located on either bank of the principal sulcus of the monkey brain differ mainly in the nature of the fourth layer; there is a marked increase in thickness and packing density in layer IV as one proceeds from the dorsal to ventral banks of this sulcus.

The ability to determine clearly the exact number of layers is also helpful for parcellation. Differences in the number of layers are the results in part of absolute numerical differences and in part to vague borders between adjacent laminae. Thus, in primitive fields such as the cingulate and insular proisocortex, the fifth and sixth layers are barely separable, resulting in a fairly homogeneous deep stratum. Furthermore, lamina IV is nearly devoid of granular neurons, and, therefore, difficult to identify. These features provide the proisocortex with a less stratified appearance. With passage across a border toward the isocortex proper, lamina IV fills in and layers V and VI become clearly separable.

It is important to stress that a given architectonic field is not perfectly homogeneous in appearance, i.e., there are small fluctuations within its borders. This probably reflects issues of columnar organization, clustering of neuronal groups, and even features of microvascular architecture. Attention to such minute focal variation may lead to the identification of "too many" fields. However, such trivial changes usually do not reflect themselves in all layers, as do reliable borders; they do not persist beyond a few cell diameters; and they tend to repeat several times within an architectonic field, often exhibiting a pattern of repetition which in itself represents an architectonic characteristic of the area.

A word of caution should be mentioned about the columnar characteristics of a given field. Investigators have often relied heavily on these architectonic properties. However, in these authors' experience, columnar features are particularly dependent on plane of section and cannot be relied upon for consistency of border setting. In lissencephalic brains this is less often a significant problem, but in highly folded cortices such as in human and whale brains, reliance on columnar features may amount to a significant hindrance in reliable and reproducible parcellation.

Folding of the cortex tends to distort the architectonic appearance and often results in "too many" areas. Both laminar and cellular distortions, however, assume predictable patterns which have been specified by Bok (1959). To summarize briefly, the layers in the superficial stratum are compressed and the deeper layers increase in depth at the tops of gyri. At the bottom of sulci there occurs the reverse effect: the superficial layers are widened whereas the deep layers are compressed. Layer IV changes the least. Cells lying in those layers undergo the predictable changes, i.e., in layers that increase in depth the pyramids are elongated in the direction perpendicular to the pial surface, whereas those lying in compressed layers are flattened longitudinally. It is possible to parcellate true sulcal fields when it is noted that the relative widths of the layers and shapes of the neurons violate the predicted folding artifacts. One example of such a field is found in the depth of the central sulcus of the brains of primates, where a small field (the intersensory motor area) separates the rostrally lying motor area from the caudally located somesthetic koniocortex. Passing from the somesthetic koniocortex to the sulcal field, layers V and VI broaden instead of flattening, heralding the transition to the internodense primary motor cortex.

The confirmation of architectonic borders is made easier if the opportunity arises for checking borders against those obtained by different stains. One useful staining alternative to the cellular stains outlined in Nissl preparations is provided by myelin stains. In myelin preparations attention is paid to the patterns of intracortical myelinated fibers and to the general density of myelin in the area. Fields differ in the patterns of vertical and horizontal myelinated axons. The differences may be in the number of fiber bundles as well as in the density of fiber staining within and between the bundles. Thus, a field may have one or two horizontal stripes of Baillarger (cingulostriate and bistriate, respectively), or may be altogether astriate. Occasionally a third horizontal stripe, the stripe of Kaes–Bechterew, may be visible in the superficial portion of layer III (see Chapter 3). There are several patterns of the radial fibers as well, having to do mainly with their length of extension toward the pial surface. Myeloarchitectonics is less useful than cellular (cyto) architectonics in our hands. This results from the difficulty in achieving adequate intracortical myelin staining especially in primitive brains lacking well-developed horizontal fiber plexuses, as well as in primitive regions of advanced brains.

6. References

Allman, J. M., and Kaas, J. H., 1971, A representation of the visual field in the caudal third of the middle temporal gyrus of the owl monkey, *Brain Res.* **31**:85.

Bailey, P., and von Bonin, G., 1951, *The Isocortex of Man,* University of Illinois Press, Urbana.

Bailey, P., von Bonin, G., and McCulloch, W. S., 1950, *The Isocortex of the Chimpanzee,* University of Illinois Press, Urbana.

Baillarger, J.-G.-F., 1840, Recherches sur la structure de la couche corticale des circonvolutions du cerveau, *Mém. Acad. R. Med.* **8**:149.

Berlin, R., 1858, Beitrag zur Strukturlehre der Grosshirnwindungen, cited in Schlapp (1898).

Betz, W., 1874a, Die Untersuchungmethode des Centralnervensystems des Menschen, *Centralbl. Med. Wiss.* **1874**:4.

Betz, W., 1874b, Anatomischer Nachweis zweier Gehirncentra, *Centralbl. Med. Wiss.* **1874**:578.

Betz, W., 1874c, Anatomischer Nachweis zweier Gehirncentra, *Centralbl. Med. Wiss.* **1874**:595.

Betz, W., 1881a, Ueber die feinere Struktur der Gehirnrinde des Menschen, *Centralbl. Med. Wiss.* **1881**:193.

Betz, W., 1881b, Ueber die feinere Struktur der Gehirnrinde des Menschen, *Centralbl. Med. Wiss.* **1881**:209.

Betz, W., 1881c, Ueber die feinere Struktur der Gehirnrinde des Menschen, *Centralbl. Med. Wiss.* **1881**:231.

Bok, S. T., 1959, *Histonomy of the Cerebral Cortex,* Elsevier, Amsterdam.

Bolton, J. S., 1900, The exact localization of the visual area of the human cerebral cortex, *Philos. Trans. R. Soc. London Ser. B* **193**:165.

Braak, H., 1980, *Architectonics of the Human Telencephalic Cortex,* Springer, Berlin.

Brodmann, K., 1903a, Beiträge zur histologischen Lokalisation der Grosshirnrinde: Die Regio Rolandica, *J. Psychol. Neurol.* **2**:79.

Brodmann, K., 1903b, Beiträge zur histologischen Lokalisation der Grosshirnrinde: Der Calcarinatypus, *J. Psychol. Neurol.* **2**:133.

Brodmann, K., 1903c, Zwei neue Apparate zur Paraffinserientechnik, *J. Psychol. Neurol.* **2**:206.

Brodmann, K., 1905a, Beiträge zur histologischen Lokalisation der Grosshirnrinde: Die Rindenfeldern der niederen Affen, *J. Psychol. Neurol.* **4**:177.

Brodmann, K., 1905b, Beiträge zur histologischen Lokalisation der Grosshirnrinde: Die Riesenpyramidentypus und sein Verhalten zu den Furchen bei den Karnivoren, *J. Psychol. Neurol.* **6**:108.

Brodmann, K., 1906, Beiträge zur histologischen Lokalisation der Grosshirnrinde: Über den allgemeinen Bauplan des Cortex pallii bei den Mammaliern und Zwei homologe Rindenfelder im Besonderen. Zugleich ein Beitrag zur Furchenlehre, *J. Psychol. Neurol.* **6**:275.

Brodmann, K., 1908a, Beiträge zur histologischen Lokalisation der Grosshirnrinde: Die Cortexgliederung des Menschen, *J. Psychol. Neurol.* **6**:231.

Brodmann, K., 1908b, Beiträge zur histologischen Lokalisation der Grosshirnrinde: Die cytoarchitektonische Cortexgliederung der Halbaffen (Lemuriden), *J. Psychol. Neurol.* **10**:287.

Brodmann, K., 1909, *Vergleichende Lokalisationlehre der Grosshirnrinde,* Barth, Leipzig.

Brodmann, K., 1912, Neue Ergibnisse über die vergleichende Lokalisation der Grosshirnrinde mit besonderer Berücksichtigung des Stirnhirns, *Anat. Anz. Suppl.* **41**:157.

Brodmann, K., 1914, Physiologie des Gehirns, in: *Neue Deutsche Chirurgie,* Vol. 11 (P. von Brun, ed.), pp. 85–426, Enke, Stuttgart.

Campbell, A. W., 1905, *Histological Studies on the Localization of Cerebral Function,* Cambridge University Press, London.

Caviness, V. S., Jr., 1975, Architectonic map of neocortex of the normal mouse, *J. Comp. Neurol.* **164**:247.

Flechsig, P., 1920, *Anatomie des menschlichen Gehirns und Rückenmarks auf myelogenetischer Grundlage,* Thieme, Leipzig.

Fritsch, G., and Hitzig, E., 1870, Über die elektrische Erregbarkeit des Grosshirns, *Arch. Anat. Physiol. Wiss. Med.* **1870**:300.

Galaburda, A. M., and Pandya, D. N., 1982, Role of architectonics and connections in the study of primate brain evolution, in: *Primate Brain Evolution: Methods and Concepts* (E. Armstrong and D. Falk, eds.), pp. 203–216, Plenum Press, New York.

Gennari, F., 1782, *De Peculiari Structura Cerebri Nonnullisque Eius Morbus,* Parma.

Gurewitsch, M., and Chatschaturian, A., 1928, Zur Cytoarchitektonik der Grosshirnrinde der Feliden, *Z. Anat. Entwicklungsgesch.* **87**:100.

Hammarberg, C., 1895, *Studien über Klinik und Pathologie der Idiotie, nebst Untersuchungen über die normale Anatomie der Hirnrinde,* Druck der akademischen Buchdruckerei, Upsala.

Hubel, D. H., and Wiesel, T. N., 1965, Receptive fields and functional architecture in two nonstriate visual areas (18 and 19) of the cat, *J. Neurophysiol.* **28**:229.

Jones, E. G., and Burton, M., 1976, Areal differences in the laminar distribution of thalamic afferents in cortical fields of the insular, parietal and temporal regions of primates, *J. Comp. Neurol.* **168**:197.

Jones, E. G., and Powell, T. P. S., 1970, An anatomical study of converging sensory pathways within the cerebral cortex of the monkey, *Brain* **93**:793.

Kaes, T., 1907, *Die Grosshirnrinde des Menschen in ihren Massen und in ihrem Fasergehalt,* Fischer, Jena.

Krieg, W. J. S., 1946, Connections of the cerebral cortex. I. The albino rat. A topography of the cortical areas, *J. Comp. Neurol.* **84**:221.

Lashley, K. S., and Clark, G., 1946, The cytoarchitecture of the cerebral cortex of *Ateles:* A critical examination of architectonic studies, *J. Comp. Neurol.* **85**:223.

Leonard, C. M., 1969, The prefrontal cortex of the rat. I. Cortical projections of the mediodorsal nucleus. II. Efferent connections, *Brain Res.* **12**:321.

Lewis, B., 1877, A new freezing microtome for the preparation of sections of brain and spinal cord, *J. Anat. Physiol.* **11**:537.

Lewis, B., 1879a, On the comparative structure of the cortex cerebri, *Brain* **1**:77.

Lewis, B., 1879b, Application of freezing methods to the microscopic examination of the brain, *Brain* **1**:348.

Lewis, B., 1880, III. Researches on the comparative structure of the cortex cerebri, *Philos. Trans. R. Soc. London* **171**:35.

Lewis, B., and Clarke, H., 1878, The cortical lamination of the motor area of the brain, *Proc. R. Soc. London* **27**:38.

Lorente de Nó, R., 1933, Studies on the structure of the cerebral cortex. I. The area entorhinalis, *J. Psychol. Neurol.* **45**:381.

Lorente de Nó, R., 1938, Cerebral cortex: Architecture, intracortical connections, motor projections, in: *Physiology of the Nervous System* (J. F. Fulton, ed.), 3rd ed., pp. 291–325, Oxford University Press, London.

Mallory, F. B., 1938, *Pathological Technique: A Practical Manual for Workers in Pathological Histology including Directions for the Performance of Autopsies and for Microphotography*, Saunders, Philadelphia.

Merzenich, M. M., and Brugge, J. F., 1973, Representation of the cochlear partition on the superior temporal plane of the macaque monkey, *Brain Res.* **50**:275.

Mesulam, M.-M., and Mufson, E. J., 1982, Insula of the Old World monkey. I. Architectonics in the insulo-orbito-temporal component of the paralimbic brain, *J. Comp. Neurol.* **212**:1.

Meynert, T., 1867, Der Bau der Grosshirnrinde und seine örtlichen Verschiedenheiten, nebst einen pathologisch-anatomischen Corollarium, *Vierteljahresschr. Psychiatr.* **1**:77.

Meynert, T., 1869, Der Bau der Grosshirnrinde und seine örtlichen Verschiedenheiten, nebst einen pathologisch–anatomischen Corollarium, *Vierteljahresschr. Psychiatr.* **2**:88.

Meynert, R., 1872, The brain of mammals, in: *Manual of Histology*, Vol. 2 (S. A. Stricker, ed.), pp. 650–766, Wood, New York.

Nissl, F., 1894, Ueber die sogenannten Granula der Nervenzellen, *Neurol. Centralbl.* **13**:781.

Oswaldo-Cruz, E., and Rocha-Miranda, C. E., 1968, *The Brain of the Opossum (Didelphis marsupiales): A Cytoarchitectonic Atlas in Stereotaxic Coordinates,* Univ. Federal do Rio de Janeiro, Rio de Janeiro.

Pandya, D. N., and Sanides, R., 1973, Architectonic parcellation of the temporal operculum in rhesus monkey and its projection pattern, *Z. Anat. Entwicklungsgesch.* **139**:123.

Powell, T. P. S., and Mountcastle, V. B., 1959, The cytoarchitecture of the postcentral gyrus of the monkey *Macaca mulatta, Bull. Johns Hopkins Hosp.* **105**:108.

Rose, J. E., and Woolsey, C. N., 1948, Structure and relations of limbic cortex and anterior thalamic nuclei in rabbit and cat, *J. Comp. Neurol.* **89**:279.

Rose, J. E., and Woolsey, C. N., 1949, The relations of thalamic connections, cellular structure and evocable electrical activity in the auditory region of the cat, *J. Comp. Neurol.* **91**:441.

Sanides, F., 1972, Representation in the cerebral cortex and its area lamination patterns, in: *Structure and Function of Nervous Tissue*, Vol. 1 (G. A. Bourne, ed.), pp. 329–453, Academic Press, New York.

Sarkissov, S. A., Filimonoff, I. N., Kononowa, E. P., Preobraschenskaja, I. S., and Kukuew, L. A., 1955, *Atlas of the Cytoarchitectonics of the Human Cerebral Cortex*, Medgiz, Moscow.

Schlapp, M., 1898, Der Zellenbau der Grosshirnrinde des Affen *Macacus cynomolgus, Arch. Psychiatr. Nervenkr.* **30**:583.

Seltzer, B., and Pandya, D. N., 1978, Afferent cortical connections and architectonics of the superior temporal sulcus and surrounding cortex in rhesus monkey, *Brain Res.* **149**:1.

Smith, G. E., 1901, Notes upon the natural subdivisions of the cerebral hemispheres, *J. Anat. Physiol.* **35**:431.

Smith, G. E., 1907, A new topographical survey of the cerebral cortex: Being an account of the distribution of the anatomically distinct cortical areas and their relationship to the cerebral sulci, *J. Anat.* **41**:237.

Soemmering, S. T., 1788, *Vom Hirn und Ruckenmark*, Mainz, Winkopp.

Ulinski, P. S., 1974, Cytoarchitecture of cerebral cortex in snakes, *J. Comp. Neurol.* **158**:243.

van Bogaert, L., and Théodoridès, J., 1979, *Constantin von Economo (1876–1931): The Man and the Scientist*, Österreichischen Akademie der Wissenschaften, Vienna.

Vicq d'Azyr, F., 1786, *Traité d'anatomie et de physiologie*, Didot, Paris.

Vogt, O., 1910, Die myeloarchitektonische Felderung des menschlichen Stirnhirns, *J. Psychol. Neurol.* **15**:221.

Vogt, O., 1911, Die Myeloarchitektonik des Isocortex parietalis, *J. Psychol. Neurol.* **18**:379.

Vogt, O., 1927, Architektonik der menschlichen Hirnrinde, *Allg. Z. Psychiatr.* **86**:247.

Vogt, C., and Vogt, O., 1919, Allgemeinere Ergebnisse unserer Hirnforschung, *J. Psychol. Neurol.* **25**:279.

von Bonin, G., and Bailey, P., 1947, *The Neocortex of Macaca mulatta*, University of Illinois Press, Urbana.

von Economo, C., and Koskinas, G. N., 1925, *Die Cytoarchitectonik der Hirnrinde des erwachsenen Menschen*, Springer, Berlin.

Walker, A. E., 1938, *The Primate Thalamus*, University of Chicago Press, Chicago.

Zeki, S. M., 1978, Functional specialization in the visual cortex of the rhesus monkey, *Nature (London)* **274:**423.

Zilles, K., Schleicher, A., and Kretschmann, H. J., 1978, A quantitative approach to cytoarchitectonics. I. The areal pattern of the cortex of *Tupaia belangeri, Anat. Embryol.* **153:**195.

Zilles, K., Rehkämper, G., Stephan, H., and Schleicher, A., 1979, A quantitative approach to cytoarchitectonics. IV. The areal pattern of the cortex of *Galago demidovii, Anat. Embryol.* **157:**81.

Zilles, K., Zilles, B., and Schleicher, A., 1980, A quantitative approach to cytoarchitectonics. VI. The areal pattern of the cortex of the albino rat, *Anat. Embryol.* **159:**335.

3

Architectonics as Seen by Lipofuscin Stains

HEIKO BRAAK

1. Introduction

Most types of neurons forming the brain of the human adult contain a large amount of pigment. Moreover, the human brain appears particularly strongly pigmented, differing in this respect markedly from brains of many subhuman mammalian species.

The pigment in nerve cells differs from that stored in glial cells or endothelial cells. There is also evidence for considerable variation in its chemical and morphological characteristics (Braak, 1971; Schlote and Boellaard, 1983). Most types of intraneuronal pigment can be stained by aldehyde fuchsin. The staining reaction probably depends on the amount of sulfur contained in the granules which is transformed into strongly acidic–SO_3H groups by means of an oxidation with performic acid. At low pH of the staining solution, the basic dye aldehyde fuchsin binds more or less selectively only to the pigment granules. After appropriate processing the technique stains only the pigment stored in nerve cells. Lipofuscin deposits in glial cells or endothelial cells remain more or less unstained.

The varying amount of intraneuronal pigment, its size and shape, stainability, and pattern of distribution can generally serve as an excellent criterion for the determination of various types of nerve cells (Obersteiner, 1903, 1904; Vogt and Vogt, 1942; Mannen, 1955; H. Braak, 1980). The amount of intraneuronal pigment increases slowly with advancing age (Leibnitz and Wünscher,

HEIKO BRAAK • Anatomical Institute, 6000 Frankfurt/Main 70, Federal Republic of Germany.

1967; Mann and Yates, 1974; Brizzee *et al.*, 1975a,b; Glees and Hasan, 1976; Mann *et al.*, 1978; West, 1979). This change does not markedly affect the other characteristics of the pigment so that most types of nerve cells retain a characteristic pigmentation throughout a lifetime (Braak, 1978a).

2. Pigmentation of Isocortical Cell Types

The telencephalic cortex is a heteromorphic gray, i.e., it is composed of different types of nerve cells. For pigmentoarchitectonic investigations it is therefore necessary to first study the characteristic pattern of pigmentation of each of the various neuronal types present. This calls for a thorough study of Golgi-impregnated nerve cells showing all the minute details of the cellular processes. The main advantage of the Golgi technique is that it makes it possible to produce a scrupulous and unequivocal classification of neuronal types. Nevertheless, the silver precipitation techniques have drawbacks. They are capricious and stain only a small number of the cells present. Moreover, certain types of nerve cells are frequently impregnated, whereas others are stained only rarely. Therefore, quantitative estimates of the frequency of the various types of nerve cells cannot be obtained from an analysis of Golgi-impregnated material.

2.1. The Combined Golgi–Pigment Staining Technique

Golgi-impregnated neurons are densely filled with an opaque precipitation of silver chromate, rendering an examination of cytoplasmic details impossible. These difficulties can be overcome by using a newly developed modification of the Golgi technique that permits lixiviation of most of the undesired precipitate, converting the remnants to a transparent coating stable enough to withstand various counterstaining procedures (Braak, 1983). In this way, cytoplasmic inclusions such as intracellular pigment deposits within individual nerve cells can readily be seen, for the cell body and the cellular processes are transparent (Figs. 1 and 2). The method can be used for the silver chromate Golgi techniques (Braitenberg *et al.*, 1967; Valverde, 1970; Schierhorn and Nagel, 1977; Millhouse, 1981). Nerve cells which can clearly be classified on account of the typical features of their cellular processes are selected for photographic documentation (Fig. 1A). Sections are then transferred into a weak aqueous solution of ammonia, in which lixiviation of most of the silver chromate precipitations occurs. Only a fine scattering of particles remains, leaving the cells translucent, but brownish in color. They still show all the fine details of the cellular processes (Fig. 1B). In the following step the coating is stabilized and becomes transparent when the sections are placed in a solution of potassium ferricyanide (Fig. 1C). To demonstrate intraneuronal lipofuscin deposits, preparations can now be processed by oxidation with performic acid and staining with aldehyde fuchsin (H. Braak, 1980), so that the particular features of pigmentation may then be related to the characteristics of the cellular processes (Figs. 1D and 2).

The main conclusion to be drawn from such combined Golgi–pigment studies is that the characteristics of the pattern of pigmentation are indicative of the neuronal type (Braak and Braak, 1982a,b).

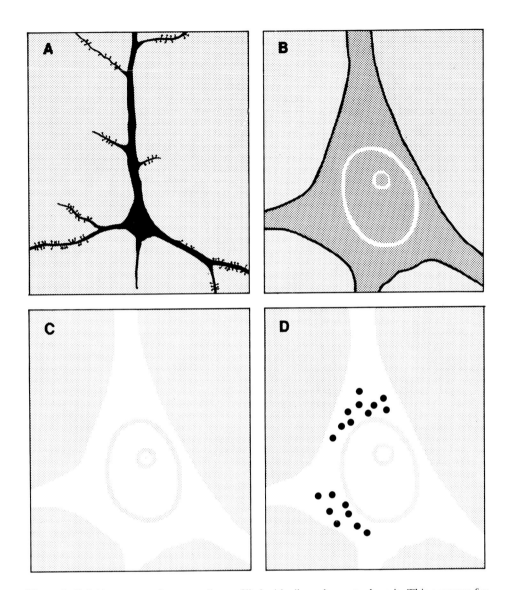

Figure 1. Golgi-impregnated nerve cells are filled with silver chromate deposit. This accounts for their dark appearance when studied with the transmission light microscope. Thus, cytoplasmic components of impregnated neurons cannot be studied (A). With the newly developed deimpregnation technique, most of the deposit is dissolved by a weak solution of ammonia. A fine scattering of particles remains, giving impregnated cells a brownish appearance (B), and these cells become transparent after oxidation with potassium ferricyanide. The coating is stable enough to withstand various counterstaining procedures (C). Afterwards the pigment deposits can be stained by the performic acid–aldehyde fuchsin technique. Hence, this modified Golgi technique enables one to perceive the characteristic pattern of pigmentation within the cell body and the cellular processes of impregnated neurons (D).

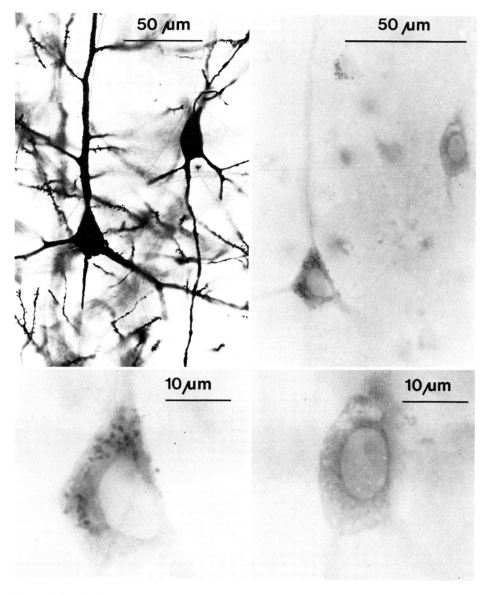

Figure 2. A typical pyramidal cell and stellate cell of the isocortex (layer IIIab) as seen in the Golgi impregnation (left side) and after deimpregnation and counterstaining with performic acid–aldehyde fuchsin (right side). The lower portion of the figure shows higher-magnification photographs of both cortical nerve cells. The pyramidal cell shows a finely granulated and widely dispersed pigment within the cell body while the stellate cell is devoid of pigment.

2.2. Isocortical Cell Types

Most of the nerve cells forming the telencephalic cortex can be classified as either pyramidal cells or stellate cells (Fig. 3). The axons of most of the various types of pyramidal cells and "modified pyramidal cells" (H. Braak, 1980) enter the white matter and terminate in subcortical centers or in other parts of the cortex. Cells of this type may also be called "projection cells." The axons of the various types of stellate cells, however, split up into their terminal ramification close to the parent soma. These cells may be referred to as "local-circuit" neurons." Figure 3 gives a diagrammatic representation of both classes of cortical neurons and their typical patterns of pigmentation.

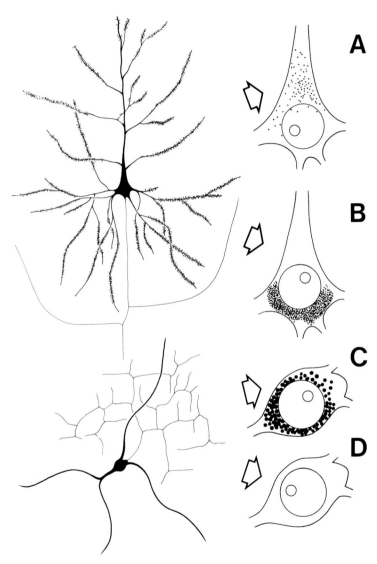

Figure 3. Diagrammatic representation of the two main classes of cortical nerve cells and their basic pattern of pigmentation. The pyramidal cells generally contain fine pigment granules that are widely distributed throughout the cell body. The pigment has only a moderate capacity to be stained by aldehyde fuchsin (A). Only a few types of large pyramidal cells, which are by no means frequent in the isocortex, contain dense agglomerations of pigment (B). Conversely, the stellate cells are either filled with coarse and intensely stained pigment granules (C) or are devoid of pigment (D).

2.3. Pigmentation of Cortical Projection Cells

In pyramidal cells, the pigment is usually randomly dispersed throughout the cell body. Some types of pyramidal cells even show a small number of pigment granules in the proximal parts of their apical dendrites (see Fig. 16C; Braak, 1974a). The axon hillock and the axon itself are normally devoid of pigment (E. Braak, 1980; Braak et al., 1980). The pigment in the pyramidal cells is finely granulated and can only be weakly stained by aldehyde fuchsin (Figs. 2 and 3A).

Only a few types of pyramidal cells show dense aggregations of pigment in the form of large clumps (Fig. 3B). These types are the Betz pyramidal cells of layer Vb and another type of large pyramidal cell residing within the lower portion of layer III. Both types of special pyramids are by no means general components of the isocortex but occur in only a few areas. Betz cells are encountered in various parts of the precentral and postcentral gyri, in some areas buried in the depth of the cingulate sulcus (Braak, 1976a; Braak and Braak, 1976), and in the anterogenual region of the proisocortex (Braak, 1979c). Large pigment-laden IIIc pyramids are typical components of some association areas such as the temporal magnopyramidal region, which is probably the morphological counterpart of the speech center of Wernicke (Braak, 1978b), the inferofrontal magnopyramidal region which probably corresponds to the speech center of Broca, and the superofrontal magnopyramidal region, which includes wide parts of the first frontal gyrus and contains the "supplementary" motor cortex (Braak, 1979b). All the other varieties of isocortical pyramidal cells show a more or less scattered distribution of pigment, the amount and stainability of which depends on the type of pyramidal cell and its location within the various cortical layers (Braak, 1978a).

2.4. Pigmentation of Cortical Local-Circuit Neurons

Local-circuit neurons show a pattern of pigmentation that differs markedly from that of pyramidal cells. They either are filled with coarse and intensely stained pigment granules or lack pigmentation (Figs. 3C, D). Those stellate cells that are devoid of pigment or show only a small amount are most common in the isocortex (Fig. 2). They are encountered in all cellular layers. In contrast, the pigment-laden varieties are mainly located in the corpuscular layer (layer II) and the multiform layer (layer VI).

The deep stellate cells which are rich in pigment are relatively large and only occur in great numbers in the "older" parts of the isocortex adjoining the allocortical core. The superficial pigment-laden stellate cells, however, are small and mostly encountered in phylogenetically "younger" parts of the cortex, such as the "association" areas spreading over the opercula of the lateral cerebral sulcus (Braak, 1978a; Schlegelberger and Braak, 1982). In the temporal magnopyramidal areas, they attain such a density that they form a dark band in pigment preparations.

The small pigment-laden stellate cells of the corpuscular layer (layer II) and subjacent portions of the pyramidal layer (layer III) are probably specific components of the human isocortex. They have not yet been shown to occur in the

subhuman mammalian brain. Because of their high concentration in phylogenetically advanced portions of the isocortex, one might be tempted to consider
that these small local-circuit neurons have a particular significance for the "higher"
functions of the human brain (Braak, 1974b; E. Braak, 1976).

2.5. The Combined Nissl–Pigment Staining Technique

The characteristics of intraneuronal pigmentation allow one to clearly classify a given nerve cell as belonging to either the group of pyramidal cells or the
group of stellate cells. In this regard the pigment preparation is superior to the
Nissl preparation and a simple combination of a pigment and Nissl stain provides
a remarkably increased amount of information. Preparations processed in this
way allow a meticulous classification of cortical neurons. They furthermore permit quantitative analyses of the various types of projection cells and local-circuit
neurons. Also, since projection cells and local-circuit neurons may respond differently to diseases and aging, the combined pigment–Nissl preparations will
probably be of value in the analysis of pathologically altered brain tissue (Braak
and Goebel, 1978, 1979).

3. Pigmentoarchitectonic Analysis of the Isocortex

The isocortex not only shows a horizontal pattern of cortical laminae but it
also displays vertical patterns, so that pigment preparations clearly show the
borders of both the laminae and the areas. The fact that the aldehyde fuchsin
technique demonstrates only a single cytoplasmic component allows one to considerably increase the thickness of the sections. This is a clear advantage over
the possibilities offered by the Nissl preparations, for Nissl preparations become
increasingly indistinct with increasing section thickness, on account of the great
number of glial and endothelial cell nuclei that obscure the picture of the nerve
cell assemblies. Depending on the size and complexity of the structure to be
investigated, a section thickness between 400 and 1000 μm is recommended for
pigment preparations. In these sections the pigment deposit of an individual
nerve cell almost recedes into the background and appears as only a tiny spot,
a great number of which superimpose each other to clearly show the borders
and internal organization of the subcortical nuclei and cortical areas (Braak,
1978a, 1980).

The analysis of brain architectonics is a field of research that essentially fills
the gap between macroscopic and microscopic investigations. Accordingly, the
thick pigment preparations are especially useful for low-power examination with
the stereomicroscope. Furthermore, the sections can be tilted under the stereomicroscope in such a manner that obliquely cut portions of the cortex appear
as if cut perpendicular to the surface. This is a definite advantage for parcellation
of cortices with many gyri. In general, the numerous superimposed dots, seen
at a glance, permit easy recognition and reliable determination of the boundaries
of both the cortical layers and the cortical areas.

4. Horizontal Pattern of Isocortical Laminae

The general scheme of isocortical lamination pattern as seen in the Nissl preparation, the myelin preparation, and the pigment preparation is given in Fig. 4.

4.1. Cytoarchitectonics

The basis of cytoarchitectonics is the Nissl preparation, which shows homotypical isocortical areas to be formed of six laminae. The nomenclature recommended by Vogt and Vogt (1919) is applied in the following descriptions. The isocortical layers are designated by Roman numerals and named from the surface toward the white matter: the molecular layer (I), the corpuscular layer

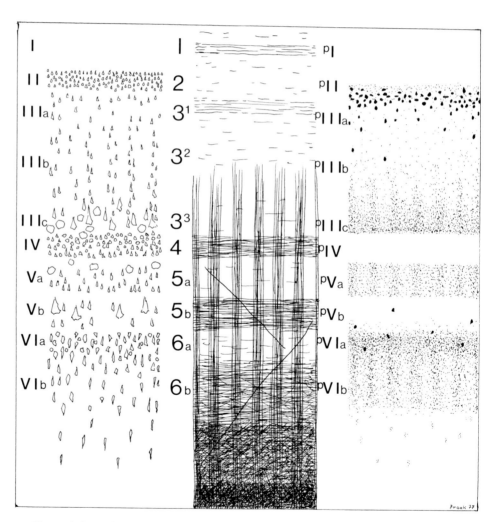

Figure 4. Synopsis of the fundamental cyto-, myelo-, and pigmentoarchitectonic schemes.

(II), the pyramidal layer (III), the granular layer (IV), the ganglionic layer (V), and the multiform layer (VI). Differences in size, shape, and packing density of the pyramidal cells mainly account for the fact that cortical laminae can be distinguished in cell-stained preparations. Glial cells are more or less randomly dispersed throughout the cortex. Unlike the various types of pyramidal cells, the various types of stellate cells are not confined to specific cortical layers (E. Braak, 1982).

The nomenclature of Vogt and Vogt permits a short and precise characterization of the different cortical areas. For example, the term *magnopyramidal* refers to an isocortical area with large pyramidal cells in layer III, whereas the term *gigantoganglionic* refers to an area with outstandingly large pyramids in layer V. A broad layer IV, densely filled with small nerve cells, distinguishes the *hypergranular* cortex. A *magnocellular* or *parvocellular* cortex has a predominance of either large or small nerve cells. In places, layer IIIc is broader than layer V and well-filled with large pyramidal cells. This gives the field the *externocrassior* character. It should be emphasized that the term *granule cell* is derived from the small size of the cells and in the isocortex it does not refer to a specific neuronal type, so that isocortical *granule cells* may be small pyramidal cells, small stellate cells, or an admixture of both.

4.2. Myeloarchitectonics

The basis of myeloarchitectonics is the myelin preparation, which also reveals a lamination pattern that can be compared with the set of laminae seen in cell-stained material. To distinguish them from the cellular layers, the myeloarchitectonic laminae are marked by Arabic numerals and named from the pial surface inwards: the tangential layer (1), the dysfibrous layer (2), the suprastriate layer (3), the external stria (outer stripe of Baillarger) (4), the intrastriate layer and internal stria (inner stripe of Baillarger) (5), and the substrate and limiting layer (6).

The tangential plexus of myelinated fibers in layer 1 shows considerable variation from one area to another. It is particularly dense in primary motor and sensory areas. Layer 2 is almost devoid of myelinated fibers. The deeper plexus in the superficial portion of layer 3—the stripe of Kaes–Bechterew—is well developed only in a few areas and these are mainly the paraconiocortical fields, i.e., areas that surround the primary sensory centers (see Fig. 5). Layers 4 and 5b generally contain clearly delimited bands of tightly packed myelinated fibers—the outer and inner stripe of Baillarger—which are mainly formed by myelinated axon collaterals of pyramidal cells residing in layers 3 and 5a, respectively (Clark and Sunderland, 1939; Braitenberg, 1962, 1978; Fisken *et al.*, 1975).

The clarity of the stripes of Baillarger define the *astriate, unistriate,* or *bistriate* characteristic of a cortical area. A denser outer stripe is noted as typus *externodensior*. An *extremostriate* cortex contains the stripe of Kaes–Bechterew in addition to the lines of Baillarger. The *typus dives* or *typus pauper* refers to a high or low average myelin content of the cortex, and it is interesting that the evolutionary elaboration of the cortex is accompanied by a general increase in its myelin content (Bishop and Smith, 1964; Sanides, 1970).

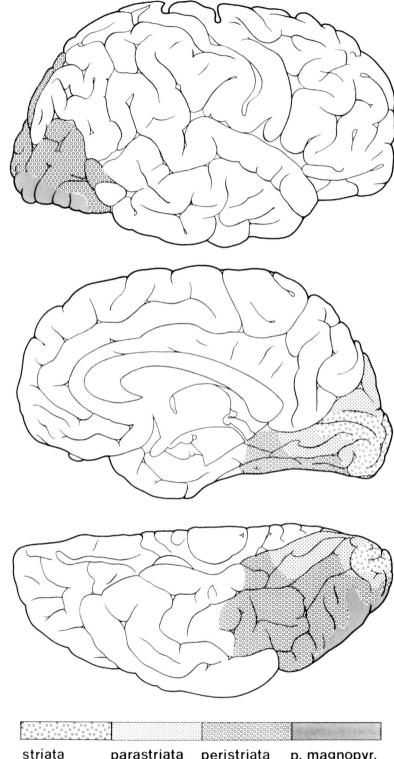

striata   parastriata   peristriata   p. magnopyr.

4.3. Pigmentoarchitectonics

The basis of pigmentoarchitectonics is the pigment preparation, which again shows a clear lamination pattern that is often more easily recognized than that seen in Nissl preparations. To distinguish them from cyto- and myeloarchitectural laminae, the set of layers discernible in pigment preparations is characterized by a prefixed "p" and Roman numerals. Differences in the amount of pigment stored in pyramidal cells mainly account for the fact that cortical laminae can be distinguished in pigment preparations. The majority of isocortical stellate cells are devoid of pigment and only the pigment-laden varieties of stellate cells add some features to the typical appearance of the isocortex in a pigment preparation.

The molecular layer (PI) is almost devoid of pigmented neurons while the corpuscular layer (PII) is mainly composed of very sparsely pigmented small pyramidal cells. The packing density of the small pigment-laden stellate cells in the lower zone of the corpuscular layer and subjacent portions of the pyramidal layer varies from one isocortical area to another. The pigment content in the pyramidal layer (PIII) generally increases from top to bottom. Only the primary sensory and primary motor fields show the reverse pattern, with the pigmentation decreasing from the superficial to the deeper portions of the layer. Two lightly pigmented stripes follow, and these are referred to as the external and internal teniae (PIV and PVb), which are separated from each other by the weakly pigmented pyramidal cells of layer PVa. The internal tenia is set off from the white matter by the multiform layer (PVI) which is generally rich in pigment.

The breadth and location of the two light bands generally correspond to the breadth and location of the stripes of Baillarger. Some areas, however, may display clear teniae but show insignificant or nonexistent lines of Baillarger. Most types of cortical pyramidal cells lying within a thick plexus of axonal ramifications do not accumulate lipofuscin deposits even in old age, and at present there is no plausible hypothesis to explain this phenomenon. Whatever the conditions for the development of the pallid teniae may be, in the pigment preparations they correspond to the location and breadth of the axonal plexus, which may or may not be myelinated. Consequently, the pigment preparation may well serve as a supplement to a myelin preparation which displays only those plexuses which are rich in myelinated fibers. In this sense, pigment preparations give much the same information as a combination of cell-stained and fiber-stained preparations, for they show a certain proportion of the nerve cells which are made evident by their pigment deposits, and at the same time the main tangential fiber plexuses are indicated by the pallid teniae.

Different areas of the cortex may show both teniae, only the outer one, or neither the outer nor the inner band. These patterns are referred to as *biteniate*, *uniteniate*, or *ateniate*. A field with an outer tenia that is broader than the inner

---

Figure 5. Map of the main structurally different territories of the human occipital lobe. Note the small surface spread of the striate area. The visual core field is completely surrounded by the parastriate area. The peristriate region covers the rest of the occipital lobe and also extends into inferior portions of the temporal lobe. The magnopyramidal peristriate area is located at the edge of the superolateral and inferior surface of the hemisphere.

one is *externoteniate*. The *typus obscurus* and *typus clarus* define areas with high and low average pigment content. Normally, a high myelin content corresponds to an overall sparse pigmentation, and vice versa.

5. Vertical Pattern of Isocortical Areas

The isocortex of higher primates and man shows highly elaborate sensory and motor core fields—or primary fields—that are surrounded by somewhat less specialized fields forming the "belt" areas or secondary fields. These in turn are separated from each other by the homotypical cortex, which is particularly extended in the human brain. The territories outside the core and the belt are frequently referred to as "association" cortex. Myelogenetically, the core fields differentiate early. They are followed by the belt areas and much later by the association areas (Conel, 1939–1967; Jacobson, 1963; Yakovlev and Lecours, 1967; Holloway, 1968).

As pointed out by Brodmann (1909), the occipital lobe of the human brain can be divided into three large zones of different structure. These zones correspond to the aforementioned general tripartition into a core, a belt, and a surrounding association cortex (Figs. 5 and 13). Hence, the occipital fields can be used to illustrate the basic principles of isocortical architectonics. Furthermore, pigment preparations of the three main cortical types of the occipital lobe—the striate area (field 17 of Brodmann), the parastriate area (field 18 of Brodmann), and the peristriate region (field 19 of Brodmann)—show peculiarities in their structure that cannot be seen with the aid of either the Nissl or the myelin techniques. Herein clearly lies the value of pigmentoarchitectonic analysis.

5.1. The Striate Area

The extent of the striate area is easy to delineate. The disappearance of the line of Gennari that abruptly occurs on passing from the core to the belt area permits delineation of the striate area even with the unaided eye. Its extent on the free surface of the brain is almost limited to the medial surface of the hemisphere (Fig. 5).

For a better understanding of pigmentoarchitectonics, it seems advisable to first give a short description of the characteristics which appear in the Nissl and the myelin preparations.

The heterotypical cortex is small and in the Nissl preparations it is extremely parvocellular (= koniocortex). The lamination pattern is largely obscured by a predominance of tiny nerve cells, which in the Nissl preparations cannot reliably be classified as either pyramidal or stellate cells (Fig. 6). Approximately eight

Figure 6. Nissl preparation of the striate area of the human brain. The cortex is narrow and parvocellular. The pattern of lamination is not easily recognizable. In particular, the broad band of small cells—generally referred to as layer IVc—seems to be uniformly composed of tiny "granule" cells. Layer V contains a scattered population of large pyramidal cells of Meynert (pM). Cresyl violet, 15 μm.

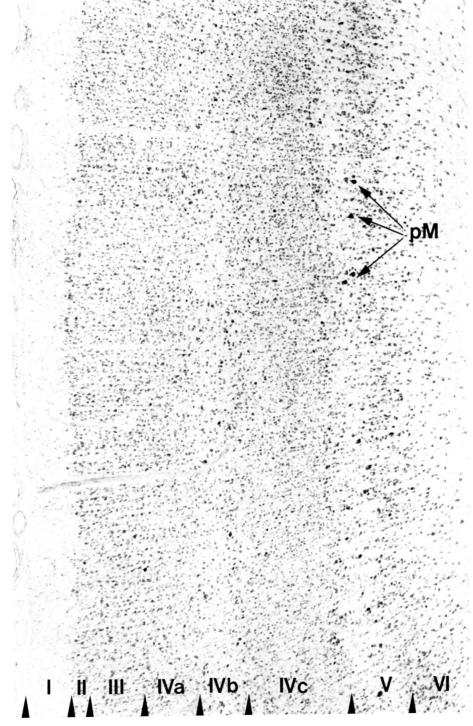

72

CHAPTER 3

laminae can be distinguished. These laminae cannot readily be compared to laminae found in the visual cortex of subprimate mammalian species (Sanides, 1972). The primary visual field of subhuman primates, nevertheless, generally shows a comparable pattern of lamination, but the nomenclature used by various authors differs markedly (Hassler and Wagner, 1965; Billings-Gagliardi *et al.*, 1974; Valverde, 1977). To avoid confusion, a synopsis of the various nomenclatures used is given in Table I.

The molecular layer (I) is fairly broad and contains a few scattered nerve cells.

The corpuscular layer (II) and the pyramidal layer (III) are mainly composed of small pyramidal cells and the border between these layers is indistinct. The pyramidal cells in layer III are slightly larger than those of the corpuscular layer and they are more widely separated from one another.

The subjacent layer IVa shows a higher density of nerve cells than the pyramidal layer. It is followed by a cell-sparse zone, layer IVb, with a scattered population of somewhat larger nerve cells, the "solitary" cells of Ramón y Cajal (1909–1911). These are polygonal neurons with a few stout processes extending in various directions. In general, the "solitary" cells lack an apical dendrite, and they contain some scattered clumps of basophilic material that extend into the

Table I. Pattern of Lamination in the Striate Area of Man and Various Subhuman Primates According to Various Authors[a]

Ramón y Cajal (1909–1911)	Brodmann (1909)	von Economo and Koskinas (1925)	Rose (1935)	Bailey and von Bonin (1951)	Garey (1971)	Lund and Boothe (1975)	Braak (1976b)
1	I	I	I	i	I	I	I
2	II	II	II	ii	II	II	II
	III	III	III	iiia	IIIa	IIIA IIIB	IIIa,b
3	IVa	(IIIb)	IVa	iiib	IIIb	IVA	IIIc–IVa
4	IVb	(IIIc)	IVbα	iva	IIIc	IVB	IVb
	IVb	IV	IVbβ	ivbα	IIIc	IVCα	IVcα
5	IVc	IV	IVc	ivbα	IV	IVCβ	IVcβ
6	IVc	Va	Va	ivbβ	V	VA	IVd / Va
7	V	Vb	Vb	v	V	VB	Vb
8	VIa	VI	VI	via	VI	VI	VIa
9	VIb	VI	VII	vib	VI	VI	VIb

[a] The gray area gives the approximate location of the line of Gennari.

proximal dendrites (E. Braak, 1982). The next layer, IVc, is very broad and contains a great number of small nerve cells packed tightly together, and in Nissl preparations a further subdivision of layer IVc is barely recognizable. The enormous breadth of the granular layer (IVa–c) gives the cortex a hypergranular character.

The ganglionic layer (V) is a cell-sparse zone with some very large Meynert pyramidal cells scattered throughout (Fig. 6). The Meynert pyramidal cells are a feature of the striate area (Clark, 1942; Shkol'nik-Yarros, 1971; Chan-Palay *et al.*, 1974; Palay, 1978; Braitenberg and Braitenberg, 1979; E. Braak, 1982). The initial portions of their basal dendrites are often thicker than those of the apical dendrites and the cells contain coarse clumps of basophilic material that extend into the dendrites.

The multiform layer (VI) is rich in medium-sized cells and may be subdivided into a cell-rich VIa and a cell-sparse VIb.

In myelin preparations, the striate area appears as an intensely stained field (typus dives) (Figs. 7 top, 8).

The tangential layer (1) reveals a thick plexus of myelinated fibers running more or less parallel to the cortical surface and the striate area shares this feature with other isocortical core fields. The association cortex which develops late in ontogeny is far less richly endowed with myelinated fibers in layer 1.

The dysfibrous layer (2) is almost devoid of myelinated fibers.

The suprastriate layer (3) shows a moderately dense plexus of fibers that mostly are of delicate calibre, and the myelinated radii, i.e., the fiber bundles that are arranged perpendicular to the surface, extend up to the boundary between sublaminae 3^2 and 3^3. This pattern can be referred to as the euradiate characteristic. The radii are thin and mainly composed of fine to medium-sized fibers.

The outer stripe of Baillarger in the striate area is extremely broad and dense, and in this area it is frequently referred to as the line of Gennari, in honor of the investigator to whom we owe the first description of this band (1782) and implicitly, the insight that the cortex as a whole is not a uniformly built structure. The line of Gennari corresponds to layer IVb and the upper portions of layer IVc in Nissl preparations. It is composed of a dense mesh of fibers, mainly of fine calibre, intertwining in all directions, and whereas the upper boundary is relatively sharply drawn, the lower one appears slightly blurred.

The relatively pallid intrastriate layer (4c and 5a) corresponds in position with the small-celled layer IVc of the Nissl preparation. It contains a narrow zone of tightly packed and horizontally aligned myelinated fibers. This is frequently not seen in thin (30-μm) myelin preparations processed according to the commonly used, but less precise, staining techniques of Heidenhain–Woelcke or Loyez. In contrast, sufficiently thick (100-μm) frozen sections cut perpendicular to the cortical surface and stained with an appropriate technique clearly reveal the existence of the narrow line (4d). The line is unique to the striate area and does not occur in any other isocortical field.

A definite inner line of Baillarger cannot be reliably identified in the striate area, although in certain places a weak line with blurred boundaries is recognizable (Vogt and Vogt, 1919; Kawata, 1927; Kirsche and Kirsche, 1962). The absence of the inner line would give the cortex the seldom-occurring *singulostriate*

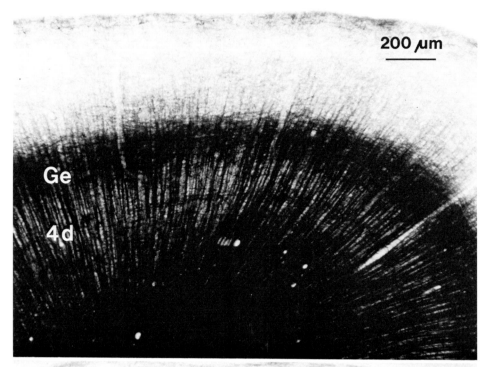

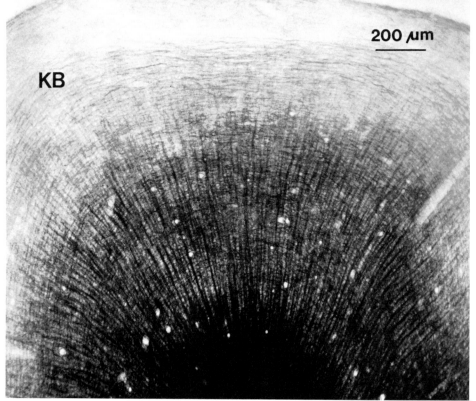

characteristic (Sanides and Gräfin Vitzthum, 1965a; Gräfin Vitzthum and Sanides, 1966; Sanides, 1972). The presence of a broad, dense outer line and a weak blurred inner one is denoted as an extremely *externodensior* type.

The substriate and limiting layer (6) contains about the same amount of myelin as the zone of the blurred inner line of Baillarger.

In pigment preparations the striate area shows few lipofuscin deposits (typus clarus). The field nevertheless discloses a very clear lamination (Fig. 9) and 12 layers can be distinguished.

The molecular layer (^{P}I) is almost devoid of pigment although it contains a moderate number of pigmented astrocytes, most of which lie immediately underneath the narrow and pallid external glial layer (Niessing, 1936; Ramsey, 1965; Lopes and Mair, 1974; Braak, 1975).

The corpuscular layer (^{P}II) contains a large number of small pyramidal cells with very fine and weakly stained pigment granules.

The outer parts of the pyramidal layer (^{P}IIIab) also harbor small and sparsely pigmented pyramidal cells. A large number of pigment-laden stellate cells are scattered about the supragranular layers and they are packed most dense in the lower portions of the corpuscular layer. In the striate area, pigment-laden stellate cells are also encountered in the subjacent pyramidal layer, even in its deeper portions (Fig. 9).

The following layer (^{P}IIIc–IVa) is moderately densely pigmented and shows blurred upper and lower borders. Its constituents are the relatively large pyramidal cells characteristic of layer IIIc and polygonal cells which lack apical dendrites and are characteristic components of layer IV. The layer is therefore termed ^{P}IIIc–IVa. It corresponds to layer IVa of Nissl preparations.

The outer tenia is extremely broad and appears almost devoid of pigment. As one would anticipate, its location and extent correspond to the location and extent of the line of Gennari.

The most distinct part of the striate area in pigment preparations lies below the outer tenia. Here, the broad and apparently homogeneously composed layer IVc of Nissl preparations is resolved into four narrow and distinctly delimited layers, ^{P}IVcα, ^{P}IVcβ, ^{P}IVd, and ^{P}Va. ^{P}IVcα is a moderately pigmented lamina with a blurred upper border. Deep portions of the line of Gennari partially extend into this layer, possibly accounting for its blurred upper border.

The subjacent layer ^{P}IVcβ is clearly demarcated and richly pigmented, and Golgi preparations reveal that it is composed of a homogeneous population of small polygonal cells with slender and relatively short dendrites endowed with a moderate number of spines (Lund, 1973; Lund and Boothe, 1975; Braak, 1976b; E. Braak, 1978, 1982; Lund *et al.*, 1981). Neurophysiological investigations, carried out on primates, have shown that these cells receive the bulk of

Figure 7. (Top) Myelin preparation of the striate area of the human brain. Note the thick plexus of myelinated fibers in the tangential layer. The radii extend up to the border between layers 3^2 and 3^3. The broad line of Gennari (Ge) is a hallmark of the visual core field. The narrow myelin-rich stripe, 4d, is also characteristic of the striate area and does not occur in any other isocortical area. (Bottom) Myelin preparation of the parastriate area of the human brain. Note the plexus of myelinated fibers in the upper portion of the suprastriate layer, well above the radii piercing layer 3^3. This plexus forms the line of Kaes–Bechterew (KB) and gives the parastriate area the extremostriate characteristic. Schroeder's lithium hematoxylin, 100 μm.

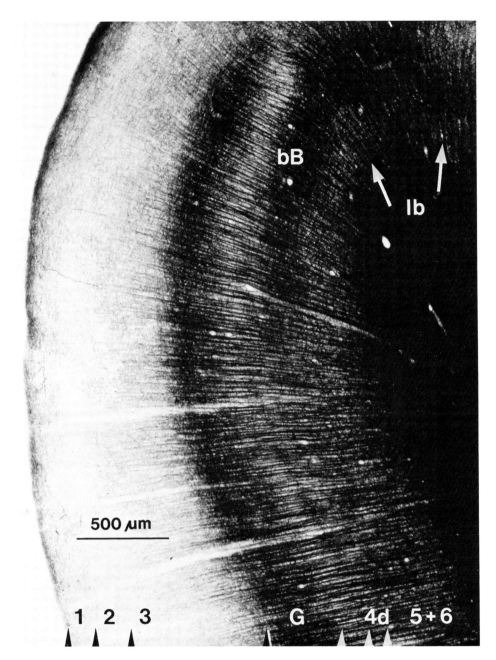

Figure 8. The striate and parastriate demarcation area (limes striatus and limes parastriatus). Note the particular wealth of myelinated fibers in the tangential layer (1) in both demarcation areas. The bridging line of Baillarger (bB) gives the striate demarcation area a bistriate character. The radii are particularly thick in the parastriate demarcation area (limiting bundles, 1b). Note that the narrow line 4d does not fuse into the bridging line of Baillarger. Schroeder's lithium hematoxylin, 100 μm.

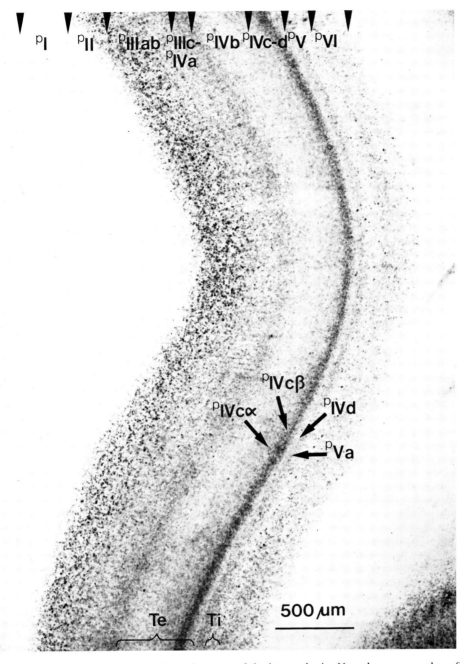

Figure 9. Pigment preparation of the striate area of the human brain. Note the great number of pigment-laden stellate cells in the supragranular layers (ᴾII and ᴾIII). Four narrow and distinctly delineated laminae correspond to the broad cell-rich stripe termed layer IVc of Nissl preparations. Layer ᴾIVcβ is particularly conspicuous in pigment preparations and is a unique feature of the visual core field. Aldehyde fuchsin, 800 μm.

the projection fibers originating from the parvocellular lamellae of the lateral geniculate body (Hubel and Wiesel, 1972, 1977; Lund, 1973). One advantage of the pigment staining technique is that this main entrance of the visual radiation into the cortex can be seen.

Similar to laminae ^{P}IVcα and ^{P}IVcβ, the subsequent layers ^{P}IVd and ^{P}Va are also composed of very small nerve cells. In contrast to layer ^{P}IVcβ, their main components are tiny pyramidal cells which are regularly aligned and possess thin threadlike apical dendrites. In layer ^{P}IVd these pyramidal cells are devoid of pigment and they are only modestly pigmented in layer ^{P}Va.

Layer ^{P}IVd is a feature unique to the striate area and does not occur in any other isocortical field. The existence of a dense fiber plexus probably accounts for the conspicuous pallor of its cellular components. In fact, the extent and location of the narrow plexus of myelinated fibers apparent in the myelin-stained preparations (4d, Figs. 7 top and 8) exactly correspond to the extent and location of layer ^{P}IVd. One could hypothesize that the fiber plexus is mainly composed of myelinated axon collaterals generated from axons of the small polygonal cells located in layer ^{P}IVcβ. This has not yet been demonstrated, but the possible existence of regularly aligned collaterals of IVcβ neurons would certainly influence the development of ideas concerning intrastriate connections, in particular the manner in which the input from the lateral geniculate body is distributed within the striate area.

The inner tenia (^{P}Vb) is only a narrow band and it corresponds to the cell-sparse layer V of Nissl preparations. Its presence gives the field a biteniate character. The cell bodies of the Meynert pyramidal cells contain only a few fine pigment granules and these are only faintly stained by aldehydefuchsin. Comparison between the two teniae shows that the striate area is one of the extremely externoteniate areas, a feature it shares with all other isocortical core fields.

The multiform layer (^{P}VI) is more or less clearly split into a densely pigmented upper portion (^{P}VIa) and a weakly pigmented lower one (^{P}VIb).

In summary, the lamination of the striate area is more clearly visible in pigment preparations than in Nissl-stained material. The cell-rich layer IVc of Nissl preparations is composed of different varieties of uniformly small cells arranged in distinct laminae. The presence of an orderly array within an accumulation of equally sized small cells may easily be overlooked in Nissl preparations. This is a typical pitfall if cortical analysis is based only on Nissl-stained material.

The Striate Border (Limes Striatus)

A change in structure occurs close to the boundary between the striate area and the parastriate area (Fig. 8) for the inner line of Baillarger abruptly becomes recognizable. This forms the "bridging stripe of Baillarger" (Sanides and Gräfin Vitzthum, 1965b). The narrow line 4d remains well above the clearly demarcated inner line of Baillarger, and thus, layer 4d cannot be interpreted as a remnant of the inner line of Baillarger. Hence, the small marginal zone of the striate area with its bistriate character is different from the central portion. It may therefore be delineated as an independent area, the striatal demarcation area (limes striatus).

5.2. The Parastriate Area

79

ARCHI-
TECTONICS
AS SEEN BY
LIPOFUSCIN
STAINS

The parastriate area adjoins the visual core field throughout its circumference. In the human brain, the extent of this area over the free surface is almost restricted to the medial surface of the hemisphere (Fig. 5), and anterior portions of the field are buried in the common trunk of the parieto-occipital and the calcarine sulcus.

The cortex of the visual belt area is thicker than that of the core field, and in Nissl preparations a predominance of medium-sized pyramidal cells gives the cortex a mediocellular character (Fig. 10 top).

The supragranular layers I, II, and IIIab do not show remarkable differences from the corresponding laminae in the striate area (Valverde, 1978).

The main constituents of the lower pyramidal layer (IIIc) are medium-sized to large pyramidal cells, but in contrast to the visual core field, the parastriate area shows the normal pattern of the third layer, with pyramidal cells increasing in size from top to bottom.

The granular layer (IV) is well developed and contains a large number of small and tightly packed pyramidal cells. This field is therefore of the eugranular type.

The ganglionic layer (V) can be subdivided into Va, a thin layer harboring relatively small pyramidal cells, and Vb, which is cell-sparse and has somewhat larger pyramidal cells scattered throughout.

The cell density of the multiform layer (VI) is highest at the top of the layer, decreasing continually toward the white matter, and the lower portion of the layer gradually merges with the white substance.

In Nissl preparations, layer IIIc is the most conspicuous portion of the parastriate area. The predominance of layer IIIc over layer V gives the belt area an externocrassior character.

In myelin preparations, the parastriate area shows an overall high content of myelinated fibers (typus dives).

The tangential layer (1) still contains a broad and dense plexus of myelinated fibers running parallel to the cortical surface but the plexus is less accentuated than in the striate area.

The dysfibrous layer (2) is a narrow zone almost devoid of myelinated profiles.

The upper portions of the suprastriate layer (3) display a fair number of thick, horizontally aligned, myelinated fibers forming the line of Kaes–Bechterew. This attribute gives the belt area an extremostriate character. The radiate bundles extend up to the boundary between layer IIIab and layer IIIc. The line of Kaes–Bechterew lies well above this borderline as is depicted in the lower half of Fig. 7.

Both lines of Baillarger (4 and 5b) as well as the intrastriate layer contain a large number of myelinated horizontal fibers. Subsequently, two individual lines are barely recognizable, for the lines seem to merge. The parastriate area can therefore be classified with the conjunctostriate fields.

The substriate and limiting layer (6) is a relatively fiber-sparse zone and resembles that of the striate area.

In pigment preparations, the belt area is usually still sparsely endowed with

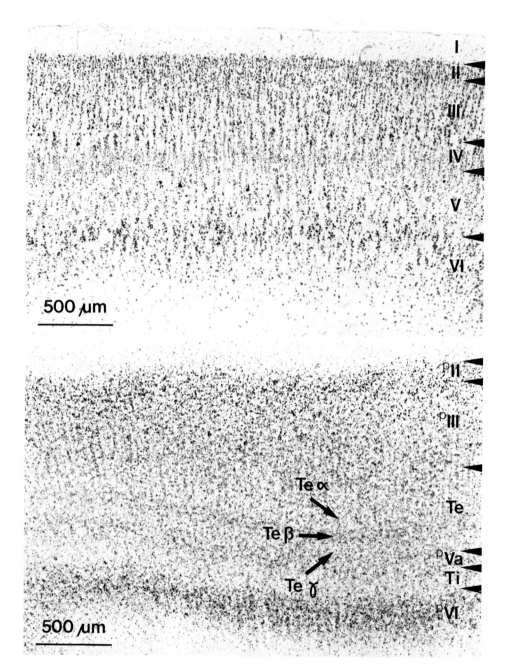

Figure 10. (Top) Nissl preparation of the parastriate area of the human brain. The eugranular field shows a clear-cut granular layer (IV). Cresyl violet, 35 μm. (Bottom) Pigment preparation of the same area. On the average, the belt area is relatively lightly pigmented. Note the tripartition of the external tenia (Teα, Teβ, Teγ). This is a hallmark of the parastriate field and allows clear delineation of the border between the parastriate area and the peristriate region. Aldehyde fuchsin, 800 μm.

pigment (typus clarus) but not quite as pronounced as the core field (Fig. 10 bottom).

The small pyramidal cells of layers ^{P}II and ^{P}IIIab are particularly poorly pigmented but large numbers of pigment-laden stellate cells are densely distributed over the lower portions of the corpuscular layer and these extend into the subjacent portions of the pyramidal layer (IIIab).

The upper portions of the third layer are typically well pigmented, with a slight increase in pigment content from top to bottom. A blurred zone with decreasing pigment content follows. The large pyramidal cells within the lower portion of the third layer are almost devoid of pigment.

The limits of the outer tenia do not correspond to those of the granular layer. The external tenia is a broad stripe extending not only over the granular layer but also into portions of the pyramidal layer (Teα). Deep penetration of the outer tenia into the pyramidal layer is a marked feature common to isocortical core fields and belt areas. Most conspicuous in core fields, this trait is generally less pronounced in the adjoining belt areas. The broadening of the outer tenia reverses the normal pigmentation pattern of layer ^{P}III; the overall pigment content decreases as the layer is followed from top to bottom.

In the parastriate area, the outer tenia exhibits a unique pattern in that it contains a narrow zone (Teβ) filled with moderately pigmented nerve cells. These neurons are tightly clustered and contain fine dustlike pigment granules. To clearly demonstrate this faintly pigmented stripe, a section thickness of more than 500 μm and preparations that have been cut perpendicular to the cortical surface are required (Fig. 10 bottom). For visual examination, sufficient tilting of the preparations under the stereomicroscope generally allows identification of this line. The lower portion of the outer tenia is again a pigment-sparse zone (Teγ). This marked triple layering of the outer tenia is a hallmark of the parastriate area and does not occur in any other field of the isocortex. Therefore, the border between the parastriate area and the surrounding peristriate region is well marked in pigment preparations, although it is often barely recognizable in Nissl or myelin preparations (von Economo and Koskinas, 1925; Bailey and von Bonin, 1951; Gattas *et al.*, 1981; Lund *et al.*, 1981).

Layer ^{P}Va shows blurred upper and lower limits. It is dominated by small to medium-sized pyramidal cells with a moderate amount of weakly tinged pigment.

The internal tenia (Ti = ^{P}Vb) is a bit broader than in the striate area and has a more pallid appearance than the outer tenia in the parastriate field. The outer tenia is clearly wider than the inner one, and thus the parastriate area is of the biteniate and markedly externoteniate type.

The upper border of the multiform layer (^{P}VI) is clearly marked by an abrupt increase in the average pigment content. The amount of pigment decreases gradually from top to bottom, so there is no clear boundary between the layer and the underlying white substance.

The Parastriate Border (Limes Parastriatus)

Close to the boundary toward the visual core field, the parastriate area shows changes in its structure that permit delineation of another narrow area (limes parastriatus).

In Nissl preparations, the distinguishing feature of this zone is the presence of conspicuously large pyramidal cells in layer III. They are present in small numbers, more or less evenly distributed throughout the lower portion of the layer (IIIc), and they can even be found in the granular layer (IV). Because pyramids of this size do not occur in other parts of the parastriate field, this zone has been referred to by von Economo and Koskinas (1925) as *limes parastriatus gigantopyramidalis* (OBγ).

In this region myelin preparations display particularly thick radiate fiber bundles, the "limiting bundles" (Sanides and Gräfin Vitzthum, 1965b). These bundles allow delineation of the parastriate border area as depicted in Fig. 8.

In pigment preparations, the zone is less distinct. The only conspicuous difference between it and other portions of the parastriate area is the presence of pigment-laden and intensely stained large pyramidal cells within the pallid outer tenia. These special pyramidal cells correspond to the large pyramids seen in Nissl preparations. In the parastriate area, most pyramidal cells in layer IIIc are devoid of pigment. Hence, the unusually large pigment-laden IIIc pyramidal cells in the border zone are by no means normal constituents of the third layer. Instead, this special type of pyramidal cell occurs only in certain regions of the isocortex.

It seems well established that the parastriate border zone has a particular functional significance for connecting neighboring points of the visual field on both sides of the vertical meridian (Vogt, 1929; Myers, 1962, 1965; Sanides and Gräfin Vitzthum, 1965b; Zeki, 1970; Glickstein and Whitteridge, 1974; Shoumura *et al.*, 1975; Shoumura, 1981).

5.3. The Peristriate Region

The parastriate area is surrounded by the peristriate region which is composed of many areas with a common structural pattern. The peristriate region spreads over all portions of the occipital lobe not occupied by the visual core and belt. Medially, and superolaterally, its peripheral border coincides with the confines of the occipital lobe. Inferiorly, the peristriate region extends considerably into basal portions of the temporal lobe (Fig. 5).

The Magnopyramidal Peristriate Area

A detailed description of the various peristriate areas is not within the scope of the present text. It seems advisable to describe only the magnopyramidal peristriate field, which appears to be the most highly differentiated portion of the homotypical peristriate association cortex. The magnopyramidal portion of the peristriate region spreads over the edge, between the inferior facies and the superolateral facies of the hemisphere, as is shown in Fig. 5. Anteriorly, it extends to the preoccipital incisure (Braak, 1977).

The Nissl preparations show a homotypical cortex with balance between layers dominated by pyramidal cells and "granule" cells (Fig. 11).

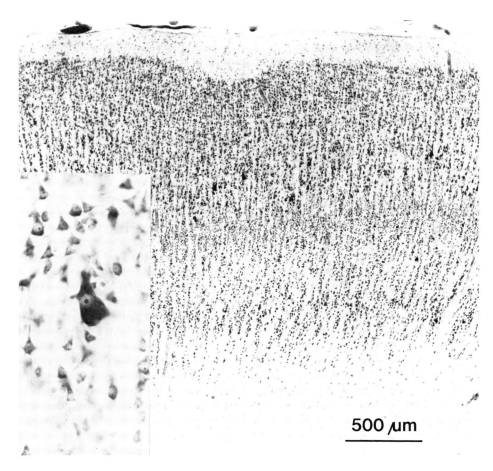

Figure 11. Nissl preparation of the magnopyramidal peristriate area. Note the large pyramidal cells within the lower reaches of the third layer (inset). Cresyl violet, 35 μm.

The supragranular layers II and IIIab remain almost unchanged compared to the corresponding laminae of the parastriate field. There is a size gradient in the pyramidal layer, with the cells near the granular layer being largest. Layer IIIc is very broad and contains many large pyramidal cells (Fig. 11). In this respect, it resembles layer IIIc in the parastriate border zone. The large pyramids give the field a clear magnopyramidal characteristic.

A well-developed granular layer (IV) indicates the eugranular nature of the field.

The ganglionic layer with its cell-rich upper (Va) and cell-sparse lower portion (Vb) is a bit broader than the corresponding layer in the parastriate area. Layer IIIc and layer V are almost equally broad (typus equocrassus).

The multiform layer (VI) does not differ markedly from that of the parastriate area.

In myelin preparations only a moderate amount of myelinated fibers can be seen. The tangential fiber plexus is clearly less well developed than in the visual core field or in the belt area. The dysfibrous layer (2) is a particularly pallid zone and the suprastriate layer (3) is also devoid of myelinated fibers. The line of Kaes–Bechterew is absent and only the myelinated radii pierce the lower portion of the layer. The peristriate cortex is of the euradiate type.

Neither line of Baillarger shows as high a myelin content as in the parastriate field. Again the intrastriate layer is richly endowed with fine "ground" fibers and therefore the lower border of the outer line, as well as the upper border of the inner line, cannot be traced with certainty. In certain places, the conjunctostriate type of the field changes into the bistriate and equodense character.

The substriate and limiting layer (6) has the same pallid appearance as in the parastriate area.

In pigment preparations, the peristriate field is neither strongly nor weakly endowed with lipofuscin deposits (Fig. 12).

The supragranular layers PI, PII, and PIIIab appear similar to those of the parastriate area although the pigment-laden stellate cells are more clustered along the border between the corpuscular layer and the pyramidal layer, so that layer PIIIab is a relatively pallid stripe.

The lower reaches of the pyramidal layer (PIIIc) are unusual in that they have a conspicuous population of large and pigment-rich pyramidal cells. These give the field a magnopyramidal character. The large pyramids are mainly located within layer PIIIc but many can also be found within subjacent portions of the outer tenia. The cells are scattered throughout the layer with relatively large distances between them (Fig. 12) and they are intermixed with a dense population of the common type of third-layer pyramidal cells, with small, moderately stained pigment granules widely dispersed throughout the cell body. These pigment-laden pyramidal cells amass lipofuscin granules in an aggregate that often forms a bowl-shaped mass with rounded contours in the vicinity of the nucleus. Most often, the pigment aggregate is contained in the basal portions of the cytoplasm, but it can also be encountered in other locations. The axon hillock always remains devoid of pigment. In spite of their dense aggregations, the individual granules do not tend to amalgamate. The pigment is more intensely stained by aldehyde fuchsin than is the pigment in the common third-layer pyramidal cells, but the staining capacity of the aggregates is less than that of the coarse granules in the pigmented stellate cells. Within the peristriate region, the existence of unusually large third-layer pyramidal cells with voluminous pigment aggregations is confined to the limits of the magnopyramidal area.

The outer and inner teniae are clearly recognizable and equally broad, and therefore the cortex is biteniate and equoteniate. In layer PVa, moderately pigmented pyramidal cells prevail. The multiform layer (PVI) shows the common pattern of relatively high pigment content decreasing gradually from the top toward the white matter.

On account of its location and structural uniqueness, it is tempting to suggest that the magnopyramidal peristriate area might serve as a visual "gnostic" field that is of particular importance for the more advanced processing of visual information.

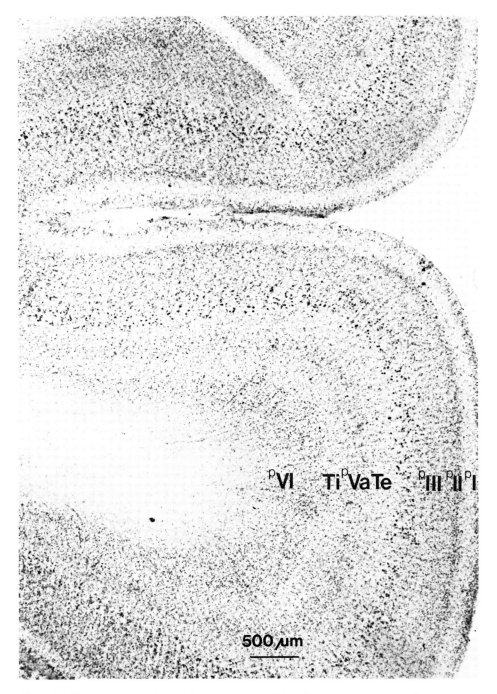

Figure 12. Pigment preparation of the magnopyramidal peristriate area. Note the dense accumulation of small pigment-laden stellate cells in layer PII forming a narrow dark line. The lower regions of the pyramidal layer are made conspicuous by the existence of unusually large pigment-laden pyramidal cells loosely scattered among a population of layer IIIc pyramidal cells with a normal pattern of pigmentation. Aldehyde fuchsin, 800 μm.

area striata

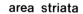

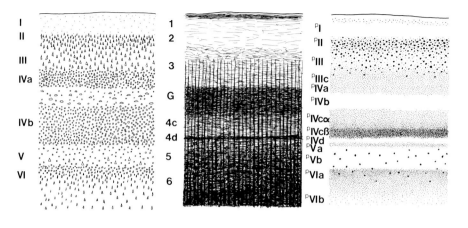

I	1	ᴾI
II	2	ᴾII
III	3	ᴾIII
IVa		ᴾIIIc
	G	ᴾIVa
		ᴾIVb
IVb	4c	ᴾIVcα
	4d	ᴾIVcß
		ᴾIVd
V	5	ᴾVa
VI	6	ᴾVb
		ᴾVIa
		ᴾVIb

area parastriata

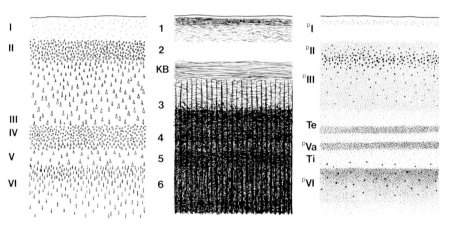

I	1	ᴾI
II	2	
	KB	ᴾII
		ᴾIII
III	3	
IV	4	Te
V	5	ᴾVa
		Ti
VI	6	ᴾVI

area peristriata magnopyramidalis

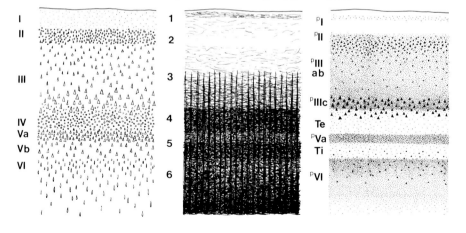

I	1	ᴾI
II	2	ᴾII
III	3	ᴾIII ab
		ᴾIIIc
IV	4	Te
Va		ᴾVa
Vb	5	Ti
VI	6	ᴾVI

5.4. General Remarks on Magnopyramidal Areas

87

ARCHI-
TECTONICS
AS SEEN BY
LIPOFUSCIN
STAINS

Pigment-laden and unusually large third-layer pyramidal cells are rarely encountered in the isocortex and occur in only a limited number of specialized association areas. Such areas have not as yet been recognized in the brains of subhuman primates. Each of the various lobes of the human brain contains a more or less extended magnopyramidal territory (Fig. 14). Within the temporal lobe a large magnopyramidal region is found extending over lateral portions of the temporal plane, i.e., the upper bank of the first temporal convolution immediately behind the transverse gyrus of Heschl. Due to its location, this structurally unique temporal magnopyramidal region can probably be considered the morphological counterpart of the speech center of Wernicke (Braak, 1978b). The parietal lobe also shows an extended magnopyramidal region covering large parts of the inferior parietal lobule. Finally, two magnopyramidal regions can be distinguished within the frontal lobe. The smaller one, the inferofrontal magnopyramidal region, spreads over portions of the fronto-parietal operculum immediately in front of the precentral gyrus. Its location coincides with that of the speech center of Broca (Braak, 1979b). The superofrontal magnopyramidal region is very extended and stretches over large portions of the superior frontal convolution, including the "supplementary" motor region. These portions of the first frontal convolution are known to be involved in the production of speech (Penfield and Rasmussen, 1949, 1950; Erickson and Woolsey, 1951; Penfield and Roberts, 1959; Talairach and Bancaud, 1966).

One feature common to all magnopyramidal areas is that they are very conspicuous in studies on regional cortical blood flow. Recently developed techniques permit fairly precise measurements of cortical blood flow either at rest or during the performance of different tasks (Ingvar and Schwartz, 1974; Ingvar, 1976, 1978; Roland and Larsen, 1976; Ingvar and Philipson, 1977; Larsen *et al.*, 1978; Lassen *et al.*, 1978; Roland *et al.*, 1980a,b). These measurements suggest a functional parcellation of the free surface of the hemispheres. The functional

←——————————————————————————————

Figure 13. Synopsis of the striate area, the parastriate area, and the magnopyramidal peristriate area as seen in Nissl-, myelin-, and pigment-stained preparations. The characteristics of the visual core, the belt area, and the magnopyramidal "association" field are listed below:

Striate area:

Parvocellular	Dives, euradiate	Clarus
Hypergranular	Singulostriate	Biteniate
Externocrassior	Externodensior	Externoteniate

Parastriate area:

Mediocellular	Dives, euradiate	Clarus
Eugranular	Conjunctostriate	Biteniate
Externocrassior	Extremostriate	Externoteniate

Magnopyramidal peristriate area:

Eugranular	Subconjunctostriate	Biteniate
Equocrassus	Equodensus	Equoteniate
Magnopyramidal	Euradiate	Magnopyramidal

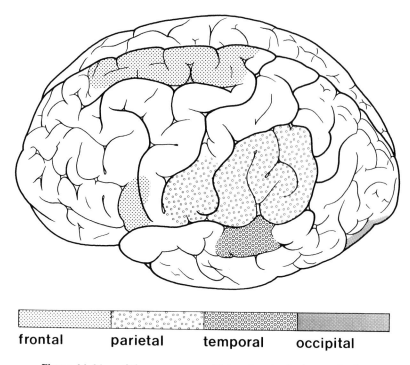

frontal   parietal   temporal   occipital

Figure 14. Map of the magnopyramidal regions in the human brain.

brain map thus achieved can be compared to anatomical landmarks. The location and extent of the diverse magnopyramidal regions outlined in Fig. 14 closely correspond to portions of the brain which show a high rate of blood flow even at rest. During speech production, the local blood flow is increased in the temporal, the inferofrontal, and the superofrontal magnopyramidal regions.

The superofrontal territory seems to be important not only in the production of speech, but also in the programming of all voluntary movements. This is indicated by an increase of cortical blood flow in some precentral motor areas and the superofrontal magnopyramidal region during execution of complex sequences of fast finger movements. During programming of the same complex motor sequences—without actually executing it—it is only the superofrontal magnopyramidal region that shows the blood flow increase, a result pointing to the particular significance of this territory for planning of voluntary movements (Roland *et al.*, 1980a).

6. Age Changes of the Isocortex

The use of pigment preparations is not restricted to anatomical studies of the horizontal lamination and the vertical parcellation of the telencephalic cortex for they also offer advantages for the examination of pathological changes. Due to superposition of numerous pigment deposits, the thick preparations show even subtle changes in the pattern of pigmentation. These changes are more marked if they are linked to a certain cell type or a certain lamina.

To demonstrate these advantages, typical age changes of the human iso-cortex will be described. In this context, it should be emphasized that very little is known about general age-related nerve cell changes of the *iso*cortex. A lot of attention has been paid to the granulovacuolar degeneration of Simchowicz (Woodard, 1962; Tomlinson and Kitchener, 1972; Ball, 1977; Ball and Lo, 1977; Mann, 1978). This degeneration, however, is retricted to *allo*cortical pyramidal cells of the hippocampus. Also the formation of Alzheimer's neurofibrillary changes is predominantly encountered in pyramidal cells of the *allo*cortex, as far as nondemented patients of old age are concerned (Alzheimer, 1907; Hirano and Zimmerman, 1962; Friede, 1966; Jamada and Mehraein, 1968; Tomlinson *et al.*, 1968, 1970; Dayan, 1970a,b; Hirano, 1970; Tomlinson, 1972, 1977; Mor-imatsu *et al.*, 1975; Ball, 1976, 1977, 1978; Ball and Nuttall, 1981; Mann and Yates, 1981; Perry *et al.*, 1981). The changes described here are confined to the limits of the isocortex. They are layer specific and occur in all isocortical fields. In the human brain, the isocortex covers a major portion of the telencephalon. Hence, even a subtle change of a single isocortical layer will affect a considerable proportion of the total number of nerve cells.

6.1. Loss of Supragranular Pigment-Laden Stellate Cells

The supragranular layers undergo the most severe structural changes with age. Specifically, the small pigment-laden stellate cells show a considerable nu-merical decrease as age advances and this is well shown in the striate area. The pigment-laden stellate cells normally form a broad band in this area and this band stands out against the very sparsely pigmented pyramidal cells of layer ^{P}II and ^{P}IIIab (Fig. 15). Accordingly, a loss of this type of local-circuit neurons can easily be seen (Fig. 15). There may nevertheless be some difficulties in recog-nizing the first stages of this cell loss since in addition to the pigment accumu-lations in small stellate cells, a fair number of extraneuronal pigment deposits of about the same size may be present. The staining capacity of these deposits is comparable to that of the pigment in stellate cells, so that these dots can easily be misinterpreted if preparations are only studied under the low-power stereo-microscope. Combined Nissl–pigment preparations reveal that these pigment deposits are stored within astrocytes. Normally, glial cells of the corpuscular and pyramidal layers do not contain pigment that can be intensely stained by alde-hydefuchsin, and the occurrence of extraneuronal lipofuscin deposits within the supragranular layers is a characteristic feature of an age-changed isocortex. It is probable that the atypical astrocytic pigment deposits may be due to neuron-ophagia of pigment-laden stellate cells. Extraneuronal pigment clumps may re-main within these layers for several years, but they will finally disappear.

Very little is known about the functional significance of the small pigment-laden stellate cells, but whatever their function may be, a numerical decrease of a single component of the isocortex will probably more severely impair cortical function than a comparable overall loss of cortical nerve cells.

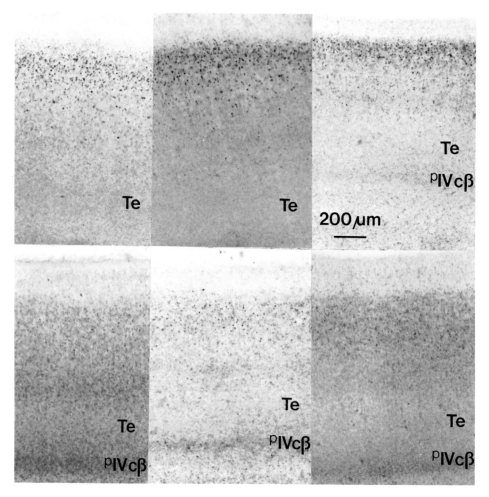

Figure 15. Loss of pigment-laden stellate cells during aging. Pigment preparations of the striate area. (Top) Left: 34-year-old man, endocarditis; middle: 38-year-old man, suicide: right: 45-year-old man, cardiac infarction. (Bottom) Left: 80-year-old man, tuberculosis; middle: 85-year-old woman, suicide; right: 88-year-old man, pulmonary embolism. The external tenia (Te) and, when apparent, layer $^{p}IVc\beta$ are indicated at the right margin. Aldehyde fuchsin, 800 μm.

6.2. Axonal Enlargements of Supragranular Pyramidal Cells

Certain types of pyramidal cells exhibit another change that becomes increasingly prominent with advancing age. In normal pyramidal cells the pigment is finely granulated and widely dispersed, but is contained only within the cell body (Fig. 16A). Also the pigment aggregates in large layer IIIc and layer Vb pyramidal cells are confined to the limits of the cell body (Fig. 16B). Only a few types of allocortical pyramidal cells show pigment accumulations extending into proximal portions of the apical dendrite (Fig. 16C, pyramidal cells of the ammonshorn).

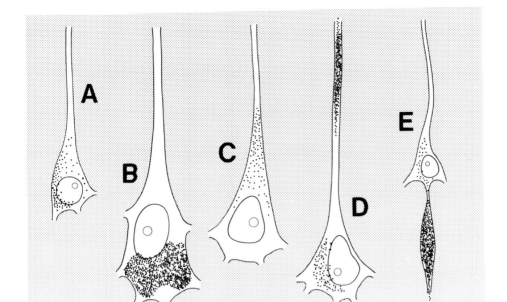

Figure 16. Diagrammatic representation of the various locations of pigment in cortical pyramidal cells. (A) Normal pyramidal cell with lipofuscin granules widely dispersed within the cell body. (B) The pigment aggregates in large layer IIIc and layer Vb pyramidal cells are also confined to the limits of the cell body. (C) Pyramidal cells of the ammonshorn show pigment extending into proximal portions of the apical dendrite. (D) Outer pyramidal cells of the subiculum are conspicuous in that they contain spindle-shaped accumulations of pigment within circumscribed portions of their apical dendrites. (E) Pathological accumulation of pigment within the proximal axon of layer III pyramidal cells.

Pigment accumulations within cellular processes can be considered as a pathological change. There are only a few exceptions to this rule.

Pigment in *dendrites* is seen only rarely. Some subcortical nuclei show accumulation of lipofuscin at this strange location (Braak, 1972b), and the Purkinje cells of the cerebellar cortex occasionally display small pigment deposits at branching points of their coarser dendrites. In the telencephalic cortex, it is only the outer pyramidal cells of the subiculum (allocortex) that normally develop large and spindle-shaped lipofuscin aggregations within circumscribed portions of the stem of their apical dendrites (Braak, 1972a). The pigment is never found in basal dendrites or in side branches of the apical dendrite (Fig. 16D). The dendritic pigment is a characteristic unique to the subiculum and so it can be used for reliable delineation of this allocortical center. Questions regarding the characteristic location of the dendritic pigment spindles and the conditions of their development remain unanswered. It is also unknown whether the dendritic pigment accumulations might ever reach such a size as to impair the vitality of the dendritic tree distal to the spindle. None of the various types of stellate cells or isocortical pyramidal cells normally contains pigment within their dendrites.

As a general rule, the *axon* and the *axon hillock* are also devoid of pigment. Lipofuscin granules do not normally develop within the various portions of the axon and nor are they transported from the cell body into the axon. The morphological substrate which prevents lipofuscin granules from passing beyond the limits of the axon hillock is unknown as yet although other fine particles, such as mitochondria, obviously pass beyond the axon hillock. Appearance of pigment within the axon represents a pathological change, and this can be observed in the senescent brains which show a great number of pyramidal cells with pigment accumulations in the initial portions of their axons (Fig. 16E). The change is mainly confined to the pyramidal cells of layer PIIIab (Fig. 17). Hence, the process is layer specific. It affects only a certain type of pyramidal cell and has never been observed in local-circuit neurons (Braak, 1979a). In particular, the slender and sparsely pigmented pyramidal cells of layer PIIIab develop dilations of their axonal initial segment, and the size and shapes of these expansions vary considerably (Figs. 17e–k). Frequently, the axon hillock is filled with pigment and only a perpendicularly arranged row of a few granules indicates the position of the axon itself (Fig. 17k). The axon hillock may also appear expanded, but generally a tight constriction between the basal portion of the cell body and the axonal expansion is encountered. The axonal enlargements may become quite large, and sometimes the volumes of the spindles considerably exceed that of the parent soma.

Figure 18 displays Golgi-impregnated layer IIIab pyramidal cells which were close to each other in the frontal isocortex. On the left, an obviously unchanged pyramidal cell shows a well-developed skirt of basal dendrites and many side branches of the apical dendrite. These processes are richly endowed with spines, and the axon gives off a fair number of recurrent collaterals. On the right, a IIIab pyramidal cell with an enlarged initial segment is depicted, and as can be seen, the dendritic arbor and the average spine density of the pyramidal cells with dilated axons exhibit no apparent changes.

Electron microscopical studies reveal that the normal initial segment of layer IIIab pyramidal cells shows an incomplete undercoating of the axolemma with gaps not only at synaptic contacts (Palay *et al.*, 1968; Peters *et al.*, 1968; Jones and Powell, 1969) but also opposite to the processes of the asrocytes (E. Braak, 1980). In this regard, it bears a certain resemblance to the initial segment of immature nerve cells. The pigment-filled expansions display an axolemma devoid of undercoating (Fig. 18) even though there is no loss of synaptic contacts or marked alteration of adjacent profiles. Synaptic contacts on the soma of pyramidal cells are rare (Colonnier, 1968), but they are frequently encountered at the axon hillock and initial axonal segment (Jones and Powell, 1969). The large number of synaptic contacts along the fusiform dilations supports the assumption that the expanded process is indeed the proximal axon. The soma membrane apparently does not contribute to the development of the spindle. In contrast, the similarly shaped swellings that have been reported to occur in feline GM_1 gangliosidosis have been interpreted as pathological processes of the soma which displace the axonal initial segment distally (Purpura and Baker, 1978; Purpura *et al.*, 1978; Walkley *et al.*, 1980, 1981). The incomplete undercoating of the normal initial segment in IIIab pyramidal cells of the human

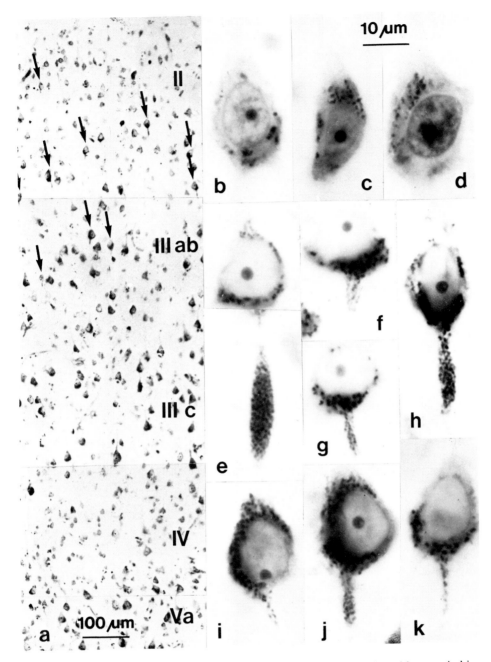

Figure 17. Axonal enlargements of supragranular pyramidal cells. (a) Prefrontal homotypical iso-cortex, 70-year-old man. Arrows indicate layer IIIab pyramidal cells with pigment-filled proximal axon. The layers are indicated at the right-hand margin. (b–d) Typical pattern of pigmentation of layer IIIab pyramidal cells of the same area in a brain of a 36-year-old man. (e–k) Senescent layer IIIab pyramidal cells of a 70-year-old man. Combined pigment–Nissl preparation, aldehyde fuch-sin–methylene blue, 10 μm.

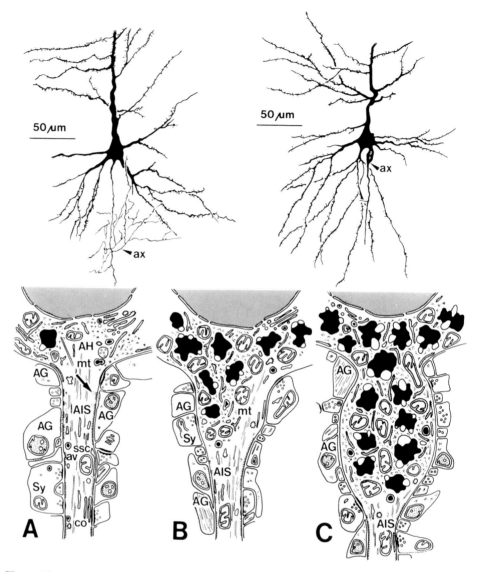

Figure 18. (Top) Camera lucida drawings of layer IIIab pyramidal cells. First frontal gyrus, 70-year-old man. The cell on the left shows the normal appearance of pyramidal cells at this location. The cell on the right displays a spindle-shaped enlargement of its proximal axon (ax). (Bottom) Schematic representation of the development of axonal dilations. (A) Normally, the axon hillock (AH) and the initial segment (AIS) are devoid of pigment and rough endoplasmic reticulum cisterns. The initial segment is characterized by fasciculated microtubules (mt) and a dense undercoating (arrow). The undercoating shows gaps at synaptic contacts (Sy), at sites where subsurface cisterns (ssc) and cisternal organelles (co) are closely apposed to the membrane, or where alveolated vesicles (av) open upon the membrane. In addition, gaps can be seen opposite to the processes of the astrocytes (AG). (B) The changes begin at the junction between the axon hillock and initial segment. Here, the cytoplasm becomes invaded by lipofusein granules and rough endoplasmic reticulum cisterns, and the fasciculated microtubules (mt) are pushed aside. Only remnants of the undercoating can be seen. (C) At an advanced level of alteration, the proximal axon is dilated and filled with lipofuscin granules and rough endoplasmic reticulum cisterns. The membrane is devoid of an undercoating. The axon at the distal end of the enlargement shows the characteristic features of the initial segment.

adult may contribute to the particular vulnerability of this type of isocortical nerve cell (E. Braak, 1980; Braak *et al.*, 1980).

Because of the regular alignment of cortical pyramidal cells, axonal dilations can easily be recognized and counted in pigment preparations, and Fig. 19 displays the frequency of these dilations in a series of 30 nondemented females. None of the patients had a history of neurological disorder. The pigment-filled axonal dilations have been counted in an area of constant width and depth (9.4 mm², 100-μm depth) comprising portions of layers II–III in the homotypical frontal isocortex covering the banks of the olfactory sulcus (Braak and Bumann, 1981). Despite a marked variation between individuals, the results show a striking increase in the number of the spindles with increasing age.

The change is by no means confined to the frontal cortex but occurs to about the same extent in all other isocortical territories of both hemispheres.

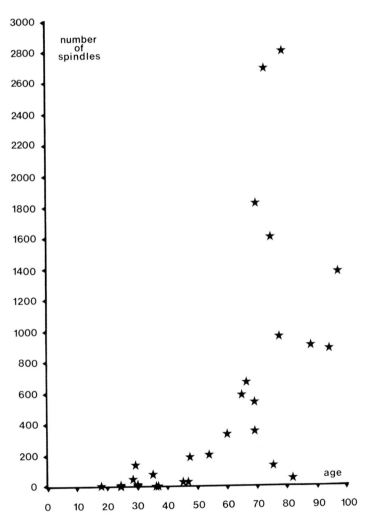

Figure 19. Diagram showing the numerical increase of pigment-filled axonal spindles with growing age.

There are also no apparent differences between males and females (Braak, 1979a) and the change seems to be unique to the human brain, for pigment-laden enlargements of the initial segments of the third-layer pyramidal cells have not been reported to occur in the senescent subhuman mammalian brain.

6.3. Neuronal Ceroid Lipofuscinosis

This set of changes, i.e., loss of supragranular pigment-laden stellate cells and development of axonal dilations of layer III pyramidal cells, bears a close resemblance to structural alterations that have been reported to occur in the brains of patients afflicted with juvenile neuronal ceroid lipofuscinosis (Braak and Goebel, 1978, 1979).

In this storage disease (Zeman, 1976), the supragranular layers are severely depleted of pigment-laden stellate cells. Only a few dots of densely packed extraneuronal pigment accumulations point to the breakdown of pigmented nerve cells and neuronophagia (Fig. 20).

The slender pyramidal cells in the upper regions of the third layer accumulate an only modest amount of ceroid-type lipopigment within their cell bodies but show large to giant fusiformly swollen initial axonal segments (Fig. 20). The axon hillock is often dilated as well, giving the pigment-filled portion of the axon the shape of an hourglass. The storage material found in such axonal segments is generally more finely granulated and less intensely stained than that in the cell body. Conversely, the large pyramidal cells forming the lower regions of the third layer store huge amounts of ceroid-type lipopigment within their cell bodies but rarely display dilated axons. The local-circuit neurons which are normally devoid of pigment also contain some storage material, but this again leads only to an expansion of their cell bodies.

The granular layer (IV) appears almost unchanged, but the ganglionic layer is markedly attenuated due to a loss of pyramidal cells in layer Va. Pigment preparations generally display the granular layer (IV) as well as the lower portions of the ganglionic layer (Vb) as pale stripes—the outer and inner teniae. These can clearly be recognized in Fig. 21 which shows a part of the densopyramidal area in the peristriate region (Braak, 1977). This field represents a homotypical cortex with equally broad teniae and well-developed layer Va. Figure 20 displays the same field from a patient afflicted with juvenile ceroid lipofuscinosis. As a result of the almost complete disappearance of layer PVa, the two light teniae fuse to form a broad band. The subjacent layer PVb seems less eroded

———————————————————————————————→

Figure 20. (Top) Pigment preparation of the densopyramidal peristriate area from a 17-year-old patient afflicted with juvenile neuronal ceroid lipofuscinosis. Note the fusion of the two light teniae brought about by cell loss in layer PVa. Note also the almost complete disappearance of small pigment-laden stellate cells in the supragranular layers and the great number of pigment-filled axonal enlargements of layer IIIab pyramidal cells. Layer IIIc pyramidal cells store huge amounts of ceroid-type lipopigment within their cell bodies. Aldehyde fuchsin, 800 μm. (Bottom) Higher-magnification photographs of layer IIIab pyramidal cells with large pigment-filled dilations of their proximal axons. The arrow points to an intensely stained extraneuronal accumulation of pigment. Aldehyde fuchsin, 100 μm.

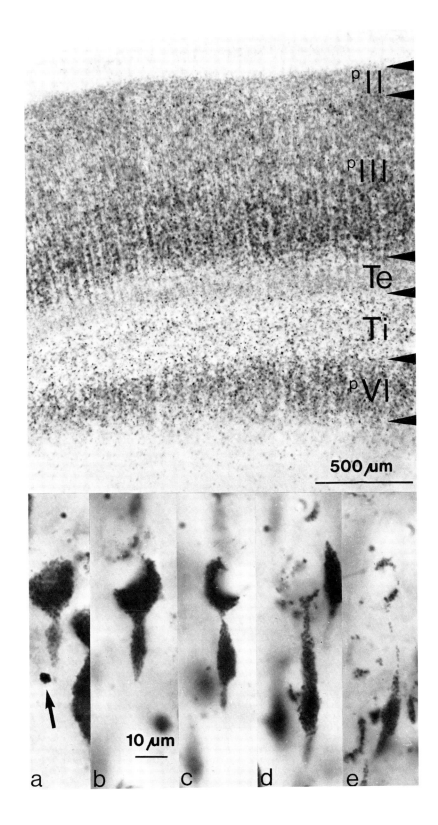

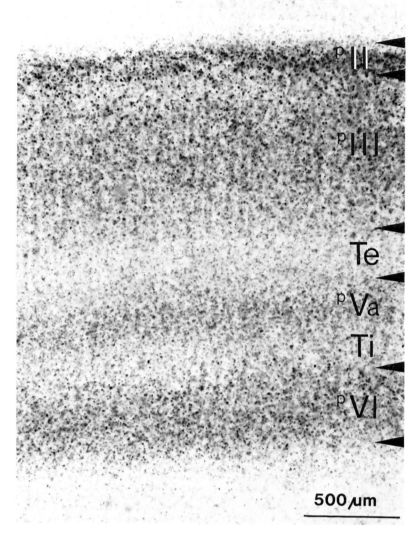

Figure 21. Pigment preparation of the densopyramidal peristriate area of the human brain (45-year-old man). The lamination is indicated at the right hand-margin. Note the two light teniae with the moderately pigmented layer Va squeezed in between. Aldehyde fuchsin, 800 μm.

and the multiform layer (PVI) contains nerve cells which store a great amount of ceroid-type lipopigment within their cell bodies. Storage material within cellular processes can only rarely be encountered.

In the juvenile neuronal ceroid lipofuscinosis, layer-specific changes which have been described can be found in all isocortical areas, only slightly modified by the architecture of the respective field.

There is also evidence of an almost identical set of architectonic pathology in the isocortex of patients suffering from the *adult* type of neuronal ceroid lipofuscinosis. In general, the changes are less severe than in the *juvenile* type; specifically, the cell loss in layer ᴾVa is far less pronounced. Furthermore, the change is not evenly distributed over the entire isocortex but is prominent in the frontobasal and temporopolar regions, while the occipital cortex shows identical but markedly fewer abnormalities.

Partly due to poor definition, there has been a long debate as to whether or not an *adult* type of neuronal ceroid lipofuscinosis exists. Pigmentoarchitectonic analysis permits clear diagnosis indicating its value for recognition of layer-specific alterations (Goebel *et al.*, 1982).

In a sense, the juvenile and adult types of neuronal ceroid lipofuscinosis mimic the changes revealed by the *senescent* isocortex. Because there are animal models of this disease which display similar cortical changes (Koppang, 1973–1974), the question arises as to whether neuronal ceroid lipofuscinosis could be a useful model for the effects of aging (Zeman, 1971). This would allow for more systematic investigations on the conditions responsible for the development of the described layer-specific alterations. In neuronal ceroid lipofuscinoses, the development of axonal enlargements precedes other signs of neuronal degeneration (Williams *et al.*, 1977) and the extent of the pathological change parallels the clinical course of the disease (Purpura and Suzuki, 1976). The development of pigment-filled dilations of the proximal axon is also an inevitable consequence of growing old and the extent of this cortical change closely parallels the course of aging.

ACKNOWLEDGMENT. This study was supported by the Deutsche Forschungs-
gemeinschaft.

7. References

Alzheimer, A., 1907, Über eine eigenartige Erkrankung der Hirnrinde, *Centralbl. Nervenheilk. Psychiatr.* **30**:177–179.

Bailey, P., and von Bonin, G., 1951, *The Isocortex of Man*, University of Illinois Press, Urbana.

Ball, M. J., 1976, Neurofibrillary tangles and the pathogenesis of dementia: A quantitative study, *Neuropathol. Appl. Neurobiol.* **2**:395–410.

Ball, M. J., 1977, Neuronal loss, neurofibrillary tangles and granulovacuolar degeneration in the hippocampus with ageing and dementia—A quantitative study, *Acta Neuropathol.* **37**:111–118.

Ball, M. J., 1978, Topographic distribution of neurofibrillary tangles and granulovacuolar degeneration in hippocampal cortex of ageing and demented patients: A quantitative study, *Acta Neuropathol.* **42**:73–80.

Ball, M. J., and Lo, P., 1977, Granulovacuolar degeneration in the ageing brain and in dementia, *J. Neuropathol. Exp. Neurol.* **36**:474–487.

Ball, M. J., and Nuttall, K., 1981, Topography of neurofibrillary tangles and granulovacuoles in hippocampi of patients with Down's syndrome: Quantitative comparison with normal ageing and Alzheimer's disease, *Neuropathol. Appl. Neurobiol.* **7**:13–20.

Billings-Gagliardi, S., Chan-Palay, V., and Palay, S. L., 1974, A review of lamination in area 17 of the visual cortex of *Macaca mulatta*, *J. Neurocytol.* **3**:619–629.

Bishop, G. H., and Smith, J. M., 1964, The sizes of nerve fibers supplying cerebral cortex, *Exp. Neurol.* **9**:483–501.

Braak, E., 1975, On the fine structure of the external glial layer in the isocortex of man, *Cell Tissue Res.* **157**:367–390.

Braak, E., 1976, On the fine structure of the small, heavily pigmented non-pyramidal cells in lamina II and upper lamina III of the human isocortex, *Cell Tissue Res.* **169:**233–245.

Braak, E., 1978, On the structure of the human striate area: Lamina IV cβ, *Cell Tissue Res.* **188:**217–234.

Braak, E., 1980, On the structure of lamina IIIab-pyramidal cells in the human isocortex: A Golgi and electron microscopical study with special emphasis on the proximal axon segment, *J. Hirnforsch.* **21:**439–444.

Braak, E., 1982, On the structure of the human striate area, in: *Advances in Anatomy, Embryology, and Cell Biology,* Vol. 77 (F. Beck, W. Hild, J. van Limborgh, R. Ortmann, J. E. Pauly, and T. H. Schiebler, eds.), pp. 1–87, Springer, Berlin.

Braak, E., Braak, H., Strenge, H., and Muhtaroglu, U., 1980, Age-related alterations of the proximal axon segment in lamina IIIab-pyramidal cells of the human isocortex: A Golgi and fine structural study, *J. Hirnforsch.* **21:**531–535.

Braak, H., 1971, Über das Neurolipofuscin in der unteren Olive und dem Nucleus dentatus cerebelli im Gehirn des Menschen, *Z. Zellforsch. Mikrosk. Anat.* **121:**573–592.

Braak, H., 1972a, Zur Pigmentarchitektonik der Großhirnrinde des Menschen. II. Subiculum, *Z. Zellforsch. Mikrosk. Anat.* **131:**235–254.

Braak, H., 1972b, Ober die Kerngebiete des menschlichen Hirnstammes. V. Das dorsale Glossopharyngeus- und Vagusgebiet, *Z. Zellforsch. Mikrosk. Anat.* **135:**415–438.

Braak, H., 1974a, On the structure of the human archicortex. I. The cornu ammonis: A Golgi and pigmentarchitectonic study, *Cell Tissue Res.* **152:**349–383.

Braak, H., 1974b, On pigment-loaded stellate cells within layer II and III of the human isocortex. A Golgi and pigmentarchitectonic study, *Cell Tissue Res.* **155:**91–104.

Braak, H., 1976a, A primitive gigantopyramidal field buried in the depth of the cingulate sulcus of the human brain, *Brain Res.* **109:**219–233.

Braak, H., 1976b, On the striate area of the human isocortex: A Golgi and pigmentarchitectonic study, *J. Comp. Neurol.* **166:**341–364.

Braak, H., 1977, The pigment architecture of the human occipital lobe, *Anat. Embryol.* **150:**229–250.

Braak, H., 1978a, On the pigmentarchitectonics of the human telencephalic cortex, in: *Architectonics of the Cerebral Cortex* (M.A.B. Brazier and H. Petsche, eds.), pp. 137–157, Raven Press, New York.

Braak, H., 1978b, On magnopyramidal temporal fields in the human brain—Probable morphological counterparts of Wernicke's sensory speech region, *Anat. Embryol.* **152:**141–169.

Braak, H., 1979a, Spindle-shaped appendages of IIIab-pyramids filled with lipofuscin: A striking pathological change of the senescent human isocortex, *Acta Neuropathol.* **46:**197–202.

Braak, H., 1979b, The pigment architecture of the human frontal lobe. I. Precentral, subcentral, and frontal region, *Anat. Embryol.* **157:**35–68.

Braak, H., 1979c, Pigment architecture of the human telencephalic cortex. V. Regio anterogenualis, *Cell Tissue Res.* **204:**441–451.

Braak, H., 1980, Architectonics of the human telencephalic cortex, in: *Studies of Brain Function,* Vol. 4 (H. B. Barlow, E. Florey, O. J. Grüser, and H. Van der Loos, eds.), pp. 1–147, Springer-Verlag, Berlin.

Braak, H., 1983, Transparent Golgi impregnations: A way to examine both details of cellular processes and components of the cell body, *Stain Technol.* **58:**91–95.

Braak, H., and Braak, E., 1976, The pyramidal cells of Betz within the cingulate and precentral gigantopyramidal field in the human brain: A Golgi and pigmentarchitectonic study, *Cell Tissue Res.* **172:**103–119.

Braak, H., and Braak, E., 1982a, Neuronal types in the claustrum of man, *Anat. Embryol.* **163:**447–460.

Braak, H., and Braak, E., 1982b, Neuronal types in the striatum of man, *Cell Tissue Res.* **227:**319–342.

Braak, H., and Bumann, K., 1981, Morphological changes of the third isocortical layer in the senescent brain and in Alzheimer's disease, *Gerontology (Basel)* **27:**101.

Braak, H., and Goebel, H. H., 1978, Loss of pigment-laden stellate cells: A severe alteration of the isocortex in juvenile neuronal ceroid-lipofuscinosis, *Acta Neuropathol.* **42:**53–57.

Braak, H., and Goebel, H. H., 1979, Pigmentoarchitectonic pathology of the isocortex in juvenile neuronal ceroid-lipofuscinosis: Axonal enlargements in layer IIIab and cell loss in layer V, *Acta Neuropathol.* **46:**79–83.

Braitenberg, V., 1962, A note on myeloarchitectonics, *J. Comp. Neurol.* **118:**141–156.

101

ARCHI-
TECTONICS
AS SEEN BY
LIPOFUSCIN
STAINS

Braitenberg, V., 1978, Cortical architectonics: General and areal, in: *Architectonics of the Cerebral Cortex* (M.A.B. Brazier and H. Petsche, eds.), pp. 443–465. Raven Press, New York.

Braitenberg, V., and Braitenberg, C., 1979, Geometry of orientation columns in the visual cortex, *Biol. Cybern.* **33**:179–186.

Braitenberg, V., Guglielmotti, U., and Sada, E., 1967, Correlation of crystal growth with the staining of axons by the Golgi procedure, *Stain Technol.* **42**:277–283.

Brizzee, K. R., Harkin, J. C., Ordy, J. M., and Kaack, B., 1975a, Accumulation and distribution of lipofuscin, amyloid, and senile plaques in the aging nervous system, in: *Aging*, Vol. 1 (H. Brody, D. Harman, and J. M. Ordy, eds.), pp. 39–77, Raven Press, New York.

Brizzee, K. R., Kaack, B., and Klara, P., 1975b, Lipofuscin: Intra- and extraneuronal accumulation and regional distribution. in: *Neurobiology of Aging* (J. M. Ordy and K. R. Brizzee, eds.), pp. 463–484, Plenum Press, New York.

Brodmann, K., 1909, *Vergleichende Lokalisationslehre der Großhirnrinde*, Barth, Leipzig.

Chan-Palay, V., Palay, S. L., and Billings-Gagliardi, S. M., 1974, Meynert cells in the primate visual cortex, *J. Neurocytol.* **3**:631–658.

Clark, W. E. L., 1942, The cells of Meynert in the visual cortex of the monkey, *J. Anat.* **76**:369–376.

Clark, W. E. L. and Sunderland, S., 1939, Structural changes in the isolated visual cortex, *J. Anat.* **73**:563–574.

Colonnier, M., 1968, Synaptic patterns on different cell types in the different laminae of the cat visual cortex: An electron microscope study, *Brain Res.* **9**:268–287.

Conel, J. L., 1939–1967, *The Postnatal Development of the Human Cerebral Cortex*, Vols. I–VIII, Harvard University Press, Cambridge, Mass.

Dayan, A. D., 1970a, Quantitative histological studies on the aged human brain. I. Senile plaques and neurofibrillary tangles in "normal" patients, *Acta Neuropathol.* **15**:85–94.

Dayan, A. D., 1970b, Quantitative histological studies on the aged human brain. II. Senile plaques and neurofibrillary tangles in senile dementia (with an appendix on their occurrence in cases of carcinoma), *Acta Neuropathol.* **16**:95–102.

Erickson, T. C., and Woolsey, C. N., 1951, Observations on the supplementary motor area of man, *Trans. Am. Neurol. Assoc.* **76**:50–56.

Fisken, R. A., Garey, L. J., and Powell, T. P. S., 1975, The intrinsic, association and commissural connections of area 17 of the visual cortex, *Philos. Trans. R. Soc. London Ser. B.* **272**:487–536.

Friede, R. L., 1966, The histochemical architecture of the ammonshorn as related to its selective vulnerability, *Acta Neuropathol.* **6**:1–13.

Garey, L. J., 1971, A light and electron microscopic study of the visual cortex of the cat and monkey, *Proc. R. Soc. London Ser. B* **179**:21–40.

Gattas, R., Gross, C. G., and Sandell, J. H., 1981, Visual topography of V2 in the macaque. *J. Comp. Neurol.* **201**:519–539.

Glees, P., and Hasan, M., 1976, Lipofuscin in neuronal aging and diseases, in: *Normale und pathologische Anatomie*, Vol. 32 (W. Bargmann and W. Doerr, eds.), pp. 1–68, Thieme, Stuttgart.

Glickstein, M., and Whitteridge, D., 1974, Degeneration of layer III pyramidal cells in area 18 following destruction of callosal input, *Anat. Rec.* **178**:362–363.

Goebel, H. H., Braak, H., Seidel, D., Doshi, R., Marsden, C. D., and Gullotta, F., 1982, Morphological studies on adult neuronal–ceroid lipofuscinosis (NCL), *Clin. Neuropathol.* **1**:151–162.

Gräfin Vitzthum, H., and Sanides, F., 1966, Entwicklungsprinzipien der menschlichen Sehrinde, in: *Evolution of the Forebrain* (R. Hassler and H. Stephan, eds.), pp. 435–442, Thieme, Stuttgart.

Hassler, R., and Wagner, A., 1965, Experimentelle und morphologische Befunde über die vierfache corticale Projektion des visuellen Systems, *8th Int. Congr. Neurol.* **3**:77–96.

Hirano, A., 1970, Neurofibrillary changes in conditions related to Alzheimer's disease, in: *Alzheimer's Disease: A Ciba Foundation Symposium* (G. E. W. Wolstenholme and M. O'Connor, eds.), pp. 185–201, Churchill, London.

Hirano, A., and Zimmerman, H. M., 1962, Alzheimer's neurofibrillary changes: A topographic study, *Arch. Neurol.* **7**:227–242.

Holloway, R. L., 1968, The evolution of the primate brain: Some aspects of quantitative relations, *Brain Res.* **7**:121–172.

Hubel, D. H., and Wiesel, T. N., 1972, Laminar and columnar distribution of geniculo-cortico fibers in the macaque monkey. *J. Comp. Neurol.* **146**:421–450.

Hubel, D. H., and Wiesel, T. N., 1977, Ferrier Lecture. Functional architecture of macaque monkey visual cortex, *Proc. R. Soc. London Ser. B* **198**:1–59.

Ingvar, D. H., 1976, Functional landscapes of the dominant hemisphere, *Brain Res.* **107**:181–197.

Ingvar, D. H., 1978, Localization of cortical functions by multiregional measurements of the cerebral blood flow, in: *Architectonics of the Cerebral Cortex* (M.A.B. Brazier and H. Petsche, eds.), pp. 235–243, Raven Press, New York.

Ingvar, D. H., and Philipson, L., 1977, Distribution of cerebral blood flow in the dominant hemisphere during motor ideation and motor performance, *Ann. Neurol.* **2**:230–237.

Ingvar, D. H., and Schwartz, M. S., 1974, Blood flow patterns induced in the dominant hemisphere by speech and reading, *Brain* **97**:273–288.

Jacobson, S., 1963, Sequence of myelination in the brain of the albino rat. A. Cerebral cortex, thalamus and related structures, *J. Comp. Neurol.* **121**:5–29.

Jamada, M., and Mehraein, P., 1968, Verteilungsmuster der senilen Veränderungen im Gehirn: Die Beteiligung des limbischen Systems bei hirnatrophischen Prozessen des Seniums und bei Morbus Alzheimer, *Arch. Psychiatr. Nervenkr.* **211**:308–324.

Jones, E. G., and Powell, T. P. S., 1969, Synapses on the axon hillocks and initial segments of pyramidal cell axons in the cerebral cortex, *J. Cell Sci.* **5**:495–507.

Kawata, A., 1927, Zur Myeloarchitektonik der menschlichen Hirnrinde, *Arb. Neurol. Inst. Univ. Wien* **29**:191–225.

Kirsche, W., and Kirsche, K., 1962, Zur Fibrilloarchitektonik des Neocortex von *Macaca mulatta Zimmermann, J. Hirnforsch.* **5**:83–125.

Koppang, N., 1973–1974, Canine ceroid-lipofuscinosis—A model for human neuronal ceroid-lipofuscinosis and aging, *Mech. Ageing Dev.* **2**:421–445.

Larsen, B., Skinhoj, E., and Lassen, N. A., 1978, Variations in regional blood flow in the right and left hemispheres during automatic speech, *Brain* **101**:193–209.

Lassen, N. A., Larsen, B., and Orgogozo, J. M., 1978, Les localisations corticales vues par la gamma-caméra dynamique: Une nouvelle approche en neuropsychologie, *Encephale* **4**:233–249.

Leibnitz, L., and Wünscher, W., 1967, Die lebensgeschichtliche Ablagerung von intraneuronalem Lipofuscin in verschiedenen Abschnitten des menschlichen Gehirns, *Anat. Anz.* **121**:132–140.

Lopes, C. A. S., and Mair, W. G. P., 1974, Ultrastructure of the outer cortex and the pia mater in man, *Acta Neuropathol.* **28**:79–86.

Lund, J. S., 1973, Organization of neurons in the visual cortex, area 17, of the monkey *(Macaca mulatta), J. Comp. Neurol.* **147**:455–496.

Lund, J. S., and Boothe, R. G., 1975, Interlaminar connections and pyramidal neuron organization in the visual cortex, area 17, of the macaque monkey, *J. Comp. Neurol.* **159**:305–334.

Lund, J. S., Hendrickson, A. E., Ogren, M. P., and Tobin, E. A., 1981, Anatomical organization of primate visual cortex area VII, *J. Comp. Neurol.* **202**:19–45.

Mann, D. M. A., 1978, Granulovacuolar degeneration in pyramidal cells of the hippocampus, *Acta Neuropathol.* **42**:149–151.

Mann, D. M. A., and Yates, P. O., 1974, Lipoprotein pigments—Their relationship to ageing in the human nervous sytem. I. The lipofuscin content of nerve cells, *Brain* **97**:481–488.

Mann, D. M. A., and Yates, P. O., 1981, The relationship between formation of senile plaques and neurofibrillary tangles and changes in nerve cell metabolism in Alzheimer type dementia, *Mech. Ageing Dev.* **17**:395–401.

Mann, D. M. A., Yates, P. A., and Stamp, J. E., 1978, The relationship between lipofuscin pigment and ageing in the human nervous system, *J. Neurol. Sci.* **37**:83–93.

Mannen, H., 1955, La cytoarchitecture due système nerveux central humain regardée au point de vue de la distribution de grains de pigments jaunes contenant de la graisse, *Acta Anat. Nipp.* **30**:151–174.

Millhouse, O. E., 1981, The Golgi methods, in: *Neuroanatomical Tract-Tracing Methods* (L. Heimer and M. J. Robards, eds.), pp. 311–344, Plenum Press, New York.

Morimatsu, M., Hirai, S., Muramatsu, A., and Yoshikawa, M., 1975, Senile degenerative brain lesions and dementia, *J. Am. Geriatr. Soc.* **23**:390–406.

Myers, R. E., 1962, Commissural connections between occipital lobes of the monkey, *J. Comp. Neurol.* **118**:1–16.

Myers, R. E., 1965, Organization of visual pathways, in: *Functions of the Corpus Callosum* (E. G. Ettlinger, ed.), pp. 133–138, Churchill, London.

103

ARCHI-
TECTONICS
AS SEEN BY
LIPOFUSCIN
STAINS

Niessing, K., 1936, Über systemartige Zusammenhänge der Neuroglia im Großhirn und über ihre funktionelle Bedeutung, *Gegenbaurs Morphol. Jahrb.* **78**:537–584.

Obersteiner, H., 1903, Über das hellgelbe Pigment in den Nervenzellen und das Vorkommen weiterer fettähnlicher Körper im Centralnervensystem, *Arb. Neurol. Inst. Wien* **10**:245–274.

Obersteiner, H., 1904, Weitere Bemerkungen über die Fett-Pigment Körnchen im Centralnervensystem, *Arb. Neurol. Inst. Wien* **11**:400–406.

Palay, S. L., 1978, The Meynert cell, an unusual cortical pyramidal cell, in: *Architectonics of the Cerebral Cortex* (M.A.B. Brazier and H. Petsche, eds.), pp. 31–42, Raven Press, New York.

Palay, S. L., Sotelo, C., Peters, A., and Orkand, P. M., 1968, The axon hillock and the initial segment, *J. Cell Biol.* **38**:193–201.

Penfield, W., and Rasmussen, T., 1949, Vocalization and arrest of speech, *Arch. Neurol. Psychiatry* **61**:21–27.

Penfield, W., and Rasmussen, T., 1950, *The Cerebral Cortex of Man*, Macmillan Co., New York.

Penfield, W., and Roberts, C., 1959, *Speech and Brain—Mechanisms*, Princeton University Press, Princeton, N. J.

Perry, E. K., Blessed, G., Tomlinson, B. E., Perry, R. H., Crow, T. J., Cross, A. J., Dockray, G. J., Dimaline, R., and Arregui, A., 1981, Neurochemical activities in human temporal lobe related to aging and Alzheimer-type changes, *Neurobiol. Aging* **2**:251–256.

Peters, A., Proskauer, C. C., and Kaiserman-Abramof, I. R., 1968, The small pyramidal neuron of the rat cerebral cortex: The axon hillock and initial segment, *J. Cell Biol.* **39**:604–619.

Purpura, D. P., and Baker, H. J., 1978, Meganeurites and other aberrant processes of neurons in feline G_{M1}-gangliosidosis: A Golgi study, *Brain Res.* **143**:13–26.

Purpura, D. P., and Suzuki, K., 1976, Distortion of neuronal geometry and formation of aberrant synapses in neuronal storage diseases, *Brain Res.* **116**:1–21.

Purpura, D. P., Pappas, G. D., and Baker, H. J., 1978, Fine structure of meganeurites and secondary growth processes in feline G_{M1}-gangliosidosis, *Brain Res.* **143**:1–12.

Ramón y Cajal, S., 1909–1911, *Histologie du Système Nerveux de l'Homme et des Vertébrés* (translated by L. Azoulay), Maloine, Paris.

Ramsey, H. J., 1965, Fine structure of the surface of the cerebral cortex of human brain, *J. Cell Biol.* **26**:323–333.

Roland, P. E., and Larsen, B., 1976, Focal increase of cerebral blood flow during stereognostic testing in man, *Arch. Neurol.* **33**:551–558.

Roland, P., Larsen, B., Lassen, N. A., and Skinhoj, E., 1980a, Supplementary motor area and other cortical areas in organization of voluntary movements in man, *J. Neurophysiol.* **43**:118–136.

Roland, P. E., Skinhoj, E., Lassen, N. A., and Larsen, B., 1980b, Different cortical areas in man in organization of voluntary movements in extrapersonal space, *J. Neurophysiol.* **43**:137–150.

Rose, M., 1935, Cytoarchitektonik und Myeloarchitektonik der Großhirnrinde, in: *Handbuch der Neurologie*, Vol. 1 (O. Bumke and O. Förster, eds.), pp. 588–778, Springer, Berlin.

Sanides, F., 1970, Functional architecture of motor and sensory cortices in primates in the light of a new concept of neocortex evolution. in: *Advances in Primatology*, Vol. I (C. Noback and W. Montagna, eds.), pp. 137–208, Meredith, New York.

Sanides, F., 1972, Representation in the cerebral cortex and its areal lamination patterns, in: *Structure and Function of Nervous Tissue*, Vol. 1 (G. A. Bourne, ed.), pp. 329–453, Academic Press, New York.

Sanides, F., and Gräfin Vitzthum, H., 1965a, Zur Architektonik der menschlichen Sehrinde und den Prinzipien ihrer Entwicklung, *Dtsch. Z. Nervenheilkd.* **187**:680–707.

Sanides, F., and Gräfin Vitzthum, H., 1965b, Die Grenzerscheinungen am Rande der menschlichen Sehrinde, *Dtsch. Z. Nervenheilkd.* **187**:708–719.

Schierhorn, H., and Nagel, I., 1977, Qualitativer Vergleich der Impregnationsresultate verschiedener Golgi-Techniken: Untersuchungen am Neocortex adulter Albinoratten, *J. Hirnforsch.* **18**:345–356.

Schlegelberger, T., and Braak, H., 1982, The packing density of supragranular pigment-laden stellate cells in phylogenetically older and newer portions of the human telencephalic cortex, *J. Hirnforsch.* **23**:49–54.

Schlote, W., and Boellaard, J. W., 1983, The role of lipopigment during aging of nerve and glial cells in the human central nervous system, in: *Brain Ageing*, Vol. 21 (J. Cervos-Navarro and B. L. Strehler, eds.), pp. 27–74, Raven Press, New York.

Shkol'nik-Yarros, E. G., 1971, *Neurons and Interneuronal Connections of the Central Visual System*, Plenum Press, New York.

Shoumura, K., 1981, Further studies on the size specificity of commissural projecting neurons of layer III in areas 17, 18, 19 and the lateral suprasylvian area of the cat's visual cortex, *Arch. Histol. Jpn.* **44:**51–70.

Shoumura, K., Ando, T., and Kato, K., 1975, Structural organization of 'callosal' OBg in human callosum agenesis, *Brain Res.* **93:**241–252.

Talairach, J., and Bancaud, J., 1966, The supplementary motor area in man (anatomo-functional findings by stereo-electroencephalography in epilepsy), *Int. J. Neurol.* **5:**330–347.

Tomlinson, B. E., 1972, Morphological brain changes in non-demented old people, in: *Ageing of the Central Nervous System* (H. M. van Praag and A. F. Kalverboer, eds.), pp. 38–57, De Erven F. Bohn N. V. Uitgevers, Haarlem.

Tomlinson, B. E., 1977, The pathology of dementia, in: *Dementia* (C. Wells, ed.), pp. 113–153, Davis, Philadelphia.

Tomlinson, B. E., and Kitchener, D., 1972, Granulovacuolar degeneration of hippocampal pyramidal cells, *J. Pathol.* **106:**165–185.

Tomlinson, B. E., Blessed, G., and Roth, M., 1968, Observations on the brain of non-demented old people, *J. Neurol. Sci.* **7:**331–356.

Tomlinson, B. E., Blessed, G., and Roth, M., 1970, Observations on the brains of demented old people, *J. Neurol Sci.* **11:**205–242.

Valverde, F., 1970, The Golgi method: A tool for comparative structural analyses, in: *Contemporary Research Methods in Neuroanatomy* (W. J. H. Nauta and S. O. E. Ebbeson, eds.), pp. 11–31, Springer-Verlag, Berlin.

Valverde, F., 1977, Lamination of the striate cortex, *J. Neurocytol.* **6:**483–484.

Valverde, F., 1978, The organization of area 18 in the monkey: A Golgi study, *Anat. Embryol.* **154:**305–334.

Vogt, C., and Vogt, O., 1919, Allgemeinere Ergebnisse unserer Hirnforschung, *J. Psychol. Neurol.* **25:**279–461.

Vogt, C., and Vogt, O., 1942, Morphologische Gestaltungen unter normalen und pathogenen Bedingungen, *J. Psychol. Neurol.* **50:**161–524.

Vogt, M., 1929, Ober fokale Besonderheiten der Area occipitalis im cytoarchitektonischen Bilde, *J. Psychol. Neurol.* **39:**506–510.

von Economo, C., and Koskinas, G. N., 1925, *Die Cytoarchitektonik der Hirnrinde des erwachsenen Menschen*, Springer, Berlin.

Walkley, S. U., Baker, H. J., and Purpura, D. P., 1980, Morphological changes in feline G_{M1}-gangliosidosis: A Golgi study, in: *Animal Models in Neurological Disease* (F. C. Rose and P. O. Behan, eds.), pp. 419–429, Pitman Medical, London.

Walkley, S. U., Wurzelmann, S., and Purpura, D. P., 1981, Ultrastructure of neurites and meganeurites of cortical pyramidal neurons in feline gangliosidosis as revealed by the combined Golgi–EM technique, *Brain Res.* **211:**393–398.

West, C. D., 1979, A quantitative study of lipofuscin accumulation with age in normals and individuals with Down's syndrome, phenylketonuria, progeria and transneuronal atrophy, *J. Comp. Neurol.* **186:**109–116.

Williams, R. S., Lott, I. T., Ferrante, R. J., and Caviness, V. S., 1977, The cellular pathology of neuronal ceroid-lipofuscinosis, *Arch. Neurol.* **34:**298–305.

Woodard, J. S., 1962, Clinicopathological significance of granulovacuolar degeneration in Alzheimer's disease, *J. Neuropathol. Exp. Neurol.* **21:**85–91.

Yakovlev, P. J., and Lecours, A. R., 1967, The myelogenetic cycles of regional maturation of the brain, in: *Regional Development of the Brain in Early Life* (A. Minkowski, ed.), pp. 3–70, Blackwell, Oxford.

Zeki, S. M., 1970, Interhemispheric connections of prestriate cortex in monkey, *Brain Res.* **19:**63–75.

Zeman, W., 1971, The neuronal ceroid lipofuscinoses–Batten–Vogt syndrome: A model for human aging?, *Adv. Gerontol. Res.* **3:**147–170.

Zeman, W., 1976, The neuronal ceroid-lipofuscinoses, in: *Progress in Neuropathology*, Vol. III (H. M. Zimmerman, ed.), pp. 203–223, Grune & Stratton, New York.

II

Neurons

4

Classification of Cortical Neurons

ALAN PETERS and EDWARD G. JONES

1. Introduction

The purpose of this chapter is to give a general introduction to the topic of neuronal classification, and to serve as a background for the subsequent chapters in this section.

Over the years a number of attempts have been made to classify neurons of the cerebral cortex, but none of the classification schemes has gained wide acceptance. It is now generally agreed, however, that a broad morphological separation of cortical neurons into pyramidal and nonpyramidal types is acceptable, for there is relatively little controversy about which features distinguish pyramidal cells from the rest (Fig. 1). The main problem has been how to classify the cell types that are not pyramids, and what names to assign them. Though they are frequently referred to as *stellate cells* (Sholl, 1956), there is debate about whether this is the more appropriate name for them, or whether it would be better to call them *nonpyramidal cells*. The reason is that many of these neurons are not star-shaped. Consequently, there seems to be little reason to retain the term *stellate cell*, except perhaps for those particular neuronal types which have dendrites radiating out in all directions from their cell bodies.

ALAN PETERS • Department of Anatomy, Boston University School of Medicine, Boston, Massachusetts 02118. EDWARD G. JONES • James L. O'Leary Division of Experimental Neurology and Neurological Surgery and McDonnell Center for Studies of Higher Brain Function, Washington University School of Medicine, Saint Louis, Missouri 63110.

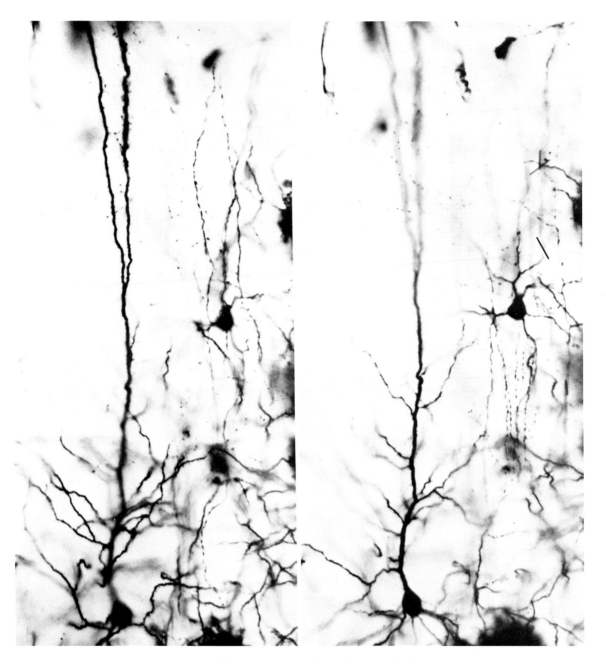

Figure 1. Two photographs, taken at different depths of focus, of Golgi-impregnated pyramidal and nonpyra- midal cells lying side by side in monkey somatic sensory cortex.

To examine the overall morphology of neurons, preparations impregnated by the Golgi technique are still most commonly used. This technique, first applied to the nervous system by Golgi (1873, 1882) and employed so effectively by Ramón y Cajal (1909–1911), has had a resurgence in recent years as investigators have become more interested in the detailed morphology of neurons. It is the technique that most readily shows the shapes and morphological characteristics of large numbers of cells. Consequently, it is the preferred technique for ascertaining how many varieties of neurons are present in a particular area of cerebral cortex, and the descriptions of neurons which are derived from studying Golgi-impregnated material serve as a point of reference to which information about neurons derived from other methods is referred. For example, when the electron microscope is used to define the cytological features of a neuron, the types of junctions made by its axon terminals, and the types of synapses made by axon terminals synapsing with its cell body and dendrites, this new information is incorporated into the basic corpus of knowledge derived from Golgi preparations of that neuronal system. Electron microscopic data add an entirely new dimension to the information available about a neuronal type, for on the basis of the kinds of synapses made by its axon terminals when they are visualized in thin sections, suggestions can be made about whether that particular type of neuron plays an excitatory or an inhibitory role. Such postulations need, of course, to be confirmed by physiological studies, although at present, little functional data of this type are available for the cerebral cortex. Nevertheless, information is accumulating about the receptive field properties of cortical neurons, and about how neurons in the sensory areas respond to stimuli presented peripherally (e.g., Martin and Whitteridge, 1982). It is now apparent that cortical neurons can be grouped into several functional classes (e.g., Hubel and Wiesel, 1977). Initially, it was not known which morphological types of neurons were to be included in these functional classes, but the correlation between function and morphological characteristics is now being made by some neurophysiologists. This is done by first recording from neurons and then injecting them with intracellular markers such as horseradish peroxidase (HRP) so that they can be visualized (e.g., Gilbert and Wiesel, 1979, 1981; Lin *et al.,* 1979). This technique, although practiced by only a few, has not only served to make important correlations between function and morphology, but has also allowed for better morphological descriptions of some neuronal types. This is because when compared to the image seen in Golgi preparations, more of the neuron, and especially its axonal plexus, is often visualized by intracellular staining. Further, since only a few, isolated neurons are filled, their processes can be followed from section to section to obtain more complete reconstructions than is normally possible from Golgi preparations. In addition, as will be discussed in a later section of this chapter, electron microscopy of individual neurons filled with HRP or chosen from specially prepared Golgi preparations (e.g., Fairén *et al.,* 1977), enables their synaptic connections with afferent inputs and with other neurons in their near vicinity to be identified and characterized. Such data are particularly important in determining synaptic differences among neurons.

HRP and various other axoplasmically transported markers have also had an impact on other aspects of neuronal classification. For example, following the retrograde transport of these markers, it has been possible, in a number of areas of the cerebral cortex, not only to show that pyramidal cells are the main or only source of efferent axons, but also to define the laminar distributions of pyramidal cells projecting to different sites (e.g., Jones, 1981). Further, by using retrograde labeling in combination with anterograde labeling or degeneration of another axon system, the afferent connections of a particular output cell can be examined electron microscopically (e.g., Hornung and Garey, 1980; Hendry and Jones, 1980; White and Hersch, 1981, 1982).

More recently, immunocytochemistry has been employed as a means of localizing some of the neurotransmitters and related substances contained within various populations of cortical neuronal types. In particular, the distribution of GABA and certain peptides has been examined (e.g., Ribak, 1978; Emson and Hunt, 1981). This technique is still in its infancy and the significance of some of the data is far from clear, but there are already indications that not only do some of the morphologically definable groups of neurons contain specific neurotransmitters, but that some of these morphologically defined types contain subpopulations with a different neurotransmitter. This is especially true in terms of the distribution of peptides.

Another approach to determining the neurotransmitters used by neurons is to employ autoradiography to ascertain which types of neurons accumulate various tritiated neurotransmitters (e.g., Chronwall and Wolff, 1980; Hendry and Jones, 1981). Some of the data obtained by this approach supplement the data obtained through the use of immunocytochemistry, but in other cases there is no alternative to using tritiated autoradiography, for antisera are not yet available to enzymes involved in the synthesis of many putative neurotransmitters in cortex, such as aspartate, glutamate, and glycine.

2. Golgi Preparations

In Golgi-impregnated material, neurons are traditionally examined in sections cut at a thickness of 100 to 150 μm, and in the vertical plane of orientation. This is at right angles to the pial surface, and generally neurons chosen for detailed examination are ones situated in the center of the section. In many cases, even this section thickness and the position of the neuron within the section is inadequate to allow all of the processes of a neuron to be seen in the single section, so that frequently a search has to be made in adjacent sections for those missing portions of processes that have been cut by the microtome.

2.1. Pyramidal Neurons

Pyramidal neurons are those which possess a dominant apical dendrite that passes from the cell body of the neuron to extend vertically, toward the pial surface (see Chapter 5). Typically, the cell body of a pyramidal neuron is conical and other dendrites, the basal ones, radiate out from the base of the cell body (Fig. 1). All of the dendrites of pyramidal cells bear spines, and although these spines may be absent from the proximal portions of the apical and basal dendrites, they cover the more distal portions of these primary dendrites, as well as the secondary and tertiary dendrites which are formed as the dendrites branch. The distribution of spines is not even, for their concentration reaches a maximum some 80 μm away from the cell body (Fig. 2) and then declines again distally. It is also characteristic for the axons of pyramidal cells to arise from the base of the cell body, or from one of the basal dendrites close to the cell body, and then to descend vertically toward the white matter, usually giving off horizontal or gently recurrent collaterals as they do so.

These features are characteristic of what we may call typical pyramidal neurons which are present in layer III and in layer V. The apical dendrites of these neurons ascend toward the pial surface, giving off a number of branches (sometimes at selective levels) as they pass through the overlying layers toward layer I, where they usually form a spray of terminal branches. Indeed, most of the dendrites contained within layer I are derived from pyramidal cells (see Chapter 14).

In addition to these typical pyramidal cells, however, there are other cells which are modified in form, but nonetheless are easily recognized as having pyramidal features. Among these modified pyramidal cells are those of layer II. The apical dendrites of these neurons are very short, divaricated, or even absent, so that the layer I terminal tuft arises directly from the apex of the soma, which

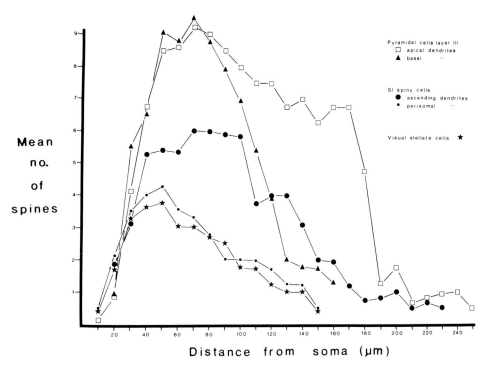

Figure 2. Numbers of spines per 10-μm segment of dendrite on spiny stellate cells of layer IV of monkey visual cortex compared with those on small layer III pyramidal cells and on the ascending and perisomal dendrites of "star pyramids" in layer IV of monkey somatic sensory cortex. From data illustrated in Jones (1975).

in every other way resembles that of a typical pyramid. Other obvious modified pyramidal cells are some of those in layer VI, which have apical dendrites that extend from one side of the cell body or arise from a basal dendrite and then bend to attain a vertical trajectory after they have passed laterally for some distance. The apical dendrites of these neurons may only reach as far as layer IV, and the ones ending there or in higher layers may or may not form a terminal tuft. It is not infrequent for the other dendrites of layer VI cells to be polarized to one side of the cell body, or for them to descend toward the white matter, giving the neurons a fusiform appearance (O'Leary, 1941). Further, some of the pyramidal neurons in layer VI may have thin apical dendrites, which bear only few spines and give off few branches as they ascend to other layers.

Another modified pyramidal neuron is frequently encountered in layer IV. These pyramidal neurons differ from the typical ones in having very thin apical dendrites as compared with the tapering and thicker apical dendrites with stout bases which extend from the pyramidal neurons with cell bodies in layer V and in layer III. Further, the cell bodies of these layer IV pyramids have rather oval shapes and instead of the other dendrites arising from the base of the cell body they radiate out in all directions. This radiation of the dendrites has resulted in these layer IV cells being termed *star pyramids* (Lorente de Nó, 1949), a name which reflects their similarity to both pyramidal cells and to the common spiny nonpyramidal cell of layer IV (see Chapter 7).

2.2. Nonpyramidal Neurons

The morphological features of typical and modified pyramidal neurons have been stressed because neurons described as being "nonpyramidal" in type are so-called because they lack the features of pyramidal cells (Fig. 1). They cannot be defined by the possession of features common to the group, so the definition is a negative one. They appear in all sizes and have a variety of dendritic field shapes, but none of them has a dominant, single, apical dendrite which is much longer than the other dendrites arising from the cell body. In addition, many nonpyramidal cells have no dendritic spines or, at least, many fewer dendritic spines than pyramidal cells; at least one variety, however, can have dendrites which bear almost as many spines as pyramidal cells.

Having decided that particular Golgi-impregnated neurons lack the features of pyramidal cells, the problem then arises about how to classify them. Whatever approach is decided upon, it is clearly necessary to examine many preparations of the particular cortical area and to use a number of variations of the Golgi technique to impregnate the material. It is only by making many preparations that one can be assured of seeing examples of all of the different kinds of nonpyramidal cells present, and of being able to collect enough examples of each kind to attempt a classification.

The basic approach to the classification of nonpyramidal cells is to first determine how many types show distinct and identifiable differences in terms of the shapes and sizes of their somata; the number, distribution, length, and branching patterns of their dendrites; the presence or absence of dendritic spines; and the form and distribution patterns of the axonal ramifications (Jones, in distinguishing one type from another, and to accept a greater or lesser degree of variability within a particular type. Feldman and Peters (1978) suggested that at least a preliminary classification can be made on the basis of the distribution patterns of the dendrites and the frequency with which spines arise from the dendrites. Thus, on the basis of the forms of their dendritic trees, neurons can be classified as being multipolar, bitufted, or bipolar. The dendrites of multipolar neurons arise from any part of the surface of the cell body, so that they have no preferred site of origin, and they radiate out in all directions. Bitufted cells, on the other hand, have dendrites extending from two opposite poles of the soma, which are usually ovoid or spindle-shaped. When the long axis of the cell body is oriented vertically, the dendrites form ascending and descending tufts, and when the cell body has the long axis oriented parallel to the pial surface, the dendrites extend horizontally. In contrast to bitufted cells, bipolar neurons have single dendrites extending from the opposite poles of the soma to give rise to elongated, and markedly narrow, dendritic trees.

In addition to the form of the dendritic tree, the abundance of dendritic spines can be specified. Thus, neurons can be further classified as being spinous (spiny), sparsely spinous, or smooth (spine-free). Spinous neurons have dendrites with a density of spines approaching or even matching that of most pyramidal cells. At the other extreme are those neurons with smooth dendrites, from which protruding spines are extremely uncommon, but rarely completely absent. Intermediate between these two extremes are the sparsely spinous neurons, and this category contains neurons with a wide range of spine densities. It is important to note, however, that the spine densities on the dendrites of many of these nonpyramidal neurons can be relatively high in infant animals, and can decline with age.

Using the criteria of dendritic patterns and spine densities, it is possible to effect a basic classification of nonpyramidal cells in rat visual cortex (Feldman and Peters, 1978) and in rat cingulate cortex (Vogt and Peters, 1981). The approach has also been useful for classifying cells in cat visual cortex (Peters and Regidor, 1981), but in this cortex, as well as the cortex of the monkey (Valverde, 1971; Lund, 1973; Jones, 1975), other criteria, such as cell size, dendritic length, and, in particular, axonal characteristics, have to be added to achieve a comprehensive classification. One reason for this is that cells with totally different axonal ramifications can have very similar dendritic fields. Another is that in primates, the number of different kinds of nonpyramidal cells in the cortex seems to increase, and many are best recognized by the characteristics of their axonal distribution patterns and the forms of the terminals of the axonal plexus.

Exactly how many different morphological types of nonpyramidal cells can be distinguished as clear-cut entities, reproducible from study to study, is not clear. The obvious reasons why this information is not available are the following. First, there are few thorough Golgi studies of neurons in specific areas of the cerebral cortex of single species. Second, it is often difficult to correlate the descriptions of nonpyramidal neurons presented by different authors expecially when only some of the morphological criteria mentioned above have been used. Third, it is not possible to ascertain if all of the nonpyramidal cell types present have been encountered in any given study. Nevertheless, it is apparent that a number of readily recognizable nonpyramidal cell types do exist, and these particular cell types are the subjects of the following chapters.

Spiny stellate cells (Chapter 7) are characteristic of layer IV in a number of species. They are usually multipolar neurons, and the density of spines extending from their dendrites can approach that of the pyramidal cells. These are the only truly spiny nonpyramidal cells in the cerebral cortex. Their major axonal system is an ascending one.

There are many varieties of smooth and sparsely spinous multipolar nonpyramidal cells. One of them is the *basket cell* (Chapter 8), so-called because of the participation of the axon in the formation of weaves of preterminal axons that surround the cell bodies of pyramidal cells and form axosomatic synapses with them. The basket cells of layers III–VI are the largest nonpyramidal neurons. They have long, smooth or sparsely spinous dendrites, and this contrasts with many of the smooth or sparsely spinous multipolar cells with axons that form a variety of plexuses and have at least part of the axonal plexus overlapping the dendritic tree in distribution. These *local plexus neurons* (Chapter 13) have not been well classified and may consist of several types. One type of local plexus neuron, the *neurogliaform cell* (Chapter 12), is quite distinct, however, for it has rather short dendrites and an extensive local axonal plexus resembling a branching thread that interweaves with the thin dendrites. The other local plexus neurons have less rich axonal plexuses.

Chandelier cells (Chapter 10) are also often multipolar and have sparsely spinous dendrites, but some of them are bitufted. Consequently, these neurons are difficult to distinguish from other types on the basis of their dendritic features. Fortunately, these cells have very distinctive axonal plexuses, in which the axons end in short vertical strings of boutons which are readily recognized in Golgi preparations.

Bipolar cells (Chapter 11) are also distinctive since, as pointed out, they typically have single dendrites extending from each end of the cell body, to form a vertically oriented and narrow dendritic tree. This dendritic tree is much narrower than that of *double bouquet cells* (Chapter 9), for as the name *double bouquet* implies, these are often bitufted neurons, but the most distinguishing feature of double bouquet cells is their vertically oriented arrays of axonal branches.

All of these specific types of nonpyramidal cells are present in layers II through V of the neocortical areas of the cerebral cortex (see Chapter 6). Layers I and VI contain rather different types of nonpyramidal cells, many of which have horizontally oriented dendrites. Consequently, the neurons in these layers are considered in separate chapters (Chapters 14 and 15). One reason why the neurons in layers I and VI are somewhat different from those present in the intervening layers is suggested by Marin-Padilla (1971, 1978). Marin-Padilla (1971, 1978) shows that the wall of the embryonic cerebral vesicle contains a layer of primitive neurons, and calls it the *primordial plexiform layer*. He suggests that during development, this layer becomes split by the formation of the cortical plate, so that in the mature neocortex, layer I and lower layer VI are the derivatives of the primordial plexiform layer, and the intervening layers the derivatives of the more newly formed cortical plate.

Electron microscopy has led to a better understanding of neuronal structure (e.g., Peters *et al.*, 1976). Among other things, it has helped us to appreciate the nature of the organelles that are contained within the cell bodies of neurons of the cerebral cortex. It has shown the cytological differences between axons and dendrites, and has revealed the nature of dendritic spines. But perhaps the greatest contribution of electron microscopy has been in the elucidation of the form of synapses in the cortex and the distribution of synapses over the surfaces of different types of cortical neurons.

In the cerebral cortex the most commonly encountered types of synapses are chemical ones that use neurotransmitters. Other types of synapses, the so-called electrical synapses, at which the plasma membranes of the pre- and post-synaptic elements come together to form gap junctions, have only been very infrequently described in the cerebral cortex (Peters, 1980). Consequently, it is not known whether they play a significant role in the functioning of the cerebral cortex.

With few exceptions (e.g., Sloper, 1982; Sloper and Powell, 1978), in the cerebral cortex the presynaptic components of the conventional chemical synapses are axon terminals, which are recognized in electron microscopic preparation by their content of lucent synaptic vesicles among which may be a few dense core vesicles. The postsynaptic element can be a dendrite, dendritic spine, neuronal soma, or axon initial segment but never, apparently, another axon terminal. Two types of chemical synapses (Figs. 3 and 4) can be recognized on the basis of their morphology, as first shown by Gray (1959). Some of the synapses are described as being asymmetric (Colonnier, 1968) or type I (Gray, 1959) synapses, which have a rather wide cleft of about 80 μm between the pre- and postsynaptic membranes. This cleft is bisected by a layer of dense material, and there are other accumulations of dense material on the cytoplasmic faces of the pre- and postsynaptic membranes. Of these, the accumulation beneath the postsynaptic membrane is the most prominent and this is what leads to such synapses being called asymmetric, although the difference between the amount of dense material associated with the pre- and postsynaptic membranes depends somewhat on the nature of the postsynaptic component. Thus, synapses involving dendritic spines display the greatest amount of postsynaptic dense material, while asymmetric synapses involving dendritic shafts and neuronal somata have less of a postsynaptic density associated with them and, consequently, a less obvious asymmetry. A second important feature of asymmetric synapses is that the synaptic vesicles in the presynaptic profile are usually spherical in aldehyde-fixed material.

The other chemical synapses are described as being symmetric or type 2 synapses. In comparison with the asymmetric synapses (see Figs. 3 and 4), the symmetric ones have a narrower synaptic cleft in which a bisecting layer of dense material is less obvious. In addition, the synaptic junction often has the pre- and postsynaptic dense material confined to patches against which the synaptic vesicles cluster, and the postsynaptic dense material is not obviously more prominent

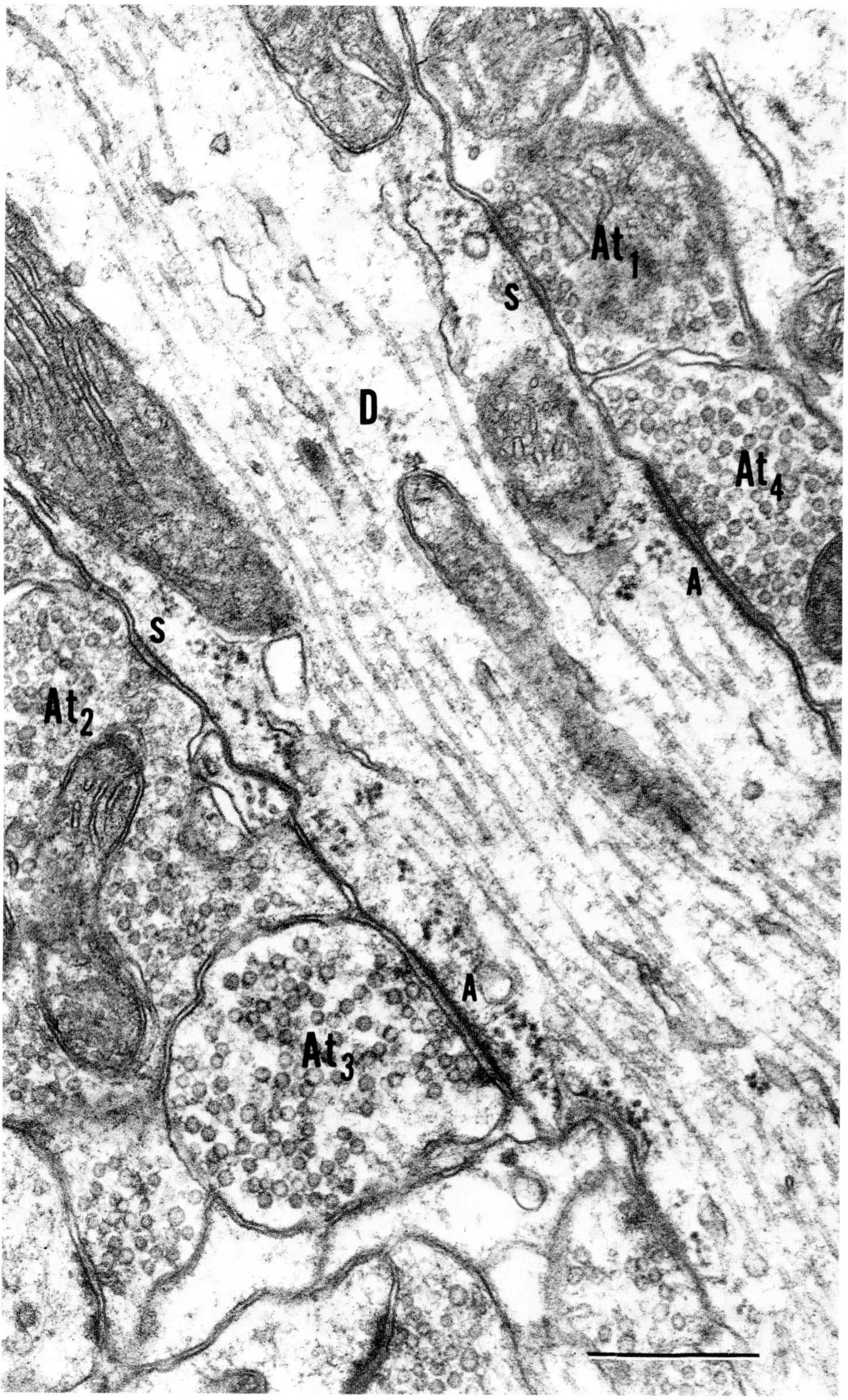
At1
S
D
At4
A
S
At2
A
At3

than the presynpatic material, so that the synaptic junction is symmetric in appearance. Another feature of symmetric synapses is that after fixation of cortical tissue by aldehydes, some of the synaptic vesicles in the presynaptic element may become elongated or ellipsoidal, and even the ones which remain spherical are smaller than those contained within axon terminals forming asymmetric synapses (Figs. 3 and 4).

As will become apparent in later chapters, there is accumulating evidence that in the cerebral cortex, asymmetric synapses have an excitatory function, while symmetric synapses are inhibitory. It is also important to mention that as far as can be determined, all of the synapses formed by the axon terminals of a given neuron are of the same morphological type.

This latter information, as well as the data about how asymmetric and symmetric synapses are distributed over the surfaces of neurons can be obtained by first determining the morphology of a neuron in the light microscope and then studying that same neuron in the electron microscope. Nowadays this usually means that the neurons are filled with a substance that allows its cell body and processes to be visualized in both the light and electron microscopes. There are two means of achieving this end. One is to fill the neuron intracellularly with a marker such as HRP that can then be reacted to produce an electron-dense deposit within the cell. The second is to impregnate the neuron with the Golgi technique, so that it becomes filled with silver chromate. However, there are difficulties in examining Golgi-impreganted neurons directly in the electron microscope for the silver chromate deposit produced by the Golgi reaction is so dense that it masks the cytological features of the neuron to be examined. A number of attempts have been made to alleviate this problem (see Blackstad, 1982), and one solution is to substitute gold for the silver chromate deposit (e.g., Fairén *et al.*, 1977). Of these two combined light and electron microscopic approaches, the intracellular filling of cortical neurons has hardly been used, and there are few electron microscope studies of Golgi-impregnated neurons, so that these techniques are still in their infancy. Nevertheless, results of the studies that have been published, coupled with the numerous studies of cortical tissue prepared for conventional electron microscopy, enable some conclusions to be drawn.

One conclusion is that pyramidal neurons receive only symmetric synapses on their cell bodies, while their dendritic shafts receive both symmetric and asymmetric synapses; symmetric axodendritic synapses are most common on the surfaces of proximal dendrites (Chapter 5). It is also evident that the spines projecting from the dendrites of pyramidal cells probably all receive at least one asymmetric synapse, though, in addition, some may receive a symmetric synapse. The terminals of the axons of pyramidal neurons both in and outside the cortex all form asymmetric synapses.

These same synaptic features also seem to be possessed by the spiny non-

←

Figure 3. The dendrite (D) of a smooth nonpyramidal cell is forming symmetric synaptic junction(s) with two axon terminals (At$_1$ and At$_2$), and asymmetric synaptic junctions (A) with two other axon terminals (At$_3$ and At$_4$). Note the round vesicles in the axon terminals forming asymmetric synapses and the smaller elongated vesicles in the axon terminals forming the symmetric synapses. Rat visual cortex. The scale marker equals 0.5 μm.

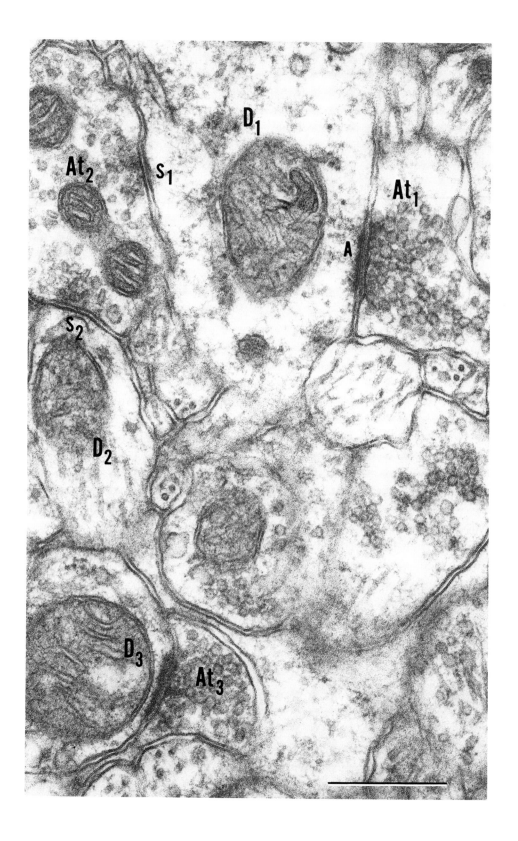

pyramidal cells, but the other types of nonpyramidal cells so far examined by combined light and electron microscope techniques are different, for they all receive both symmetric and asymmetric axosomatic synapses. This largely confirms the earlier conclusion, based on examining cortical tissue prepared conventionally for electron microscopy, that the cell bodies of pyramidal and nonpyramidal cells can be distinguished from each other on the basis of the types of synapses they form, the pyramidal cells having only asymmetric axosomatic synapses and the nonpyramidal cells having both symmetric and asymmetric axosomatic synapses. Although the spiny stellate cell seems to be the only exception to this generalization, as more neuronal types are examined, other exceptions may emerge.

No generalizations can be made about differences between pyramidal and nonpyramidal neurons on the basis of the types of synapses formed by their axons. The axons of pyramidal cells form asymmetric synapses (e.g., Winfield *et al.*, 1981), but synapses of this same type are also formed by the axons of at least the spiny stellate cells and of some bipolar cells (Peters and Kimerer, 1981); yet others may be discovered as further cell types are examined. It is assumed on this basis that the pyramidal cells, the spiny stellate cells, and some of the bipolar cells are excitatory neurons, though there is only confirmatory physiological evidence for the pyramidal cell (e.g., Phillips, 1959). The remainder of the nonpyramidal cells examined, namely the chandelier cells (Somogyi, 1977; Fairén and Valverde, 1980; Peters *et al.*, 1982), the neurons with local plexus axons (LeVay, 1973; Peters and Fairén, 1978; Peters and Proskauer, 1980), and the double bouquet cells (Somogyi and Cowey, 1981), all have axons forming symmetric synapses, suggesting that they may be inhibitory neurons.

The studies that produce this kind of information, in which a neuron is first identified in the light microscope and then examined ultrastructurally to determine its synaptology, are only just beginning. Few neuronal types have been examined, and none of these, with the possible exception of the chandelier cells, has been studied extensively enough to assess exactly where the axon terminals of the specific type of neuron make their synapses. Consequently, our information about the synaptic relationships between specific types of neurons is, to say the least, fragmentary, and because of the limited numbers of each type examined, the range of variability is unknown.

Even less is known about the neurotransmitters used by the various kinds of pyramidal and nonpyramidal cells. Nevertheless, we can be optimistic that it is only a matter of time before this information becomes available from immunocytochemical studies. The technology to derive this information is, or is becoming, available and new antisera are being continuously developed.

Ultimately, these various approaches will mean that not only will we be able to classify neurons on the basis of their morphology, but also on the basis of their physiological responses to various stimuli, their projections to other struc-

$\leftarrow$

Figure 4. A dendrite (D$_1$) is forming an asymmetric synapse (A) with one axon terminal (At$_1$) and a symmetric synapse (S$_1$) with a second axon terminal (At$_2$), which is also synapsing (S$_2$) with another dendrite (D$_2$). At the bottom of the field is an axon terminal (At$_3$) forming an asymmetric synapse with a third dendrite (D$_3$). Monkey visual cortex. The scale marker equals 0.5 μm.

tures in the central nervous system, their connections to other cortical neurons, and their transmitter characteristics. At present, we are far from the goal of having all of these data available about even one neuronal type, and it is not clear that functional differences will always be reflected in morphological differences or vice versa. But clearly, the techniques are available, and as the information accumulates, it will lead to a better understanding of how the various areas of the cortex process information.

4. References

Blackstad, T. W., 1982, Tract tracing by electron microscopy of Golgi preparations, in: *Neuroanatomical Tract Tracing Methods* (L. Heimer and M. J. RoBards, eds.), pp. 407–440, Plenum Press, New York.

Chronwall, B. M., and Wolff, J. B., 1980, Prenatal and postnatal development of GABA-accumulating cells in the occipital neocortex of the rat, *J. Comp. Neurol.* **190:**187–208.

Colonnier, M., 1968, Synaptic patterns on different cell types in the different laminae of the cat visual cortex: An electron microscope study, *Brain Res.* **9:**268–287.

Emson, P. C., and Hunt, S. P., 1981, Anatomical chemistry of the cerebral cortex, in: *The Organization of the Cerebral Cortex* (F. O. Schmitt, F. G. Worden, G. Adelman, and S. G. Dennis, eds.), pp. 325–346, MIT Press, Cambridge, Mass.

Fairén, A., and Valverde, F., 1980, A specialized type of neuron in the visual cortex of cat: A Golgi and electron microscope study of chandelier cells, *J. Comp. Neurol.* **194:**761–780.

Fairén, A., Peters, A., and Saldanha, J., 1977, A new procedure for examining Golgi impregnated neurons by light and electron microscopy, *J. Neurocytol.* **6:**311–337.

Feldman, M., and Peters, A., 1978, The forms of non-pyramidal neurons in the visual cortex of the rat, *J. Comp. Neurol.* **179:**761–794.

Gilbert, C. D., and Wiesel, T. N., 1979, Morphology and intracortical projections of functionally characterised neurones in the cat visual cortex, *Nature (London)* **280:**120–125.

Gilbert, C. D., and Wiesel, T. N., 1981, Laminar specialization and intracortical projections in cat primary visual cortex, in: *The Cerebral Cortex* (F. O. Schmitt, F. G. Worden, G. Adelman, and S. G. Dennis, eds.), MIT Press, Cambridge, Mass.

Golgi, C., 1873, Sulla stuttura della sostanzagrigia del cervello, *Gaz. Med. Ital. Lombardia* **6:**244–246.

Golgi, C., 1882, Sulla fina anatomia degli organi centrali del sistema nervoso. 1. Note preliminari sulla struttura morfolgia e vicenderoli rapporta delle cellule gangliari, *Riv. Sper. Freniat R. Med. Leg. Alienazioni Ment.* **8:**165–195.

Gray, E. G., 1959, Axo-somatic and axo-dentritic synapses in the cerebral cortex: An electron microscopic study, *J. Anat.* **93:**420–433.

Hendry, S. H. C., and Jones, E. G., 1980, Electron microscopic demonstration of thalamic axon terminations on identified commissural neurons in monkey somatic sensory cortex, *Brain Res.* **196:**253–257.

Hendry, S. H. C. and Jones, E. G., 1981, Sizes and distributions of intrinsic neurons incorporating tritiated GABA in monkey sensory-motor cortex, *J. Neurosci.* **1:**390–408.

Hornung, J. P., and Garey, L. J., 1980, A direct pathway from thalamus to visual callosal neurons in cat, *Exp. Brain Res.* **38:**121–123.

Hubel, D. H., and Wiesel, T. N., 1977, Functional architecture of macaque monkey visual cortex, *Proc. R. Soc. London Ser. B.* **198:**1–59.

Jones, E. G., 1975, Varieties and distribution of non-pyramidal cells in the somatic sensory cortex of the squirrel monkey, *J. Comp. Neurol.* **160:**205–268.

Jones, E. G., 1981, Anatomy of cerebral cortex: Columnar input–output relations, in: *The Cerebral Cortex* (F. O. Schmitt, F. G. Worden, G. Adelman, and S. G. Dennis, eds.), pp. 199–235, MIT Press, Cambridge, Mass.

LeVay, S., 1973, Synaptic patterns in the visual cortex of the cat and monkey: Electron microscopy of Golgi preparations, *J. Comp. Neurol.* **150:**53–86.

Lin, C.-S., Friedlander, M. J., and Sherman, S. M., 1979, Morphology of physiologically identified neurons in the visual cortex of the cat, *Brain Res.* **172**:344–348.

Lorente de Noó, R., 1949, Cerebral cortex: Architecture, intracortical connections, motor projections, in: *Physiology of the Nervous System* (J. F. Fulton, ed.), 3rd ed., pp. 288–313, Oxford University Press, London.

Lund, J. S., 1973, Organization of neurons in the visual cortex, area 17, of the monkey *(Macaca mulatta)*, *J. Comp. Neurol.* **147**:455–496.

Marin-Padilla, M., 1971, Early prenatal ontogenesis of the cerebral cortex (neocortex) of the cat *(Felis domestica)*: A Golgi study, *Z. Anat. Entwicklungsgesch.* **134**:117–145.

Marin-Padilla, M., 1978, Dual origin of the mammalian neocortex and evolution of the cortical plate, *Anat. Embryol.* **152**:100–126.

Martin, A. E., and Whitteridge, D., 1982, The morphology, function and intracortical projections of neurones in area 17 of the cat which receive monosynaptic input from the lateral geniculate nucleus (LGN), *J. Physiol. (London)* **328**:37–38P.

O'Leary, J. L., 1941, Structure of the area striata of the cat, *J. Comp. Neurol.* **75**:131–164.

Peters, A., 1980, Morphological correlates of epilepsy: Cells in the cerebral cortex, in: *Antiepileptic Drugs: Mechanisms of Action* (G. H. Glaser, J. K. Penny, and D. M. Woodbury, eds.), pp. 21–48, Raven Press, New York.

Peters, A., and Fairén, A., 1978, Smooth and sparsely-spined stellate cells in the visual cortex of the rat: A study using a combined Golgi–electron microscope technique, *J. Comp. Neurol.* **181**:129–172.

Peters, A., and Kimerer, L. M., 1981, Bipolar neurons in rat visual cortex: A combined Golgi–electron microscope study, *J. Neurocytol.* **10**:921–946.

Peters, A., and Proskauer, C. C., 1980, Smooth or sparsely spined cells with myelinated axons in rat visual cortex, *Neuroscience* **5**:2079–2092.

Peters, A., Palay, S.L., Webster, H. D., 1976, *The Fine Structure of the Nervous System: The Neurons and Supporting Cells*, Saunders. New York.

Peters, A., and Regidor, J., 1981, A reassessment of the forms of nonpyramidal neurons in area 17 of cat visual cortex, *J. Comp. Neurol.* **203**:685–716.

Peters, A., Proskauer, C. C., and Ribak, C. E., 1982, Chandelier cells in rat visual cortex, *J. Comp. Neurol.* **206**:397–416.

Phillips, C. G., 1959, Actions of antidromic pyramidal volleys on single Betz cells in the cat, *Q. J. Exp. Physiol.* **44**:1–25.

Ramón y Cajal, S., 1909–1911, *Histologie du Système Nerveux de l'Homme et des Vertébrés* (translated by L. Azoulay), Vol. II, Maloine, Paris.

Ribak, C. E., 1978, Aspinous and sparsely-spinous stellate neurons in the visual cortex of rats contain glutamic acid decarboxylase, *J. Neurocytol.* **7**:461–478.

Sholl, D. A., 1956, *The Organization of the Cerebral Cortex*, Mathews, London.

Sloper, J. J., 1972, Gap junctions between dendrites in the primate neocortex, *Brain Res.* **44**:641–646.

Sloper, J. J., and Powell, T. P. S., 1978, Gap junctions between dendrites and somata of neurons in the primate sensori-motor cortex, *Proc. R. Soc. London Ser. B.* **203**:39–47.

Somogyi, P., 1977, A specific axo-axonal interneuron in the visual cortex of the rat, *Brain Res.* **136**:345–350.

Somogyi, P., and Cowey, A., 1981, Combined Golgi and electron microscopic study on the synapses formed by double bouquet cells in the visual cortex of the cat and monkey, *J. Comp. Neurol.* **195**:547–566.

Valverde, F., 1971, Short axon neuronal subsystems in the visual cortex of the monkey, *Int. J. Neurosci.* **1**:181–197.

Vogt, B. A., and Peters, A., 1981, Form and distribution of neurons in rat cingulate cortex: Areas 32, 24 and 29, *J. Comp. Neurol.* **195**:603–625.

White, E. L., and Hersch, S. M., 1981, Thalamocortical synapses of pyramidal cells which project from SmI to MsI cortex in the mouse, *J. Comp. Neurol.* **198**:167–181.

White, E. L., and Hersch, S. M., 1982, A quantitative study of thalamocortical and other synapses involving the apical dendrites of corticothalamic projection cells in mouse SmI cortex, *J. Neurocytol.* **11**:137–157.

Winfield, D. A., Brooke, R. N. L., Sloper, J. J., and Powell, T. P. S., 1981, A combined Golgi–electron microscopic study of the synapses made by the proximal axon and recurrent collaterals of a pyramidal cell in the somatic sensory cortex of the monkey, *Neuroscience* **6**:1217–1230.

5

Morphology of the Neocortical Pyramidal Neuron

MARTIN L. FELDMAN

1. Introduction

It is now well over 100 years since the appearance of the earliest accounts and illustrations of specific cell types in the cerebral cortex. The observations which derive from this early period emphasized the pyramidal neuron, although in later years, and particularly recently, the study of nonpyramidal cells came to occupy an increasingly important place in cortical research. In retrospect, the reasons for the historical emphasis on pyramidal cells are easy to discern. They include the relatively large sizes of the cells, their abundance and ubiquity in the cortex, and their striking form and arrangements. Historically, then, the pyramidal neuron came to be considered the principal cell of the cortex, in much the same loose way that the Purkinje cell came to be thought of as the principal cell of the cerebellum. That this emphasis was well founded is indicated by the fact that we can now define cerebral cortex in histological terms by its complement of pyramidal cells, in addition to its laminar arrangement. Further, recent quantitative work has made it clear that the pyramidal neurons are indeed the numerically dominant cell type of the neocortex (Polyakov, 1956; Braitenberg, 1978; Sloper *et al.*, 1979; Winfield *et al.*, 1980). That they may be overwhelmingly

MARTIN L. FELDMAN • Department of Anatomy, Boston University School of Medicine, Boston, Massachusetts 02118.

so is suggested by the probability that the quantitative studies have classified as pyramidal only the more obvious, or typical, cases of pyramidal neurons.

The present chapter provides an overview of the major morphological aspects of the neocortical pyramidal cell. Critical historical landmarks in the development of our knowledge of the pyramidal cell are reviewed. The development of pyramidal cells and their characteristic morphological features are discussed and the kinds of variations that occur in cell form are indicated. Principal emphasis throughout is placed upon light microscopic observations, although these are frequently supplemented by ultrastructural data when available and directly relevant.

It is the aim of this presentation to furnish a broad background for understanding the general morphological status of the pyramidal cell as a cortical element and for interpreting the many highly detailed studies which have been carried out on this cell type. The treatment leaves to a study of the primary literature the task of exhaustive documentation of such things as specific cell variants and regional and species differences, although an indication of the range of available information in such areas is given.

Finally, a word needs to be said concerning the definition of a pyramidal neuron. Customary practice would suggest that the term ought to designate those elements to which it was first applied. However, the case of the pyramidal cell is one in which original usage of the term *pyramidal* differs from present usage. With the histological techniques available in the early period of cortical investigation, little else beyond the outline of the cell body could be seen with any clarity. The term, then, as first applied, designated cell bodies with a pyramid-shaped profile. The later analysis of these cells using the Golgi methods, which revealed the neuronal processes emanating from the cell bodies, made it clear that the earlier category of "pyramidal" cells really included cells of more than one fundamental "type." Thus, there occurred a gradual shift in the meaning of the term. Out of the growing number of Golgi analyses, many classification schemes evolved to demarcate pyramidal from nonpyramidal cells. Perikaryal size and geometry, dendritic arborization pattern, spine density, and axonal trajectory all have served as differentiating criteria in these schemes. While there did develop universal agreement concerning the pyramidal or nonpyramidal nature of certain "classical" cell forms (Globus and Scheibel, 1967a; Colonnier, 1968; Jones and Powell, 1970; Peters, 1971), many neurons were shown to exist which presented difficulties for one or another of most of the proposed criteria. One thinks in this regard of cells such as nonpyramidal cells which are larger than most pyramidal cells, or of nonpyramidal cells whose axons project into the white matter, or of so-called spiny stellate cells. However, of all the differentiating criteria which have been used, one, the existence of an apical dendrite, has managed to survive serious objection, and this criterion appears to be sufficient to unequivocally separate the two major classes of cortical neurons. Accordingly, pyramidal cells may be defined as those cortical neurons which possess an apical dendrite (Figs. 1–6). It is, of course, to be hoped that continued work along modern lines will establish the existence of additional definitive criteria. One potential such criterion, the extent and nature of the axosomatic synaptic ensemble, appears particularly promising in this respect, and further advances in fields such as neurochemistry may be anticipated.

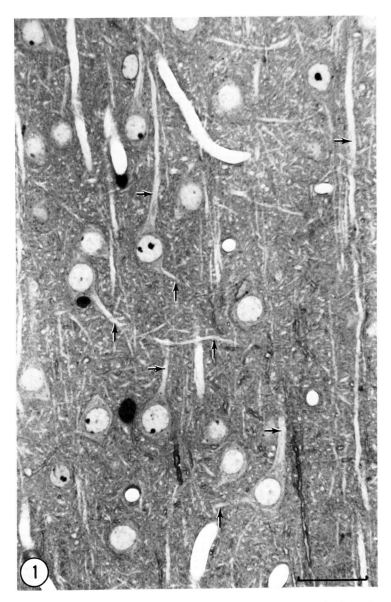

Figure 1. Pyramidal neurons in layers II/III of rat visual cortex, 1-μm plastic section oriented approximately parallel to the apical dendrites (horizontal arrows). Basal dendrites are indicated by vertical arrows. Calibration line, 25 μm.

2. Historical Perspective

In the era before the advent of electron microscopy, unquestionably the most dramatic advances in our knowledge of pyramidal cell morphology came with the application of the impregnation method discovered by Golgi near the end of the last century. Prior to that development, inadequacies of histological

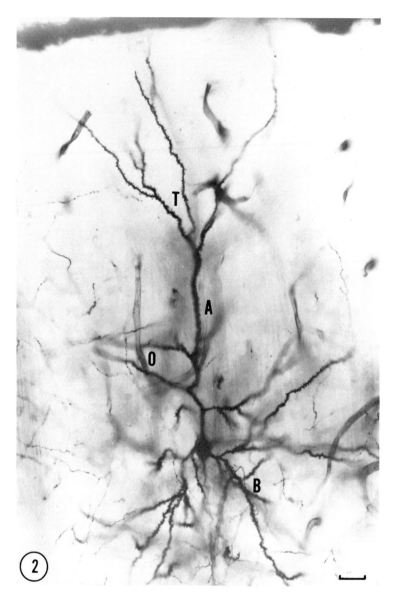

Figure 2. Layer II/III pyramidal neuron in rat area 39 (Krieg, 1946), Golgi rapid preparation. A, apical dendrite; B, basal dendrites; O, oblique branch dendrites; T, terminal tuft. Calibration line, 25 μm.

technique did not allow a clear appreciation of pyramidal cell form to emerge. Nevertheless, to that pre-Golgi period belong the first definite observations and descriptions of pyramidal cells, or at least of their cell bodies. Examples of historically relevant illustrations of pyramidal cells are given in Chapters 1 and 2 of this volume.

Among the early observations of what seem obviously to be neocortical pyramidal cell bodies are the sketches produced by von Kölliker, which appeared

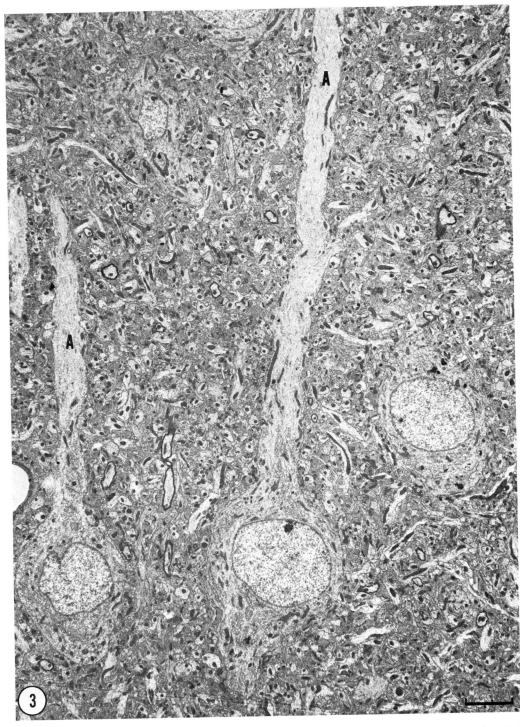

Figure 3. Pyramidal neurons in rat visual cortex as visualized in a thin section oriented parallel to the apical dendrites (A). Calibration line, 5 μm.

in his textbook of human histology published in the middle of the last century (Kölliker, 1850–1854), and which were followed shortly by similar observations by Berlin (1858). It was probably Berlin who used the term *pyramidal* for the first time.

There then followed the important work of Meynert, who described the distribution of various types of pyramidal cell bodies (Meynert, 1867). While much of Meynert's emphasis, following Baillarger, was on cortical lamination patterns, this was firmly grounded in cytological considerations. He thus developed a rather clear understanding of the differential distribution of pyramidal cells of various sizes, noting, for example, the occurrence of giant cells in his fourth and sixth layers of the eight-layered cortex of the occipital lobe, and their absence in the five-layered cortex of the hippocampus. In the light of later knowledge, it is probable that many of the large fourth-layer cells in Meynert's carmine-stained preparations were actually nonpyramidal cells. The distinction was to be clarified by Ramón y Cajal, leaving only the giant layer V pyramids as the true solitary cells of Meynert.

Examining Meynert's illustrations of pyramidal cells, little detail is seen beyond somal size and shape. No detail is seen in the perikaryal cytoplasm and the nuclei are typically, and inaccurately, drawn with angular contours that parallel the triangular sides of the cell body surface. But established once and for all was the principle of regional and laminar specificity of at least some pyramidal cells, most notably the large cells now bearing his name.

The second major contribution to the principle of specificity was the discovery by Betz (1874) of the large pyramidal cells which he localized in the precentral gyrus. These he described as giant cells—"Riesenpyramiden"—occurring in nests of two, three, or more cells, and being present in man, chimpanzee and other primates, and dog. He also provided quantitative descriptions of somal size, number of dendrites, and internest separations, to which he added the intriguing observation that the cells are more numerous and apparently larger on the right side of the brain. By reference to the physiological findings which had recently been reported by Fritsche and Hitzig, Betz correctly deduced the motor function of these cells.

Further advances in the study of pyramidal cells were, in many cases, linked to developments in tissue preparation and staining that went beyond the Gerlach carmine technique used by the majority of early workers. Lewis, for example, described the use of osmium tetroxide followed by the dye aniline black, and the use of the ether freezing microtome for the study of fresh cortical tissue. From material thus prepared, Lewis published numerous drawings of pyramidal cells (Lewis and Clarke, 1878; Lewis, 1879, 1881; see Chapter 2). In these, the shapes of the cells are clear and the origins of the apical and the basal dendrites

Figure 4. Pyramidal neurons in rat visual cortex, Golgi rapid impregnation. The impregnated cell bodies at the bottom of the figure are layer V pyramidal neurons whose long apical dendrites (A) ascend toward the pial surface (P). Between the layer V neurons and the pial surface is a horizontal stratum containing numerous layer II/III pyramidal neurons. The terminal tufts of both sets of neurons form a dense dendritic mat in layer I. Calibration line, 50 μm.

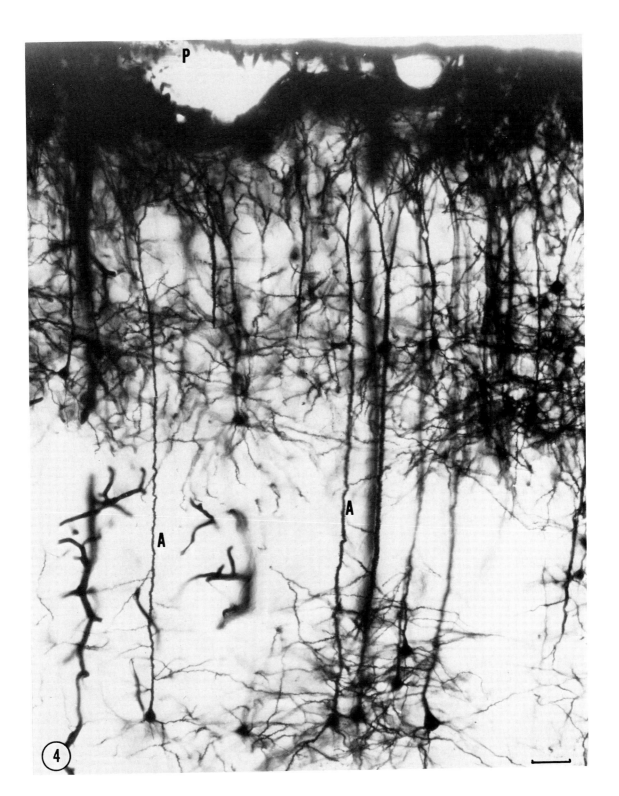

from the cell bodies are evident, although occasionally cells are depicted as though the orientation of the apical dendrites were random. As in previous work, there is no consistent indication of the origin of the pyramidal cell axon. In the joint publication with Clarke, descriptions were given of human pyramidal cells in what was becoming a relatively well-studied cortical area, the precentral gyrus. Among the findings presented were figures of pyramidal cells cut in the tangential (surface-parallel) plane, clearly illustrating the radially symmetrical spread of the basal dendrites from the soma. In the subsequent papers, the observations were expanded to include other brain regions, and tissue from cat, sheep, pig, and monkey. In confirmation of earlier work, pyramidal cells were shown to vary in size from lamina to lamina within a cortical region. Somal dimensions, number of dendrite origins, and other factors such as nuclear/cytoplasmic ratios were studied quantitatively. The giant cells described by Betz were also observed and measured, the values obtained being generally comparable to those arrived at by Betz. Of considerable interest to Lewis was his observation that the reported topographic specificity of Betz cells, i.e., their restricted locus in the prefrontal gyrus, was apparently more precise than had been imagined. What Lewis found was that the cells were not homogeneously dispersed over the gyrus but were disposed in large groups which, he felt, corresponded to the specific motor subareas described by Ferrier. Further, there appeared to be a gradient of cell size, with the largest Betz cells being found at the longitudinal fissure, and the remaining cells becoming progressively smaller as the lower extremity of the convolution is approached. A final feature of interest in Lewis' work is his explicit attention to the question of differences between species in pyramidal cell morphology. He noted carefully, for example, the unusually large number of cell bodies in the individual nests of Betz cells in the sheep brain. And in the 1879 article, he presented, in a single "Table of Measurements," parallel columns for man, cat, and sheep showing, lamina by lamina, pyramidal cell sizes in specific brain regions.

The years just prior to the turn of the century saw the increasing adoption of the new dyes introduced principally by Nissl. In the hands of Schlapp (1898) and others, dyes such as thionin and methylene blue, coupled with improving methods of fixation, were beginning to make their contribution to the morphological picture of the pyramidal cell (see Chapter 2, Fig. 4). The Betz cell shown at the right of Fig. 6 in Hammarberg's monograph (1895), for example, has a strikingly contemporary look compared to the sketchy, vaguely featureless depictions of most earlier workers. Clear Nissl bodies dot the perikaryal cytoplasm and extend into the bases of the larger dendrites. To the right of the nucleus, a small cytoplasmic patch suggests the appearance of a lipofuscin deposit. The

Figure 5. Two layer V pyramidal neurons in rat area 39, Golgi rapid impregnation. The apical dendrites (A) give rise to numerous oblique branch dendrites (O) over the proximal third of their length and then ascend, with little further branching, to form terminal tufts (T) in the vicinity of the layer I/II border. The proximal portions of the apical dendrites are shown at higher magnification in Fig. 11. Calibration line, 50 μm.

Figure 6. Upper portion of apical dendrite (A) of a layer VI pyramidal neuron in rat area 39, Golgi rapid impregnation. The apical dendrites of a number of deeply situated pyramidal neurons do not reach layer I but terminate at midcortical levels. In this example, the terminal tuft illustrated (T) is formed in layer IV. Calibration line, 25 μm.

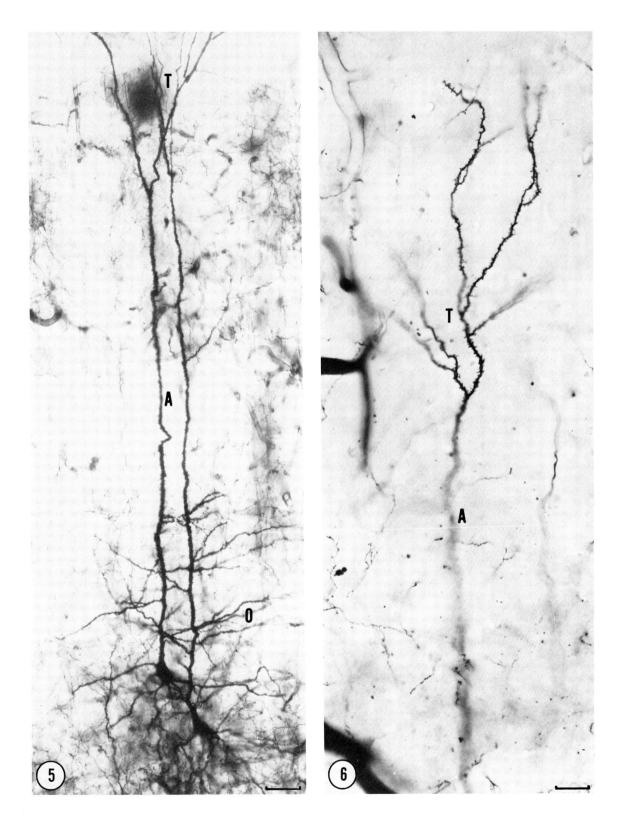

nucleus itself is a definite oval shape and contains a distinct nucleolus. Each individual dendrite origin is shown as a gradually tapering process. An appreciable length of the initial portion of the apical dendrite is shown, and the origin of oblique branches from it is clear. Hammarberg presents very many additional pyramidal cells, from both normal and mentally defective cases, at a similar level of detail. It may be noted, incidentally, that Hammarberg's work represented the first systematic attempt to understand a clinical entity such as idiocy in neurocytological terms.

The type of results obtained in the work outlined above may be thought of as "pre-Golgi," although in fact the two lines of research overlapped for about 25 years. Golgi's first mention of his new impregnation technique appeared in 1873, but it was not until considerably later that a detailed description of the method was published. Virtually all of Golgi's work was published in Italian, and it was probably this that kept his methods and results unfamiliar to the great majority of non-Italian workers for over a decade (Ramón y Cajal, 1937). It was only with the appearance of the "Sulla fina anatomia degli organi centrali del sistema nervoso" (Golgi, 1882–1885) that a translation into French (Golgi, 1883) was undertaken.

Prior to the widespread appreciation of the contributions of the Golgi technique, a considerable amount had been learned about the pyramidal cell. The range of perikaryal sizes and shapes was known, and the basic dyes had afforded the first tentative glimpses of the structures populating the somal interior. It was known that pyramidal cell bodies of essentially similar form were distributed over the whole cortex and were found in a wide variety of species. At the same time it was clear that a fine-grain analysis, taking into account such factors as cell dimensions and packing densities, revealed differences in laminae, regions, and species. But what was lacking above all was an appreciation of the overall form of the cell, and specifically the form of its processes. The true extent of these processes could only be guessed at, based upon observations using the newly developed silver stains, such as that of Ramón y Cajal, and the few examples, provided by Deiters and others, of more or less intact neurons which had been teased free from macerated pieces of tissue. There thus existed morphological questions of the most fundamental nature. How did the dendrites end? Did dendritic patterns correlate with the size and position of the cell body? Did all cells have an axon? What was the relationship between the axon and the nerve fibers and tracts of the neuropil? To all of these questions, and more, the results obtained with the Golgi method provided or contributed an answer.

The extraordinary usefulness of the method has continued to the present time, although not without occasional periods of questioning the genuineness of the impregnation images. That such concerns were in large part ill-founded was first evident in Ramón y Cajal's demonstration (1954, 1955) that Golgi-type images could also be obtained by the use of a completely independent technique, Ehrlich's methylene blue. In the modern era, several developments (e.g., Fairén *et al.*, 1977) have verified the accuracy of the method. Particularly convincing is the indistinguishability of Golgi images and those observed following intracellular filling of neurons by injected horseradish peroxidase (see, e.g., Figs. 4–8 of Donoghue and Kitai, 1981).

The beautiful drawings executed by Golgi himself—full of fine detail, with the axons drawn in red, and presented in large foldout plates—were the first renderings of relatively complete pyramidal cells. The examples in the 1882–1885 work are of cells at various depths in the precentral gyrus and the occipital and frontal cortices of human brains and from the occipital and frontal cortices of dog brains. Many of the cells depicted have what by modern standards would be judged as completely impregnated axons. These often exhibit extensive collateral branching. For at least some clearly pyramidal neurons the main branch of the axon is shown exiting from the cortex in a more or less directly vertical fashion to enter the underlying white matter. Such axons were associated with Golgi's type I cells, and were characterized by him as having a relatively small complement of collaterals and as transforming directly into myelinated nerve fibers. In other cases, however, cells which also appear to be pyramidal, such as cells 2 and 8 in plate I, exhibit axons which ramify locally and do not appear to exit from the cortex. These axons were associated with Golgi's type II cells, and were characterized as being highly ramified and as entering into "una rete nervosa estresa a tutti gli strati di sostanza grigia." With respect to the dendrites of the pyramidal cells, the principal points of interest in Golgi's drawings are the clear illustrations of the apical, oblique branch, and basal dendrites, and on the negative side the absence of dendritic spines and of terminal tufts of apical dendrites. In general, the dendrites were believed by Golgi to serve a nutritive function, and, accordingly, to have functional contacts with blood vessels.

These inaccuracies were soon to be corrected by the work of Ramón y Cajal. His first encounter and subsequent extensive experimentation with the Golgi method are described in his *Recuerdos* (1937), and his principal findings on the cerebral neocortex are summarized in Chapters 24–27 and 34–35 of the second volume of *Histologie* (1955), a work which appeared in the original Spanish during the period 1899–1904. Relying principally on the Golgi method, but with supplementary data from the use of Nissl stains, Ehrlich's methylene blue, reduced silver nitrate, and fiber stains, Ramón y Cajal's observations represented the largest single step forward in the history of our knowledge of pyramidal cell form. The descriptions and illustrations established a standard of morphological precision against which all future Golgi studies were to be judged. Collectively, the work embraced a wide variety of species—human, rodents, rabbit, cat, dog, birds, reptiles, frog, and fish—and was carried out upon numerous regions of the cortex. Among the many contributions was the discovery, and establishment of the true nature, of the pyramidal dendritic spines (1891). These were to play a significant role in Ramón y Cajal's advancement of the doctrine of "neuronismo" (1954). What distinguished this work above all was a wealth of detail concerning individual cells, extended invariably to a consideration of broader issues of neural function. Contributing to this detail was the correlation of results from the various staining methods applied. Thus, for particular classes of Golgi-impregnated pyramidal cells, it was possible to specify relationships to cell layers, fiber systems, and glial elements, and the interiors of the cell bodies and their processes could be described in terms of neurofibrillar and other components.

In comparing Ramón y Cajal's illustrations with those of Golgi, perhaps the most striking difference is not the greater completeness in Ramón y Cajal's drawings of individual cells, but rather a difference in cellular context. Whereas Golgi's plates give the impression of showing collections of isolated cells, Ramón y Cajal's (which almost certainly were also composites from a number of separate preparations) emphasized the interplay among neurons by including varieties of cells in their appropriate local relationships. There is a strong feeling for the complexity of the neuropil, and one can readily appreciate the extent of potential interaction among cellular elements, for example, the spatial overlap between the basal dendritic arborization of a pyramidal cell and the axonal collaterals of a nearby nonpyramidal cell. There is also in Ramón y Cajal a much stronger emphasis on the distinctiveness of pyramidal cells in different brain regions and at different levels. That this distinctiveness is less pronounced in Golgi's work is to be expected, as it reflected his view that specificity of function in a cortical region depends not on the intrinsic organization of the cortex but on the specificity of external connections (Golgi, 1882–1885). This "unicist" view, to use Ramón y Cajal's term (1899), minimizing the significance of structural diversity in the cortex, contrasted sharply with Ramón y Cajal's own belief. It is important to add, however, that built into his "pluralist" doctrine was a "factor of general order," that is to say, a principle of structural commonality that was shared by all cortical regions. This general factor, for him, was represented by the molecular layer and by the layers of small and large pyramidal cells (1899). These are, however, global features, and his recognition of their constancy was not incompatible with his attempts to define structural peculiarities of pyramidal cells in specific loci. Very much the same pluralist theme, rich cytological variation superimposed on an "elementary cortical pattern," was expressed in the extension of Ramón y Cajal's Golgi work by Lorente de Nó (1943).

A final historical development, and one that is also of contemporary significance, was the movement toward a systematic quantitative analysis of pyramidal cell structure. This movement, in a sense the antithesis of the individual-cell approach of Golgi analysis, was initiated by Bok (1936, 1959) but found its most influential exponent in Sholl (1953, 1956). It was not that Sholl's work was more detailed than Bok's—quite the reverse was true. In fact, it was the minuteness of detail in Bok, probably seen at the time as bordering on the trivial, that impeded widespread appreciation of his work. It must have been difficult, for example, 50 years ago, to know what to do with the information that the nuclear volume of pyramidal cells in the superior temporal gyrus is proportional to the square of its distance from the pial surface (Bok, 1934). From the standpoint of pyramidal cell morphology, the most significant aspect of Sholl's work was his statistical approach to the analysis of the dendritic tree. Considering a sample of cortical neurons of all types and sizes, Sholl demonstrated that the number of dendritic branches is unrelated to either the size of the cell body or its depth below the pial surface. He then considered the extent of dendritic arborization as a function of distance from the cell body, quantifying this relationship by counting the number of intersections between dendritic branches and a set of equally spaced concentric spheres centered on the soma. This analysis carried out for basal dendritic trees was found to yield a linear function when the log of the number of intersections was plotted against distance from the cell body. Sholl then went on to consider the implications that this mode of analysis had for synaptic connectivity. He postulated the existence of a cuff-shaped "connective zone" surrounding the individual dendrites at a distance of 0.5 μm, and made the assumption that "any axon lying within this zone may 'make a contact'."

What was envisioned was an analysis in which knowledge about the extent and rate of decay of a dendritic field's connectivity potential would provide valuable information about "the extent to which a single neuron may be influenced by impulses travelling in its neighborhood." By extension, it might then be possible to develop a mathematical approach to the connectivity of the cortex as a whole. Just how thoroughgoing Sholl's belief in this possibility was is indicated by his analogy between the visual cortex and "a statistical machine with a random input" (1953). In the light of more modern work demonstrating the high degree of specificity of synaptic relationships, Sholl's statistical assumptions about synaptic connectivity are open to serious criticism. However, his quantitative approach to the characterization of the dendritic arborizations of pyramidal and other neurons gave rise to a significant amount of modern work and remains a valuable contribution.

3. The Typical Adult Pyramidal Cell

This section reviews the morphology of those structural features shared by the large majority of typical adult pyramidal neurons. Examples of such generalized elements are the characteristic origin and disposition of the basal dendrites, the form and distribution of dendritic spines, and the dense undercoating of the axolemma. In certain cases, such as the presence of dendritic spines, the features discussed are not the exclusive property of neurons of the pyramidal type, but they will be described in terms of data derived from studies of pyramidal cells.

Considering the long history of the study of pyramidal neurons, it is surprising that we still lack a comprehensive scheme of classification of pyramidal cell types, although efforts in this direction have been made (Lorente de Nó, 1943; Sholl, 1956; Globus and Scheibel, 1967a; Braak, 1980). In part, this lack is attributable to the fact that close examination of large numbers of pyramidal cells reveals a picture of great diversity both within and across species. Inevitably, therefore, departures from the type of account given here will be encountered in any systematic examination of a wide range of pyramidal cells. In some instances, such variations are sufficiently fundamental to warrant independent treatment. These cases, which include forms such as the Betz cells and inverted pyramids, will be discussed in Section 4 of this chapter.

3.1. The Cell Body

Morphologically, the pyramidal neuron is a highly polarized cell. Its axis of polarization is linear, spans the thickness of the cortex, and is oriented normal to the plane of the pial surface. As seen in a Golgi preparation sectioned parallel to the cellular axis, the three main elements contributing to the linear orientation are the apical dendrite, extending from the cell body toward the pial surface; the vertically elongate cell body; and the axon, whose main process extends from the base of the cell body downward toward the white matter that underlies the cortex. The cell body is thus interposed at some level along the mid-course of the cellular axis.

Pyramidal cell somata may be situated in all of the cellular laminae of the cortex (layers II through VI). In some loci, progressive increases in somal size are encountered in successively deeper layers (von Economo and Koskinas, 1925; von Bonin and Bailey, 1947; Tömböl, 1974), although numerous exceptions to this generalization exist. In many cortices, such as area 17 of the rat (Peters, 1981), the cell bodies are particularly prominent in layers II/III and V. In cortices with a well-developed granular layer IV, such as the primary sensory cortices, the pyramidal cell bodies of this layer are characteristically quite small.

As mentioned previously, the term *pyramidal* originally denoted a cell body of small or large size which exhibited a triangular profile in sectioned material and which was believed to have the three-dimensional form of a pyramid or, more accurately, a cone. But with the revelation of the processes of individual neurons in Golgi preparations, it became clear that the triangular-appearing cell bodies shared with many nontriangular cells certain basic features, most notably an apical dendrite (Figs. 1–6) and, in most cases, an axon that descended vertically into the white matter (see Fig. 15). With this new information, the importance attached to the shape of the soma diminished. Golgi himself (1882–1885), while referring to certain neurons as "cellule piramidali," saw the fundamental dichotomy between cortical cell types not as being between pyramidal and nonpyramidal cells, but as being between cells with two basically different forms of arborization of the axon, Type I cells having a long projecting axon that exited from the cortex and Type II cells a locally ramifying axon.

There is today widespread acceptance of the fact that pyramidal cells may possess a variety of somal shapes (Figs. 2, 4, 11, 14, 15). In fact, it is not uncommon in studying neocortical pyramidal neurons in Golgi preparations to find that cells with triangular cell bodies are outnumbered by those displaying other shapes (e.g., Vaughan, 1977). These include spherical, ovoid, rhomboidal, and irregular forms. Nevertheless, it remains generally true that most large cell bodies with a distinctly triangular outline are classifiable as pyramidal neurons, that is, they display an apical dendrite emerging from the pial vertex of the triangle. For this reason, the cell bodies of what we presently conceptualize as "classical pyramidal cells" are triangular in profile.

Granting the existence of a spectrum of pyramidal cell body forms, one may ask whether or not the cell bodies of nonpyramidal cells have a completely different spectrum of shapes or perhaps of sizes. In an explicit study of this question in the various laminae of rat visual cortex (Feldman and Peters, 1978), the traced perikaryal silhouettes of Golgi-impregnated pyramidal and nonpyramidal cells were compared. It was found that neither perikaryal size nor shape reliably discriminates between pyramidal and nonpyramidal neurons. Two general exceptions to this finding were noted: the large triangular perikarya of "classical" pyramidal form and the largest perikarya of layer V. These were consistently pyramidal in type. One conclusion that can be drawn from the data is that studies which presume to discriminate pyramidal and nonpyramidal cells on the basis of cell body size and shape need to be interpreted with caution.

The sizes of pyramidal cell bodies vary widely, and are subject to progressive alteration with advancing age (Feldman, 1976; Vaughan and Vincent, 1979). In normal young adult individuals, perikaryal sizes run the gamut from very small cells on the order of 12 μm in width in, for example, layer IV of sensory cortices (Lund *et al.*, 1981) up to the giant cells of Betz (Betz, 1874), whose width may reach 60 μm. An indication of the range of sizes that may be observed is given in Sholl's data for the visual and motor cortices of the cat (1953). Expressing perikaryal size in terms of surface area, the pyramidal cells in the various laminae of the visual cortex were found to range between 470 and 3870 μm², and those of the motor cortex to range between 310 and 6384 μm². In cat somatosensory cortex, Mungai (1967) reported a considerably narrower but still appreciable range, 616 to 1257 μm². These somal values represented less than 5% of the total surface areas of the cell bodies plus their processes.

The fine structure of the pyramidal cell body has been well studied in a variety of species and cortical loci. Among the early complete accounts is that of Peters and Kaiserman-Abramof (1970) dealing with layer II/III pyramids in rat parietal cortex. As illustrated in that study, the perikaryal surface is rather smooth-contoured, although exceptionally, spines in small numbers are encountered protruding from it. The nucleus is large and spherical. Its size, in the examples studied, limits the perikaryal cytoplasm to a relatively thin rim. While the nuclear surface is typically smooth, deep infoldings are occasionally encountered. The nucleoplasm is pale and rather homogeneous, with only scanty condensations of chromatin being present either under the nuclear envelope or scattered in the nucleoplasm. The nucleolus is large and single. Occasionally, intranuclear rods (Siegesmund *et al.*, 1964; Sotelo and Palay, 1968; Feldman and Peters, 1972) are present, as they are in pyramidal neurons elsewhere in rat cortex (Vaughan and Vincent, 1979). Within the perikaryal cytoplasm, a notable feature is the relative sparsity of aggregated rough endoplasmic reticulum (RER). The cisternae that are present are only moderately studded with ribosomes, the majority of ribosomes being present free in the cytoplasm, typically in polyribosomal form. The observed paucity of highly aggregated accumulations of RER correlates well with the pallid appearance of the pyramidal cell perikaryon in light microscopic preparations stained with basic dyes (Fig. 1). One common locus of the Nissl substance that is present is at the origin of dendrites, and particularly the apical dendrite, from the perikaryon. The apically situated Nissl substance, when evident, frequently appears to cap the top of the nucleus and often extends into the base of the dendrite. Occasionally, peripherally located perikaryal cisternae of RER are observed to give rise to subsurface cisterns (Peters *et al.*, 1976), frequently arranged in stacks of two or more parallel cisternae. These have very narrow or closed lumina and are separated by gaps containing a rather dense flocculent material. Ribosomes are found only on the innermost surface of the organelle. One common location for subsurface cisternae is at sites of apposition between adjacent pyramidal cell somata (Jones and Powell, 1970). Like the RER, the Golgi apparatus is sparse, but tends to be found at the bases of the dendrites, and again particularly the apical dendrite, and also at the axon hillock. Also present in the perikaryal cytoplasm are oval and round profiles of mitochondria as well as many microtubules and a few neurofilaments. Where the cytoplasm is limited to a thin layer, the microtubules generally appear to run in a circumnuclear orientation. Typical lysosomal elements are found within the perikaryon, together with lipofuscin granules in varying degrees of abundance.

In all essential respects, Peters and Kaiserman-Abramof's account of normal pyramidal cell bodies has been corroborated in studies of other species and cortices. There is, for example, a high degree of agreement with the ultrastructural findings of Jones and Powell (1970) in somatic sensory cortex and the findings of Garey (1971) and Tömböl (1974) in visual cortex.

The various constituents of the pyramidal cell body remain for the most part unchanged throughout the adult life span (see Vaughan and Vincent, 1979). However, with advancing age there occurs an accumulation of several types of elements. Chief among these is the material generally referred to as lipofuscin, although this material actually occurs in heterogeneous forms (Vaughan and Peters, 1974; Siakotos and Munkres, 1981). The age-related accumulation of lipofuscin pigment by pyramidal cells has received extensive attention, and is reviewed in Brizzee's chapters in Sohal's book (1981). In recent years, Braak (see Chapter 3, this volume) has developed an important new technique for studying intracytoplasmic pigment. In addition to its utility in studying pigment per se and in the delineation of cytoarchitectonic boundaries, Braak's method represents a significant contribution to the laminar and regional classification of pyramidal cell types.

The universality of pigment accumulation by pyramidal and other neuronal types has led to the conclusion that it is, in essence, a benign morphological change (Feldman and Peters, 1974b), and probably does not play a major role in the age-related death of cortical neurons (Brody, 1976). By contrast, other morphological elements of the aging perikaryon bear a quantitative relationship to the development of dementing processes in man. Among these elements is the neurofibrillary tangle (Alzheimer, 1907), whose detailed structure has been described by Terry and Wiśniewski (1970) and by Wiśniewski et al. (1976). In light microscopic sections of aged cortex stained by silver techniques such as that of Bodian or von Braunmühl, tangles appear as dense, often flame-shaped inclusions which in pyramidal neurons may extend up into the proximal portion of the pyramidal apical dendrite (Scheibel and Scheibel, 1975). Whether the tangles are confined to neurons of the pyramidal type has not been established with certainty. In the electron microscope, the tangles appear as packed bundles of aligned filaments whose structure suggests a *de novo* formation in aged cells, rather than an alteration of preexisting microtubules or neurofilaments. Analysis at high magnification has led Wiśniewski and colleagues (1976) to the conclusion that the component filaments are organized in the form of helically wound pairs.

3.2. The Dendrites

The morphological hallmark of the pyramidal neuron is the apical dendrite (Figs. 1–6). This is a single process which typically arises from the apex of the cell body. It is distinguished from the remaining dendrites of the cell by its very gradually tapering origin from the cell body, its relatively large diameter, and its long, straight course toward the pial surface.

Apart from the apical dendrite, three additional dendritic systems (Figs. 2, 5, 11, 14)—not aligned in the radial axis of orientation of the cell as a whole—typify the pyramidal neuron. The first of these, the terminal tuft, is the subpial dendritic spray formed by the branching of the distal end of the apical dendrite. Characteristically, the terminal tuft originates as a bifurcation of the apical dendrite in the vicinity of layer II. The second dendritic system consists of the oblique branch dendrites. These extend as collaterals from the shaft of the apical dendrite. They are the least highly branched of the three dendritic systems. Finally, the system of basal dendrites extends outward from the lower portion of the pyramidal cell body. The individual dendritic trunks emerge in radial fashion, somewhat like the ribs of an umbrella. While the basal dendrites, like the apical dendrite, originate from the cell body by means of tapering cytoplasmic cones, the gradualness of the taper is not as pronounced as is the case with the apical dendrite. Consequently, the line of demarcation between the cell body and the basal dendrites can usually be ascertained without difficulty. The line of demarcation in the case of the apical dendrite, on the other hand, is often exceptionally ambiguous. This is of importance in quantitative studies in which, for example, the height of the cell body is to be measured.

Some writers have referred to the three dendritic systems just described as the horizontal elements of the pyramidal cell, as distinct from the vertically aligned apical dendrite and main axonal process. It is important to note, however, that each of the three classes of nonapical dendrites ramifies in highly variable planes, with varying degrees of obliquity. Cases of convincing surface-parallel orientation can be found, for instance, in the large basal dendrites of Betz cells (Scheibel and Scheibel, 1978) or the ends of certain terminal tuft dendrites coursing just below the pial surface, but these are the exception and not the rule.

The morphological features of the apical dendrite mentioned above make these processes readily recognizable in the electron microscope and in semithin sections examined light microscopically. Sections cut in a plane parallel to the dendritic axis, i.e., perpendicular to the pial surface, often reveal many long profiles of apical dendrites issuing from the upper poles of pyramidal cell bodies (Fig. 3). In many cases, isolated profiles of apical dendrites, if cut in an approximately axial plane of section (Fig. 12), can be recognized by virtue of their large diameter and their straight and highly oriented trajectories. Apical dendrites are also apparent in the tangential, or surface-parallel, plane of section (Figs. 8–10). Viewed in this plane, the relatively large diameter of the apical dendrites and their preferential aggregation in dendritic clusters (see below) provide the chief criteria by means of which they are recognized. In rat visual cortex (Figs. 8, 9) the measured diameters of apical dendrites in clusters range from 1 to over 3 μm, with the proportions of small, medium, and large dendrites shifting with advancing age (Feldman and Dowd, 1975; Feldman, 1976).

An account of the ultrastructure of the apical dendrite, as it appears in rat parietal cortex, has been given by Peters and Kaiserman-Abramof (1970). Their observations of the origin of the apical dendrite show that microtubules funnel from the perikaryon into the base of the dendrite by passing around the cisternae of the RER and Golgi apparatus typically present in that region. Within the dendrite, the microtubules quickly assume a longitudinal orientation parallel to the dendritic axis (Fig. 12). Also commonly observed at the base of the dendrite are lysosomal elements, multivesicular bodies, and aggregations of free ribosomes; occasionally, a centriole is encountered in this region as well. The prevalence of the RER becomes progressively diminished over the first 50 μm or so of the apical dendrite. The elements that are present are preferentially located beneath the plasma membrane, often in bulges of the dendritic surface. Commonly, multiple cisternae of the Golgi apparatus are found in the center of the proximal portion of the dendrite. Similar aggregations are also found more distally at the origins of oblique branch dendrites. Elsewhere in the dendrite, isolated cisternae of SER are occasionally encountered, and again are often found beneath the plasma membrane. Those cisternae which are more centrally located tend to be oriented parallel to the long axis of the dendrite, and the same is true of the elongated mitochondria wihin the dendritic cytoplasm. In transverse sections of the more distal regions of the apical dendrite, the most prominent cytoplasmic feature is the array of microtubules. These are disposed in an ordered pattern within the dendrite, with a center-to-center spacing between adjacent microtubules of 200 to 400 nm. Scattered in the cytoplasm among the microtubules is a rather electron-dense flocculent material that often appears to extend between the microtubules. At the origins of oblique branch dendrites, some of the microtubules from the proximal portion of the oblique dendrite curve into the distal portion of the oblique dendrite. There thus exist populations of microtubules which appear to course entirely between dendritic segments, without a connection with the perikaryon.

Presumably, microtubules play a role in the maintenance of dendritic form. Purpura *et al.* (1982) have recently described a microtubular alteration in frontal pyramids of children with progressive behavioral abnormalities of neurological origin. The apical and basal dendrites of over 90% of the pyramids examined exhibited pronounced varicosities and spine loss. Ultrastructurally, the microtubules in affected regions were observed to be in disarray, having lost their longitudinality and their parallel relationships with one another. While it is difficult to specify the sequence in which the changes take place, Purpura and colleagues hypothesize that it is the microtubular disorganization that is involved in the disturbance of dendritic form and the subsequent dendritic dystrophy.

Many of the ultrastructural features of the apical dendrite are also encountered in the trunks of the basal dendrites, although on a reduced scale, owing presumably to the smaller diameter of these processes (Peters and Kaiserman-Abramof, 1970). The more distal segments of the basal dendrites, as well as the remaining dendritic branches of the pyramidal cell, do not display any distinctive ultrastructural characteristics. Electron microscopic images of these smaller dendrites, as identified following Golgi deimpregnation by gold substitution (Fairén *et al.*, 1977), typically reveal little else beyond microtubules and occasional mitochondria.

In a serial section study of layer I rat parietal cortex, Vaughan and Peters (1973) reconstructed the form of the tips of spinous dendrites that they interpreted as terminal tuft dendrites. The tips described end bluntly. They are approximately 0.5 μm in diameter and display a very slight expansion of their final 1 μm. One or two asymmetric synapses occur at the tip but do not encompass it. The terminal cytoplasm is not distinctive, and contains the tip of a single axial mitochondrion, a very small number of microtubules, and one or two profiles of SER in either cisternal or vesicular form.

The straight, radial course of the apical dendrite shafts might at first suggest that they project toward the pial surface as rather uniformly scattered individual elements. Underlying such a view, however, is the assumption that the cell bodies of origin are themselves homogeneously dispersed in the tangential plane. That such is not the case, at least in some regions of cortex, is well established (von Economo, 1929; Lorente de Nó, 1943; Jones and Powell, 1970). Consideration of this fact prompts the alternative suggestion that apical dendrites might be aggregated in ensembles of some sort as they ascent through the cortex. This in fact is true, as has been demonstrated in primates by von Bonin and Mehler (1971) and by Peters and Walsh (1972) in a study of rat somatic sensory cortex. In the latter work, the examination of tangentially oriented plastic sections clearly revealed the bundling of apical dendrites into vertically oriented dendritic clusters (Figs. 7, 8). This important feature of cortical organization has been shown to have wide regional and species generality (Fleischhauer *et al.*, 1972; Feldman and Peters, 1974a; Fleischhauer, 1974; Winkelmann *et al.*, 1975). The exact signficance of the clusters has, however, not yet become apparent. It is not known, for example, whether or not there is a specific relationship between the clusters and the vertical bundles of axons which traverse the cortex (Kaes, 1907), or between the clusters and the larger columnar elements which have been identified by physiological techniques (Mountcastle, 1957; Hubel and Wiesel, 1963, 1969). It does seem clear, however, that the arrangement of the dendrites into clusters provides the opportunity for simultaneous activation of groups of dendrites and the segregation of inputs to discrete groups. One anatomical feature of the clusters that may enhance the opportunity for simultaneous activation is the fact that in the intracluster neuropil the spines of adjacent apical dendrites freely interdigitate (Feldman, 1975).

That the existence of clusters escaped notice for so long is attributable to two main factors. The first is the fact that the detailed course of the apical dendrites was only able to be studied in Golgi preparations. Because the selectivity of impregnation with this technique is such that contiguous elements are infrequently impregnated (Ramón-Moliner, 1970), it was not possible to visualize sufficient numbers of adjacent dendrites to reveal the cluster pattern. The second factor was the historical predilection for examining sections of cortex in either one of the cardinal planes of section or in sections that were vertically oriented with respect to the pial surface. Relatively little attention was paid to the examination of sections cut in the tangential plane. This is the one plane in which the clusters stand out with unmistakable clarity, although with experience, elements of the clusters can be identified in other planes of section as well.

The principal components within the clusters are the apical dendrites of layer V pyramidal neurons. When viewed in tangential sections at the level of layer IV (Fig. 7), the individual clusters are frequently observed to contain from three to nine apical dendrites and to be separated by distances which are variable but which often range from 30 to 50 μm (Feldman and Peters, 1974a; Fleischhauer *et al.*, 1972). The exact values of these measures vary significantly within and across species. Within a given cortical region, the primary determinants are the distribution and packing density of the pyramidal cell bodies and the exact depth of the tangential plane examined. At progressively more superficial levels, the number of dendrites per cluster increases as the apical dendrites of layer IV and layer III pyramidal neurons join the peripheral margins of the clusters. These additions also account for the fact that the discreteness of the clusters, as viewed in tangential sections, diminishes as the plane of section ascends from layer IV toward the pial surface.

Viewed at low magnification, the chief elements defining the dendritic clusters are the large apical dendrites of layer V pyramidal neurons. It is these which are encountered in numbers varying from three to nine per cluster. Closer examination, however, reveals that a number of smaller transversely sectioned dendrites are scattered in and among the large clustered dendrites and also in the intercluster neuropil (Fig. 7). Within the clusters, these small dendritic profiles often equal or exceed in number the large-diameter apical dendrites. The origin of the small dendrites has not been ascertained. While they may originate from small pyramidal neurons of layers V and VI, the possibility that some of them are nonpyramidal cannot be ruled out.

Among the reported variations in cluster patterning is an unusual feature noted by Fleischhauer (1974) in cat sensorimotor cortex. There, the layer V pyramids in the posterior sigmoid gyrus give rise to apical dendrites which have a primary bifurcation in close proximity to the cell body. The secondary apical branches diverge, curving only gradually toward the pial surface, so that in the vicinity of layer IV, instead of vertical clusters one encounters numerous examples of obliquely interlacing dendrites. It is only at the approximate level of layer III that these dendrites assume a vertical orientation and bundle together with other similar dendrites to form clusters.

When apical dendrites are examined individually in Golgi preparations, small numbers of oblique branch dendrites, typically two to five, are observed extending from each apical dendrite. The oblique branch origins appear at first to be randomly distributed along the apical shaft. However, specific study of this point involving large collections of apical dendrites indicates that many of the points of oblique branch origin are subject to preferential laminar specificity (Lorente de Nó, 1943; O'Leary, 1941). The layer IV pyramids Lorente de Nó designated as "star pyramids," for example, were distinguished from "ordinary" pyramids by the fact that numerous oblique branches were given off within layer IV but none in layers II and III. What appears to correlate best with the particular laminar pattern observed is the layer in which the parent cell body is situated (Lund and Boothe, 1975). The significance of this factor may in turn hinge upon the laminar specificity of the various presynaptic elements present within the cortex (Lorente de Nó, 1943; Lund and Boothe, 1975).

Figure 7. Apical dendritic clusters as visualized in a tangentially oriented 2-μm plastic section at the level of layer IV of rat visual cortex. One cluster is indicated by open arrows. Calibration line, 25 μm.

Figure 8. The large profile is a transversely sectioned apical dendrite within a dendritic cluster, as visualized in a tangential section through layer IV of rat visual cortex. The round mitochondrial profiles and the regular arrays of microtubules are characteristic of apical dendrites in this plane of section. At S, a dendritic spine extending from the apical dendritic shaft and containing a spine apparatus (arrow) forms an asymmetric synapse with an axon terminal. Calibration line, 0.5 μm.

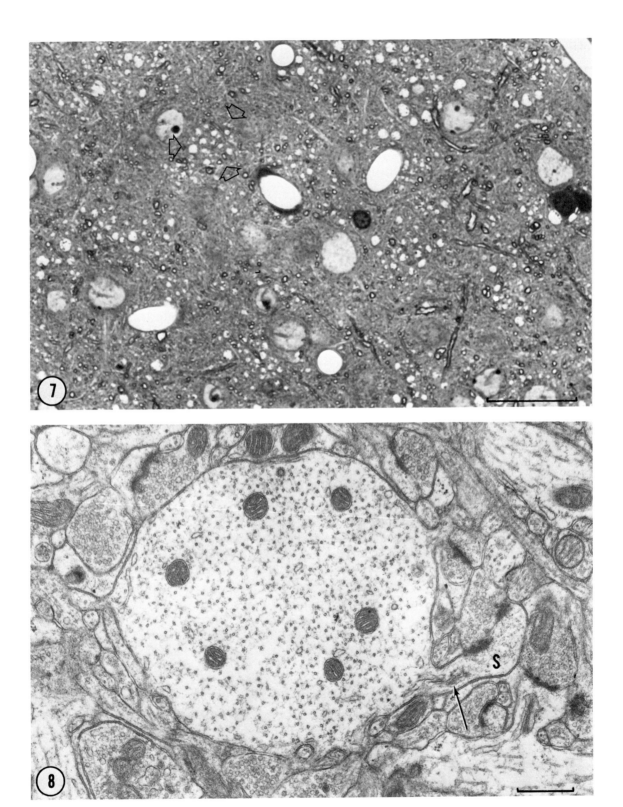

A similar sort of specificity appears to apply to the length of the apical dendrite as a whole. Although it is generally true that pyramidal apical dendrites extend to layer I, there have long been known to exist pyramidal neurons whose apical dendrites terminate in a variably developed terminal tuft deeper within the cortex (Shkol'nik-Yarros, 1971; Parnavelas *et al.*, 1977a; Braak, 1980; and Fig. 6). Among the early well-known descriptions of variants of this sort is that of Lorente de Nó (1943). He described pyramids of a "medium" and "short" type, cells of layers V and VI whose apical dendrites terminated within or below layer IV. In rat visual cortex, it is common to find layer VI pyramids with apical dendrites terminating in the vicinity of layer IV (Fig. 6).

A detailed and comprehensive study which underscores the nonrandomness of apical dendrite features is that of Lund and Booth (1975) in macaque visual cortex. This study is particularly valuable because it includes pyramidal cells of each of the cellular sublaminae of the cortex, with the exception of the two strata forming the authors' layer IVc, in which no pyramidal cell bodies have been detected (Lund, 1973). Based on Golgi observations, the authors describe categories of cells, defined according to the laminar depth of the cell bodies and the laminae or sublaminae in which the apical dendrite tips, the oblique branches, and the axonal collateral terminations are located. Twelve distinct patterns of pyramidal apical dendrite arborization are described. Five of these involve pyramidal cells whose apical dendrites do not reach layer I, the distal tips of individual types ramifying in various laminae between midlayer IV and layer II. These short pyramids originate from cell bodies situated deep in the cortex, in layer VI and, in one case, lower layer V. The arborization patterns described include apical dendrite patterns which have from zero to four oblique branch projections extending outward into specific laminae. The cells devoid of oblique branch projections are a population of deep layer V pyramids whose apical dendrites terminate in layer II or the upper portion of layer III. Among the cells with relatively few oblique branch projections are those whose apical dendrites terminate short of layer I. Two categories of cells characteristically exhibit four sets of oblique branches. The first category consists of layer IVb pyramids, with oblique branch ramifications in layers IVb, IIIb, IIIa, and II. The second category consists of the very large pyramids of lower layer V, which have oblique branch projections into layers Vb, Va, the upper portion of IVc, and IVb. With two exceptions, all laminae receive oblique branch projections, although the four sublaminae of layer IV are somewhat infrequently provided in this respect. The two laminae which are devoid of apical dendrite oblique branches are the upper and lower sublaminae of layer IV, the two strata in which the input from the parvocellular layers of the dorsal lateral geniculate body terminates (Hubel and Wiesel, 1972; Lund, 1973). By contrast, the dendritic projections into layers VI, Va, and IIIa appear to be abundant.

Just what functional significance may be attached to the observed dendrite–lamina associations is difficult to determine, although it seems reasonable to speculate that the observed specificity relates to preferential input to the cortical pyramidal cells from lamina-specific afferent axons, such as those arising from the magnocellular and parvocellular regions of the lateral geniculate. Presumably, certain associations are more significant than others in influencing the function of specific pyramidal neuron types. From an anatomical standpoint, an important step forward would be quantitative study of the frequency and extent of the various types of dendritic projection patterns. Such information might reasonably be expected to focus attention on those patterns which represent particularly significant aspects of intracortical circuitry.

As mentioned above, the basal dendrites of the classical pyramidal cell extend radially outward from the base of the perikaryon in skirtlike fashion. In Golgi preparations, three to five basal dendritic trunks per cell are typically seen, although it is important to recognize that the opacity of the Golgi precipitate makes it difficult to visualize dendrites which extend from the cell body in either direction along the visual axis. Explicit quantitative study of the numbers of origins per cell in vertical sections led Sholl (1953) to conclude that in cat visual and motor cortex the number is never less than four and seldom greater than seven. When basal dendrite origins are observed in tangential section (Figs. 9, 10), it is apparent that some pyramidal neurons may have as many as 10, or even more, basal dendrites (Vaughan, 1977). On the other hand, some pyramidal neurons, particularly in primate cortices, may exhibit only one well-developed basal dendrite (Braak, 1980). The number of dendrites, as well as their extent, is subject to alteration during later stages of the life span (Scheibel *et al.*, 1975; Scheibel and Scheibel, 1975; Feldman, 1977; Vaughan, 1977; Buell and Coleman, 1979).

A number of the basal dendrites of typical pyramidal neurons (Figs. 1, 2, 9, 10, 14, 15) extend out laterally from the perikaryon, with secondary and tertiary branches that may either ascend or descend. Other dendrites follow obliquely descending courses, while still others have a predominantly downward course, toward the white matter. The descending basal dendrites are often of sufficient length to cross laminar borders. Basal dendrites of many layer III pyramids, for example, may be frequently observed to extend into layer IV. This means that pyramidal cell bodies not only have apical dendritic fields that ramify through more superficial layers of the cortex, but also basilar fields that may extend their dendritic surfaces into at least one deeper-lying lamina. A general consideration of the basilar dendritic system as a whole suggests that the overall form of its territory is approximated by a hemisphere whose flat upper surface is centered on the cell body. This geometry is characteristic for the idealized classical pyramidal neuron, in which the basal dendrite origins emerge from the periphery of the broad base of the perikaryon. In addition to such dendrites, however, it is a common observation that dendrites, usually fewer in number than those just described, may also emerge from other perikaryal positions. These include the center of the base of the cell body and regions high up along the sides of the cell body, near the apical dendrite. Such origins are frequently seen in cases where the cell body is not of the classical pyramidal shape. In many instances, the dendrites originating from the upper portion of the perikaryon follow an obliquely ascending course, terminating at levels well above that of the cell body. These dendrites obviously do not ramify within the hemispherical zone mentioned above. While it may not be strictly correct to refer to dendrites of this type as basal dendrites, no specific term for them has been applied.

Basal dendrites branch rather freely, and are of variable length (Table I). Commonly, a positive association is observed between perikaryal size and the extent of the dendritic field. Recent observations indicate that this extent may be a significant feature of pyramidal cell function, since neurons with large dendritic fields display large receptive fields when studied physiologically (Gilbert and Wiesel, 1979). Basal dendrite lengths for a given cell (from somal origin to distal tip) typically range from a length about equal to that of the oblique branch dendrites to lengths which may be two or three times greater (Kemper *et al.*, 1973; Winkelmann *et al.*, 1973). Basal dendrite lengths are also somewhat greater than the lengths of terminal tuft dendrites (Winkelmann *et al.*, 1973). Selected examples of length measurements from the literature are presented in Table I.

In addition to the measurement of dendritic fields as a whole, there has developed a significant technical literature dealing with the detailed morphometric analysis of individual dendrite length, branching pattern, and branching angle. For a treatment of this subject, the reader is referred to the papers of Berry *et al.* (1972), Lindsay and Scheibel (1974), Hollingworth and Berry (1975), Smit and Uylings (1975), Uylings and Smit (1975), and Cupp and Uemura (1980).

The quantitative work on dendritic fields referred to above has for the most part been carried out in the light microscope on Golgi-impregnated material, and this necessitates recognition of several cautionary methodological points. Among these is the need to appreciate the relationship between neuronal geometry and section thickness. The majority of studies dealing with dendritic length have been confined to measurement of dendrites that are entirely or almost entirely contained within the thickness of single sections. It would appear to be inevitable that such measurements underestimate the true magnitude of dendritic lengths, since the extent of pyramidal cell dendritic spread frequently exceeds the section thickness. This results in a selection bias favoring shorter dendrites. The extent of error may be compounded in those cases where preferential planes of dendritic arborization are not taken into account. One solution to this problem is the more widespread adoption of measurement systems (e.g., Paldino and Harth, 1977b) which trace impregnated processes across sectioned ends into adjacent sections. A second concern in quantitative Golgi analyses is perhaps more disturbing, since it relates to the nature of the Golgi impregnation itself. At issue is the question of the completeness of impregnation of neuronal processes. As a working assumption, it has generally proven to be productive to assume that the distal end of an impregnated process coincides with the point at which the impregnation is seen to terminate. It should be realized, however, that the validity of this assumption is far from established. Mostly unpublished observations during the course of electron microscopic study of deimpregnated gold-substituted neurons that were judged to be well impregnated have made it clear that there do exist instances of only partial filling of neuronal processes with visible Golgi precipitate (see Peters and Proskauer, 1980). Cell bodies, too,

$\longrightarrow$

Figure 9. Tangentially sectioned layer V pyramidal neuron in rat visual cortex, Golgi rapid impregnation. In this plane of section, the basal dendrites are seen to extend radially from the cell body. Calibration line, 25 μm.

Figure 10. Tangentially sectioned layer III pyramidal neuron in rat visual cortex. The plane of section passes through two basal dendrite origins (B). At the perikaryal surface, several axosomatic synapses are evident (arrows) as well as a region of apposition with a neighboring pyramidal cell body (P). A, apical dendrite of a deeper-lying pyramidal neuron. Calibration line, 2 μm.

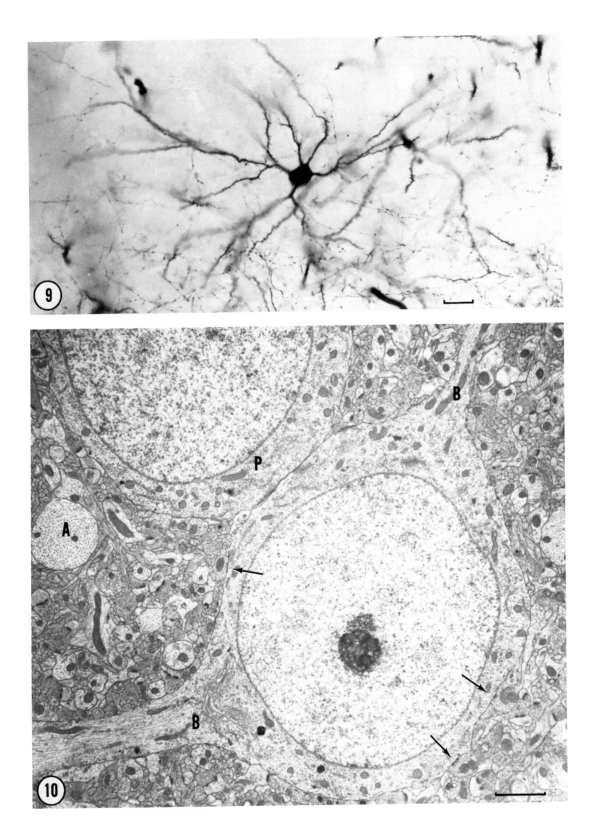

Table I. Sizes of Pyramidal Cell Dendritic Fields

Dendritic system	Cortex	Location of cell body (lamina)	Dendritic field radius (µm)[a]	Reference
Terminal tuft	Rat, sensory	V	161	Winkelmann *et al.* (1973)
	Macaque, visual	—	125	Lund (1981)
Oblique branch	Macaque, motor	II	116	Kemper *et al.* (1973)
		IIIa	187	
		IIIb	191	
		IIIc	182	
		V	181[b]	
		VI	198[b]	
Basal	Macaque, motor	II	134	Kemper *et al.* (1973)
		IIIa	195	
		IIIb	225	
		IIIc	221	
		V	263[b]	
		VI	268[b]	
	Macaque, visual	II/III	92	Lund (1981)
		V	130–340	
		VI	117–385[c]	
	Cat, visual	—	100–182	Sholl (1953)
	Cat, motor	—	120–282	Sholl (1953)
	Cat, somatosensory	—	189–251[d]	Mungai (1967)
	Rat, sensory	V	185	Winkelmann *et al.* (1973)
	Rabbit, visual	V	140	Globus and Scheibel (1967c)

[a] Values measured from the axis of the cell (apical dendrite or center of the cell body) to the dendritic tips; values are means unless ranges are given.
[b] Excludes largest pyramidal cells.
[c] Includes Meynert cells.
[d] Longest dendrites.

may on occasion fail to impregnate fully (Peters and Fairén, 1978). An important, though unanswered, question is the frequency of the partial impregnation phenomenon. There are several possible approaches to the resolution to this question. One is the specific comparison of processes which have been Golgi impregnated and similar processes as they are revealed after being intracellularly labeled. A second approach is the systematic electron microscopic study of terminal impregnation regions following deimpregnation and gold-toning. Finally,

$\longrightarrow$

Figure 11. Higher magnification of the proximal portions of the apical dendrites seen in Fig. 5. Note the initial spine-free portion of the apical dendrite (A). The apical dendritic spines begin to appear in substantial numbers approximately at the level of the arrow, although occasional isolated spines are evident more proximally. B, basal dendrite; O, oblique branch dendrite. Calibration line, 25 µm.

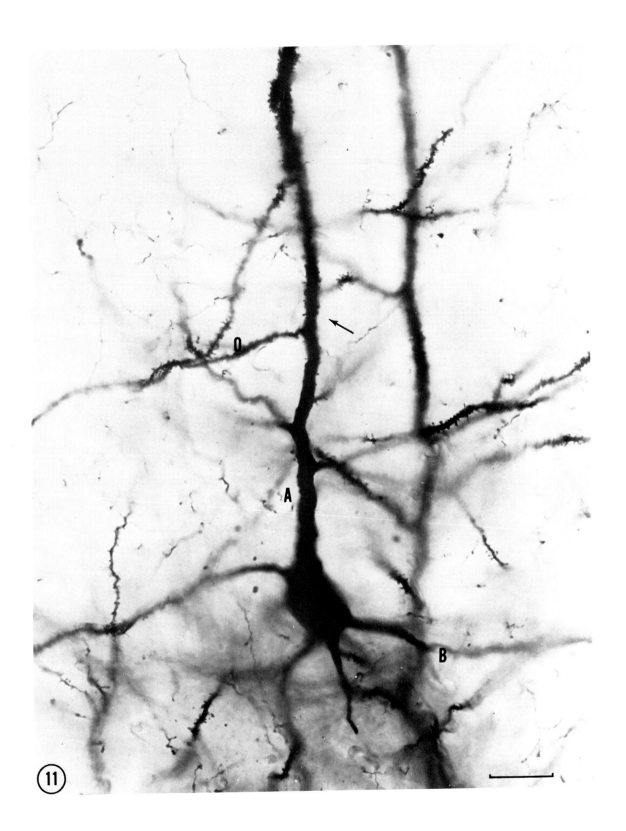

there is a need for further methodological studies such as that of Williams *et al.* (1978). It should be emphasized that the factors cited above are probably not of major significance in most quantitative Golgi studies, but not enough information is yet available to know what importance should be attached to them. It seems reasonable, however, to assume that the major conclusions which have been arrived at in the quantitative work are valid, although the absolute accuracy of the numerical values reported may require careful critical interpretation.

The radial outgrowth of the basal dendrites from the perikaryon has prompted several investigators to study the basal dendrite projections of individual pyramidal cells in Golgi-impregnated sections cut in the tangential plane (Figs. 9, 10). The first careful study of such preparations was carried out on rat, cat, and monkey visual cortex by Colonnier (1964), and was followed by the reports of Wong (1967) on cat auditory cortex and Mungai (1967) on cat somatic sensory cortex. In Colonnier's work, pyramidal basal dendrite fields were examined in all of the cellular layers of the cortex with a view towards determining the shapes of the dendrite fields. Elongate fields were defined as those whose major diameter was more than 1.5 times longer than the minor diameter; remaining fields were defined as circular. Both circular and elongate fields were observed, but circular fields were more common, especially in layer III. Among the circular fields, two subtypes were present, one in which the basal dendrites radiated in all directions in nonpreferential fashion, and one in which they tended to concentrate in two orientations, at right angles to each other, in cruciate form. In the relatively small number of cells exhibiting elongate basal dendrite fields, the long axes of the various fields were observed to be oriented in all directions. Elongated fields of various cells in a localized region were frequently seen to be oriented at various angles to one another, and to be scattered among cells with circular fields. Significantly, however, a population analysis revealed that there did exist preferential axes of orientation of the elongated fields. In the rat and cat, there was a tendency for the axes to be directed in an anterior–posterior orientation. In the monkey, the preferred axis of orientation was parallel to the lunate sulcus, in a medial–lateral orientation. Colonnier observed that these axes corresponded in each species to the axis of vertical vision, that is, the preferred axis corresponded to the cortical representation of the axis extending from the lower to the upper part of the retinal field. The orientation axes of terminal tufts were also examined, and again both circular and elongated axes were apparent. Not enough data were available to arrive at a conclusion about which form predominates in the terminal tufts, or whether there was a preferred axis of orientation, but it was clear that there was no relationship between the orientation of the terminal tuft field and the orientation of the basal dendrite field for the same individual layer II pyramid. For a given cell, both might be circular, both might be elongate, or one of each pattern might be present. If both were elongate, there was no observed similarity in the two axes of orientation.

The results of the subsequent studies by Mungai (1967) and Wong (1967) are basically in agreement with Colonnier's findings. Both, for instance, reported a great preponderance of circular over elongated pyramidal dendrite fields, with some of the circular fields displaying the cruciate pattern.

More recent work has tended to focus on cases of directional selectivity of pyramidal dendritic fields. In Fleischhauer's (1978) study of cat area 4, tangential

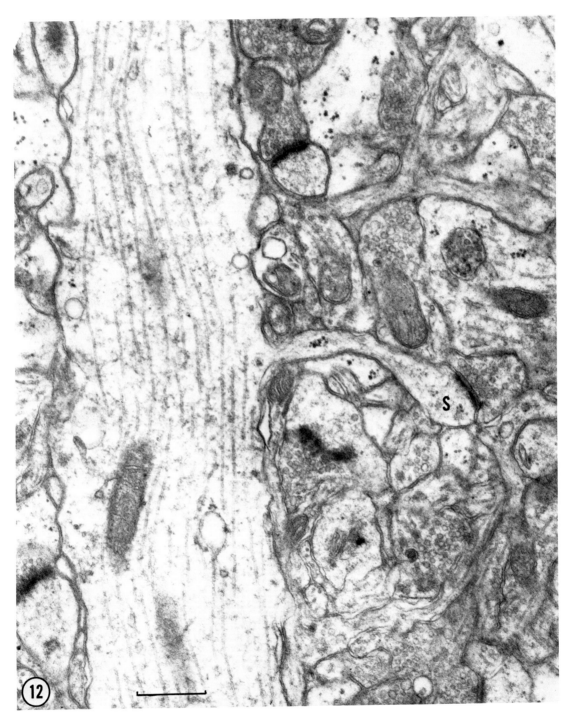

Figure 12. Longitudinal section of an apical dendrite in rat visual cortex. A spine emerges from the dendritic shaft and forms an asymmetric synapse at its terminal enlargement (S). The prominent cytoplasmic constituents of the dendritic shaft are the axially oriented microtubules. Calibration line, 0.5 μm.

Bodian as well as Golgi sections were studied. The findings reveal a prominent preferential orientation of both cell bodies and dendrites. The majority of the perikaryal profiles of layer V pyramids viewed in the tangential plane are oval, and the long axes of these ovals are preferentially oriented in one direction, roughly parallel to the ansate sulcus. Furthermore, the bifurcating apical dendrites of this cortex mentioned earlier in conjunction with dendritic clusters (Fleischhauer, 1974) are seen to have a preferential plane of bifurcation that is oriented parallel to the long axes of the cell bodies. In the auditory cortex of the cat, Glaser *et al.* (1979) examined the geometry of basal dendrite projection preferences not only in the tangential plane but also in the vertical plane. In the latter plane, a preferential dorsoventral orientation was observed, and evidence was presented that the preferred axes might be aligned with local isofrequency contours, defined physiologically. In a further study of this possibility, Glaser and McMullen (1980) explicitly correlated physiological and anatomical results in layer IV of rabbit auditory cortex. The data were consistent with the earlier study in suggesting that the pyramidal basal dendrites share the same alignment preference as the isofrequency contours.

Further evidence supporting the functional significance of pyramidal dendritic field orientation has recently been furnished by Tieman and Hirsch (1982). In cats reared under conditions in which only vertical or horizontal lines were viewed, analysis of dendrite fields of layer III pyramidal cells of the visual cortex disclosed shifts in the distribution of the field orientations that were correlated with the rearing condition. This result is in good agreement with earlier findings of dendritic shifts in both nonpyramidal (Coleman and Riesen, 1968; Valverde, 1968) and pyramidal neurons (Valverde, 1970) consequent upon manipulation of visual stimulation.

In summary, then, all of the dendritic systems of the pyramidal cell may have patterns of arborization which exhibit preferential rather than random orientations or geometries. Considerably more still remains to be done in this area, however. Anatomically, it will be particularly important to investigate further the significance of the pattern in terms of the details of intracortical connectivity, and the degree of consistency of the patterns both from cell to cell within given cortical regions and among the various dendritic systems of individual cells.

3.3. The Dendritic Spines

A major morphological feature of pyramidal cell dendrites is the presence of dendritic spines (Figs. 8, 11, 12, 14). Although by no means confined to neurons of the pyramidal type (Feldman and Peters, 1978), spines are present in abundance on the various dendrites of all typical pyramidal cells, where they function as the primary postsynaptic structures of the cell (Colonnier, 1968; Colonnier and Rossignol, 1969; Peters *et al.*, 1976). In considerably smaller numbers, spinelike structures are also occasionally encountered projecting from the cell body and axon of pyramidal cells. It is usually assumed that the latter are pre- rather than postsynaptic structures. Whether or not the spines have a functional significance beyond their status as simple postsynaptic structures is an issue of some neurobiological interest, but one which at the present time is also largely speculative (see Peters *et al.,* 1976; Schüz, 1978; Swindale, 1981).

The story of the controversy following Ramón y Cajal's original descriptions of the dendritic spines has been frequently recounted (Marin-Padilla, 1967; Scheibel and Scheibel, 1968). It was a controversy that persisted, stubbornly, until 1959, when Gray's electron microscopic observations of rat occipital cortex established unequivocally that spines were true protrusions of dendritic cytoplasm, enveloped by an extension of the plasma membrane of the dendritic shaft (Fig. 12).

Since the appearance of Gray's report, numerous accounts of spine ultrastructure have appeared. Among these is the description provided by Peters and Kaiserman-Abramof (1970) based on examination of layer II/III pyramids in rat parietal cortex. The spines described contain a wispy floccular material, similar to that observed between dendritic microtubules, in both the stalk and end bulb of the spine, so that the cytoplasmic matrix of the spine appears slightly darker than that of the parent dendrite (Fig. 12). Very occasionally, small numbers of ribosomes and round vesicles, some coated, are present. In the bulbs of larger spines a few microtubules may be encountered. Many spines, particularly the larger ones, contain a spine apparatus (Fig. 8), a cisternal organelle similar in form to one that may also be present in the axon initial segment (Peters *et al.,* 1968) and dendritic trunk (Kaiserman-Abramof and Peters, 1972) of pyram-

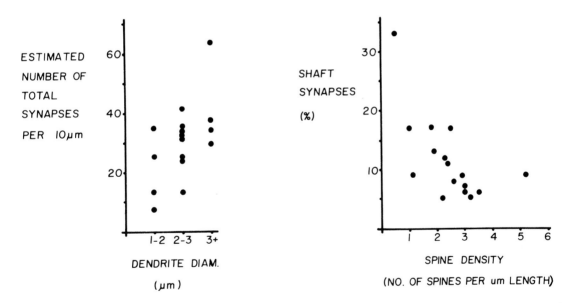

Figure 13. (Left) Estimated numbers of total synapses (on spines plus on shafts) per 10-μm length of apical dendrite as a function of apical dendritic diameter. Numbers of spine synapses are based on an average of 1.1 axospinous synapses per spine (about every 10th spine forms two synapses). Data points represent apical dendrites of 16 layer V pyramidal neurons. The data derive from reconstruction and analysis of tangentially oriented serial thin sections through layer IV in rat visual cortex. (Right) Percentage of synapses on apical dendritic shafts as a function of spine density. Shaft synapse percentages are calculated as number of synapses formed with the apical dendritic shaft divided by the total number of synapses formed with the dendrite (number of shaft synapses plus the estimated number of axospinous synapses). Data points and source of data as for previous graph.

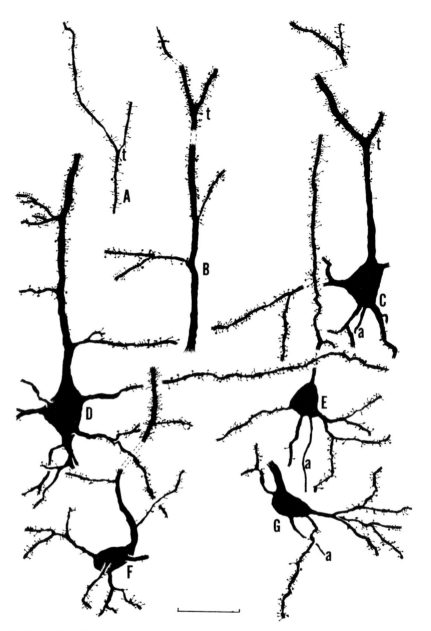

Figure 14. Examples of spine distributions on various pyramidal cell dendrites. Tracings from rat visual cortex, Golgi rapid impregnation. A, thin apical dendrite bifurcating into its terminal tuft (t). B, apical dendrite of deep layer II/III pyramid showing its initial spine-free portion; connected to this segment by dotted lines is the terminal tuft bifurcation (t) of the same dendrite; this is connected by dotted lines to a tracing of the tip of one of the terminal tuft dendrites. C, upper layer II/III neuron; note that the apical dendrite forms very few spines before the terminal tuft bifurcation (t); the dotted line connects to a tracing of a more distal segment of the terminal tuft. D, layer V pyramidal neuron. E, layer IV pyramidal neuron. F, G, layer VI pyramidal neurons. The dotted lines on the apical dendrite of cell F connect to a tracing of a segment of the same apical dendrite in layer V. The ventrally directed dendrite from cell G projects into the white matter. Calibration line, 25 μm.

idal neurons. The spine apparatus appears as originally described by Gray (1959), being composed of a variable number of flattened sacs, separated by 30- to 50-nm gaps containing thin dense laminae. On serial reconstruction, the sacs can be shown to be folds of a single complex cistern (see also Fairén and Valverde, 1973). Usually, the long axes of the sacs are oriented parallel to the length of the spine stalk. In many cases, the spine apparatus appears to be in continuity with the SER of the dendritic shaft. A number of spines, particularly the smaller ones, appear to lack a spine apparatus, as is also true in the cat (Colonnier, 1968). At the other extreme, the largest spines can have two or three apparently independent spine apparatuses.

In the light microscope, spines are commonly studied in Golgi preparations. A number of the investigations which have been carried out have involved quantitative assessment of the numbers of visible spines present along a given length of dendrite. Examples of obtained spine densities are given in Table II. As visualized in Golgi material, several types of spines are apparent. The classical dendritic spine of the cerebral cortex, and the type most commonly encountered, is of the stalk-and-bulb variety, termed *thin spines* in the account given by Peters and Kaiserman-Abramof (1970). The stalk of such a spine is approximately 0.5 μm or less in diameter, with the thinnest examples approaching the limits of resolution of the light microscope. The stalk extends outward, usually with some degree of curvature, from the dendritic shaft for a distance of from 0.5 to 4 μm. Despite this large range, the dimensions of the majority of these spines are reasonably constant (Jacobson, 1967), with an average length, in Peters and Kaiserman-Abramof's study, of 1.7 μm. Although occasional spines display forked stalks, with two bulbs, single stalks are the rule. The terminal bulb of the typical spine averages 0.5 to 1 μm in diameter, with diameters greater than 1 μm occurring only rarely.

As first pointed out by Jones and Powell (1969a), one of the sources of variation in the dimensions of thin spines of pyramidal neurons is the diameter of the parent dendrite, an observation consistent with the situation in hippocampal granule cells (Laatsch and Cowan, 1966). Large-diameter dendrites tend to have relatively small spines, while small-diameter dendrites tend to have, among their spine complement, a number of spines with both relatively long stalks and somewhat enlarged terminal bulbs. In the case of the smallest dendrites, the diameter of the bulb may exceed that of the dendritic shaft. A consequence of the inverse relationship between dendrite diameter and spine length is that there exists a tendency toward equalization of the diameters of the dendritic receptive zones, as measured from a spine tip to the tip of a spine on the opposite side of the dendrite, of small and large dendrites.

In addition to the thin spines, two additional types exist. Characteristic of the first of these are large terminal bulbs, up to about 1.5 μm in diameter. These spines are termed *mushroom-shaped spines* by Peters and Kaiserman-Abramof. They have a somewhat thicker stalk than the thin spines and constitute only a small proportion of the total spine complement. A final spine variety, the stubby spines, are quite short and thick, appearing as blunt nubbinlike projections which lack a discriminable stalk. These spines are also relatively infrequent, though they are somewhat more prevalent than the mushroom-shaped spines. They are often present in very small numbers as the most proximal spines of the apical

Table II. Examples of Densities of Visible Dendritic Spines as Observed in Normal Golgi-Impregnated Pyramidal Cells

Cortex	Dendrite measured	Typical spine density (spines/μm)[a]	Reference
Mouse, visual	Apical[b]	0.90	Valverde (1967)
Rat, visual	Apical	1.43	Feldman and Dowd (1974, 1975)
	Terminal tuft	0.74	
	Oblique br.	1.26	
	Basal	0.82	
Rat, visual	Apical[b]	0.73	Parnavelas *et al.* (1973)
	Terminal tuft[b]	0.58	
	Oblique br.[b]	0.67	
	Basal[b]	0.57	
Rat, visual	Apical[b]	1.12	Fifková (1970)
Rat, visual	Apical	0.65–0.75	Winkelmann *et al.* (1976)
Rat, sensory	Apical[b]	0.84	Kunz *et al.* (1972)
Hamster, frontal/parietal	Apical[b]	0.77	Marin-Padilla and Stibitz (1968)
Rabbit, visual	Apical	0.54	Globus and Scheibel (1967c)
	Terminal tuft	0.26	
	Oblique br.	0.40	
	Basal	0.32	
Macaque, motor	Apical	0.53–0.97	Kemper *et al.* (1973)
	Terminal tuft	0.29–0.54	
	Oblique br.	0.29–0.49	
	Basal	0.29–0.45	
Human, supramarginal gyrus	Apical[b]	0.62	Valverde (1970)
Human, motor	Apical[b]	1.03	Marin-Padilla (1967)

[a] Values reported in the original publications have been normalized in all cases to number of spines per 1-μm length of dendrite.
[b] Value given is for the region of the dendrite having the highest density of spines.

dendrite (Jones and Powell, 1969a; Peters and Kaiserman-Abramof, 1970). A point of interest concerning this specific spine type is the recent demonstration that its numbers in the rat are selectively affected by both housing conditions and aging. At 20 months of age, the density of this spine type is elevated in rats reared alone as compared with rats raised three per cage (Connor and Diamond, 1982). In addition, between the age of young adulthood and 21 months of age, the density of nubbinlike spines increases steadily (Connor *et al.*, 1980). In conjunction with the report of an overall spine loss with age (Feldman and Dowd, 1975), the latter finding might suggest that nubbinlike spines are altered or degenerative forms. However, at the present time good evidence for this proposition is completely lacking. One fact that is established, however, is that at least some of these spines form normal-appearing synapses (Jones and Powell, 1969a;

Figure 15. Upper layer II/III pyramidal neuron in rat area 39, Golgi rapid impregnation. The axon gives rise to a number of axon collaterals (arrows) which branch and ramify widely in various orientations through layer II/III. Calibration line, 25 μm.

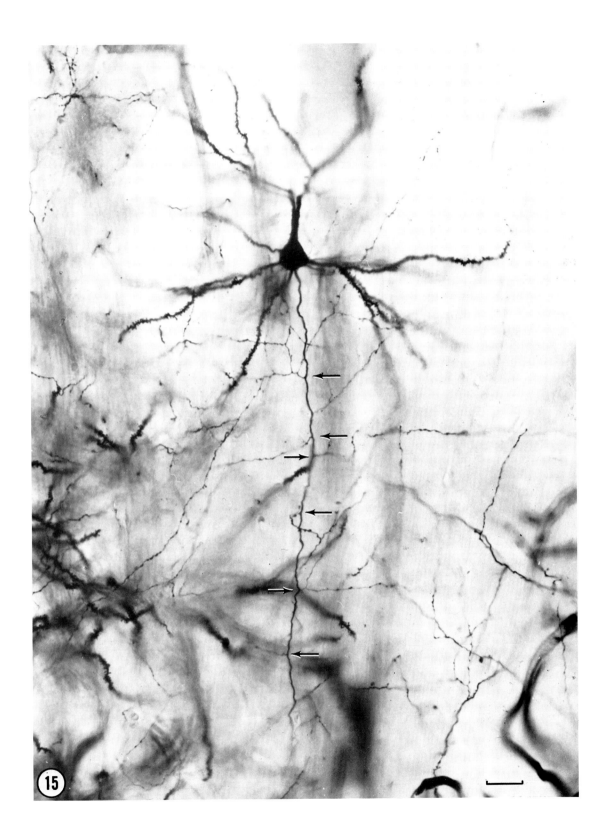

15

Peters and Kaiserman-Abramof, 1970). Whether spines in general undergo alterations in form under normal *in vivo* conditions is a question of great interest but one which remains unanswered at present. It does seem to be the case that changes in spine dimensions can be induced under experimental conditions, such as electrical stimulation (e.g., Fifková and Van Harreveld, 1977). Furthermore, certain populations of spine appear to contain actin (Fifková and Delay, 1982; Landis and Reese, 1982) and therefore to be at least potentially capable of form modulation.

Characteristically, the proximal dendritic trunks emanating from the pyramidal cell body are devoid of spines (Figs. 11, 14). This spine-free dendritic segment is longer in the case of the apical dendrite than in the case of the basal dendrites. At distances which range from 15 to 75 μm from their origins, the dendrites begin to acquire spines. These rapidly increase in number, with relatively high spine densities being maintained over the remainder of the dendritic tree. Quantitative study of the spine populations of entire apical dendrites has demonstrated that the spines are not distributed with uniform density in all regions of the dendrite (Table II and Fig. 14). For layer V cells of mouse visual cortex (Valverde, 1967), there occurs a general increase in mean spine density with increasing distance along the dendritic shaft. For most of the length of the apical dendrite, the increase is roughly exponential in form, the values approaching asymptote about halfway along the course of the dendrite. Studies on layer V pyramids in other species also reveal an orderly variation in spine density along the apical dendrite, although the form of the curve differs somewhat from the distribution described in the mouse in that the asymptotic level is not maintained over the distal half of the dendrite (see, for example, Fig. 11 in Valverde, 1970). In rat sensory cortex (Kunz *et al.*, 1972), an exponential increase is observed over the proximal third or so of the dendrite, reaching a peak at the level of layer IV. From that peak, however, there is a conspicuous decrease in spine density in successively more distal segments of the dendrite. In hamster frontal and parietal cortex (Marin-Padilla and Stibitz, 1968), the form of the distribution is similar, but there occurs a secondary peak around the midpoint of the dendrite. After an exponential rise in spine density and an asymptote at the layer III/IV border, the small secondary peak brings the spine density to a maximum in lower layer III. There then occurs a gradual linear decrease along the remainder of the dendrite. The same three components of the spine density curve, with a similar peak in lower layer III, are seen in cells of the human motor, somesthetic, and auditory cortices (Marin-Padilla, 1967; Marin-Padilla *et al.*, 1969). Analysis of the complex form of the distributions for the human and hamster data led Marin-Padilla and his co-workers to consider the possibility that the shape of the function results from the summation of several spine distribution curves, each with a Gaussian distribution. It was determined that in each species there did in fact exist a set of curves whose superposition produced a function quite close in form to the function originally obtained by spine-counting. In the hamster, four such curves were found, the highest peaking in layer III approximately coincident with the peak of the original distribution, and the remainder peaking in layer I, layer IV, and at the layer IV/V border. In the human, five curves were presented, the additional curve exhibiting a peak in layer II. The two sets of curves represent intriguing models which suggest an explanation of the observed regional variations in spine density. Within each set of curves, the individual component curves hypothetically represent relatively independent populations of spines. The curve peaking within layer IV, for example, would represent a population of spines that is postsynaptic to a population of axons which preferentially terminate in layer IV, such as the specific thalamic afferents. The other component curves would represent other spine populations, each associated with an afferent axonal system. Thus, the model would predict that the observed variations in spine density along the apical dendrite as a whole would be lamina-specific and would ultimately reflect the differential laminar patterning in the distribution of the various populations of afferent axons. These speculations are consistent with observed data showing examples of spine density changes which occur at the borders of laminae having discrete axonal inputs. In monkey visual cortex, for example, apical dendrite spines are reduced in number within the lower portion of layer IVc, and the point at which the spines begin on the apical dendrites of large layer Vb neurons is situated at the entrance of the dendrite into the upper portion of layer IVc (Lund, 1973).

As a general rule, spine densities on terminal tufts, oblique branches, and basal dendrites (Table II) are not as high as those seen on the densely spined portions of the apical dendrite (Globus and Scheibel, 1966, 1967b; Feldman and Dowd, 1975; Parnavelas *et al.*, 1977a), although the various spine densities may be correlated for individual neurons (Schüz, 1978). Whether the spine densities on the nonapical dendrites exhibit regular sequential changes along their lengths as has been reported for apical dendrites is not yet established with certainty. In addition to dendritic locus, other factors which influence spine density are cortical depth and dendrite diameter. In rat (Parnavelas *et al.*, 1977a), rabbit (Globus and Scheibel, 1966, 1967b), and primate cortex (Kemper *et al.*, 1973), spine densities appear to be higher on more superficially situated pyramidal cells. In the primate study, this was observed to be true of all of the dendritic systems—terminal tufts, apical dendrite shafts, oblique branches, and basal dendrites—of comparable pyramids. With respect to the influence of shaft diameter on spine density, several relevant studies have been done on rat visual cortex. In one, apical dendrites were reconstructed from serial thin sections (Feldman, 1975), and in a second, spine counts were carried out on normal Golgi material (Feldman and Dowd, 1975). In both sets of observations, a clear positive relationship between spine density and dendrite diameter was noted (Fig. 13). Results consistent with this conclusion have since been reported for populations of aged rats by Connor and Diamond (1982) and for young adult animals by Rothblat and Schwartz (1979). Linear regression analyses done by the latter authors indicate that for normal cortex, approximately 50% of the variance in spine density can be related to dendrite diameter. Diameter therefore needs to be regarded as a significant variable in quantitative spine studies.

In almost all of the studies referred to above, the numbers of dendritic spines have been quantified on Golgi-impregnated dendrites. Such enumerations, consisting of counts of the total number of visible spines, inevitably underestimate the true number of spines present in the dendritic length examined. This is true because only a portion of the existing spines will be visible by virtue of their extension into the clear area flanking the margins of the dendritic shaft.

Many, and in some cases most, of the spines will not be visible and hence will remain uncounted since they will be hidden from view either in front of or behind the opaque dendritic shaft. This circumstance has been recognized by many workers (e.g., Chan-Palay *et al.,* 1974; McConnell and Berry, 1978) but there has been little appreciation of the magnitude of the underestimation, and equally important, its variability from dendrite to dendrite and from segment to segment of the same dendrite. This question has been directly addressed in a study carried out by Feldman and Peters (1979). They point out that the degree of underestimation may be as little as 20% or as much as 70%. It is therefore possible for two dendrite segments to yield visible spine counts which, in terms of spine number per unit length, are equal but which represent true spine numbers that differ significantly. This places a very serious restriction on the comparability of visible spine counts within or between dendrite populations. The two major variables governing the magnitude of the underestimation are dendrite shaft diameter and the length of the spines. The greater the diameter of the shaft segment studied and the shorter the average spine length, the higher the proportion of spines that will be obscured. For example, in the determination of spine density along the course of an apical dendrite shaft, it may be found that the shaft diameter will decrease along a proximodistal gradient, and that along the same gradient spine length will increase (e.g., see Jones and Powell, 1969a). Under these conditions, visible spine counts in proximal segments of the dendrite may seriously underrepresent the true spine population present, whereas counts done on distal segments may more closely approximate the true spine density of the segment. Thus, what is required for the most accurate analysis and comparison is a method of estimating true spine density that takes the above factors into account. Such a method, with an independent confirmation of its accuracy, is presented by Feldman and Peters (1979).

While accurate comparison of dendritic spine numbers in Golgi material requires recognition of the factors just discussed, it is nevertheless true that appreciable differences in spine numbers will be revealed by simple enumeration of visible spines. Therefore, in Golgi studies which focus on differences in visible spine counts, there should ordinarily be little question concerning the existence of reported differences that are relatively large, although in all cases the absolute values of the various spine densities need to be interpreted with considerable caution.

In recent years, the differences in observed spine densities which have received the most attention are those which are useful in differentiating neuronal types and those which are observed on pyramidal neurons that are not typical of the normal young adult cortex. Cells in the latter category are those which have undergone alteration as a result of factors such as advancing age, pathogenetic and hereditary abnormalities, and experimental manipulations. That such factors may be reflected in altered spine densities was discovered in the period immediately following Ramón y Cajal's description of spines (Monti, 1895; Demoor, 1898; Querton, 1898; Soukhanoff, 1898a,b). Among the variables explored in this early work were chemical stimulation, sleep state, and food intake. Work in the modern period has been extensive and wide-ranging. Included in the specific entities to which spine density has been reported to be sensitive are experimentally produced deafferentation, alteration of sensory input by surgical or environmental manipulation, undernutrition, X-irradiation, chromosomal abnormalities such as the trisomies, and senile dementia. No attempt will be made here to review this literature. For references, the reader is referred to the papers by Feldman and Dowd (1975), Huttenlocher (1975), Ryugo *et al.* (1975a,b), Mehraein *et al.* (1975), Marin-Padilla (1976), Winkelmann *et al.* (1976, 1977), Parnavelas (1978), Rothblat and Schwartz (1979), Brizzee *et al.* (1980), Connor *et al.* (1980), Salas (1980), and Heumann and Rabinowicz (1982).

3.4. The Axon and Its Projections

As visualized in Golgi preparations, the typical pyramidal cell axon emerges from the base of the cell body by means of a small conical protrusion of the perikaryon, the axon hillock. Somewhat less frequently, the axon originates either by means of a common stem with a basal dendrite or from the trunk of a basal dendrite. In the latter instances, the axon origin is often located at a distance of 5–10 μm from the cell body, although distances up to 30 μm have been encountered (Sloper and Powell, 1979).

The study of axonal trajectories in Golgi preparations from adult material is hampered by the fact that a majority of the axons are impregnated for only a short distance beyond their origin. Commonly, this distance corresponds to the length of the proximal unmyelinated portion of the axon, or initial segment, which in monkey cortex measures 23–55 μm (Sloper and Powell, 1973, 1979). While most pyramidal cell axons do acquire a myelin sheath, there are some which appear to remain unmyelinated (Peters, 1981; Winfield *et al.*, 1981).

In cases in which the full extent of the axon is impregnated (Fig. 15), enabling it to be followed through the cortex, its main process can be seen to project downward into the white matter. The orientation of its trajectory parallels that of the apical dendrites. Along the intracortical course of the axon, collateral branches are given off (Fig. 15). These run in a variety of directions and vary widely in extent and degree of ramification. In comparison with the appearance of the dendrites of the pyramidal cell, the axon is thin, nontapering, and smooth-surfaced. While occasional spinelike protrusions from the axonal surface may be visible, these are never as densely distributed as the spines studding the dendrites. Observations of axonal thicknesses frequently reveal diameters in the range of 0.5–1 μm, and when large numbers of pyramidal cells of various sizes are examined, there appears to be a general positive relationship between somal size and axon diameter (Shkol'nik-Yarros, 1971; Sloper and Powell, 1979).

The extension of the pyramidal cell axon down into the white matter appears to be a feature common to most but not all pyramidal neurons, since a number of indpendent reports have described cells whose axons remain entirely intracortical. Examples of such neurons are the pyramids described by Ramón y Cajal (1899) in cat and human cortex, Shkol'nik-Yarrows (1971) in monkey and human, and Gilbert and Wiesel (1982) in cat. In Sholl's (1956) classification of cell types in cat cortex, such cells form one of the four categoreis of pyramidal cells, the "P4" cell. In Lund and Boothe's (1975) study in the monkey, cells which have only recurrent axons are described in each of the two sublaminae of layer V. In both strata the cells have a poorly developed apical dendrite and have axons which curve in recurrent fashion to ramify in the supragranular layers. As illustrated by Lund and Boothe, the axons of these cells leave the cell body and head down toward the white matter for distances of approxiamtely 35 and 50 μm before exhibiting a sharp upward bend. In addition to pyramidal cells with intrinsic axons, it is of interest to note that there also exist nonpyramidal neurons whose axons do project into the white matter (e.g., Ramón y Cajal, 1899; Lund *et al.*, 1975; Segraves and Rosenquist, 1982). One thing that seems clear from these examples is that axonal projection to the white matter is not an infallible criterion in the differential classification of pyramidal and nonpyramidal neurons.

Several studies have examined the ultrastructure of the initial portion of the axon. The first complete report that focused on the pyramidal cell was that of Peters *et al.*, (1968) in which the axon hillock and initial segment of layer II/III pyramids in rat parietal cortex were described. The principal findings have since been confirmed in other cortices (e.g., Sloper and Powell, 1979). As described in the rat, the plasma membrane of the axon is lined by an electron-dense undercoating (Palay *et al.*, 1968) approximately 10 nm thick. The undercoating begins at the distal narrowing of the axon hillock and defines the proximal boundary of the initial segment. In instances where the axon arises from a dendrite, the undercoating begins at the point of axon origin. The undercoating continues as far as the point at which the axon acquires a myelin sheath. In certain specific cell types, the normally continuous nature of the undercoating may display periodic interruptions as a characteristic feature (Braak *et al.*, 1980). But as a general rule, only occasional gaps are seen and these occur in highly specific positions, either at postsynaptic sites or in regions where cisternal organelles lie in close proximity to the plasma membrane. These cisternae tend to be peripherally located in the axoplasm and, in their most typical form, consist of several longitudinally aligned flattened sacs. The sacs are separated by gaps which are 40 nm in width and which contain plates of dense material.

A further characteristic of the initial segment described by Peters and colleagues is the presence of longitudinally oriented fascicles of microtubules. The fascicles originate within the axon hillock as aggregates of three or four microtubules. As these funnel down into the initial segment, additional microtubules join the aggregations. As a result, within the initial segment proper, there commonly exist five to seven fascicles, the number depending to some extent on axon diameter (Peters *et al.*, 1976), each containing approximately 6–12 microtubules. In the case of axon origins from dendrites rather than from a perikaryal axon hillock, the microtubular fascicles entering the intital segment originate only in the dendritic cytoplasm at the side from which the axon arises. As seen in transverse sections of the initial segment, the microtubules within a fascicle are arrayed in a row, with individual microtubules connected to their neighbors by thin crossbridges. In longitudinal sections, the crossbridges between two neighboring microtubules are seen as a series of linear elements arranged like the rungs of a ladder.

Within the axon hillock, the number of ribosomes, both free and attached to cisternae of endoplasmic reticulum, is diminished by comparison with the remainder of the perikaryon. Additional ribosomes in quite small numbers may be scattered through the initial segment, and only very occasionally are small

cisternae of RER encountered. These features account for the absence of ba-
sophilia, and hence the paleness of staining, in the axon hillock and initial
segment when examined in the light microscope after staining with basic dyes.
Among the other organelles present are mitochondria and neurofilaments, and
these tend to assume a longitudinal orientation within the initial segment. Many
initial segments have been observed to bear spinelike protrusions. These, in the
primate, vary from small sessile pegs to large pedunculated forms lined by a
continuation of the axolemmal undercoating which projects into them (Sloper
and Powell, 1979). It is probable that these protrusions are pre- rather than
postsynaptic structures.

A feature of interest concerning the proximal portion of the axon is its
specific involvement in several neuropathological processes. In aged human
tissue, a number of pyramidal cells of the third layer develop spindle-shaped
enlargements (Braak, 1979; Braak et al., 1980; see Chapter 3). These begin as
slight conical swellings and develop into giant spindles containing many lipofuscin granules but bearing normal synapses. The microtubular fascicles are
either lacking or pushed aside, and the axolemma lacks the dense undercoating,
particularly in regions adjacent to lipofuscin granules. At the distal end of the
dilation, a normal-appearing length of axon initial segment emerges and sub-
seqeuntly gives rise to typical axonal collaterals. A second example of abnormal
enlargement of the intial segment results from defects in the activity of specific
lysosomal hydrolases, producing neuronal storage diseases such as Tay–Sachs.
The enlargements have been seen both in affected humans and in a feline model,
and have been referred to by Purpura as meganeurites (Purpura and Suzuki,
1976; Walkley et al., 1981). The enlargements are fusiform, globular, or irregular, and may significantly exceed the cell body in size. Their proximal ends
may be adjacent to the base of the cell body or as much as 60 μm from it. They
may possess numerous spines, and in some cases filopodia, and they receive
synapses, although at least some of these are abnormal (Purpura and Suzuki,
1976; Purpura et al., 1978). The interiors of the meganeurites, presumably the
sites of storage of undigested substrates, are densely packed with spherical lamellar bodies. Although the enlargements emerge from the base of pyramidal
cell bodies and are continued distally by axons that appear to be normal in Golgi
preparations, the nature of the surface of the meganeurite has led Purpura and
co-workers to emphasize the "dendritelike" nature of the structures. Examinaton
of the dendritic arborizations and spines of affected neurons does not reveal
any abnormality.

Careful study of light microscopic preparations in which axonal arborizations are well impregnated has, in recent years, given rise to an enhanced appreciation of the intracortical distribution of pyramidal cell axon collaterals (Fig.
15). This has come about in part because of the ability of newer techniques such
as intracellular marker injections or retrograde filling with horseradish peroxidase to reveal axonal branch distributions (White et al., 1980). These methods
afford a very advantageous supplement to the Gogli impregnation approach.
Additionally, they appear in many cases to fully stain the entire collateral system,
and they afford some degree of experimental control over the location of the
cell body whose axon is to be studied. It is also pertinent to observe that the
extent of collateralization of intracellularly labeled axons often appears to be

appreciably greater than that revealed in Golgi studies. This point will be discussed more fully below. A second reason for the increased interest in pyramidal intracortical projections is the discovery in the cortex of discrete assemblies of neurons in which the component cellular elements share particular functional properties. The vertical organization of some of these assemblies in columnar or slablike arrays (Mountcastle, 1957; Hubel and Wiesel, 1963, 1969) has focused attention on anatomical features which could serve as links uniting the elements of the assemblies. Among such features, which include afferent axons of subcortical origin and the axons of intrinsic nonpyramidal neurons, are the axon collaterals of the pyramidal neurons. Of these, an obvious candidate for a role in vertical interlinking are the collaterals of the so-called recurrent variety, which ascend through the cortex in a vertical orientation. In addition to such recurrent collaterals, it has long been known that many pyramidal axon collaterals ramify in an oblique or predominatly horizontal trajectory (Lorente de Nó, 1943). Branches of this type are also of current interest in veiw of their potential role in influencing receptive field and lamina-specific functional properties of cortical units (Gilbert and Wiesel, 1979).

Surveys of intracortical collaterals of pyramidal cell axons reveal a wide range of collateral lengths, branching patterns, and orientations. That this variation in collateralization may not be haphazard was recognized by Lorente de Nó (1943), who expressed the belief that the cortical distribution of the axonal branches was as systematic as that of the dendrites. Much of the recent anatomical work in this area has been directed toward the substantiation of this proposition.

In Lund and Boothe's (1975) Golgi study of macaque visual cortex, systematic data are presented for the axon collaterals of pyramidal neurons in various cortical laminae. The collateralization patterns of such lamina-specific neurons are related to particular patterns of dendritic arborization of the same cells and to some of the major afferent projections to the cortex. For the most part, the data are limited to primarily vertical, or interlaminar, connections formed by the collateral branches. In some cases, however, it is clear that there exist important axonal projections in the horizontal plane. For example, the axons of pyramids of layers IVa and IVb provide lateral branches which contribute to the horizontal fiber plexus of layer IVb. One of the interesting points to emerge from the data of Lund and Boothe is the finding that almost all pyramidal neurons have recurrent collaterals that arborize in one or more laminae above the level of the cell body. For this reason, there is a particularly abundant pyramidal collateral input to the upper reaches of the cortex, in layers II and III, although collateral terminations in layer I do not appear to be present. In addition, the pyramidal axons have further collaterals that branch from the main descending axon to innervate specific laminae below the cell body. One exception to this latter generalization is the class of pyramids in layer Va which have a very poorly developed apical dendrite. These cells may lack a descending axonal projection. For certain cells, the descending axonal pattern is characterized as much by an absence of collateralization in certain laminae as by its presence. Layer II and IIIa pyramids, for example, are conspicuously devoid of branches to any of the sublaminae of layer IV, although in cat visual cortex, Tömböl (1975) has noted the projection of layer III cell axon collaterals into layer IV. Typically, pyramidal axons, in addition to their ascending and descending projections, provide local collaterals that arborize in the lamina of the cell body. In some cases, this is an extensive input. Local pyramidal collateralization within layer VI, for example, is reported by Lund and Boothe to constitute the most prolific source of axon terminals in that lamina. Similarly, it would appear that in the adult monkey, the pyramidal axon contribution to layer IV arises primarily or only from neurons whose cell bodies are situated within that layer. Individual pyramidal cell axons may collateralize within as many as seven of the cortical sublaminae, providing innervation to regions widely distributed through the thickness of the cortex. Individual layer IVb pyramids, for example, may provide recurrent collateral arborizations to layers II, IIIa, and IVb; further branches near the cell body may collateralize locally in layer IVb; and branches from the descending axons may project into the upper half of layer IVc and into layers Vb and VI. In other cases, relatively few collaterals are observed. The axons of layer II pyramids, and upper layer III pyramids, after initially giving rise to a local arborization, descend through the cortex largely unbranched, giving rise to collaterals only within layer Vb. Parenthetically, Lund and Boothe note that the descending axon trunks of the layer II pyramids often exhibit profusely spinous surfaces as they pass through layers II and III. The authors favor the view that these spines are postsynaptic structures. A final observation that may be cited from this study is the existence of instances of coextensive arborization of the axon collaterals and the dendrites of the same pyramidal neurons. For example, axon collaterals of the layer II and IIIa pyramids, and of certain layer VI pyramids observed in young animals, ramify among their own apical dendritic arborizations. Instances of similar interdigitations have also been reported in other studies (e.g., Gilbert and Wiesel, 1981).

In a recent quantitative study of squirrel monkey visual cortex, Tigges and Tigges (1982) have reported on the axon collaterals of layer II and III pyramids in young animals. In a population of 115 axons, 705 collateral branches were observed. This represents an average of approximately six collaterals per axon, a figure in reasonable agreement with the figure of eight per axon in rat visual cortex (Paldino and Harth, 1977a). The observed distribution of these collaterals strongly reinforces the principle of specificity of pyramidal cell axon collateralization. Of the 705 branches studied, 47% were local collaterals, originating within layers II/III, and 49% had their origins in layer V. This latter projection is one that has repeatedly been observed qualitatively (Lorente de Nó, 1922; O'Leary, 1941; Spatz et al., 1970; Gilbert and Wiesel, 1981). Tigges and Tigges also observed that the axons of layer V pyramids gave rise to recurrent collaterals projecting upward to layers II/III. The two levels of the cortex, layer V and layers II/III, thus appear to be reciprocally connected by pyramidal axon collaterals, a finding in good agreement with the results of Lund and Boothe (1975). As in Lund and Boothe's study, Tigges and Tigges did not emphasize the horizontal extent of the collateral branches observed. They did, however, point out that the collaterals arising in layer V typically give rise to a number of branches and are oriented horizontally, i.e., parallel to the cortical laminae.

As in the case of the analysis of dendritic fields, one approach that has been taken to the study of Golgi-impregnated intracortical pyramidal axon collaterals is the use of computer-assisted morphometric techniques. Such studies are aimed at defining the topographic characteristics of axonal arborizations in geometrical terms. Because this is an area which has not been extensively investigated, the results of one such study, that of Paldino and Harth (1977a), will be described. In this study, 39 axons of layer III and IV pyramidal cells of rat visual cortex were analyzed in single sections, i.e., the cut ends of axonal branches were not followed into adjacent sections. The axons studied gave rise to a total of 315 intracortical collateral branches. Examination of the angles the initial segments of these collaterals form with the vertical axes of their cells reveals a strong preference for 90%, indicating an initial horizontal course oriented perpendicularly to the parent axon. Also investigated was the angular direction in which the individual initial segments of the collaterals projected as they left the parent axon. In terms of azimuth (measured in a plane parallel to the pial surface), these angular directions are nonrandom, the collaterals apparently favoring extension in the sagittal plane. It is important to bear in mind, however, that only single sections, of 100-μmm thickness, were examined in this study and that these sections were cut in the sagittal plane. When whole axons, each with all of its collateral branches, are considered, various azimuthal projection patterns are observed. For some axons, the azimuthal distribution patterns of collateral endpoints is isotropic. In other words, if one were to look down upon the main axonal stem from a vantage point at the cell body, the endpoints of the collateral branches of that axon would be seen to be randomly distributed over the full 360°. In other cases, the collateral endpoints are confined to either one relativley narrow sector, which may be as small as 50°, or two narrow sectors approximately 180° apart. In still other cases, the endpoints have a wide azimuthal distribution but there are restricted void sectors into which no collaterals project. From the same perikaryal vantage point, it is possible to measure the average horizontal distance from the main axonal stem to the collateral endpoints. This yields an average radius for the columnar regions into which the axon collaterals extend. For the axonal fields studied, this figure is 64 μm, a value similar to the 100-μm radius found by Chiang (1973) for pyramidal cells located in layers II–IV.

Published measurements of the horizontal spread of Golgi-impregnated axon collaterals within the cortex have varied widely. However, it is only within the past several years that the great extent of some of these intracortical collaterals has been appreciated (Scheibel and Scheibel, 1970; Landry *et al.*, 1980). Among the long trajectories reported is the figure of 6–8 mm for a pyramidal neuron in cat visual cortex observed by Gilbert and Wiesel (1979). The pyramidal neuron described is one which was physiologically determined to be a standard complex cell in lower layer V and whose axon was filled by postrecording injection with horseradish peroxidase. In addition to an axonal process entering the white matter and an obliquely oriented collateral projecting upward into layers II/III, the long collateral illustrated by Gilbert and Wiesel extends horizontally to one side of the cell body. There is one branch point near its origin, but no further branching is apparent for several hundred micrometers. The terminals to which the collateral gives rise occur primarily in layer VI, with a smaller number being present in layer V. The projection, in spite of its great length, remains within area 17, although it extends over an area of cortex which represents a far greater area of the visual field than the field area of the parent cell. In a subsequent study (Gilbert and Wiesel, 1982), pyramidal cells with comparably long intracortical collaterals were found in superficial (layers II/III) as well as deep laminae of the cortex. The long horizontal axonal branches of the layer II/III neurons gave rise to axon collaterals both in layers II/III and in layer V. Interestingly, these collaterals were given off in clusters, and in one case the superficial set of clusters was superimposed directly over the clusters of layer V.

A second example of a site in which long horizontal collaterals have been observed is in the visual cortex of the tree shrew (Rockland *et al.*, 1982). In this species, in which the cortex is smaller than that of the cats studied by Gilbert and Wiesel, collateral extents of over 1 mm are present. The collaterals arise from the axons of small and medium pyramidal neurons high in layer II. They appear to be sparsely branched compared with those in the cat and are distributed within layers I and II.

Electron microscopic examination of Golgi preparations has demonstrated that the typical intracortical collaterals of pyramidal axons give rise to asymmetric synapses. These principally involve both dendritic spines and dendritic shafts (LeVay, 1973; Parnavelas *et al.*, 1977b; Somogyi, 1978; White *et al.*, 1980; Lund, 1981; Winfield *et al.*, 1981). Unfortunately, the precise cell types giving rise to these postsynaptic structures are for the most part unknown. Their identity will undoubtedly represent an important advance in our understanding of the functional organization of the cortex. Recently, Schüz *et al.* (1982) have reconstructed from serial thin sections a 70-μm length of Golgi-impregnated pyramidal axon collateral in mouse cortex in order to analyze the distribution of the synapses it formed. The collateral gave rise to 17 synapses, an average of one every 4 μm, although it was found that the synapses were not evenly distributed. Rather they were concentrated along the distal 44 μm of the reconstructed segment, very few synapses arising from the proximal third of the segment beginning at its origin from the parent axon. Whether or not this pattern is characteristic is not yet known, but the findings are consistent with the hypothesis that synapses arising from at least some axon collaterals may occur in clusters with preferential locations that may depend on distance from the branch point. It would seem at least equally plausible that the sites of synaptic concentrations may be a function of the types of postsynaptic elements occurring in the various regions through which the collateral courses.

In a related study, carried out in primate somatic sensory cortex, Winfield *et al.* (1981) reconstructed from a series of about 600 serial thin sections the proximal axon and collaterals of a small pyramidal cell that had been Golgi-impregnated. The cell body was situated at the layer II/III border, and the axon, which was unmyelinated, originated from one of the basal dendrites. The reconstruction of the main stem of the axon covered the first 700 μm of its length, which represented a vertically downward extension to upper layer V. Along this course three types of collateral structures were observed and reconstructed. The first of these consisted of a group of three upwardly curving collaterals that arose at distances of 50–80 μm from the cell body. These collaterals were about 100 μm in length and extended obliquely up to layer I, ramifying within the cell's dendritic field but not making contact with the dendrites. A second group of collaterals consisted of four horizontally disposed branches, each 25–50 μm in length, which arose 350–450 μm from the cell body. At least one of these branches was not completely impregnated over its entire actual length. Finally, many spinelike side branches, 2–10 μm in length, were observed on the main stem and on the collaterals. Like typical dendritic spines, these processes had narrow stalks with bulbous terminal enlargements approximately 1 μm in diameter. They were separated from one another by an average distance of 10 μm along the main axon and 16 μm along the collaterals. In all, 62 synapses, all asymmetric, were identified, 49 formed by the main axon and 13 by the collaterals. Almost all of these were formed by the spinelike structures. In one case, two nonadjacent spines each formed one synapse with a dendritic spine and a second synapse with a spine-free dendritic shaft. While the various axonal shafts exhibited varicosities, in only one instance was such a varicosity observed to form a synapse. At sites where the main axon was apposed to the perikaryon of another neuron, no evidence of a synapse was seen. Analysis of the postsynaptic components of the synapses formed showed that 40% of them were dendritic spines of unidentified origin and 60% spine-free dendritic shafts. This proportion was the same for the synapses formed by the spines of the main axon and the spines of the axon collaterals. About half of the postsynaptic spine-free dendritic shafts were of small or medium diameter, were only rarely seen to receive other synapses, were not varicose, and could not be identified as arising from a particular cortical cell type. The remaining postsynaptic shafts formed many symmetric and asymmetric synapses, were slightly varicose in outline, contained abundant mitochondria and ribosomes, and ran in straight-line courses for considerable distances. One cell type in primate somatic sensory cortex with dendritic features similar to this description is a large nonpyramidal cell (Sloper *et al.,* 1979).

After giving rise to its intracortical collateral arborizations, the main axonal stem typically projects into the white matter underlying the cortex. Three destinations are possible: Intrahemispheric, to other regions of cortex on the same side of the brain; interhemispheric, to the contralateral cortex, usually via the corpus callosum; and subcortical, to terminal areas which may extend as far caudally as the spinal cord. Many of the details of these projections are discussed in Chapter 16 of the present volume and will not be reviewed here. There are, however, several features of general interest that deserve emphasis.

In recent years, the study of pyramidal extracortical projections has received renewed impetus from the development of techniques such as those involving horseradish peroxidase and tritiated amino acids. The use of modern tracing techniques has not only broadened our knowledge of the specific projections (e.g., Wise and Jones, 1977; Jones *et al.,* 1979; Lund *et al.,* 1981) but is leading to an appreciation of the interactions that occur among projections (Goldman-Rakic and Schwartz, 1982). A clear principle which has emerged from this work is the laminar specificity of the pyramidal cell populations giving rise to the various extracortical projections from given regions (Gilbert and Kelly, 1975; Lund *et al.,* 1975) The pyramids in the various sublaminae of layer V of monkey sensory motor cortex, for example, each give rise to different subcortical projections to the striatum, brain stem, and spinal cord (Jones *et al.,* 1977). Further, the multiple projections from given cortical regions may involve different proportions of the pyramidal cells in the specific laminae of origin (Gilbert and Kelly, 1975; Segraves and Rosenquist, 1982). An additional dimension of the specificity principle is introduced by the fact that the morphological organization of the extracortical projections may vary significantly among species and among cortical regions (Ebner, 1969; Wise, 1975; Jayaraman, 1982).

The principle of laminar specificity would suggest that different projections from a cortical region arise from entirely discrete populations of pyramidal cells. However, it is not uncommon to find some degree of overlap in the laminar boundaries demarcating different populations of projection neurons. This raises the possibility that there may exist some pyramidal cells whose axons project to more than one extracortical field. One means by which this question can be approached is through the use of two different and distinctive retrogradely transported labels. Following the injection of one of the two labels into each of the two suspected terminal fields, the observation of doubly labeled perikarya in the cortex of origin would indicate cells with dual projections. Mixed results have been obtained in the recent experiments employing this technique. In some cases, only singly labeled cells are observed (Wong and Kelly, 1981; Andersen *et al.*, 1982). In other cases, however, doubly labeled cells have been found. In Goldman-Rakic and Schwartz's (1982) studies with developing and adult macaque cortex, separate dye injections (propidium iodide, fast blue, or nuclear yellow) were made into the principal sulcus and into the intraparietal sulcus of the opposite hemisphere. In several regions of cortex, in addition to singly labeled neurons, a population of medium-sized pyramids was found to be doubly labeled. Such cells therefore appear to have axonal projections into both ipsilateral and contralateral cortical regions.

Another aspect of extracortical projections which has been of recent interest is the experimental study of axonal distribution under nonnormal conditions. In one paradigm commonly studied in loci other than neocortex, interest centers upon the sprouting of intact axons into terminal fields not normally innervated by those axons. The condition producing this abnormal sprouting is denervation of the terminal field, particularly when carried out on young animals (Liu and Chambers, 1958; Raisman, 1969; Guillery, 1972; Cotman and Lynch, 1976). In a study carried out by Mustari (1975), the projections to the tectum of pyramidal cells in rat visual cortex were examined. Normally, these projections are entirely ipsilateral. However, after removing the cortex on one side, the remaining cortex was found to project to the superior colliculus, bilaterally. Furthermore, the aberrant contralateral projection exhibited the normal pattern of topographic distribution within the colliculus. It thus appears that the denervated tectum exerts some influence on the pyramidal axons in the contralateral pathway. Whether this is due to some mechanism of attraction or to the absence of inhibitory factors, or to some other mechanism, is not known. A second approach to the experimental study of factors influencing pyramidal axonal distribution has recently been taken by Kalil and Reh (1982). They unilaterally severed the hamster pyramidal tract just rostral to its point of decussation and subseqently examined the course of the severed axons. Commonly, such a procedure when carried out in the central nervous system results in the degeneration of the axons distal to the cut, often accompanied by collateral sprouts that form inappropriate terminations (Ramón y Cajal, 1928; Bernstein and Bernstein, 1973). In Kalil and Reh's study, however, the severed axons gave rise to collaterals that formed normal connections with the dorsal column nuclei and in the spinal cord, although they decussated in an aberrant manner. It thus appears that pyramidal axons may, in certain restricted cases, regenerate following injury.

A final example of the study of pyramidal axonal projections under non-normal conditions is the work of Simmons *et al.* (1982) in the visual cortex of the Reeler mouse. In this mutant, the postmigratory pyramidal cells in the young animal come to rest in abnormal laminae of the cortex (Caviness, 1976). Nevertheless, the projection of their axons to other cortical regions was observed in this study to be indistinguishable from the situation in normal animals. The connections also exhibited the same precise retinotopicity as in normals. In comparing the results in Reeler with those in the normal mouse, Simmons and colleagues express the view that the corticocortical projection cells are the same in both forms, i.e., layer V pyramidal cells which are present in the upper strata of the Reeler cortex and small layer II/III pyramidal cells which are positioned deep in the Reeler cortex. It would thus appear that the laminar specificty of pyramidal axonal projections is not necessarily inherent, in the sense of pre-destination, in the laminae themselves under all conditions.

3.5. The Axon Terminals Synapsing with the Pyramidal Cell Surface

In Colonnier's (1968) early electron microscopic study of synaptic patterns in the cerebral cortex, it was noted that the perikarya of pyramidal neurons formed very few synapses and that these were of the symmetrical variety, with the axon terminals containing flattened vesicles. In many subsequent studies, these findings have been abundantly confirmed. In single thin sections (Fig. 10), it is usual to encounter only one to six axosomatic synapses (Peters and Kaiser-man-Abramof, 1970; Jones and Powell, 1970; Parnavelas *et al.*, 1977b), usually of the *en passant* form (Peters and Kaiserman-Abramof, 1970). In layer IV of cat visual cortex, there occurs an average of 10.8 synaptic contacts/100 μm^2 of perikaryal surface (Davis and Sterling, 1979).

The synaptic vesicles of the axosomatic axon terminals have generally been assumed to be exclusively nonspherical in shape. Recently, however, contrary evidence has been presented. Kennedy (1982), in a study of cat visual cortex, retrogradely labeled with horseradish peroxidase corticotectal pyramids in layer V. Examined in the electron microscope, the pyramidal cell bodies showed not only flat-vesicle axosomatic terminals but also terminals containing spherical vesicles. The latter endings constituted 28% of all the axosomatic endings studied, and 28% of cells examined revealed both types of synapses on the same perikaryon. It is not clear why other investigators have not encountered spherical-vesicle endings. One obvious suggestion is that such endings may be a unique feature of the corticotectal cells examined by Kennedy, or perhaps they are rarer on the more superficial pyramids which have been the ones primarily studied in the past.

Synapses are also present on the spines which project from the perikaryon. These synapses in the rat resemble those formed with the unspecialized surface of the perikaryon, and Peters and Kaiserman-Abramof (1970) have illustrated an axon terminal synapsing with both a somatic spine and the perikaryal surface. It appears, therefore, that the somatic spines are of a different nature than the dendritic spines, which typically form asymmetric synapses.

Axon terminals are commonly observed to form synapses with the axon hillock and initial segment of the pyramidal cell (Peters *et al.*, 1968; Palay *et al.*, 1968; see Chapter 10). These synapses are symmetrical, whether formed with the axonal shaft or with spinous protrusions from it, and the vesicles in the presynaptic axon terminal are nonspherical (Jones and Powell, 1969b; Sloper, 1973; Sloper and Powell, 1979). Characteristically, the dense axolemmal undercoating is absent at the sites of axoaxonic synapse, its position being occupied by the dense material of the postsynaptic fuzz. Areas of axoaxonic membranes apposition may be extensive, with the presynaptic terminal enwrapping half or more of the diameter of the postsynaptic shaft. The actual synaptic complex, frequently with an adjacent punctum adhaerens, occupies only a small portion of this contact area. Serial reconstructions in primate cortex (Sloper and Powell, 1979) have shown that the cisternal organelles within the postsynaptic axons are preferentially apposed to the plasma membrane opposite the nondifferentiated portions of synapsing axon terminals. One cisternal organelle may appose up to three separate axon terminals. Axoaxonic synapses may be present in large numbers and are distributed rather evenly over the entire axon hillock and initial segment. There is some indication that the density of axoaxonic synapses may be lamina-specific. Sloper and Powell (1979) found the synaptic density on initial segments of supragranular pyramids to be about three times that on infragranular pyramids.

The proximal, spine-free portion of the pyramidal cell dendrites forms relatively few synapses, and those that are present tend to be of the symmetric variety (Jones and Powell, 1970). Further distally along the dendrites, synapses in increased numbers are found on both the dendritic shaft and dendritic spines (Figs. 8, 12), the spines forming by far the greater number. That the total synaptic complement of neocortical pyramids becomes reduced in advanced age may be predicted from the results of quantitative neuropil analyses carried out in rat visual (Feldman, 1976) and parietal (Adams and Jones, 1982) cortex and human frontal cortex (Huttenlocher, 1979).

Synapses formed directly with the dendritic shafts of both apical and basal dendrites (Hornung and Garey, 1981; White and Hersch, 1981) are of both the symmetric and asymmetric variety. On apical dendrites, the symmetric synapses usually appear to predominate, but in many cases the proportion of asymmetric synapses increases with distance from the cell body (Parnavelas *et al.*, 1977b; Davis and Sterling, 1979; Peters, 1981).

The spine synapses are typically asymmetric, and the axon terminals contain spherical vesicles. The principal density is postsynaptic and is approximately 30 nm thick (Peters and Kaiserman-Abramof, 1969). It is also somewhat darker than the density associated with asymmetric synapses on dendritic shafts (Peters, 1981). One synapse per spine is the rule, but occasionally two synapses are present. As an exceptional circumstance, occasional cases of disynaptic spines have been reported in which one synapse is asymmetric and the other symmetric

(Vaughan and Peters, 1973; Parnavelas *et al.,* 1977b; Colonnier, 1981). While uncommon in mammalian cortex, this arrangement is common in turtle visual cortex (Ebner and Colonnier, 1975).

As described by Peters and Kaiserman-Abramof (1969) in rat parietal cortex, the appearance of the axospinous synaptic zone varies with spine size. Where the terminal enlargement of the spine is small, the pre- and postsynaptic membranes form a synaptic junction that extends for almost the entire length of their apposition. In the case of large spines, the synaptic density is often discontinuous, so that more than one synaptic complex appears to be present. In actuality, this appearance is accounted for by the fact that the generally disk-shaped synaptic region includes within it one or several patches in which the synaptic density is absent.

In one study of axodendritic synaptic topography, lengths of pyramidal apical dendrites traversing layer IV of rat visual cortex were reconstructed from serial thin sections (Feldman, 1975). Some of the results obtained are presented in Fig. 13. Given the positive relationship between dendritic shaft diameter and spine density (Feldman, 1975), and considering the fact that the majority of the axodendritic synapses are formed with the dendritic spines, it is not surprising that the total number of synapses formed with a given length of thick dendrite is greater than the number formed with a given length of thin dendrite. As shown in Fig. 13, the synaptic density on thick dendrites is something on the order of double that found on thin dendrites, with medium-diameter dendrites having an intermediate synaptic density. The range of values observed in the study for all dendrites was 7.7 to 63.2 total synapses/10-μm length of apical dendrite. Of these total synapses, those formed directly with the apical dendritic shaft ranged in density from about 1 to 6 per 10 μm of dendritic length and constituted about 5 to 30% of the total number of dendritic synapses formed with both the shaft and the spines. The proportion of synapses formed directly with the dendritic shaft decreases steadily as dendritic spine density increases. As observed in serial thin-section reconstructions, the axons forming synapses with the spines and shafts of apical dendrites are for the most part vertically oriented, running parallel to the dendritic shafts, although some of the axons run obliquely. Observation of the synaptic relationships of these axons with the dendrites within individual dendritic clusters reveals a wide variety of associations. Single axons may form synapses with the spines of two or more adjacent apical dendrites, with the spine of one apical dendrite and the shaft of another, or with an apical dendritic spine and either the shaft or a spine of a nonapical dendrite.

The exact sources of the axons synapsing with the pyramidal cell surface have been difficult to specify. The difficulty has involved the identity of the origins of both the pre- and postsynaptic components in conventional thin sections. With the advent of modern technqiues, however, such as the deimpregnation and gold-toning method of Fairén *et al.* (1977) and the use of degeneration, Golgi, and transport methods in various combinations, some of the specific details of synaptic interconnections are beginning to be revealed. Of particular interest have been the projections of presynaptic neurons whose cell bodies are located in the thalamus (see White, 1979) and in the local cortex containing the postsynaptic pyramidal cells. As observed in rat visual cortex after thalamic lesions, the geniculocortical projection terminates in part on the spines of at least some pyramidal neurons (Peters and Feldman, 1976; Peters *et al.*, 1979). This finding is in agreement with the observation of pyramidal spine losses following experimental alteration of the normal thalamocortical input (Globus and Scheibel, 1967b; Valverde, 1967; Fifková, 1970; Ryugo *et al.*, 1975a,b; Hornung and Garey, 1981). Identification of the specific postsynaptic targets of degenerating fibers by means of the Golgi deimpregnation and gold-toning technique shows that they include the spines of layer III pyramidal basal, apical, and oblique branch dendrites, and the spines of layer V apical and oblique branch dendrites (Peters *et al.*, 1979). These results are consistent with those of Somogyi (1978) and with those of White (1978) and others in other cortices (Strick and Sterling, 1974). White (1978) has shown, for example, that in mouse primary somatosensory cortex, thalamocortical axon terminals synapse with the basal dendritic spines of layer III pyramidal cells and with the spines of the apical and oblique branch dendrites of layer V pyramidal cells. In subsequent work in the same cortex, Hersch and White (1981b) examined various sizes of layer V and layer VI deimpregnated and gold-toned pyramidal neurons for evidence of differential thalamic connectivity, the thalamic terminals being labelled by lesion-induced degeneration. Considerable diversity among the cells examined was observed. Within the span from layer III through layer V, a small lower layer V pyramidal cell formed only two thalamocortical synapses, one on an apical dendritic spine and one on an oblique branch spine. A large pyramid from the same stratum synapses with only one labeled terminal; surprisingly, this synapse was formed with the apical dendritic shaft. By contrast, a medium-sized pyramid from upper layer V was involved in 42 thalamocrotical synapses, which accounted for 15% of all its axospinous synapses within the layer of apical dendrite reconstructed (Hersch and White, 1981a). A small and a large layer VI pyramid formed 6 and 34 thalamocortical synapses, respectively. While too few cells were studied to suggest what the rules might be for categorizing these variations, it seems clear from these results that the thalamocortical synaptic pattern on pyramidal neurons varies widely from cell to cell. This finding is not unexpected in view of the variable spine changes observed by Valverde, Ryugo and colleagues, and others. It is of interest to note that Ryugo *et al.* (1975a,b) found that neonatal sensory restriction produced spine losses only on deep layer V pyramidal neurons, whereas Hersch and White found the deep layer V cells to receive only sparse direct connections from the thalamus. It may thus be the case that the spine losses consequent upon early sensory restriction are not wholly mediated by direct thalamocortical fibers.

The finding that pyramidal neurons vary in the extent of their thalamic connectivity suggests that the pyramidal cells may differ in some fundamental respect from one another. One way in which they might vary is in their projection pattern. Pyramids which project callosally, for example, might differ from corticotectal cells in the extent to which they receive thalamocortical input. It thus becomes important to be able to examine the thalamocortical input to pyramidal neurons which have known projections. A satisfactory methodology for investigating this question has only been developed within the past several years. The technique consists of labeling pyramids not with Golgi impregnation but with retrogradely transported horseradish peroxidase injected in the region of the cell's axonal termination. The labeled perikaryon is then examined for synapses with axonal terminals marked by lesion-induced degeneration. In one application of this method, in cat visual cortex, Hornung and Garey (1981) determined that two callosally projecting layer III pyramids received direct thalamocortical input on their basal dendrites. In one case, the synapse was formed with a basal dendritic spine, and in the other with the dendritic shaft. In a more extensive and highly significant study in mouse primary somatosensory cortex, White and Hersch (1981) examined the thalamic connectivity in layer IV of the basal dendrites of six layer III and IV pyramidal neurons which projected to the ipsilateral motor cortex. The thalamocortical synapses observed were all of the asymmetric type and were made only with spines. The thalamocortical synapses accounted for between 1.49 (2 of 134) and 12.62% (13 of 103) of all axospinous synapses on the dendritic lengths reconstructed. In one case, a portion of apical dendrite at the layer III/IV border was reconstructed. It exhibited 5.55% (4 of 72) thalamocortical synapses. A tendency was observed for there to be a higher proportion of thalamocortical synapses on basal dendritic lengths within layer IV than for dendritic lengths just above the layer III border. Precise laminar depth may therefore be an important controlling factor in determining thalamocortical connectivity. However, cell-to-cell variability in proportion of thalamocortical synapses appears to be about as great for this population of similarly projecting cells as for previous populations with unknown projections (Hersch and White, 1981b). It is important to note, though, that certain specific populations of commonly projecting pyramidal neurons do have unique thalamocortical connectivity patterns. For example, only a very limited (0.3–0.9% of the apical dendritic synapses in layer IV) number of thalamic terminals synapse with the corticostriatal projection neurons in mouse primary somatosensory cortex (Hersch and White, 1982).

In addition to the above observations on the projection neurons to motor cortex, White and Hersch have found the axons of two of the postsynaptic pyramidal neurons to be sufficiently well labeled to follow them in the serial thin-section series. One axon acquired a myelin sheath about 20 μm from the cell body and then gave rise to an unmyelinated collateral. The second axon gave rise to an unmyelinated collateral and then becaame myelinated at a distance of about 60 μm from the cell body. Both collaterals formed only asymmetric synapses. Of the combined total of 12 postsynaptic elements identified, half were dendritic spines and half were the shafts of nonspinous dendrites which also received numerous other asymmetric and symmetric synapses. One of the postsynaptic dendritic spines was lightly labeled with horseradish peroxidase, thus suggesting the existence of direct synaptic connections between pyramidal cells showing common axonal projections. This type of connection is one which had been surmised from conventional Golgi material, in which pyramidal basal dendrites have been observed to be in contact with axon collaterals from other pyramidal neurons (Fairén and Valverde, 1973). These findings may be related to an observation of axoaxonic contact made by Butler and Jane (1977). Following thermal lesions of the superficial layers of rat visual cortex, these authors found evidence of degenerating axons on the spines and dendritic shafts of what were presumably layer V pyramidal neurons, thus suggesting the existence of direct local connections among pyramidal cells.

A further source of axon terminals forming synapses with the pyramidal cell surface is neighboring nonpyramidal neurons. One such neuron, long known from Golgi studies of the cortex (Ramón y Cajal, 1954, 1955), is the so-called basket cell (see Chapters 6 and 8). The axon collaterals of this cell type course horizontally and provide twigs to numerous pyramidal perisomatic plexuses. These plexuses are the "baskets." The basket cells have been described in Golgi studies of several cortices, including the human motor cortex (Marin-Padilla, 1969), in which the baskets envelop the cell bodies of Betz and other pyramidal cells, and the monkey somatic sensory cortex (Jones, 1975). As illustrated in classical Golgi preparations, such as those of Marin-Padilla (1969), the baskets consist of rather dense and tangled axonal meshes surrounding the cell bodies and proximal dendrites. The meshes appear to be somewhat less dense than the baskets on cerebellar Purkinje cells (Jones, 1981). Each pyramidal basket is formed by a number of basket cell axon collaterals. Individual fibers may provide only several branches to the basket, but these branches may contact all parts of the soma and proximal dendritic segments. The fiber may then continue on in a horizontal orientation to contribute to additional baskets. The basket cells observed by Marin-Padilla were invariably a distinctive type of nonpyramidal neuron of medium size, most frequently encountered around midcortical depths. Clear spines are present on the soma, and the dendrites are long and thin with a moderate spine complement. The dendritic arborization pattern is radiate, with a tendency toward vertical and horizontal trajectories. The vertically disposed dendrites may extend from layer II to layer VI. The main stem of the basket cell axon may ascend or descend, with horizontal collateral branches that may project up to 2 mm in length. According to Jones (1981), the axonal arborization is flattened in a plane at right angles to the long axes of the pre- and postcentral gyri. Numerous horizontal collaterals, at varying levels, may arise from a single main axon, each contributing to several baskets and collectively supplying baskets to perikarya in all layers of the cortex. Recent observations of basket cell axons in cat visual cortex have provided the information that in addition to the long horizontal collaterals the axon gives rise to a dense local plexus, that the synapses formed by the axon terminals are symmetrical, and that the postsynaptic neurons may include nonpyramidal as well as pyramidal cells (Fairén and DeFelipe, 1982).

It is quite possible that the basket cells are the same cells as those described in the rat as multipolar stellate cells by Peters and Proskauer in 1980 (Peters, 1981). These cells, described more fully in Chapters 6 and 13, appear to provide the majority of symmetric synapses in rat visual cortex. They give rise to multiple synaptic contacts with the perikarya and dendritic shafts of pyramidal neurons and also synapse with axon initial segments.

Among the remaining nonpyramidal neurons which provide local synaptic connections to the pyramidal cells are the chandelier cells (Somogyi, 1977; Fairén and Valverde, 1980; Peters *et al.*, 1982) and the bipolar cells (Peters and Kimerer, 1981), described in Chapters 10 and 11. In rat visual cortex, the candlelike terminations of the chandelier cell axon form highly specific symmetric synapses with the axon initial segments of layer II/III pyramidal neurons. These synapses are arranged in the forms of vertical arrays of serial boutons (see Chapter 10), the uppermost terminal being located 7–14 μm from the pyramidal cell body.

Individual pyramidal initial segments may be contacted by one or more candle-like arrays, or in some cases by none. In any event, the initial segments appear to form additional synapses which are not derived from chandelier cell axons. One potential source of these other terminations are the multipolar stellate cells referred to above. The axons of bipolar neurons typically give rise to vertically oriented branches (Feldman and Peters, 1978) which parallel the trajectories of clustered pyramidal apical dendrites. These branches form multiple asymmetrical synapses with the spines of the apical dendrites and, occasionally, with the apical dendritic shafts (see Chapter 11).

The account given above summarizes much of what is known concerning the specific sources of synaptic input to the pyramidal neuron. Obviously, many gaps in our knowledge still remain to be filled in before we can produce the kind of wiring diagram that is required for a complete anatomical specification of this cell type. More information is required concerning the synaptic relationships of the distal reaches of the dendritic tree. What, for example, are the origins of the inputs to the considerable portion of the dendritic tree in layer I? In addition, quantitative data are needed to determine the degree of generality of the synaptic patterns which have been observed. Are the described synaptic inputs to the dendritic spines sufficient to account for all of the axospinous synapses that exist, and what variations occur within and among cortical areas in various species? Many additional questions can be raised which point up further problems which remain to be faced. What anatomical interrelationships exist among the various inputs to specific pyramidal neurons? How do synaptic input patterns relate to the projections of the postsynaptic cells? What synaptic arrangements tie particular populations of cells together in ways that may be functionally meaningful? Preliminary answers, of varying degrees of completeness, are available in all of these areas. It is encouraging to note that there already exist workable techniques by means of which a much more satisfactory understanding than we presently possess can be achieved.

4. Other Pyramidal Cell Forms

Systematic accounts of pyramidal cell populations have consistently called attention to a number of types of pyramidal neurons with atypical morphological features (Globus and Scheibel, 1967a; Braak, 1980). Such cells include those with unusual dendritic arrangements and those of exceptionally large size such as the Betz and Meynert cells.

Among the cells with atypical dendritic patterns, one highly interesting case is the large entorhinal multipolar neuron described in human cortex by Braak *et al.* (1976). As visualized in the cellular islands at the surface of the parahippocampal gyrus, these neurons lack an apical dendrite, although they have densely spinous dendrites and their axon emerges from the base of the cell body and projects downward to the white matter. From their radiate dendritic form and the lack of an apical dendrite, it appears clear that these neurons, when examined in isolation, are nonpyramidal. However, by tracing the lamina in which they are situated toward the temporal isocortex, Braak and colleagues were able to demonstrate that as the depth of the collateral fissure is reached, the cell body acquires a typical pyramidal form and the dendritic arborization can be resolved with gradually increasing certainty into an apical dendrite and a set of basal dendrites. This is probably the clearest example of a transition between pyramidal and nonpyramidal cell forms in the adult brain.

Several other pyramidal cell variants also involve the apical dendrite. One of these is characteristic of the deepest stratum of the cortex, adjacent to the white matter. In this zone, pyramidal apical dendrites are frequently observed to originate from the lateral or dorsolateral, rather than the superficial, surface of the perikaryon (Lund and Boothe, 1975; Feldman and Peters, 1978). The apical dendrites may thus leave the vicinity of the cell body in a horizontal or oblique direction rather than assuming a direct course toward the pial surface (see Chapter 15). These cells may therefore be easily mischaracterized as nonpyramidal neurons in Golgi preparations unless care is taken to critically focus the course of the dendrites. Examination of adjacent sections may also be necessary to verify the existence of an apical dendrite. When this is done, the dendrite will be observed to gradually assume a vertical orientation and to ascend toward the pial surface, although it may terminate at a cortical level well below layer I (see Fig. 6).

At higher levels within the cortex there exist pyramidal cells whose apical dendrites are reduced to short slender processes. These cells are prominent in primate cortex, where they are found as the very small cells of layer IV (Braak, 1980; Lund *et al.,* 1981) or in layer V of macaque area 17 (Lund and Boothe, 1975). The apical dendrites may emit several collateral branches relatively close to the cell body. They then assume a threadlike appearance with few spines and without further branching. The axons of these cells arise basally, and after an initial descent, curve vertically upward or emit one or several stout upward collaterals. These may exceed the apical dendrite in diameter and in number of spinelike protrusions. It may be assumed, although it is not established, that such protrusions are pre- rather than postsynaptic structures.

The status of the apical dendrites of pyramidal neurons in layer II requires special comment. The proximity of these cells to the zone in which terminal tufts normally ramify occasions a marked attenuation of the length of the apical dendrite. However, the nature and the extent of this attenuation appears to be species specific and to vary among cortical regions. In an intriguing contribution to this area, Sanides and Sanides (1972) discuss from a phylogenetic viewpoint the "extraverted" neurons of layer II. Central to their argument is the notion that the primitive neurons (similar to those observed in many amphibians, for example) which gave rise to mammalian pyramidal cells received the majority of their synaptic input from the superficial layer of the cortex. This situation, they believe, is reflected in the organization of the oblique branches (Heimer, 1969) and in the strong thalamic inputs to layer I of presumably primitive cortex in the rat (Domesick, 1969) and to layer I of the neocortex in placental mammals (Ebner, 1969). Primitive pyramidal neurons are thus conceived of as being "extraverted" in form, that is, they display a well-developed superficial dendritic arborization extending up through layer I, and a relatively poorly developed or absent basal dendritic array. The primary function of the primitive apical dendrite is thus conceived of as being an extension designed to bring the pyramidal dendritic tree into the contact zone of layer I. The consequences of this, for Sanides and Sanides, are that primitive pyramidal neurons of layer II will be of the strongly extraverted type. True apical dendrites will often be absent, with the superficial dendrites frequently emanating from the perikaryon and angling widely through layer I. Occasionally, very short lengths of apical dendrites will be present, often obliquely oriented at an angle well off the vertical. Such neurons will be found commonly in species such as hedgehog and opossum, and particularly in presumably primitive cortices such as that of the hippocampus. That this in fact is the case is well illustrated by Sanides and Sanides. Quite apart from the correctness of their theory, there is no doubt that many layer II neurons of, for example, hedgehog neocortex are of the extraverted type, lacking a recognizable apical dendrite. Examples of similar neurons can also be found in rat neocortex (see also Kirsche *et al.*, 1973). In the primate, on the other hand, layer II neocortical pyramids appear to characteristically display well-balanced superficial and basal dendrites, and to regularly have at least short lengths of vertically oriented apical dendrites, presumably reflecting a decrease in the relative importance or abundance of the synaptic input from the subpial zone. The extraverted neuron thus appears to represent a case similar to Braak's entorhinal multipolar neurons described above. It is a cell which has certain features commonly associated with pyramidal neurons—densely spined dendrites and a vertically descending axon arising from the base of the cell body—but which lacks an apical dendrite. As in the case of the entorhinal cell, the decision to label it pyramidal or nonpyramidal may need to take into account broad considerations which are not apparent in the microscopic examination of individual cells.

A final type of pyramidal dendritic aberration is represented by what Van der Loos (1965) referred to as the "improperly" oriented pyramidal cell. The most extreme, and the most common, form of this cell is the inverted pyramid. Van der Loos defined these cells as those in which the perikaryal axis departed from the vertical by more than 20°, and studied them in rat, rabbit, cat, and monkey. Similar cells are also present in humans (Braak, 1980). In one sample of pyramidal neurons from rabbit cortex, Van der Loos found that 18% of the cells were improperly oriented, although in a second smaller sample only 1 of 27 pyramids was improperly oriented. Globus and Scheibel's (1967a) figure for the rabbit is 5%. The number of these cells commonly observed by others in the rat is very much less, Parnavelas *et al.* (1977a) estimating approximately 1%. In the rabbit and rat, the preferential location of inverted pyramids is in layers V and VI (Globus and Scheibel, 1967a; Parnavelas *et al.*, 1977). Apart from orientation, the dendritic systems of the improperly oriented cells are normal and are normally spined. The fact that the dendrites are arranged in an orientation appropriate to the somal axis is of some developmental interest, since it suggests that the control of dendritic orientation is intrinsic to the neuron and is not governed by the orientation of neuropil elements. The axonal origins of improperly oriented pyramidal neurons are often situated, as in normal cells, at the base of the cell body or on the proximal portion of a basal dendrite. However, instances of unconventional origins are also observed. This includes origins from the lateral surface of the perikaryon, from the transition region between the perikaryon and the apical dendrite, from the apical dendritic shaft as far away as 30 μm from the perikaryon, and even from an oblique branch dendrite (Van der Loos, 1965; Kirsche *et al.*, 1973). Regardless of the axon origin, however, the eventual course of the axon is vertically downward, toward the white matter, so that this aspect of the neuronal geometry does seem to be governed by factors extrinsic to the cell.

Several types of neocortical pyramidal cells are atypical principally by virtue of their large size. One such cell type is a giant spine-poor cell of cat auditory association cortex described by Kaplan and Scheibel (1980). The cells are sparsely distributed in layer V. They measure 40–75 μm in height and 20–25 μm in width, and are thus comparable in size to the Betz cells of the cat (Kaiserman-Abramof and Peters, 1972) and the Meynert cells of the macaque (Palay, 1978). The basal dendrites form a wide skirt, and the apical dendrite is a thick (6- to 8-μm diameter) pially directed process which is usually unbranched but which bifurcates in layer III. One interesting feature of these cells is the fact that they appear to be less abundant in 1½- to 2-year-old cats than in 12- to 18-year-old cats. However, the cells from the younger cats appear to be more densely spined. In the old cats, fewer than 10 spines occur between the origin and bifurcation of the apical dendrite, a distance which may exceed 400 μm.

Since their original description by Betz in 1874, the giant cells of the agranular frontal cortex have received extensive study, with much of the early literature reviewed by Walshe (1942). The principal area in which the classical Betz cells are found corresponds with Brodmann's area 4, although Braak (1976b) has found a field of Betz cells in layer Vb of the cingulate sulcus cortex at a level anterior to the central sulcus. The distribution in the macaque has been described by Nañagas (1922). The size of the Betz cells is quite variable, ranging from the upper values given by Betz in human cortex, 120 μm in height by 60 μm in width, to sizes that are comparable to the dimensions of the largest of the non-Betz pyramids. In part, the variation in size appears to be locus-dependent, the largest cells occurring medially, in the paracentral lobule, and the smallest laterally in the lower portion of the precentral gyrus approximately 2–4 cm above the Sylvian fissure (Walshe, 1942). The cells in cat vary from 40 × 25 μm to 110 × 60 μm (Kaiserman-Abramof and Peters, 1972). The cells occur in layer V and are either solitary or in groups of three to four cells (von Economo and Koskinas, 1925). In 24-month-old macaques, the groups are separated by approximately 380 μm (Kemper *et al.*, 1973).

In the cat (Kaiserman-Abramof and Peters, 1972), the apical dendrites of the Betz cells typically bifurcate at their bases into two or three major branches that diverge laterally as they extend toward the pial surface. The main trunk of the dendrite, prior to its bifurcation, is massive, averaging 7.5 μm in diameter, and bears few spines. The basal dendrites are prominent, and in addition there exist a number of other dendrites that extend laterally from all levels of the cell body. The dendrites bear numerous spines, including some of unusually large size. The nucleus is large and central, and with few concentrations of chromatin. The perikaryal cytoplasm contains well-developed Nissl bodies and lipofuscin granules, often concentrated at the base of the apical dendrite. A number of glial cells of all major types, but chiefly astrocytes, are associated with the perikaryon in satellite positions. Morphometric analysis of axosomatic relationships indicates that the average Betz cell perikaryon bears approximately 870 axon terminals. Where these have been observed to form synapses, these are of the symmetric type characteristic for most pyramidal neurons. In terms of surface area, the axon terminals contact about 23% of the perikaryal surface, a figure that is probably considerably higher than that commonly observed on non-Betz cells.

In the human (Braak and Braak, 1976; Scheibel and Scheibel, 1978), the total Betz cell population numbers 30,000–40,000 cells, with approximately 75% of the cells being located in motor areas supplying the muscles of the leg (Lassek, 1954). Perikaryal dimensions range from 30 to 60 μm in width and 80 to 120 μm in height (von Economo, 1929). Structurally, the cells in man resemble those in the cat. One of the striking features of these neurons is the great length of the laterally projecting dendrites. These may extend more than 2 mm from the cell body, and may in some cases exceed the length of the apical dendrite. These horizontal dendrites enter into close parallel relationships with other Betz cell dendrites to form bundles of from 3 to 10 dendritic shafts. Dendrites of other non-Betz cells may also course within the bundles. In some cells, one of the basal dendrites is quite highly developed and forms a "tap root" type of dendrite bearing many collaterals and angling down through layers V and VI. The existence of an obliquely descending tap root plus other asymmetries in the extent of the laterally projecting dendrites gives many Betz cells an unbalanced appearance when viewed in Golgi preparations cut either parallel or perpendicular to the apical dendrite. In such cells, the array of highly developed dendrites may extend for well over twice the distance of the remaining dendrites. Specific anatomical orientation preferences have not been observed, imparting to individual Betz cells a highly idiosyncratic character. This individuality is reinforced by the variation in somal form, which includes in addition to classical pyramid-shaped cell bodies globular and spindle shapes. Spines on the soma and proximal portions of the dendrites are rare in human Betz cells, although occasional somata bearing multiple spines may be encountered. The initial spine-free portions of the dendrites often measure approximately 30–50 μm in length for the basal dendrites and 80–100 μm for the apical dendrite. In one case, Scheibel and Scheibel traced a tap root dendrite for over 1 mm without sign of a spine. The distal portion of the dendritic tree is richly endowed with spines, although according to Braak and Braak the spine concentration is not uniform. On the lateral dendrites the spines often appear to be clumped, the spinous stretches of the dendrite alternating with spine-free zones. Along the apical dendrite, a conspicuous increase in spine density occurs as the upper border of layer Vb is crossed. The spine density subsequently decreases.

A final aspect of human Betz cell morphology has emerged from the pigmentoarchitectonic work of Braak. His studies have shown that, in addition to their distinctive size and dendritic arborization, it is possible to distinguish the Betz cells from other large pyramids by their densely aggregated pigment deposits (Braak and Braak, 1976; Braak, 1980). These deposits appear as large cytoplasmic blocks of fine-grained texture (see Chapter 3).

Like the Betz cells, the giant pyramidal cells of Meynert, located in the occipital cortex, display several features beyond their size that distinguish them from typical pyramidal neurons. Meynert actually described two tiers of distinctive cells. The outer tier, located at the level of the stripe of Gennari, is composed of horizontal cells with broadly ramifying lateral dendrites but without an apical dendrite (Polyak, 1957; Braak, 1976a). These cells can therefore be classified as nonpyramidal neurons. The deeper cells, however, are unmistakably pyramidal, and it is these cells which will be described.

Clearly the largest neurons of the visual cortex, the Meynert cells are located within a rather narrow band in the vicinity of the layer V/VI border, most authors designating the lamina as layer V (Polyak, 1957; Garey, 1971; Chan-Palay *et al.*, 1974; Braak, 1976a), although Lund and Boothe (1975) consider it to be layer VI. Measurements of Meynert cell perikarya in the cat and macaque indicate ranges of 20–40 μm in width and 40–50 μm in height (Garey, 1971; Palay, 1978). In man, von Economo (1929) gives upper limits of 30 μm and 60 μm. Because the cells tend to occur individually rather than in small groups, as is typically the case with Betz cells, they are often referred to as the solitary cells of Meynert.

While the cells are present in the banks of the calcarine fissure, Clark (1942) found their packing density in the macaque to be greater on the lateral occipital surface, where they are separated by an average space of 0.86 mm. In the same material, the average separation in the calcarine area was found to be 1.33 mm. Clark estimates their number in macaque visual cortex to be approximately 1300 per hemisphere. More recent estimates (Chan-Palay *et al.*, 1974) are considerably higher, and it has been speculated that Clark's animals may have been subject to age-related loss of cortical neurons (see Devaney and Johnson, 1980). This question, as Palay (1978) emphasizes, deserves careful attention, especially in view of the fact that a small number of Meynert cells in young animals appear to be pyknotic and hyperchromic. Normally, the perikaryal cytoplasm is palestaining in Nissl preparations and is almost devoid of lipofuscin in pigmentoarchitectonic studies (Braak, 1976a). In the cat, Meynert cells are evident in areas 18 and 19 as well as area 17, although they are reduced in number and, in area 19, tend to occupy a somewhat more superficial position (Garey, 1971). While there is good agreement that Meynert cells are readily identifiable in the carnivore and primate brain, their claimed existence in rodents and lagomorphs (Shkol'nik-Yarros, 1971; Parnavelas *et al.*, 1977a) is debatable.

In the macaque (Garey, 1971; Chan-Palay *et al.*, 1974; Palay, 1978), Golgi-impregnated Meynert cells exhibit a massive dendritic system. One of the cytological characteristics of the dendrites is their dense packing with neurofilaments. In this respect they differ from other visual cortical pyramids, which contain predominantly microtubules. Studied in Golgi preparations, the Meynert cell basal dendrites are only moderately branched, but extend laterally for considerable distances, often 400–500 μm but occasionally up to 700 μm. The basal dendrites also ramify downward, through layer VI. All of these branches are richly supplied with dendritic spines. Approximately three-quarters of all of the cell's spines are borne on the basal dendrites. The apical dendrite extends vertically from the perikaryon and produces a well-developed terminal tuft, about 400 μm in diameter, in layers I and II. The proximal 30–60 μm of the apical dendrite is relatively aspinous and gives rise to two or three spinous oblique branches which ramify weakly within layer V. Few additional oblique branches are evident over the remainder of the apical dendrite. Distal to the proximal segment, the apical dendrite acquires an extremely dense spine coat which is maintained for the remainder of its traverse of layer V. This densely spined segment of the apical dendrite bears approximately 10% of the spine complement of the entire dendritic tree. At the layer IV/V border there occurs an abrupt diminution of the spine density, suggesting a selective avoidance of the geniculocortical input to the visual cortex. At the junction of sublaminae IVb and IVa, the incidence of spines decreases again, and increasingly long stretches of the dendrite become devoid of spines. The apical dendrite segment between the IV/V border and the terminal tuft bears only 2.5% of the spines on the dendritic tree. The spines reappear as the terminal arborization begins in layer II, although the spine density is somewhat lower than that present on the basal dendrites. The terminal portion of the apical dendrite accounts for 8–13% of the total number of spines.

The axon of the Meynert cell originates from the basal surface of the cell body or from one of the basal dendrites. It arises from a low axon hillock and descends into the white matter. According to Tömböl (1975), several collaterals arise from the initial portion of the axon within layer V and ascend to layers II and III. The Meynert cell perikarya in the macaque are not labeled following horseradish peroxidase injections into the lateral geniculate nucleus or superior colliculus (Lund and Boothe, 1975), but they are labeled in the marmoset after injections of area MT, the middle temporal visual area (Spatz, 1975) and in the macaque after injections of cortical area STS (Lund *et al.*, 1975). The temporal visual area receives a strong projection from area 17 (Spatz *et al.*, 1970). What the direct sources of synaptic input to the Meynert cell are is not known. However, in a recent experiment in the cat, Winfield (1982) demonstrated that the cells are sensitive to visual deprivation. Following dark-rearing, there was a reduction of approximately 80% in the frequency with which Meynert cells could be distinguished in Nissl preparations. Reductions were also observed in lid-sutured animals, but the effects were considerably less dramatic. Whether the Meynert cells were actually lost or merely shrank below the threshold of detection was not determined.

5. The Emergence of Pyramidal Cell Features during Maturation

Ramón y Cajal's discovery of the excellent Golgi impregnations that could be obtained in very young animals led him inevitably to the study of cortical morphogenesis (Ramón y Cajal, 1937, 1955). Based on his Golgi observations of developing neurons, primarily in the fetal and newborn mouse, rabbit, and human, Ramón y Cajal concluded, as Vignal (1888) had, that pyramidal cell differentiation occurs first for the deeper-lying cells and then progresses with time toward the pial surface. At any one stage of development, there was also observed a gradient according to cell size, the larger pyramids exhibiting the more advanced differentiation.

Ramón y Cajal described several successive phases of differentiation, beginning with the primitive bipolar phase in the fetus, in which radial processes extending from the poles of a fusiform soma span the full thickness of the cortex. Following resorption of the original basal process (Ramón y Cajal's neuroblast phase), the pyramidal cells enter a second bipolar phase, in which the superficial process, by virtue of its orientation, thickness, somewhat varicose contour, and subpial bifurcations, begins to assume the characteristics of a mature apical dendrite. The elongating peripheral process, which is the developing axon, is also radially oriented; it gradually lengthens to the point where it can be traced down into the white matter. During this second bipolar stage, neither definitive basal dendrites nor axon collaterals are yet present. In the next phase of development, shortly before birth in the mouse and rabbit, side branches begin to emerge from the apical dendrite, at first near the cell body and then at progressively higher levels, and an elaboration of the terminal tuft is evident. The basal dendrites also begin to make their appearance. Frequently, one of the early basal dendrites is a descending process which has a short trunk in common with the origin of the axon, as subsequently described by Morest (1970). In addition, dendritic spines begin to form, initiating, for Ramón y Cajal, the functional maturation of the cell. The final developmental phase is marked by the appearance of axon collaterals. These arise at right angles from the parent axon and are initially short, with small terminal varicosities. Subsequently, increases in the length and branching of all processes, dendritic and axonal, occur. In summary, Ramón y Cajal's sequential stages of pyramidal cell maturation, beginning with the deeper-lying and larger pyramids, involve the initial elaboration of the apical dendrite and axon; then the basal dendrites, branches of the apical dendrite, and dendritic spines; and finally the axon collaterals.

An abundance of subsequent work has tended to confirm this general pattern (Rabinowicz, 1964; Poliakov, 1966; Marty and Pujol, 1966) although there are discrepant observations in specific cases, such as the finding that terminal tufts of superficial pyramidal cells mature earlier than those of deep pyramids in dog somatosensory cortex (Molliver and Van der Loos, 1970). Certainly the early observation of a general deep-to-superficial gradient of development fits nicely with the autoradiographic findings of Angevine and Sidman (1961), repeatedly confirmed, demonstrating the so-called "inside-out" sequence of neuron migration and arrival in the cortex (Rakic, 1971, 1972, 1981). Similarly, the notion that a primitive attachment process degenerates and is replaced by the definitive axon is supported by modern studies of neurogenesis such as that of Morest in the opossum (1970).

Certain forms of developing nonpyramidal neurons—the horizontally oriented cells of layer I and certain large presumably stellate cells which may ultimately reside in layer VI (Åström, 1967; Shimada and Langman, 1970; Stensaas, 1967; Marin-Padilla, 1970, 1971)—appear to undergo substantial degenerative or regressive changes in the later stages of cortical maturation. This remodeling suggests that, for such cells, certain morphological features may be required at one stage of development that are no longer required at later stages. Generally, fundamental changes in neuronal form do not occur in the case of developing pyramidal neurons once the basic form of the cell has been established. However, on a finer scale, it is clear that some of the individual dendritic processes which are elaborated relatively early in development may ultimately disappear or become more simplified in form (e.g., Stanfield and O'Leary, 1982).

From time to time, attempts have been made to arrive at generalizations concerning relative developmental tempos of pyramidal and nonpyramidal neurons (Jacobson, 1978). It is, however, important to recognize the limitations of such generalizations. The nature of these limitations is well documented in the work of Marin-Padilla (1971, 1972a) and Purpura (1975a, 1975b). For one thing, there exist problems in the unequivocal recognition of developing pyramidal cells, owing to the technical difficulties of studying cell form in early ontogenesis and to the modulations of cell form occurring during development. Second, the actual maturational timetable in any one species is dependent to a large extent on cortical locus. In addition, there may exist considerable variation, particularly in human material, in the time course of maturation from one individual to another at the same age or even from one cell to another within the same restricted locus in an individual brain. Such variations often make it exceptionally difficult to arrive at general judgements of maturational "state."

In the visual cortex of the human fetus, the most active period of pyramidal dendritic differentiation and development occurs between 6 and 8 months of gestational age. This is relatively late in comparison with the similarly active phase in the motor cortex (Marin-Padilla, 1970; Purpura, 1975a,b). In the human motor cortex, the pyramidal cells are in place at about the midpoint of the gestational period (Marin-Padilla, 1971). This occurs at approximately the same or perhaps a somewhat later stage of gestation in the cat (Marin-Padilla, 1971) and later still in the rat (Berry and Rogers, 1965; Raedler and Sievers, 1975). Purpura's (1975b) studies of the human visual cortex indicate that at the start of the active phase, at 25 weeks gestational age, the pyramidal cells exhibit apical dendritic shafts but lack true basal dendrites, showing at most a few fine, filamentous processes emanating from the somata of large pyramidal cells. Similarly, occasional processes or filopodia extend from the apical dendrites of the larger cells. Apical dendrites longer than 500 μm are seldom observed in Purpura's Golgi preparations, so that deeper-lying pyramids do not yet appear to have attained their dendritic projections to layer I. Some of the apical dendritic terminations display complex enlargements, interpreted as growth cones, indicating the future extension toward the pial surface. The apical dendritic shafts, particularly those of the small and medium pyramidal cells, are somewhat tortuous and they display lumpy enlargements and varicosities. This is less true of the deeper pyramids. True dendritic spines are absent. In spite of its rudimentary state of development, Purpura has found it possible to record visual evoked potentials from the visual cortex at this stage. It is of interest in this regard that synapses on dendritic shafts are already present at this age in at least some areas of human fetal cortex (Molliver *et al.*, 1973). At 26–27 weeks, apical dendrites increase in length and basal dendrites begin to appear on the smaller pyramidal cells. The dendrites of the large pyramids become more highly developed, although true dendritic spines are still lacking. During the ensuing 6 weeks, pronounced changes occur. In Purpura's 33-week material, developing Meynert cells are obvious. Apical dendrites have lengthened further and the superficial pyramids exhibit numerous basal dendritic sprouts as well as oblique branch sprouts from the apical dendrite. Significantly, dendritic spines are now present in abundance, with some evidence of a proximodistal gradient of spine development on the processes of the Meynert cells. The axons of the Meynert cells give rise to clear collateral branches.

The appearance of the dendritic spines is a morphogenetic event of unquestioned significance, since it signals the readiness of the pyramidal cells to begin forming a mature synaptic pattern. To what extent the axon terminals that will synapse with the developing spines are the same as or different from those initially present on the dendritic shaft (see Cotman *et al.*, 1973) is not yet clear. As is apparent from the work of Marin-Padilla (1972b), confirmed by Purpura (1975a), the earliest form of dendritic spine in human material is a long, thin process, often with conspicuous varicosities. Its trajectory may display prominent kinks or bends. In the fetal human motor cortex (Purpura, 1975a), these thin processes are detectable in small numbers at 18 weeks of gestational age. More are evident at 26 weeks, and still more at 33 weeks. While some mushroom and stubby spines (terminology of Peters and Kaiserman-Abramof, 1970) are present at this latter age, and occasionally at earlier ages, long thin processes still predominate. The transformation of the pyramidal cell spine complement to the mature morphological pattern is a protracted process, extending well into postnatal life (Poliakov, 1966; Marin-Padilla, 1972b; Purpura, 1975a). During the course of this process, the long polymorphous spines are completely replaced by—or perhaps become transformed into—the mature types of short spines (Marin-Padilla, 1967). While the formation and modulation of specific spine forms, as well as a number of other developmental changes, may occur at rather rapid rates (Schüz, 1978) during specifically timed phases of development, it is worth noting that the full development of some pyramidal cell features, e.g., axon myelination (Yakovlev and Lecours, 1967), may continue well into postnatal life (Conel, 1939–1963). In the rat, too, pyramidal axon myelination may extend over a comparably protracted time period (Berry, 1974).

In the developing neocortex of the cat, cells which are unequivocally identifiable as pyramidal neurons are first detected at about 4 weeks of gestational age. The development of pyramids of layer V has been studied between this age and birth, at about 8½ weeks, by Marin-Padilla (1972a). As illustrated in Fig. 4 of his report, the major developmental changes undergone by cat pyramidal cells in the prenatal period are as follows. At about 4 weeks of gestational age, the small fusiform somata give rise to primitive apical dendrites and short lengths of developing axon. Both are unbranched, but the distal tip of the apical dendrite exhibits several nubbinlike extensions presaging the terminal tuft. At 35 and 40 days, the cell bodies begin to enlarge and to gradually acquire their mature shapes. Basal dendrites begin to appear and the terminal tuft expands somewhat. At 45 days, oblique branches appear at the proximal end of the apical dendrite, and the terminal tuft and basal dendrites display definite secondary and tertiary branches. Short collaterals from the lengthening axon begin to be evident. These neural elaborations coincide in time with the first incursions into the cortical plate by horizontally disposed corticopetal fibers. These fibers, in the opinion of Marin-Padilla (see Chapter 14) and others (Morest, 1969b), play an important inductive role in pyramidal cell maturation (see also Wise *et al.*, 1979). Progressive development of all of the morphological features of the pyramidal cell is seen at the 50-day stage and at birth, although developmental studies beyond this period (Noback and Purpura, 1961) indicate that the progress of cellular maturation, in terms of features such as dendritic length, will continue at least into the third postnatal week.

It is at approximately the 45-day stage that the first dendritic spines are recognized (Marin-Padilla, 1972a). These are present on the proximal portion of the apical dendrite, on the basal dendrites, and on the cell body. By day 50, with the arrival of a new stratum of corticopetal fibers at about the level of the developing layer III, spines begin to appear along the middle reaches of the layer V pyramidal apical dendrites, and by birth they stud the entire dendritic surface of the cell. In the Golgi material studied by Scheibel and Scheibel (1968), a correlation was noted between the time of appearance of dendritic spines and the first observations of axonal contacts with apical dendrites.

In the developing cerebral neocortex of the rat (Berry, 1974), the major stages of pyramidal cell differentiation occur after birth, although occasional cells exhibiting pyramidal characteristics exist in the late prenatal cortex (Peters and Feldman, 1973). The morphological details of the prenatal situation have been described by Peters and Feldman (1973) and by Raedler and Sievers (1975), and the postnatal events by Eayrs and Goodhead (1959), Raedler and Sievers (1975), Miller (1981), and Miller and Peters (1981), among others. In the occipital cortex, the transition from a primitively organized cortex to one in which the beginnings of the mature lamination pattern is seen occurs between the third and seventh postnatal days, with the adult lamination pattern being largely complete by day 10 (Raedler and Sievers, 1975). In this and other developmental respects there exists a lateromedial gradient of maturation, the more lateral elements displaying the earlier development. This gradient may be superimposed on a more widespread caudorostral gradient which has been described in the mouse (Angevine and Sidman, 1962).

In general, the sequential steps of pyramidal cell maturation in this species follow those described above in other species. It is of considerable theoretical interest that this sequence is also manifest in cortical pyramidal neurons which develop in noncortical loci, i.e., within clumps of fetal cortical tissue surgically transplanted to the cerebella of neonatal hosts (Das, 1975). In normally developing pyramidal cells, as typically found at birth (Miller, 1981) or some days later (Eayrs and Goodhead, 1959), the soma is small and fusiform and the only clear dendritic process is the apical dendrite. This bears short and simple branches at its distal tip. Extending from the base of the cell body is a thin, unbranched axon. Over the course of the ensuing several weeks there occurs a steady growth in somal volume and in the length and complexity of the various dendritic systems (Miller, 1981). Certain aspects of this growth provide evidence for a more extensive development of the deeper-lying pyramids than is true of those more superficially situated (Juraska and Fifková, 1979; Wise *et al.,* 1979). One prominent feature of the developing dendrites in the rat up to 12–15 days of postnatal age is the presence of enlargements, presumably growth cones (Morest, 1969a,b; Scheibel and Scheibel, 1971), at the distal tips of the immature processes and occasionally along the more proximal portions of their shafts. Small numbers of fine filopodia extend from these enlargements. These filopodia and/or the vesicles or other membranous components within the enlargements (Del Cerro and Snider, 1968; Peters and Feldman, 1973) may constitute a reserve of membrane that is utilized in the eventual extension of the dendrite (Morest, 1969b). Each growth cone, according to Miller and Peters (1981), forms at least one symmetric synapse. Miller and Peters have also described a morphological sequence leading to the development of dendritic spines. In the scheme they propose, spines first appear as slightly raised elevations along the dendritic shaft. These elevations form symmetric synapses with axons. Gradually, the elevations elongate into stumpy protuberances and the junctional membrane thickenings take on the asymmetric character of adult axospinous synapses. Finally, the broad bases of the stumps narrow to produce spines of Peters and Kaiserman-Abramof's (1970) thin type, with an elongated, constricted neck and an expanded terminal portion which typically forms the axospinous synapse.

Eayrs and Goodhead (1959) noted that the mean numbers of basal dendritic trunks radiating from cell bodies reached adult values relatively early in postnatal development. This has since been studied quantitatively in hooded (Juraska and Fifková, 1979) and albino (Uylings and Parnavelas, 1981; Miller, 1981) rats. The interesting feature of the data published by Miller is the presence of a peak number of basal dendrite origins—at 6 days for layer V pyramids and at 9 days for layer II/III pyramids—just prior to the leveling off of the origin counts (see also Boothe *et al.,* 1979). These peak values are statistically significantly higher than the asymptotic values obtained at day 21. While not in complete agreement with Juraska and Fifková's or Uylings and Parnavelas's findings, the results reported by Miller, if confirmed, would suggest that basal dendrites may be included among those developmental features which are generated in superabundance and which decrease in number as maturation proceeds (e.g., Ramón y Cajal, 1955; Morest, 1969b; Jacobson, 1978).

The examples given above review the main features of pyramidal cell morphogenesis. For the most part, the studies which have provided this basic information have been confined to particular developmental stages, although there have been occasional efforts (e.g., Conel, 1939–1963) to extend the span of study well beyond the period during which the major cellular features emerge. Reference has already been made to studies which demonstrate that the process of pyramidal cell axon myelination may extend into the period of adulthood. Such findings suggest that there may exist quantitative, although perhaps not qualitative, changes in cellular features that occur continuously throughout the life span. It may, in other words, be inaccurate to conceive of pyramidal cell morphology as becoming immutably fixed at the termination of some perinatal period of development, with no further changes occurring in the normal individual until the initiation of the changes associated with old age.

This position has previously been argued from the point of view of aging changes of rat visual cortical pyramidal cells by Feldman and Dowd (1975). These authors noted, both within their own data and in a comparison of their own data with the results of others, evidence for the notion of a continuously changing spine population throughout the life span, including the developmental period (see also Connor *et al.,* 1980). They pointed out, however, the need for explicit quantitative study of this question, with a particular focus on the age range beginning at, in the rat, 15 days of age. Interestingly, a recent report describes such an analysis, carried out on visual cortical pyramidal cells of rats aged 15,

30, and 60 days (Juraska, 1982), thus extending the studies from the early postnatal developmental period (Juraska and Fifková, 1979) to the period of adulthood. Dendritic branching and spine density were measured for layer III and V pyramidal neurons at each age. It was found that there were no changes in the number of dendritic branches during the period studied. However, the length of certain dendritic branches did change. For example, the total length of the layer III basal dendrites, as well as the length of most of the component dendritic segments, increased significantly from 15 to 30 and from 30 to 60 days of age. The changes observed were variable and were specific to particular dendritic systems. The total length of layer III pyramidal oblique branches, for example, increased significantly from 15 to 30 days, and then decreased significantly by 60 days. Changes in visible spine density were also observed, and these too were variable. Among the changes seen were spine increases on layer V pyramidal terminal tufts and apical dendritic shafts between 15 and 30 days, and a decrease in spine density on layer III pyramidal basal dendrites between 30 and 60 days. It thus seems clear that, although the process is not simple and uniform, quantitative developmental changes in pyramidal neurons do extend into the period of adulthood in rat visual cortex. The same appears to be true in rat somatic sensory cortex (Wise *et al.*, 1979).

Similar results have also been obtained for spine and dendrite development in primates (Lund *et al.*, 1977; Boothe *et al.*, 1979). Quantitative study of spines in primate visual cortex reveals an increase in spine density to 8 weeks of postnatal age for both layer III and VI pyramids. Over the course of the next 2 months of development, this spine number may stay constant or may decrease. Both may occur in specific portions of individual cells, depending upon lamina. All neurons show further decreases in spine density between 9 months and 5–7 years of age, producing an adult spine density in the same range as observed in perinatal animals (Boothe *et al.*, 1979).

In summary, the morphological maturation of the pyramidal neuron may be considered at three levels of analysis. At the first and most general level are developmental features that appear to be common to all neocortical pyramidal cells, such as the earlier maturation of larger and deeper-lying elements, and the early elaboration of the apical dendrite. This is an area in which a considerable amount of information exists and about which there is widespread agreement. At the second level of analysis are largely qualitative studies which focus on the emergence of specific pyramidal cell features in particular species and cortical loci. This level of investigation has provided us with the majority of our practical knowledge of pyramidal cell development. At the third level of analysis are quantitative studies, dealing with such features as changes in dendritic length and spine density as a function of age. It is in this area that the least is known. But further studies at this level, in conjunction with correlated ultrastructural observations, are highly likely to provide the next significant step forward in our knowledge of mechanisms of pyramidal cell development.

ACKNOWLEDGMENTS. The preparation of this chapter was supported by Research Grant AG02123 and by Research Career Development Award AG00016, both from the National Institutes of Health; additional support was provided by Program Project Grant AG00001. The electron micrographs in this chapter were kindly furnished by Dr. Alan Peters. The author would also like to acknowledge with gratitude the many enjoyable and informative discussions of pyramidal cells with Dr. Alan Peters and Dr. Thomas L. Kemper, and the assistance provided by Andrew L. Feldman.

6. References

Adams, I., and Jones, D. G., 1982, Quantitative ultrastructural changes in rat cortical synapses during early-, mid- and late-adulthood, *Brain Res.* **239:**349–363.

Alzheimer, A., 1907, Über eine eigenartige Erkrankung der Hirnrinde, *Centralbl. Nerveneilk. Psychiatr.* **18:**177–179.

Andersen, R. A., Asanuma, C., and Cowan, W. M., 1982, Observations on the callosal and associational cortico-cortical connections of area 7A of the macaque monkey, *Soc. Neurosci. Abstr.* **8:**210.

Angevine, J. B., and Sidman, R. L., 1961, Autoradiographic study of cell migration during histogenesis of cerebral cortex in the mouse, *Nature (London)* **192:**766–768.

Angevine, J. B., and Sidman, R. L., 1962, Autoradiographic study of histogenesis in the cerebral cortex of the mouse, *Anat. Rec.* **142:**210.

Åström, K. E., 1967, On the early development of the isocortex in fetal sheep, in: *Developmental Neurology*, Progress in Brain Research, Vol. 26 (C. G. Bernhard and J. P. Schadé, eds.), pp. 1–59, Elsevier, Amsterdam.

Berlin, R., 1858, *Beitrag zur Strukturlehre der Grosshirnwindungen* (Inauguralabh.), Junge, Erlangen.

Bernstein, M. E., and Bernstein, J. J., 1973, Regeneration of axons and synaptic complex formation rostral to the site of hemisection in the spinal cord of the monkey, *Int. J. Neurosci.* **5:**15–26.

Berry, M., 1974, Development of the cerebral neocortex of the rat, in: *Aspects of Neurogenesis*, Studies on the Development of Behavior and the Nervous System, Vol. 2 (G. Gottlieb, ed.), pp. 7–67, Academic Press, New York.

Berry, M., and Rogers, A. W., 1965, The migration of neuroblasts in the developing cerebral cortex, *J. Anat.* **99:**691–709.

Berry, M., Anderson, E. M., Hollingworth, T., and Flinn, R. M., 1972, A computer technique for the estimation of the absolute three-dimensional array of basal dendritic fields using data from projected histological sections, *J. Microsc. (Oxford)* **95:**257–267.

Betz, V., 1874, Anatomischer Nachweis zwei Gehirncentra, *Centralbl. Med. Wiss.* **12:**578–580, 595–599.

Bok, S. T., 1934, Messungen an den Ganglienzellen der Grosshirurinde. I. Die Einheitlichkeit der einzelnen Hauptzonen, *Z. Mikrosk. Anat. Forsch.* **36:**645–650.

Bok, S. T., 1936, A quantitative analysis of the structure of the cerebral cortex, *Verh. K. Akad. Wet. Amsterdam* **35:**1–55.

Bok, S. T., 1959, *Histonomy of the Cerebral Cortex*, Elsevier, Amsterdam.

Boothe, R. G., Greenough, W. T., Lund, J. S., and Wrege, K., 1979, A quantitative investigation of spine and dendrite development of neurons in visual cortex (area 17) of *Macaca nemestrina* monkeys, *J. Comp. Neurol.* **186:**473–490.

Braak, H., 1976a, On the striate area of the human isocortex. A Golgi- and pigmentarchitectonic study, *J. Comp. Neurol.* **166:**341–364.

Braak, H., 1976b, A primitive gigantopyramidal field buried in the depth of the cingulate sulcus of the human brain, *Brain Res.* **109:**219–233.

Braak, H., 1979, Spindle-shaped appendages of IIIab pyramids filled with lipofuscin: A striking pathological change of senescent human isocortex, *Acta Neuropathol.* **46:**197–202.

Braak, H., 1980, *Architectonics of the Human Telencephalic Cortex*, Springer-Verlag, Berlin.

Braak, H., and Braak, E., 1976, The pyramidal cells of Betz within the cingulate and precentral gigantopyramidal field in the human brain: A Golgi and pigmentarchitectonic study, *Cell Tissue Res.* **172:**103–119.

Braak, H., Braak, E., and Strenge, H., 1976, Gehören die Inselneurone der Regio entorhinalis zur Klasse der Pyramiden—oder der Sternzellen? *Z. Mikrosk. Anat. Forsch.* **90:**1017–1031.

Braak, E., Braak, H., Strenge, H., and Muhtaroglu, U., 1980, Age-related alterations of the proximal axonal segment in lamina IIIab pyramidal cells of the human isocortex: A Golgi and fine structural study, *J. Hirnforsch.* **21**:531–535.

Braitenberg, V., 1978; Cortical architectonics: General and areal, in: *Architectonics of the Cerebral Cortex* (M. A. B. Brazier and H. Petsche, eds.), pp. 443–465, Raven Press, New York.

Brazier, M. A. B., 1968, Architectonics of the cerebral cortex: Research in the 19th century, in: *Architectonics of the Cerebral Cortex* (M. A. B. Brazier and H. Petsche, eds.), pp. 9–29, Raven Press, New York.

Brizzee, K. R., Ordy, J. M., Kaack, M. B., and Beavers, T., 1980, Effects of prenatal ionizing radiation on the visual cortex and hippocampus of newborn squirrel monkeys, *J. Neuropathol. Exp. Neurol.* **39**:523–540.

Brody, H., 1976, An examination of cerebral cortex and brainstem aging, in: *Aging*, Vol. 3 (R. D. Terry and S. Gershon, eds.), pp. 177–181, Raven Press, New York.

Buell, S., and Coleman, P. D., 1979, Dendrite growth in the aged human brain and failure of growth in senile dementia, *Science* **206**:854–856.

Butler, A. B., and Jane, J. A., 1977, Interlaminar connections of rat visual cortex: An ultrastructural study, *J. Comp. Neurol.* **174**:521–534.

Caviness, V. S., Jr., 1976, Patterns of cell and fiber distribution in the neocortex of the Reeler mutant mouse, *J. Comp. Neurol.* **170**:435–448.

Chan-Palay, V., Palay, S. L., and Billings-Gagliardi, S. M., 1974, Meynert cells in the primate visual cortex, *J. Neurocytol.* **3**:631–658.

Chiang, B., 1973, The organization of the visual cortex (Ph.D. dissertation, Syracuse University), cited by Paldino and Harth, 1977a.

Clark, W. E. L., 1942, The cells of Meynert in the visual cortex of the monkey, *J. Anat.* **76**:369–376.

Coleman, P. D., and Riesen, A. H., 1968, Environmental effects on cortical dendritic fields. I. Rearing in the dark, *J. Anat.* **102**:363–374.

Colonnier, M., 1964, The tangential organization of the visual cortex, *J. Anat.* **98**:327–344.

Colonnier, M., 1968, Synaptic patterns on different cell types in the different laminae of the cat visual cortex, *Brain Res.* **9**:268–287.

Colonnier, M., 1981, The electron microscopic analysis of the neuronal organization of the cerebral cortex, in: *The Organization of the Cerebral Cortex* (F. O. Schmitt, F. G. Worden, G. Adelman, and S. G. Dennis, eds.), pp. 125–152, MIT Press, Cambridge, Mass.

Colonnier, M., and Rossignol, S., 1969, On the heterogeneity of the cerebral cortex, in: *Basic Mechanisms of the Epilepsies* (H. Jasper, A. Pope, and A. Ward, eds.), Little, Brown, Boston.

Conel, J. L., 1939–1963, *The Postnatal Development of the Human Cerebral Cortex*, 6 volumes, Harvard University Press, Cambridge, Mass.

Connor, J. R., and Diamond, M. C., 1982, A comparison of dendritic spine number and type on pyramidal neurons of the visual cortex of old adult rats from social or isolated environments, *J. Comp. Neurol.* **210**:99–106.

Connor, J. R., Diamond, M. C., and Johnson, R. E., 1980, Aging and environmental influences on two types of dendritic spines in the rat occipital cortex, *Exp. Neurol.* **70**:371–379.

Cotman, C. W., and Lynch, G. S., 1976, Reactive synaptogenesis in the adult nervous system: The effects of partial deafferentation on new synapse formation, in: *Neuronal Recognition* (S. H. Barondes, ed.), pp. 69–108, Plenum Press, New York.

Cotman, C. W., Taylor, D., and Lynch, G., 1973, Ultrastructural changes in synapses in the dentate gyrus of the rat during development, *Brain Res.* **63**:205–213.

Cupp, C. J., and Uemura, E., 1980, Age-related changes in prefrontal cortex of *Macaca mulatta*: Quantitative analysis of dendritic branching patterns, *Exp. Neurol.* **69**:143–163.

Das, G. D., 1975, Differentiation of dendrites in the transplanted neuroblasts in the mammalian brain, in: *Physiology and Pathology of Dendrites*, Advances in Neurology, Vol. 12 (G. W. Kreutzberg, ed.), pp. 181–199, Raven Press, New York.

Davis, T. L., and Sterling, P., 1979, Microcircuitry of cat visual cortex: Classification of neurons in layer IV of area 17, and identification of the patterns of lateral geniculate input, *J. Comp. Neurol.* **188**:599–628.

Del Cerro, M. P., and Snider, R. S., 1968, Studies on the developing cerebellum: Ultrastructure of growth cones, *J. Comp. Neurol.* **133**:341–362.

Demoor, J., 1898, Le mechanisme et la signification de l'etat moniliforme des neurones, *Ann. Soc. R. Sci. Med. Nat. Brux.* **7**:205–250.

Devaney, K. O., and Johnson, H. A., 1980, Neuron loss in the aging visual cortex of man, *J. Gerontol.* **35**:836–841.

Domesick, V., 1969, Projections from the cingulate cortex in the rat, *Brain Res.* **12**:296–320.

Donoghue, J. P., and Kitai, S. T., 1981, A collateral pathway to the neostriatum from corticofugal neurons of the rat sensory-motor cortex: An intracellular HRP study, *J. Comp. Neurol.* **201**:1–13.

Eayrs, J. T., and Goodhead, B., 1959, Postnatal development of the cerebral cortex of the rat, *J. Anat.* **93**:385–402.

Ebner, F. F., 1969, A comparison of primitive forebrain organization in metatherian and eutherian mammals, *Ann. N.Y. Acad. Sci.* **167**:241–257.

Ebner, F. F., and Colonnier, M., 1975, Synaptic patterns in the visual cortex of turtle: An electron microscopic study, *J. Comp. Neurol.* **160**:51–79.

Fairén, A., and DeFelipe, J., 1982, Identification of basket cells in superficial layers of the cat visual cortex, *Neuroscience* **7**:S65.

Fairén, A., and Valverde, F., 1973, Centros visuales en roedores: Estructura normal y efectos de la deprivación sensorial sobre la morfología dendrítica, *Trab. Inst. Cajal Invest. Biol.* **65**:87–135.

Fairén, A., and Valverde, F., 1980, A specialized type of neuron in the visual cortex of cat: A Golgi and electron microscope study of chandelier cells, *J. Comp. Neurol.* **194**:761–779.

Fairén, A., Peters, A., and Saldanha, J., 1977, A new procedure for examining Golgi impregnated neurons by light and electron microscopy, *J. Neurocytol.* **6**:311–337.

Feldman, M. L., 1975, Serial thin sections of pyramidal apical dendrites in the cerebral cortex: Spine topography and related observations, *Anat. Rec.* **181**:354–355.

Feldman, M. L., 1976, Aging changes in the morphology of cortical dendrites, in: *Neurobiology of Aging* (R. D. Terry and S. Gershon, eds.), pp. 211–227, Raven Press, New York.

Feldman, M. L., 1977, Dendritic changes in aging rat brain: Pyramidal cell dendrite length and ultrastructure, in: *The Aging Brain and Senile Dementia* (K. Nandy and I. Sherwin, eds.), pp. 23–37, Plenum Press, New York.

Feldman, M. L., and Dowd, C., 1974, Aging in rat visual cortex: Light microscopic observations on layer V pyramidal apical dendrites, *Anat. Rec.* **178**:355.

Feldman, M. L., and Dowd, C., 1975, Loss of dendritic spines in aging cerebral cortex, *Z. Anat. Entwicklungsgesch.* **148**:279–301.

Feldman, M. L., and Peters, A., 1972, Intranuclear rods and sheets in rat cochlear nucleus, *J. Neurocytol.* **1**:109–127.

Feldman, M. L., and Peters, A., 1974a, A study of barrels and pyramidal dendritic clusters in the cerebral cortex, *Brain Res.* **77**:55–76.

Feldman, M. L., and Peters, A., 1974b, Morphological changes in the aging brain, in: *Survey Report of the Aging Nervous System* (G. J. Maletta, ed.), U.S. Department of Health, Education and Welfare, Publication (NIH) 74-296, pp. 5–22.

Feldman, M. L., and Peters, A., 1978, The forms of non-pyramidal neurons in the visual cortex of the rat, *J. Comp. Neurol.* **179**:761–794.

Feldman, M. L., and Peters, A., 1979, A technique for estimating total spine numbers on Golgi-impregnated dendrites, *J. Comp. Neurol.* **188**:527–542.

Fifková, E., 1970, The effect of unilateral deprivation on visual centers in rats, *J. Comp. Neurol.* **140**:431–438.

Fifková, E., and Delay, R. J., 1982, Cytoplasmic actin in dendritic spines as a possible mediator of synaptic plasticity, *Soc. Neurosci. Abstr.* **8**:279.

Fifková, E., and Van Harreveld, A., 1977, Long-lasting morphological changes in dendritic spines of dentate granular cells following stimulation of the entorhinal area, *J. Neurocytol.* **6**:211–230.

Fleischhauer, K., 1974, On different patterns of dendritic bundling in the cerebral cortex of the cat, *Z. Anat. Entwicklungsgesch.* **143**:115–126.

Fleischhauer, K., 1978, Cortical architectonics: The last 50 years and some problems of today, in: *Architectonics of the Cerebral Cortex* (M. A. B. Brazier and H. Petsche, eds.), pp. 99–117, Raven Press, New York.

Fleischhauer, K., Petsche, H., and Wittkowski, W., 1972, Vertical bundles of dendrites in the neo-cortex, *Z. Anat. Entwicklungsgesch.* **136**:213–223.

Garey, L. J., 1971, A light and electron microscopic study of the visual cortex of the cat and monkey, *Proc. R. Soc. London Ser. B* **179**:21–40.

Gilbert, C. D., and Kelly, J. P., 1975, The projections of cells in different layers of the cat's visual cortex, *J. Comp. Neurol.* **163**:81–106.

Gilbert, C. D., and Wiesel, T. N., 1979, Morphology and intracortical projections of functionally characterised neurones in the cat visual cortex, *Nature (London)* **280**:120–125.

Gilbert, C. D., and Wiesel, T. N., 1981, Laminar specialization and intracortical connections in cat primary visual cortex, in: *The Organization of the Cerebral Cortex* (F. O. Schmitt, F. G. Worden, G. Adelman, and S. G. Dennis, eds.), pp. 163–191, MIT Press, Cambridge, Mass.

Gilbert, C. D., and Wiesel, T. N., 1982, Clustered intracortical connections in cat visual cortex, *Soc. Neurosci. Abstr.* **8**:706.

Glaser, E. M., and McMullen, N. T., 1980, Tonotopic organization and dendrite orientation in primary auditory cortex of the rabbit, *Soc. Neurosci. Abstr.* **6**:557.

Glaser, E. M., Van der Loos, H., and Gissler, M., 1979, Tangential orientation and spatial order in dendrites of cat auditory cortex: A computer microscope study of Golgi-impregnated material, *Exp. Brain Res.* **36**:411–431.

Globus, A., and Scheibel, A. B., 1966, Loss of dendritic spines as an index of presynaptic terminal patterns, *Nature (London)* **212**:463–465.

Globus, A., and Scheibel, A. B., 1967a, Pattern and field in cortical structure: The rabbit, *J. Comp. Neurol.* **131**:155–172.

Globus, A., and Scheibel, A. B., 1967b, Synaptic loci on visual cortical neurons of the rabbit: The specific afferent radiation, *Exp. Neurol.* **18**:116–131.

Globus, A., and Scheibel, A. B., 1967c, The effect of visual deprivation on cortical neurons: A Golgi study, *Exp. Neurol.* **19**:331–345.

Goldman-Rakic, P. S., and Schwartz, M. L., 1982, Interdigitation of contralateral and ipsilateral columnar projections to frontal association cortex in primates, *Science* **216**:755–757.

Golgi, C., 1873, Sulla sostanza grigia del cervello, *Gaz Med. Ital. Lombardia* **6**:244–246 [translated by M. Santini in Santini, M. (ed.), 1975, *Golgi Centennial Symposium: Perspectives in Neurobiology*, Raven Press, New York].

Golgi, C., 1882–1885, Sulla fina anatomia degli organi centrali del sistema nervoso, *Riv. Sper. Freniatr. Med. Leg. Aliengzioni Ment.* **8**:165–195, 361–391; **9**:1–17, 161–192, 385–402; **11**:72–123, 193–220.

Golgi, C., 1883, Recherches sur l'histologie des centres nerveux, *Arch. Ital. Biol.* **3**:285–317.

Gray, E. G., 1959, Axo-somatic and axo-dendritic synapses of the cerebral cortex: An electron microscope study, *J. Anat.* **93**:420–433.

Guillery, R. W., 1972, Experiments to determine whether retinogeniculate axons can form translaminar collateral sprouts in the dorsal lateral geniculate nucleus of the cat, *J. Comp. Neurol.* **146**:407–420.

Hammarberg, C., 1895, *Studien über Klinik und Pathologie der Idiotie, nebst Untersuchungen über die normale Anatomie der Hirnrinde*, Akademischen Buchdruckerei (Edv. Berling), Upsala.

Heimer, L., 1969, The secondary olfactory connections in mammals, reptiles and sharks, *Ann. N.Y. Acad. Sci.* **167**:129–146.

Hersch, S. M., and White, E. L., 1981a, Quantification of synapses formed with apical dendrites of Golgi-impregnated pyramidal cells: Variability in thalamocortical inputs, but consistency in the ratios of asymmetrical to symmetrical synapses, *Neuroscience* **6**:1043–1051.

Hersch, S. M., and White, E. L., 1981b, Thalamocortical synapses involving identified neurons in mouse primary somatosensory cortex: A terminal degeneration and Golgi/EM study, *J. Comp. Neurol.* **195**:253–263.

Hersch, S. M., and White, E. L., 1982, A quantitative study of the thalamocortical and other synapses in layer IV of pyramidal cells projecting from mouse SmI cortex to the caudate-putamen nucleus, *J. Comp. Neurol.* **211**:217–225.

Heumann, D., and Rabinowicz, T., 1982, Postnatal development of the visual cortex of the mouse after enucleation at birth, *Exp. Brain Res.* **46**:99–106.

Hollingworth, T., and Berry, M., 1975, Network analysis of dendritic fields of pyramidal cells in neocortex and Purkinje cells in the cerebellum of the rat, *Philos. Trans. R. Soc. London Ser. B* **270**:227–264.

Hornung, J. P., and Garey, L. J., 1981, The thalamic projection to cat visual cortex: Ultrastructure of neurons identified by Golgi impregnation of retrograde horseradish peroxidase transport, *Neuroscience* **6**:1053–1068.

Hubel, D. H., and Wiesel, T. N., 1963, Shape and arrangement of columns in cat's striate cortex, *J. Physiol. (London)* **165**:559–568.

Hubel, D. H., and Wiesel, T. N., 1969, An anatomical demonstration of columns in the monkey striate cortex, *Nature (London)* **221**:747–750.

Hubel, D. H., and Wiesel, T. N., 1972, Laminar and columnar distribution of geniculo-cortical fibres in the macaque monkey, *J. Comp. Neurol.* **146**:421–450.

Huttenlocher, P. R., 1975, Synaptic and dendritic development and mental defect, in: *Brain Mechanisms in Mental Retardation* (N. A. Buchwald and M. A. B. Brazier, eds.), pp. 123–140, Academic Press, New York.

Huttenlocher, P. R., 1979, Synaptic density in human frontal cortex: Developmental changes and effects of aging, *Brain Res.* **163**:195–205.

Jacobson, M., 1978, *Developmental Neurobiology,* Plenum Press, New York.

Jacobson, S., 1967, Dimensions of the dendritic spine in the sensorimotor cortex of rat, cat, squirrel monkey, and man, *J. Comp. Neurol.* **129**:49–58.

Jayaraman, A., 1982, The cells of origin of corticostriate projection in cats, *Neuroscience* **7**:S104.

Jones, E. G., 1975, Varieties and distribution of non-pyramidal cells in the somatic sensory cortex of the squirrel monkey, *J. Comp. Neurol.* **160**:205–268.

Jones, E. G., 1981, Anatomy of cerebral cortex: Columnar input–output organization, in: *The Organization of the Cerebral Cortex* (F. O. Schmitt, F. G. Worden, G. Adelman, and S. G. Dennis, eds.), pp. 199–235, MIT Press, Cambridge, Mass.

Jones, E. G., and Powell, T. P. S., 1969a, Morphological variations in the dendritic spines of the neocortex, *J. Cell Sci.* **5**:509–529.

Jones, E. G., and Powell, T. P. S., 1969b, Synapses on the axon hillocks and initial segments of pyramidal cell axons in the cerebral cortex, *J. Cell Sci.* **5**:495–507.

Jones, E. G., and Powell, T. P. S., 1970, Electron microscopy of the somatic sensory cortex of the cat. I. Cell types and synaptic organization, *Philos. Trans. R. Soc. London Ser. B* **257**:1–11.

Jones, E. G., Coulter, J. D., Burton, G., and Porter, R., 1977, Cells of origin and terminal distribution of corticostriatal fibers arising in the sensory-motor cortex of monkeys, *J. Comp. Neurol.* **173**:53–80.

Jones, E. G., Coulter, J. D., and Wise, S. P., 1979, Commisural columns in the sensory-motor cortex of monkeys, *J. Comp. Neurol.* **188**:113–136.

Juraska, J. M., 1982, The development of pyramidal neurons after eye opening in the visual cortex of hooded rats: A quantitative study, *J. Comp. Neurol.* **212**:208–213.

Juraska, J. M., and Fifková, E., 1979, A Golgi study of the early postnatal development of the visual cortex of the hooded rat, *J. Comp. Neurol.* **183**:247–256.

Kaes, T., 1907, *Die Grosshirnrinde des Menschen in ihre Massen und ihrem Fasergehalt,* Fischer, Jena.

Kaiserman-Abramof, I. R., and Peters, A., 1972, Some aspects of the morphology of Betz cells in the cerebral cortex of the cat, *Brain Res.* **43**:527–546.

Kalil, K., and Reh, T., 1982, A light and electron microscopic study of regrowing pyramidal tract fibers, *J. Comp. Neurol.* **211**:265–275.

Kaplan, A. S., and Scheibel, A. B., 1980, Giant spine-poor pyramidal cells in auditory cortex of young and aged cats, *Soc. Neurosci. Abstr.* **6**:557.

Kemper, T. L., Caveness, W. F., and Yakovlev, P. I., 1973, The neuronographic and metric study of the dendritic arbours of neurons in the motor cortex of *Macaca mulatta* at birth and at 24 months of age, *Brain* **96**:765–782.

Kennedy, H., 1982, Types of synapses contacting the soma of corticotectal cells in the visual cortex of the cat, *Neuroscience* **7**:2159–2164.

Kirsche, W., Kunz, G., Wenzel, J., Wenzel, M., Winkelmann, A., and Winkelmann, E., 1973, Neurohistologische Untersuchungen zur Variabilität der Pyramidenzellen des sensomotorischen Cortex der Ratte, *J. Hirnforsch.* **14**:117–135.

Krieg, W. J. S., 1946, Connections of the cerebral cortex. I. Albino rat. A. Topography of the cortical areas, *J. Comp. Neurol.* **84**:221–275.

Kunz, G., Kirsche, W., Wenzel, J., Winkelmann, E., and Neumann, H., 1972, Quantitative Untersuchungen über die Dendritenspines an Pyramidenneuronen des sensorischen Cortex der Ratte, *Z. Mikrosk. Anat. Forsch.* **85**:397–416.

Laatsch, R. H., and Cowan, W. M., 1966, Electron microscope studies of the dentate gyrus of the rat. I. Normal structure with reference to synaptic organization, *J. Comp. Neurol.* **128**:359–396.

Landis, D. M. D., and Reese, T. S., 1982, Organization of filaments in presynaptic and postsynaptic cytoplasm revealed in rapidly frozen cerebellar cortex, *Soc. Neurosci. Abstr.* **8**:280.

Landry, P., Labelle, A., and Deschênes, M., 1980, Intracortical distribution of axonal collaterals of pyramidal tract cells in the cat motor cortex, *Brain Res.* **191**:327–336.

Lassek, A. M., 1954, *The Pyramidal Tract,* Thomas, Springfield, Ill.

LeVay, S., 1973, Synaptic patterns in the visual cortex of the cat and monkey: Electron microscopy of Golgi preparations, *J. Comp. Neurol.* **150:**53–86.

Lewis, W. B., 1879, On the comparative structure of the cortex cerebri, *Brain* **1:**79–86.

Lewis, W. B., 1881, Researches on the comparative structure of the cortex cerebri, *Philos. Trans. R. Soc. London* **171:**35–66.

Lewis, W. B., and Clarke, H., 1878, The cortical lamination of the motor area of the brain, *Proc. R. Soc. London* **27:**38–49.

Lindsay, R. D., and Scheibel, A. B., 1974, Quantitative analysis of the dendritic branching pattern of small pyramidal cells from adult rat somesthetic and visual cortex, *Exp. Neurol.* **45:** 424–434.

Liu, C. M., and Chambers, W. W., 1958, Intraspinal sprouting of dorsal root axons, *Arch. Neurol. Psychiatry* **79:**46–61.

Lorente de Nó, R., 1922, La corteza cerebral del ratón, *Trab. Lab. Invest. Biol. Madrid* **20:**41–78.

Lorente de Nó, R., 1949, Cerebral cortex: Architecture, intracortical connections, motor projections, in: *Physiology of the Nervous System* (J. F. Fulton, ed.), 3rd ed., pp. 288–313, Oxford University Press, London.

Lund, J. S., 1973, Organization of neurons in the visual cortex, area 17, of the monkey *(Macaca mulatta)*, *J. Comp. Neurol.* **147:**455–495.

Lund, J. S., 1981, Intrinsic organization of the primate visual cortex, area 17, as seen in Golgi preparations, in: *The Organization of the Cerebral Cortex* (F. O. Schmitt, F. G. Worden, G. Adelman, and S. G. Dennis, eds.), pp. 105–124, MIT Press, Cambridge, Mass.

Lund, J. S., and Boothe, R. G., 1975, Interlaminar connections and pyramidal neuron organisation in the visual cortex, area 17, of the macaque monkey, *J. Comp. Neurol.* **159:**305–334.

Lund, J. S., Lund, R. D., Hendrickson, A. E., Bunt, A. H., and Fuchs, A. F., 1975, The origin of efferent pathways from the primary visual cortex, area 17, of the macaque monkey as shown by retrograde transport of horseradish peroxidase, *J. Comp. Neurol.* **164:**287–304.

Lund, J. S., Boothe, R. G., and Lund, R. D., 1977, Development of neurons in the visual cortex (area 17) of the monkey *(Macaca nemestrina):* A Golgi study from fetal day 127 to postnatal maturity, *J. Comp. Neurol.* **176:**149–188.

Lund, J. S., Hendrickson, A. E., Ogren, M. P., and Tobin, E. A., 1981, Anatomical organization of primate visual cortex area V II, *J. Comp. Neurol.* **202:**19–45.

McConnell, P., and Berry, M., 1978, The effects of undernutrition on Purkinje cell dendritic growth in the rat, *J. Comp. Neurol.* **177:**159–172.

Marin-Padilla, M., 1967, Number and distribution of the apical dendritic spines of the layer V pyramidal cells in man, *J. Comp. Neurol.* **131:**475–490.

Marin-Padilla, M., 1969, Origin of the pericellular baskets of the pyramidal cells of the human motor cortex: A Golgi study, *Brain Res.* **14:**633–646.

Marin-Padilla, M., 1970, Prenatal and early postnatal ontogenesis of the human motor cortex: A Golgi study. I. The sequential development of the cortical layers, *Brain Res.* **23:**167–183.

Marin-Padilla, M., 1971, Early prenatal ontogenesis of the cerebral cortex (neocortex) of the cat *(Felis domestica):* A Golgi study, *Z. Anat. Entwicklungsgesch.* **134:**117–145.

Marin-Padilla, M., 1972a, Prenatal ontogenetic history of the principal neurons of the neocortex of the cat *(Felis domestica):* A Golgi study. II. Developmental differences and their significance, *Z. Anat. Entwicklungsgesch.* **136:**125–142.

Marin-Padilla, M., 1972b, Structural abnormalities of the cerebral cortex in human chromosomal aberrations: A Golgi study, *Brain Res.* **44:**625–629.

Marin-Padilla, M., 1976, Pyramidal cell abnormalities in the motor cortex of a child with Down's syndrome: A Golgi study, *J. Comp. Neurol.* **167:**63–82.

Marin-Padilla, M., and Stibitz, G. R., 1968, Distribution of the apical dendritic spines of the layer V pyramidal cells of the hamster neocortex, *Brain Res.* **11:** 580–592.

Marin-Padilla, M., Stibitz, G. R., Almy, C. P., and Brown, H. N., 1969, Spine distribution of the layer V pyramidal cell in man: A cortical model, *Brain Res.* **12:**493–496.

Marty, R. and Pujol, R., 1966, Maturation post-natale de l'aire visuelle du cortex cérébral chez le chat, in: *Evolution of the Forebrain* (R. Hassler and H. Stephen, eds.), pp. 405–418, Thieme Verlag, Stuttgart.

Mehraein, P., Yamada, M., and Tarnowska-Dziduszko, E., 1975, Quantitative studies on dendrites in Alzheimer's disease and senile dementia, in: *Physiology and Pathology of Dendrites* (G. W. Kreutzberg, ed.), pp. 453–458, Raven Press, New York.

Meynert, T., 1867, Der Bau der Gross-Hirnrinde und seine örtlichen Verschiedenheiten, nebst einem pathologisch–anatomischen Corollarium, *Vierteljahrsschr. Psychiatr.* **1**:77–93 (cited by Brazier, 1968).

Miller, M., 1981, Maturation of rat visual cortex. I. A quantitative study of Golgi-impregnated pyramidal neurons, *J. Neurocytol.* **10**:859–878.

Miller, M., and Peters, A., 1981, Maturation of rat visual cortex. II. A combined Golgi–electron microscope study of pyramidal neurons, *J. Comp. Neurol.* **203**:555–573.

Molliver, M. E., and Van der Loos, H., 1970, The ontogenesis of cortical circuitry: The spatial distribution of synapses in somesthetic cortex of newborn dog, *Ergeb. Anat. Entwicklungsgesch.* **42**:7–53.

Molliver, M. E., Kostovic, I., and Van der Loos, H., 1973, The development of synapses in the cerebral cortex of the human fetus, *Brain Res.* **50**:403–407.

Monti, A., 1895, Sur les altérations du système nerveux dans l'inanition, *Arch. Ital. Biol.* **24**:347–360.

Morest, D. K., 1969a, The differentiation of cerebral dendrites: A study of the post-migratory neuroblast in the medial nucleus of the trapezoid body, *Z. Anat. Entwicklungsgesch.* **128**:271–289.

Morest, D. K., 1969b, The growth of dendrites in the mammalian brain, *Z. Anat. Entwicklungsgesch.* **128**:290–317.

Morest, D. K., 1970, A study of neurogenesis in the forebrain of opossum pouch young, *Z. Anat. Entwicklungsgesch.* **130**:265–305.

Mountcastle, V. B., 1957, Modality and topographic properties of single neurons of the cat's somatic sensory cortex, *J. Neurophysiol.* **20**:408–434.

Mungai, J. M., 1967, Dendritic patterns in the somatic sensory cortex of the cat, *J. Anat.* **101**:403–418.

Mustari, M. J., 1975, An aberrant contralateral visual corticotectal pathway in albino rats, *Anat. Rec.* **181**:433.

Nañagas, J. C., 1922, Anatomical studies on the motor cortex of *Macacus rhesus, J. Comp. Neurol.* **35**:67–96.

Noback, C. R., and Purpura, D. P., 1961, Postnatal ontogenesis of neurons in cat neocortex, *J. Comp. Neurol.* **117**:291–307.

O'Leary, J. L., 1941, Structure of the area striata in the cat, *J. Comp. Neurol.* **75**:131–164.

Palay, S. L., 1978, The Meynert cell, an unusual cortical pyramidal cell, in: *Architectonics of the Cerebral Cortex* (M. A. B. Brazier and H. Petsche, eds.), pp. 31–42, Raven Press, New York.

Paley, S. L., Sotelo, C., Peters, A., and Orkand, P. M., 1968, The axon hillock and the initial segment, *J. Cell Biol.* **38**:193–201.

Paldino, A., and Harth, E., 1977a, A computerized study of Golgi-impregnated axons in rat visual cortex, in: *Computer Analysis of Neuronal Structures* (R. D. Lindsay, ed.), pp. 189–207, Plenum Press, New York.

Paldino, A., and Harth, E., 1977b, A measuring system for analyzing neuronal fiber structure, in: *Computer Analysis of Neuronal Structures* (R. D. Lindsay, ed.), pp. 59–71, Plenum Press, New York.

Parnavelas, J. G., 1978, Influence of stimulation on cortical development, in: *Progress in Brain Research*, Vol. 48 (M. A. Corner, ed.), pp. 247–259, Elsevier, Amsterdam.

Parnavelas, J. G., Globus, A., and Kaups, P., 1973, Continuous illumination from birth affects spine density of neurons in the visual cortex of the rat, *Exp. Neurol.* **40**:742–747.

Parnavelas, J. G., Lieberman, A. R., and Webster, K. E., 1977a, Organization of neurons in the visual cortex, area 17, of the rat, *J. Anat.* **124**:305–322.

Parnavelas, J. G., Sullivan, K., Lieberman, A. R., and Webster, K. E., 1977b Neurons and their synaptic organization in the visual cortex of the rat: Electron microscopy of Golgi preparations, *Cell Tissue Res.* **183**:499–517.

Peters, A., 1971, Stellate cells of the rat parietal cortex, *J. Comp. Neurol.* **141**:345–374.

Peters, A., 1981, Neuronal organization in rat visual cortex, in: *Progress in Anatomy*, Vol. 1 (R. J. Harrison, ed.), pp. 95–121, Cambridge University Press, London.

Peters, A., and Fairén, A., 1978, Smooth and sparsely spined stellate cells in the visual cortex of the rat: A study using a combined Golgi–electron microscope technique, *J. Comp. Neurol.* **181**:129–172.

Peters, A., and Feldman, M., 1973, The cortical plate and molecular layer of the late rat fetus, *Z. Anat. Entwicklungsgesch.* **141**:3–37.

Peters, A., and Feldman, M. L., 1976, The projection of the lateral geniculate nucleus to area 17 of the rat cerebral cortex, *J. Neurocytol.* **5**:63–84.

Peters, A., and Kaiserman-Abramof, I. R., 1969, The small pyramidal neuron of the rat cerebral cortex: The synapses upon dendritic spines, *Z. Zellforsch. Mikrosk. Anat.* **100**:487–506.

Peters, A., and Kaiserman-Abramof, I. R., 1970, The small pyramidal neuron of the rat cerebral cortex: The perikaryon, dendrites and spines, *Am. J. Anat.* **127:**321–356.

Peters, A., and Kimerer, L. M., 1981, Bipolar neurons in rat visual cortex: A combined Golgi–electron microscope study, *J. Neurocytol.* **10:**921–946.

Peters A., and Proskauer, C., 1980, Smooth or sparsely spined cells with myelinated axons in rat visual cortex, *Neuroscience* **5:**2079–2092.

Peters, A., and Walsh, T. M., 1972, A study of the organization of apical dendrites in the somatic sensory cortex of the rat, *J. Comp. Neurol.* **144:**253–268.

Peters, A., Proskauer, C. C., and Kaiserman-Abramof, I. R., 1968, The small pyramidal neuron of the rat cerebral cortex: The axon hillock and initial segment, *J. Cell Biol.* **39:**604–619.

Peters, A., Palay, S. L., and Webster, H. de F., 1976, *The Fine Structure of the Nervous System: The Neurons and Supporting Cells*, Saunders, Philadelphia.

Peters, A., Proskauer, C. C., Feldman, M. L., and Kimerer, L., 1979, The projection of the lateral geniculate nucleus to area 17 of the rat cerebral cortex. V. Degenerating axon terminals synapsing with Golgi impregnated neurons, *J. Neurocytol.* **8:**331–357.

Peters, A., Proskauer, C. C., and Ribak, C. E., 1982, Chandelier cells in rat visual cortex, *J. Comp. Neurol.* **206:**397–416.

Poliakov, G. I., 1966, Embryonal and postembryonal development of neurons of the human cerebral cortex, in: *Evolution of the Forebrain* (R. Hassler and H. Stephen, eds.), pp. 249–258, Thieme Verlag, Stuttgart.

Polyak, S., 1957, *The Vertebrate Visual System*, University of Chicago Press, Chicago.

Polyakov, G. I., 1956, cited in Shkol'nik-Yarros, 1971.

Purpura, D. P., 1975a, Dendritic differentiation in human cerebral cortex: Normal and aberrant developmental patterns, in: *Physiology and Pathology of Dendrites*, Advances in Neurology, Vol. 12 (G. W. Kreutzberg, ed.), pp. 91–116, Raven Press, New York.

Purpura, D. P., 1975b, Morphogenesis of visual cortex in the preterm infant, in: *Growth and Development of the Brain* (M. A. B. Brazier, ed.), pp. 33–49, Raven Press, New York.

Purpura, D. P., and Suzuki, K., 1976, Distortion of neuronal geometry and formation of aberrant synapses in neuronal storage disease, *Brain Res.* **116:**1–21.

Purpura, D. P., Pappas, G. D., and Baker, H. J., 1978, Fine structure of meganeurites and secondary growth processes in feline GM-1 gangliosidosis, *Brain Res.* **143:**1–12.

Purpura, D. P., Bodick, N., Suzuki, K., Rapin, I., and Wurzelmann, S., 1982, Microtubule disarray in cortical dendrites and neurobehavioral failure. I. Golgi and electron microscopic studies, *Dev. Brain Res.* **5:**287–297.

Querton, L., 1898, Le sommeil hibernal et les modifications des neurones cerebraux, *Ann. Soc. R. Sci. Med. Nat. Brux.* **7:**147–204.

Rabinowicz, T., 1964, The cerebral cortex of the premature infant of the 8th month, in: *Growth and Maturation of the Brain*, Progress in Brain Research, Vol. 4 (D. P. Purpura and J. P. Schadé, eds.), pp. 39–86, Elsevier, Amsterdam.

Raedler, A., and Sievers, J., 1975, The development of the visual system of the albino rat, *Adv. Anat. Embryol. Cell Biol.* **50**(Fasc. 3):1–88.

Raisman, G., 1969, Neuronal plasticity in the septal nuclei of the rat, *Brain Res.* **14:**25–48.

Rakic, P., 1971, Guidance of neurons migrating to the fetal monkey neocortex, *Brain Res.* **33:**471–476.

Rakic, P., 1972, Mode of cell migration to the superficial layers of fetal monkey neocortex, *J. Comp. Neurol.* **145:**61–84.

Rakic, P., 1981, Developmental events leading to laminar and areal organization of the neocortex, in: *The Organization of the Cerebral Cortex* (F. O. Schmitt, F. G. Worden, G. Adelman, and S. G. Dennis, eds.), MIT Press, Cambridge, Mass.

Ramón-Moliner, E., 1970, The Golgi–Cox technique, in: *Contemporary Research Methods in Neuroanatomy* (W. J. H. Nauta and S. O. E. Ebbesson, eds.), pp. 32–55, Springer-Verlag, Berlin.

Ramón y Cajal, S., 1891, Sur la structure de l'écorce cérébrale de quelques mammifères, *Cellule* **7:**125–176.

Ramón y Cajal, S., 1899, Comparative study of the sensory areas of the human cortex, in: *Clark University, Decennial Celebration* (W. E. Story and L. N. Wilson, eds.), pp. 311–382, Norwood Press, Norwood, Mass.

Ramón y Cajal, S., 1928, *Degeneration and Regeneration of the Nervous System* (translated by R. M. May), Oxford University Press, London.

Ramón y Cajal, S., 1937, *Recollections of My Life* (translated by E. H. Craigie with the assistance of J. Cano), The American Philosophical Society, Philadelphia.

Ramón y Cajal, S., 1954, *Neuron Theory or Reticular Theory? Objective Evidence of the Anatomical Unity of Nerve Cells* (translated by M. Ubeda Purkiss and C. A. Fox), Consejo Superior de Investigaciones Cientificas, Madrid.

Ramón y Cajal, S., 1955, *Histologie du Système Nerveux de l'Homme et des Vertébrés* (translated by L. Azoulay), Vol. II, Instituto Ramón y Cajal, Madrid.

Rockland, K. S., Lund, J. S., and Humphrey, A. L., 1982, Anatomical banding of intrinsic connections in striate cortex of tree shrews *(Tupaia glis), J. Comp. Neurol.* **209**:41–58.

Rothblat, L. A., and Schwartz, M. L., 1979, The effect of monocular deprivation on dendritic spines in visual cortex of young and adult albino rats: Evidence for a sensitive period, *Brain Res.* **161**:156–161.

Ryugo, D. K., Ryugo, R., and Killackey, H., 1975a, Changes in pyramidal cell spine density consequent to vibrissal removal in the newborn rat, *Brain Res.* **96**:82–87.

Ryugo, R., Ryugo, D., and Killackey, H., 1975b, Differential effect of enucleation on two populations of layer V pyramidal cells, *Brain Res.* **88**:554–559.

Salas, M., 1980, Effects of early undernutrition on dendritic spines of cortical pyramidal cells in the rat, *Dev. Neurosci.* **3**:109–117.

Sanides, F., and Sanides, D., 1972, The "extraverted neurons" of the mammalian cerebral cortex, *Z. Anat. Entwicklungsgesch.* **136**:272–293.

Scheibel, M. E., and Scheibel, A. B., 1968, On the nature of dendritic spines—Report of a workshop, *Comm. Behav. Biol. Part A* **1**:231–265.

Scheibel, M. E., and Scheibel, A. B., 1970, Elementary processes in selected thalamic and cortical subsystems—The structural substrates, in: *The Neurosciences Second Study Program* (F. O. Schmitt, ed.), pp. 443–457, Rockefeller University Press, New York.

Scheibel, M. E., and Scheibel, A. B., 1971, Selected structural–functional correlations in postnatal brain, in: *Brain Development and Behavior* (M. B. Sterman, D. J. McGuinty, and A. M. Adinolfi, eds.), pp. 1–21, Academic Press, New York.

Scheibel, M. E., and Scheibel, A. B., 1975, Structural changes in the aging brain, in: *Aging,* Vol. 1 (H. Brody, D. Harman, and J. M. Ordy, eds.), pp. 11–37, Raven Press, New York.

Scheibel, M. E., and Scheibel, A. B., 1978, The dendritic structure of the human Betz cell, in: *Architectonics of the Cerebral Cortex* (M. A. B. Brazier and H. Petsche, eds.), pp. 43–57, Raven Press, New York.

Scheibel, M. E., Lindsay, R. D., Tomiyasu, U., and Scheibel, A. B., 1975, Progressive dendritic changes in aging human cortex, *Exp. Neurol.* **47**:392–403.

Schlapp, M., 1898, Der Zellenbau der Grosshirnrinde des Affen *Macacus cynomolgus, Arch. Psychiatr.* **30**:583–607.

Schüz, A., 1978, Some facts and hypotheses concerning dendritic spines and learning, in: *Architectonics of the Cerebral Cortex* (M. A. B. Brazier and H. Petsche, eds.), pp. 129–135, Raven Press, New York.

Schüz, A., Münster, A., and Dortenmann, M., 1982, Counts of synapses on identified neurons in the mouse cortex, *Soc. Neurosci. Abstr.* **8**:209.

Segraves, M. A., and Rosenquist, A. C., 1982, The distribution of the cells of origin of callosal projections in cat visual cortex, *J. Neurosci.* **2**:1079–1089.

Shimada, M., and Langman, J., 1970, Cell proliferation, migration and differentiation in the cerebral cortex of the hamster, *J. Comp. Neurol.* **139**:227–244.

Shkol'nik-Yarros, E. G., 1971, *Neurons and Interneuronal Connections of the Central Visual System* (translated by B. Haigh), Plenum Press, New York.

Sholl, D. A., 1953, Dendritic organization in the neurons of the visual and motor cortices of the cat, *J. Anat.* **87**:387–407.

Sholl, D. A., 1956, *The Organization of the Cerebral Cortex*, Methuen, London.

Siakotos, A. N., and Munkres, K. D., 1981, Purification and properties of age pigments, in: *Age Pigments* (R. S. Sohal, ed.), pp. 181–202, Elsevier, Amsterdam.

Siegesmund, K. A., Dutta, C. R., and Fox, C. A., 1964, The ultrastructure of the intranuclear rodlet in certain nerve cells, *J. Anat.* **98**:93–97.

Simmons, P. A., Lemmon, V., and Pearlman, A. L., 1982, Afferent and efferent connections of the striate and extrastriate visual cortex of the normal and Reeler mouse, *J. Comp. Neurol.* **211**:295–308.

Sloper, J. J., 1973, The relationship of subsurface cisternae and cisternal organelles to symmetrical axon terminals in the primate sensorimotor cortex, *Brain Res.* **58:**478–483.

Sloper, J. J., and Powell, T. P. S., 1973, Observations in the axon initial segment and other structures in the neocortex using conventional staining and ethanolic phosphotungstic acid, *Brain Res.* **50:**163–169.

Sloper, J. J., and Powell, T. P. S., 1979, A study of the axon initial segment and proximal axon of neurons in the primate motor and somatic sensory cortex, *Philos. Trans. R. Soc. London* **285:**173–197.

Sloper, J. J., Hiorne, R. W., and Powell, T., P. S., 1979, A qualitative and quantitative electron microscopic study of the neurons in the primate motor and somatic sensory corticies, *Philos. Trans. R. Soc. London* **285:**141–171.

Smit, G. J., and Uylings, H. B. M., 1975, The morphometry of the branching pattern in dendrites of the visual cortex pyramidal cells, *Brain Res.* **87:**41–53.

Sohal, R. S. (ed.), 1981, *Age Pigments*, Elsevier, Amsterdam.

Somogyi, P., 1977, A specific 'axo-axonal' interneuron in the visual cortex of the rat, *Brain Res.* **136:**345–350.

Somogyi, P., 1978, The study of Golgi stained cells and of experimental degeneration under the electron microscope: A direct method for the identification in the visual cortex of three successive links in a neuron chain, *Neuroscience* **3:**167–180.

Sotelo, C., and Palay, S. L., 1968, The fine structure of the lateral vestibular nucleus in the rat. I. Neurons and neuroglial cells, *J. Cell Biol.* **36:**151–179.

Soukhanoff, S., 1898a, Contribution à l'étude des modifications que subissent les prolongements dendritiques des cellules nerveuses: Sous l'influence des narcotiques, *Cellule* **14:**50–395.

Soukhanoff, S., 1898b, L'anatomie pathologique de la cellule nerveuse, en rapport avec l'atrophie variquese des dendrites de l'écorce cérébrale, *Cellule* **14:**398–417.

Spatz, W. B., 1975, An efferent connection of the solitary cells of Meynert: A study with horseradish peroxidase in the marmoset *Callithrix*, *Brain Res.* **92:**450–455.

Spatz, W. B., Tigges, J., and Tigges, M., 1970, Subcortical projections, cortical associations and some intrinsic interlaminar connections of the striate cortex in the squirrel monkey *(Saimiri)*, *J. Comp. Neurol.* **140:**155–174.

Stanfield, B. B., and O'Leary, D. D. M., 1982, Evidence for a transitory corticospinal projection from the visual cortex during early postnatal development in the rat, *Soc. Neurosci. Abstr.* **8:**438.

Stensaas, L. J., 1967, The development of hippocampal and dorsolateral pallial regions of the cerebral hemispheres in fetal rabbits. III. Twenty nine millimeter stage, marginal lamina, *J. Comp. Neurol.* **130:**149–162.

Strick, P. L., and Sterling, P., 1974, Synaptic termination of afferents from the ventrolateral nucleus of the thalamus in the cat motor cortex: A light and electron microscope study, *J. Comp. Neurol.* **153:**77–106.

Swindale, N. V., 1981, Dendritic spines only connect, *Trends Neurosci.* September, 1981, pp. 240–241.

Terry, R. D., and Wiśniewski, H., 1970, The ultrastructure of the neurofibrillary tangle and the senile plaque, in: *Alzheimer's Disease and Related Conditions* (G. E. W. Wolstenholme and M. O'Connor, eds.), pp. 145–165, Churchill, London.

Tieman, S. B., and Hirsch, H. V. B., 1982, Exposure to lines of only one orientation modifies dendritic morphology of cells in the visual cortex of the cat, *J. Comp. Neurol.* **211:**353–362.

Tigges, J., and Tigges, M., 1982, Principles of axonal collateralization of lamina II–III pyramids in area 17 of squirrel monkey: A quantitative Golgi study, *Neurosci. Lett.* **29:**99–104.

Tömböl, T., 1974, An electron microscopic study of the neurons of the visual cortex, *J. Neurocytol.* **3:**525–531.

Tömböl, T., 1975, Collateral axonal arborizations, in: *Golgi Centennial Symposium: Perspectives in Neurobiology* (M. Santini, ed.), pp. 133–141, Raven Press, New York.

Uylings, H. B. M., and Parnavelas, J. G., 1981, Growth and plasticity of cortical dendrites, in: *Cellular Analogues of Conditioning and Neural Plasticity*, Advances in Physiological Science, Vol. 11 (O. Fehér and F. Joo, eds.), pp. 57–64, Pergamon Press, Elmsford, N.Y.

Uylings, H. B. M., and Smit, G. J., 1975, Three-dimensional branching structure of pyramidal cell dendrites, *Brain Res.* **87:**55–60.

Valverde, F., 1967, Apical dendritic spines of the visual cortex and light deprivation in the mouse, *Exp. Brain Res.* **3:**337–352.

Valverde, F., 1968, Structural changes in the area striata of the mouse after enucleation, *Exp. Brain Res.* **5:**274–292.

Valverde, F., 1970, The Golgi method: A tool for comparative structural analyses, in: *Contemporary Methods in Neuroanatomy* (W. J. H. Nauta and S. O. E. Ebbesson, eds.), pp. 12–31, Springer-Verlag, Berlin.

Van der Loos, H., 1965, The "improperly" oriented pyramidal cell in the cerebral cortex and its possible bearing on problems of neuronal growth and cell orientation, *Bull. Johns Hopkins Hosp.* **117:**228–250.

Vaughan, D. W., 1977, Age-related deterioration of pyramidal cell basal dendrites in rat auditory cortex, *J. Comp. Neurol.* **171:**501–516.

Vaughan, D. W., and Peters, A., 1973, A three dimensional study of layer I of the rat parietal cortex, *J. Comp. Neurol.* **149:**355–370.

Vaughan, D. W., and Peters, A., 1974, Neuroglial cells in the cerebral cortex of rats from young adulthood to old age: An electron microscope study, *J. Neurocytol.* **3:**405–429.

Vaughan, D. W., and Vincent, J. M., 1979, Ultrastructure of neurons in the auditory cortex of ageing rats: A morphometric study, *J. Neurocytol.* **8:**215–228.

Vignal, W., 1888, Recherches sur le developpement de la substance corticale du cerveau et du cervelet, *Arch. Physiol. Norm. Pathol. Paris Ser. IV* **2:**311–338.

von Bonin, G., and Bailey, P., 1947, *The Neocortex of Macaca mulatta*, University of Illinois Press, Urbana.

von Bonin, G., and Mehler, W. R., 1971, On columnar arrangement of nerve cells in cerebral cortex, *Brain Res.* **27:**1–10.

von Economo, C., 1929, *The Cytoarchitectonics of the Human Cerebral Cortex* (translated by S. Parker), Oxford University Press, London.

von Economo, C., and Koskinas, G. N., 1925, *Die Cytoarchitektonik der Hirnrinde des erwachsenen Menschen*, Springer, Berlin.

von Kölliker, A., 1850–1854, *Mikroskopische Anatomie, oder Gewebelehre des Menschen*, Englemann, Leipzig.

Walkley, S. U., Wurzelmann, S., and Purpura, D. P., 1981, Ultrastructure of neurites and mega-neurites of cortical pyramidal neurons in feline gangliosidosis as revealed by the combined Golgi–EM technique. *Brain Res.* **211:**393–398.

Walshe, F. M. R., 1942, The giant pyramidal cells of Betz, the motor cortex and the pyramidal tract: A critical review, *Brain* **65:**409–461.

White, E. L., 1978, Identified neurons in mouse SmI cortex which are postsynaptic to thalamocortical axon terminals: A combined Golgi–electron microscopic and degeneration study, *J. Comp. Neurol.* **181:**627–662.

White, E. L., 1979, Thalamocortical synaptic relations: A review with emphasis on the projections of specific thalamic nuclei to the primary sensory areas of the neocortex, *Brain Res. Rev.* **1:**275–311.

White, E. L., and Hersch, S. M., 1981, Thalamocortical synapses of pyramidal cells which project from SmI to MsI cortex in the mouse, *J. Comp. Neurol.* **198:**167–181.

White, E. L., Hersch, S. M., and Rock, M. P., 1980, Synaptic sequences in mouse SmI cortex involving pyramidal cells labelled by retrograde filling with horseradish peroxidase, *Neurosci. Lett.* **19:**149–154.

Williams, R. S., Ferrante, R. J., and Caviness, V. S., 1978, The Golgi-rapid method in clinical neuropathology. I. Morphologic consequences of suboptimal fixation, *J. Neuropathol. Exp. Neurol.* **37:**13–33.

Winfield, D. A., 1982, The effect of visual deprivation upon the Meynert cell in the striate cortex of the cat, *Dev. Brain Res.* **5:**53–58.

Winfield, D. A., Gatter, K. C., and Powell, T. P. S., 1980, An electron microscopic study of the types and proportions of neurons in the cortex of the motor and visual areas of the cat and rat, *Brain* **103:**245–258.

Winfield, D. A., Brooke, R. N. L., Sloper, J. J., and Powell, T. P. S., 1981, A combined Golgi–electron microscopic study of the synapses made by the proximal axon and recurrent collaterals of a pyramidal cell in the somatic sensory cortex of the monkey, *Neuroscience* **6:**1217–1230.

Winkelmann, A., Kunz, G., Winkelmann, E., Kirche, W., Neumann, H., and Wenzel, J., 1973, Quantitative Untersuchungen an Dendriten der grossen Pyramidenzellen der Lamina V des sensorischen Cortex der Ratte, *J. Hirnforsch.* **14:**137–149.

Winkelmann, E., Brauer, N., and Berger, U., 1975, Zur columnaren Organisation von Pyramiden-zellen im visuellen Cortex der Albinoratte, *Z. Mikrosk. Anat. Forsch.* **89:**239–256.

Winkelmann, E., Brauer, K., and Werner, L., 1976, Untersuchungen zu Spineveränderungen der Lamina V Pyramidenzellen im visuellen Kortex junger und subadulter Laborratten nach Dun-kelaufzucht und Zerstörung des Corpus geniculatum laterale, pars dorsalis, *J. Hirnforsch.* **17:**489–500.

Winkelmann, E., Brauer, K., and Klütz, K., 1977, Untersuchungen zur Spinedichte von Lamina V Pyramidenzellen im visuellen Kortex von Laborratten nach langdauernder Dunkelaufzucht, *J. Hirnforsch.* **18:**21–28.

Wise, S. P., 1975, The laminar organization of certain afferent and efferent fiber systems in the rat somatosensory cortex, *Brain Res.* **90:**139–142.

Wise, S. P., and Jones, E. G., 1977, Cells of origin and terminal distribution of descending projections of the rat somatic sensory cortex, *J. Comp. Neurol.* **175:**129–157.

Wise, S. P., Fleshman, J. W., and Jones, E. G., 1979, Maturation of pyramidal cell form in relation to developing afferent and efferent connections of rat somatic sensory cortex, *Neuroscience* **4:**1275–1297.

Wiśniewski, H. M., Narang, H. K., and Terry, R. D., 1976, Neurofibrillary tangles of paired helical filaments, *J. Neurol. Sci.* **27:**173–181.

Wong, D., and Kelly, J. P., 1981, Differentially projecting cells in individual layers of the auditory cortex: A double-labeling study, *Brain Res.* **230:**362–366.

Wong, W. C., 1967, The tangential organization of dendrites and axons in three auditory areas of the cat's cerebral cortex, *J. Anat.* **101:**419–433.

Yakovlev, P. I., and Lecours, A. R., 1967, The myelogenetic cycles of regional maturation of the brain, in: *Development of the Brain in Early Life* (A. Minkowske, ed.), pp. 3–70, Blackwell, Oxford.

6

Nonpyramidal Neurons

General Account

ALFONSO FAIRÉN, JAVIER DeFELIPE, and
JOSÉ REGIDOR

1. Introduction

Much information about nonpyramidal cells was available by the turn of the century, in the earliest writings by Ramón y Cajal. His contributions, based on the extensive use of the Golgi methods, are summarized in his 1911 book. This book seemed to have closed an era of an extremely promising endeavor, as Ramón y Cajal himself rather bitterly complained in 1921. His approach, in fact, was not widely followed by students of cortical architecture during the first half of the present century, although there were outstanding exceptions such as his pupil Lorente de Nó (1922, 1933, 1934, 1949) and O'Leary (O'Leary and Bishop, 1938; O'Leary, 1941). A lucid analysis of the circumstances that may have led to such a situation is given by Scheibel and Scheibel (1970). For the cerebral cortex, a significant factor was that, due to the intricacy of its neuronal circuits, no schemes of interneuronal connectivity could emerge from the analysis of Golgi preparations alone (Van der Loos, 1976), although masterly insights were

ALFONSO FAIRÉN and JAVIER DeFELIPE • Unidad de Neuroanatomia, Instituto Cajal, CSIC, Madrid 6, Spain.   JOSÉ REGIDOR • Departamento de Biología, Colegio Universitario de Las Palmas, División de Medicina, Las Palmas de Gran Canaria, Spain.   *Present address of J.DeF.:* James L. O'Leary Division of Experimental Neurology and Neurological Surgery, Washington University School of Medicine, St. Louis, Missouri 63110.

201

obtained by Lorente de Nó (1949). For a time, very simple classifications of cortical neurons, such as that by Sholl (1956), dominated the scene, but in 1966 Colonnier anticipated the real importance of reevaluating the old descriptions and, from this time on, there has been a renewed interest in Golgi studies of cortical organization. The present chapter aims at reviewing the wealth of information these studies have provided on the morphology of nonpyramidal cells in the neocortex, and at integrating these data, whenever possible, with other pieces of information that have emerged recently. In line with a recent review (Fairén and Valverde, 1979), it was deemed important to try to assemble a catalog of neuronal types to serve as a basis for the interpretation of experimental results, even if such a goal cannot be fully attained as yet. Additionally, an attempt is made at determining whether each type of nonpyramidal neuron is a constant cellular component of all areas of the neocortex and through mammalian phylogeny.

2. Methodological Considerations

This review has largely been based on the study of our own collection of Golgi preparations of young mice, rabbits, and cats. Mice were approximately 3 weeks old, and rabbits and cats 3 months. Additional material from hedgehogs, rats, and monkeys has been made available to us for comparisons, and we have examined some of the preparations of human specimens made by Ramón y Cajal himself (Cajal Museum, Madrid). Golgi drawings from the literature have constituted a second, significant source of information.

In the present account, as in most Golgi studies, a certain degree of subjectivism has been unavoidable, when defining criteria for different neuronal types (see Chapter 4). Taxonomy of neurons (Tyner, 1975; Rowe and Stone, 1977, 1980; Mann, 1979) relies on the selection of certain characteristics which may define neuronal subsets. In the present account, the choice has been to consider primarily the forms of the axonal arborizations, but other features such as the morphology of the dendritic trees have also been taken into account. Axonal geometry is, in certain cases, very distinct and facilitates comparisons with published drawings. It is obviously related to the local efferent connectivity of the cells, a feature of functional significance on which we shall dwell.

2.1. General Comments on Methodology: The Value of the Golgi Methods in Defining Nonpyramidal Cell Populations

Since most available data on morphology of nonpyramidal neurons in the cerebral cortex have derived from the use of the Golgi methods, a few comments on the powers and limitations of these procedures are pertinent. First of all, the Golgi methods, by their very nature, are unpredictable (Valverde, 1970; Scheibel and Scheibel, 1978). There are some indications that, in the Golgi–Cox method, impregnation occurs at random (Smit and Colon, 1969; Pasternak and Woolsey, 1975), but common experience with the rapid Golgi method or the Kopsch variants seems to indicate that with these techniques the impregnation is selective and bears some, as yet unclarified, relationships to the conditions in which the reaction takes place, e.g., aldehyde perfusion vs. direct immersion-fixation in the chromating solution, and duration of chromation and silvering. If impregnation is selective, it follows that negative findings, such as absence of a given cell type in a given cortex, are meaningless. Additionally, selectivity of impregnation makes the Golgi method not ideally suited to study distribution, or frequency of occurrence, of neurons in a given brain area.

Completeness of impregnation was generally believed to be related to the overall quality of the impregnations, but Golgi–electron microscope studies have made us aware of the fact that incomplete impregnations are not rare (e.g., Peters and Fairén, 1978) and confirmed the suspected fact that myelinated axons do not stain (e.g., Somogyi, 1978; Peters and Proskauer, 1980a,b; Peters and Kimerer, 1981). Recent studies using intracellular injections of markers (e.g., Gilbert and Wiesel, 1979) have also suggested that axonal impregnation may be incomplete in Golgi preparations. The use of young specimens permits better axonal impregnations but the possibility of synaptic rearrangements during early postnatal life must be considered (e.g., Somogyi et al., 1982; see Section 3.3.2).

Whether local synaptic connections may be predicted from Golgi observations has been a matter of controversy, but fortuitous contacts may be occasionally seen, the Golgi impregnation revealing both the pre- and postsynaptic elements; and the real synaptic nature of some of these contacts has been confirmed recently (e.g., Peters and Proskauer, 1980a; Peters and Kimerer, 1981; Fairén et al., 1982). However, light microscopy alone is unreliable as a means of identifying synaptic relationships.

Computer technology has offered a complementary approach to the study of Golgi-stained material (Glaser and Van der Loos, 1965; Garvey et al., 1973; Wann et al., 1973; Llinás and Hillman, 1975; and see Jones and Hartman, 1978, and Woolsey and Dierker, 1982, for reviews). The use of these procedures has been useful in defining the general trends of the tangential distribution of neuronal processes in the cerebral cortex (e.g., Glaser et al., 1979; Steffen and Van der Loos, 1980; but also see Colonnier, 1964, and Wong, 1967). Their application to the characterization of nonpyramidal cell groups (Marin-Padilla and Stibitz, 1974; Jones, 1975; Marin-Padilla, 1975; Woolsey et al., 1975; Valverde, 1976, 1978; Fairén and Valverde, 1980; Peters and Regidor, 1981) shows promise, but the potential of these methods to quantitatively define dendritic (e.g., Woolsey et al., 1975; Uylings et al., 1981) and axonal branching patterns, as an aid to classification of nonpyramidal cells in the cerebral cortex, has not been fully exploited.

2.2. Novel Approaches to Nonpyramidal Cell Organization

Many of the uncertainties associated with a Golgi analysis can often be resolved through the application of techniques which allow correlations of morphology, pharmacology, and physiology of nonpyramidal cells in the cerebral cortex. These include electron microscopy, transmitter localization, and intracellular recording and are dealt with in Chapter 4.

2.2.1. The Ultrastructural Features of Nonpyramidal Neurons

A basic dichotomy in synaptic organization between spine-free or sparsely spined and spine-laden cell types (comprising both pyramidal cells and layer IV spiny stellate cells) was established by LeVay (1973) in the visual cortex. Subsequent studies have clearly established that spine-free or sparsely spined cells do not constitute a unique category. With a single exception, the efferent synapses formed by the axonal arborizations of these cells are of the type II (Gray, 1959) or symmetrical type (Colonnier, 1968), as established by LeVay (1973) and Parnavelas *et al.* (1977b), but subtle variations seem to exist among the different types of neurons in the morphologies of these synapses (Peters and Fairén, 1978; Peters and Proskauer, 1980a; Somogyi and Cowey, 1981). In addition, the distribution of efferent synapses made by individual cell types is often very distinct, as will emerge below. It is also important to note that the relative proportions of afferent synapses from different sources can also vary among the different types of nonpyramidal neurons (Davis and Sterling, 1979; Hersch and White, 1981a; White and Rock, 1980, 1981).

Golgi–electron microscope studies, by correlating geometrical aspects revealed by the Golgi stain with these different patterns of synaptic connections, have established a firm basis for characterizing a number of nonpyramidal cell groups on morphological grounds, though not all classes have yielded to this sort of analysis yet.

2.2.2. Localization of Neurotransmitters in Nonpyramidal Neurons

Immunocytochemical studies have shown that many nonpyramidal cells contain material which cross-reacts with antibodies against glutamic acid decarboxylase (GAD), vasoactive intestinal polypeptide (VIP), cholecystokinin (CCK), avian pancreatic polypeptide (APP), or somatostatin (SRIF).

GABAergic neurons, demonstrated by GAD immunocytochemistry (Ribak, 1978; Ribak *et al.*, 1979, 1982; Emson and Hunt, 1981; Hendrickson *et al.*, 1981; Hendrickson, 1982; Hendry *et al.*, 1983a; Houser *et al.*, 1983) or the selective uptake of [^{3}H]-GABA (Hökfelt and Ljungdahl, 1972; Chronwall and Wolff, 1978, 1980; Hendry and Jones, 1981; Somogyi *et al.*, 1981a,b; Wolff and Chronwall, 1982), constitute a heterogeneous population, but all of them are intrinsic neurons (Hendry and Jones, 1981) and, as we will show, some correlations can be made with morphological types (see also Chapters 8–10, and Chapter 3 in Volume 2).

Immunocytochemical identification of peptide-containing nonpyramidal neurons may give clues to the interpretation of certain nonpyramidal cell groups which have not been sufficiently defined in Golgi-based studies (see McDonald *et al.*, 1982a; also Chapter 11, and Chapters 8 and 9 in Volume 2). In addition, coexistence of peptides in cortical neurons (e.g., APP and SRIF; see Vincent *et al.*, 1982a,b) must be taken into account to evaluate the presence of a given peptide as a defining characteristic of a certain neuronal population.

Nonpyramidal neurons which cross-react with antisera to VIP (Lorén *et al.*, 1979; Fahrenkrug, 1980; Sims *et al.*, 1980; Emson and Hunt, 1981; McDonald *et al.*, 1982a; Morrison 1982) are morphologically similar to bipolar neurons of the rat visual cortex (Feldman and Peters, 1978; Peters and Kimerer, 1981), but other VIP-containing neurons are multipolar. CCK has been localized to certain nonpyramidal neurons (Emson and Hunt, 1981; McDonald *et al.*, 1982b; Hendry *et al.*, 1983b; Peters *et al.*, 1983) which are bitufted or bipolar in form; multipolar morphologies are also found.

More extensive studies on the localizations, overall morphologies, and synaptology of immunoreactive neurons to VIP and CCK are sorely needed, since these data may provide effective clues to fully understand the organization of certain types of neurons, reviewed in Section 3.2, in which interspecific homologies have proven to be particularly difficult to establish.

3. A Comparative Overview of Nonpyramidal Cells in the Neocortex

During the preparation of the present account, our main concern has been to try to define homologies between comparable populations of nonpyramidal neurons in different cortical areas of different mammalian species. We were painfully aware of the fact that sound criteria are largely nonexistent. Nevertheless, we have tried to assemble the sets of data available with the hope that our comments, tentative as they are, will stimulate future research into the organization of nonpyramidal neurons. The rationale of our intent has not been followed customarily. It is based on the consideration of the nonpyramidal neurons as entities that may have essential features independent of the particular context (i.e., layer and area) where they happen to occur. Obviously, nonpyramidal neurons entirely comparable on the basis of a number of criteria will differ radically in their connectivities if they are located in different cortical areas or in different cortical layers and the functional roles they accomplish may necessarily be different. What we will try to analyze are the intrinsic properties of the pieces of a puzzle. How these pieces are to be assembled together in order to complete a picture of the local circuitry of a given cortical area is another concern.

The review that follows is restricted to the nonpyramidal neurons located in layers II through V of the cerebral cortex, where our best Golgi impregnations have occurred and give us a basis for comparisons with the contributions made by other authors.

A definition of the term *nonpyramidal* has been deliberately avoided. It must be pointed out, however, that nonpyramidal cells are not always nonprojecting neurons (see Section 3.5) and, on the other hand, that certain pyramidal cells may possess exclusively intracortical axons (Ramón y Cajal, 1899b, 1911; Lorente de Nó, 1949; Valverde, 1971; Lund *et al.*, 1979), but these neurons have not been considered in the present review.

To present our data, we had to choose a classification of nonpyramidal neurons. Dendritic arborizations may suitably be described on the basis of the terminology devised by Feldman and Peters (1978). How to compare axonal arborizations has posed more problems and, finally, we have adopted a descriptive classification which has its roots in Lorente de Nó (1949) and is not dissimilar to some of the ones proposed in recent studies (Jones, 1975; Norita and Kawamura, 1981; Powell, 1981). It is recognized that a *morphological* classification of nonpyramidal neurons of universal applicability is far outside the present possibilities. It is not our intention, therefore, to propose a new classification; that which we have used is a frame of reference on which to tie together the data available on nonpyramidal cell types in order to enhance both differences and similarities along a phylogenetic scale. Nonpyramidal cells have been segregated into two main groups, depending on the presence or absence of dendritic spines. Then, the nonspiny group has been further divided into four principal classes, some of which are subdivided further.

In the discussions that follow, references have been made to certain graphic representations of neurons which have been made in the literature and we have attempted to bridge the gap between the earliest contributions based on Golgi descriptions and the more recent ones. The references that have been chosen are ones that clearly illustrate current concepts about certain cell groups and in which interpretations were easy to make. Our interpretations, however, are not necessarily coincident with the ones advanced by the authors. Additionally, examples drawn from our own material are presented when they can clarify discrete points, but they are not aimed at covering all cell groups exhaustively.

3.1. Cells with Ascending Axons

This group is made up of varieties of cells with axons arborizing in laminae above their cell bodies of origin. The axons form a variable local arborization close to their origins and ascend singly, without forming a defined columnar pattern.

One type is made up of cells whose axons arborize in layer I. The first mention of these cells was by Martinotti (1889, 1890), who described a type of multipolar neuron with an ascending, nonbifurcated axon that reaches layer I, where it ramifies. His observations were soon confirmed by Ramón y Cajal (1891), who added new details to the description of what he chose to call Martinotti cells, a name which has been retained in the modern literature.

Martinotti cells have been more frequently found in layers V and VI, but they are also present in superficial layers. They are smooth or sparsely spinous, multipolar or bitufted cells that show, in some instances, a preferred development of the dendrites emanating from the lower aspect of the perikaryon (Ramón y Cajal, 1911, his Fig. 373C; Ruiz-Marcos and Valverde, 1970, their Fig. 1; Shkol'nik-Yarros, 1971, her Fig. 16). Some of the cells with ascending axons described by Ramón y Cajal are bipolar in form, and some of these (e.g., the ones illustrated in Fig. 6b of his 1891 report) are undoubtedly Martinotti cells, but in some cases (e.g., Figs. 373E and 395A in Ramón y Cajal, 1911) the axon is not shown to reach layer I. Whether these cells are bipolar cells, as defined by Feldman and Peters (1978) and Peters and Kimerer (1981), is not known.

The axon of a Martinotti cell is distinctive: it originates either from the upper surface of the cell body or from an ascending dendrite, follows a straight ascending course toward the lower tier of layer I where it ramifies in a terminal arborization that may have either a fanlike shape (Martinotti, 1889, 1890; Ramón y Cajal, 1891; Marin-Padilla, 1970a, 1972; Marin-Padilla and Marin-Padilla, 1982) or simply form long horizontal collaterals (Lorente de Nó, 1922). Occasional descending branches have also been described. In addition to this terminal arborization, it is not infrequent to observe a relatively dense local plexus originating from the initial portion of the axon (Ruiz-Marcos and Valverde, 1970; Valverde, 1976; Fairén and Valverde, 1979), which, occasionally, may be rather rich (Valverde, 1976, his Fig. 6). But, given the possibility of incomplete impregnations, it is difficult to judge how extensive a local axonal arborization should be before it can be considered characteristic. It is of interest to note that, as already suggested by Ramón y Cajal (1921, 1922), the axons of Martinotti cells may be myelinated in adult specimens.

Martinotti cells seem to be present in many species and in many cortical areas. Reports include the mouse somatosensory (Lorente de Nó, 1922) and visual cortices (Ruiz-Marcos and Valverde, 1970; Valverde, 1976, his type II axons; Fairén and Valverde, 1979); the rat visual (Feldman and Peters, 1978, their Fig. 20c) and cingulate cortices (Vogt and Peters, 1981); the rabbit visual cortex (O'Leary and Bishop, 1938; Shkol'nik-Yarros, 1971); the cat visual cortex (Ramón y Cajal, 1921, 1922; O'Leary, 1941) and other neocortical areas in the cat (Marin-Padilla, 1972, 1978); and the human somatosensory (Ramón y Cajal, 1911) and motor cortices (Marin-Padilla, 1970a: Marin-Padilla and Marin-Padilla, 1982). On the basis of these reports, it can be concluded that Martinotti cells are ubiquitous components of the mammalian neocortex. Their role in the cortical circuitry remains unknown, although it is clear, since they must represent an important synaptic input to layer I neuropil, that information on the connectivity of these cells must be obtained. There is the suggestion by Szentágothai (1978) that Martinotti axons might contribute asymmetrical synapses to the dendritic spines in layer I.

To complete the group of cells with ascending axons entering layer I, we will refer to a type of cell that Ramón y Cajal described, for the first time, in the human sensory motor cortex (1899c). In his Fig. 9G, he illustrates a "corpúsculo estrellado enano," a small multipolar or bitufted cell located in layer II, possessing an ascending axon which arborizes profusely in the suprajacent layer I. The term *axon tuft cell* coined by Szentágothai (1975) expresses accurately the essential features of this neuronal variety. Drawings of layer II cells with the axon arborizing in layer I are given by Lorente de Nó (1922) in the somatosensory (his Fig. 7H) and entorhinal cortices of the mouse (Lorente de Nó, 1933, his Fig. 4, *1*); these cells, however, do not form the typical dense axonal tufts. A recent example is given by Lund (1973) in her account of the monkey area 17 (her Fig. 30X). According to Szentágothai (1975), axon tuft cells would form symmetrical synapses on dendritic spines in layer I, but more direct evidence is necessary to substantiate this proposal.

A second conspicuous variety of cells with ascending axons may be recognized; two examples from the cat auditory cortex are shown in Fig. 1. These are large bitufted or multipolar cells, located in layers III–V; in some cases (as in cell B of Fig. 1),* the perikaryon has the form of an inverted triangle. As in

---

* In this figure, as in the other original Golgi drawings, the axons (in solid black) have been drawn in such a way that all their collaterals appear as if they were superficial to the dendritic arborization. This has been done in order to enhance the patterns of axonal distribution. To facilitate comparison of sizes, all the original illustrations of Golgi-stained cells have been reproduced at the same final magnification, with the exception of Fig. 8A.

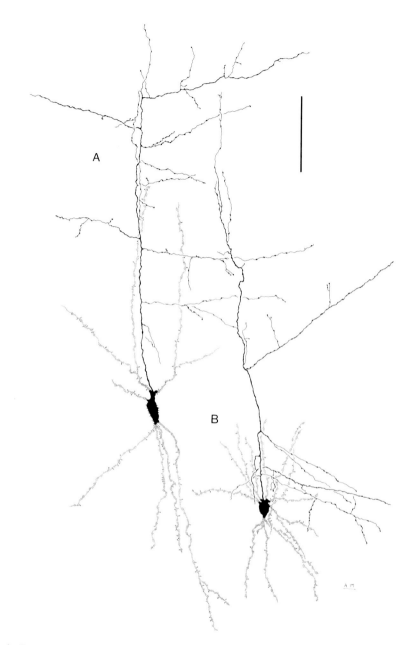

Figure 1. Two nonpyramidal neurons from the first auditory cortex of the cat. They show an ascending axonal trunk which gives rise to horizontal axonal collaterals with short side branches. Cell A is located on the upper tier of layer V and its ascending axon reaches layer III. The perikaryon of cell B is in deep layer III. The calibration bar (= 100 μm) serves for all the original Golgi drawings, with the exception of Fig. 8A.

the case of Martinotti cells, the axon stems from the upper aspect of the cell body or from the base of a dendrite and then ascends, occasionally, to layer I. One differential characteristic, however, is the presence of conspicuous, long horizontal collaterals which give origin, in turn, to short vertical branches. This neuronal variety has been known since the earliest studies of Ramón y Cajal on the cerebral cortex of the mouse (1891, his Fig. 6c) but, according to that author, they are also present in the human visual cortex (1911, his Fig. 384D*). Other examples found in the earliest literature are from the somatosensory cortex of the mouse [Lorente de Nó (1922) describes them there as "células colosales," gigantic cells, in his Figs. 11A, B, F]. They have also been seen in the rabbit visual cortex (O'Leary and Bishop, 1938, their Figs. 9-2 and 14-3) and the visual cortex of the cat (O'Leary, 1941, his Fig. 9-8). These data, obtained in rather different species, seem to indicate that such cells might be present in all mammalian cortices. It is remarkable that, with some exceptions, modern reports do not mention the existence of such nonpyramidal neurons. In their account of the rat visual cortex, Parnavelas *et al.* (1977a) illustrate, in their Fig. 6, a cell that may be comparable. Another example is the cell shown by Valverde (1976) in his Fig. 6, which has been commented on above. Since, in this latter case, the axon arborizes within layer I, it must be considered as a Martinotti cell, but the great number of horizontal branches in layers III and IV induces one to consider this cell as different. However, there are, at present, no valid arguments to justify a separation of these cells into a well-defined group, different from Martinotti cells. What must be considered, nevertheless, is the morphology of the axonal plexus, excluding the layer I component. In fact, it resembles the axonal arborization of the classical basket cells (see Section 3.4).

Other neurons with ascending axons do not project to layer I. An outstanding variety is represented by cells with a bitufted or, less frequently, multipolar morphology, located in the middle or lower layers of the cortex. They form an axon that usually bifurcates into thick, ascending branches, which end in layer II–III in the form of a dense plexus. Abundant examples are found in the earliest literature: Ramón y Cajal (1911) depicted them in layer IV of the human visual cortex (e.g., his Fig. 384, reproduced here as Fig. 4, cell B) and in the cortex of the temporal lobe (his Fig. 401M); Lorente de Nó (1922, his Figs. 22B, D) in the mouse somatosensory cortex; O'Leary and Bishop (1938, their Figs. 13-3, 13-5, and 14-5) in the visual cortex of rabbits. In these figures, a relatively sparse local plexus is observed and, in addition, an axonal tuft in lamina II–III, whose richness varies in the different renditions. It is our opinion, however, that these differences merely represent an effect of the varying qualities of the Golgi impregnation. If this is true, the sparsely spinous bitufted cell shown in Fig. 2 of the present report might be included in this category. In this example taken from the cat auditory cortex, the axon originates from the lower aspect of the perikaryon and initially descends; then it soon turns upwards to end in layer II–III.

Although similar cells are not frequently reported in recent papers, there are examples illustrated by Lund *et al.* (1979) which deserve mention. Perhaps, the most typical example is shown in their Fig. 5 (cell labeled B), but cell A in

---

* This figure has been reproduced as Fig. 4 in the present account.

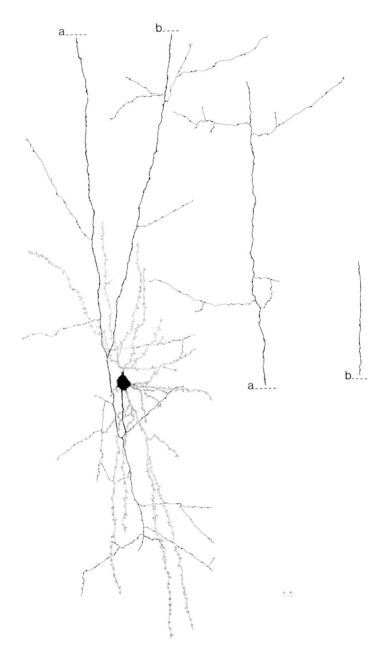

Figure 2. Sparsely spinous bitufted neurons from the first auditory area of the cat. The perikaryon is located in layer V and gives rise to a descending axon which soon recurves and, during its ascent, bifurcates to distribute sparsely in the middle of layer II–III. The two main ascending branches are continuous at a and b.

their Fig. 4, though possessing a denser, local axonal plexus, might be considered comparable. The suggestion put forward by Lund (1973) and Lund *et al.* (1979), and earlier by Lorente de Nó (1949), that some types of nonspiny stellate cells might establish highly specific interlaminar connections justifies the necessity for systematic studies of the axonal geometry and synaptology of these cells.

3.2. Cells with Columnar Axons: Double Bouquet and Bipolar Cells

A distinct population of nonpyramidal cells have axonal arborizations which distribute themselves within narrow, radially oriented columns of cortical tissue. These cells have commonly been referred to as *double bouquet cells,* a term which only defines the forms of the dendritic arborizations. A review of the pertinent literature reveals that neurons of rather variable dendritic morphology, even somewhat multipolar in form, have been considered to be double bouquet cells, on the basis of their columnar axonal plexuses. Therefore, a search for the origin of the term may be worthwhile, as it is to explore whether the cells so named constitute a homogeneous population.

The description of double bouquet cells by Ramón y Cajal (1911, pp. 538–541, and his Fig. 348, reproduced here as Fig. 3) is well known and has been summarized, notably by Colonnier (1966) and Szentágothai (1973). The difficulty, however, arises from the fact that Ramón y Cajal, in 1911, described additional, distinct varieties of neurons under the common denomination of double bouquet cells (Jones, 1975; Peters and Regidor, 1981; see Chapter 1). It seems that not only are there cells with apparently comparable axonal arborizations, but showing different dendritic morphologies (see, e.g., in Ramón y Cajal, 1911, his Fig. 384, reproduced here as Fig. 4, cell labeled E), but there are others whose axonal arborizations do not fit at all with his first descriptions of double bouquet cells (Ramón y Cajal, 1899a,d). In these earlier writings, it is evident that while the essential trait was the axonal distribution, their dendritic morphology was considered by Ramón y Cajal to be consistent. The axonal pattern he defines is a very distinctive one (Fig. 3), formed of extremely thin and very long collaterals (Ramón y Cajal states that only one-third of their total vertical span is represented in his figure), which are both ascending and descending. On the other hand, the dendritic patterns, identical in cells A and B of Fig. 3, justify the name of *células bipenachadas*—literally, bitufted cells—given by Ramón y Cajal (1899a). However, these neurons have two polar dendrites as do bipolar cells defined in the rat visual cortex by Feldman and Peters (1978) and Peters and Kimerer (1981). In fact, Peters and Regidor (1981) have considered the cells in the figure by Ramón y Cajal (Fig. 3) as being bipolar in nature.

Aiming to clarify the concept of the double bouquet cell, we have thoroughly examined original preparations made by Ramón y Cajal himself, preparations which were made available to us at the Cajal Museum in Madrid. In Fig. 5, we represent two examples; in A, a layer III cell (human somatosensory cortex) with two long dendritic tufts which span from layers II to V. In B, also taken from layer III of the human somatosensory cortex has a larger cell body but the dendritic morphology is comparable to that of cell A; however, the vertical span is more limited (layers II–III). The axon also forms a vertical plexus, but

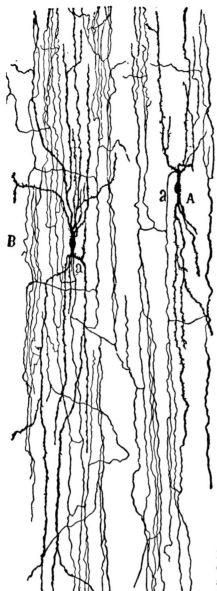

Figure 3. Reproduction of Fig. 348 from Ramón y Cajal (1911), showing two double bouquet cells with ascending and descending axonal collaterals (Section 3.2.1).

it is principally constituted by descending collaterals which make it similar to a horsetail (Szentágothai, 1973). In addition, axonal side branches are conspicuous. Cell A shows characteristics which are compatible with those shown by cells in Fig. 3. Cell B, on the other hand, has an axonal arborization more similar to those shown by cells E and F in Fig. 4, and may correspond to some of the cells analyzed by Somogyi and Cowey (1981) (see Chapter 9).

To give an idea of the excellent preservation of cells in these preparations, in Fig. 6 we present a photomontage of part of cell B in Fig. 5. Incidentally, in this photomicrograph some axonal branches are seen to approach the apical

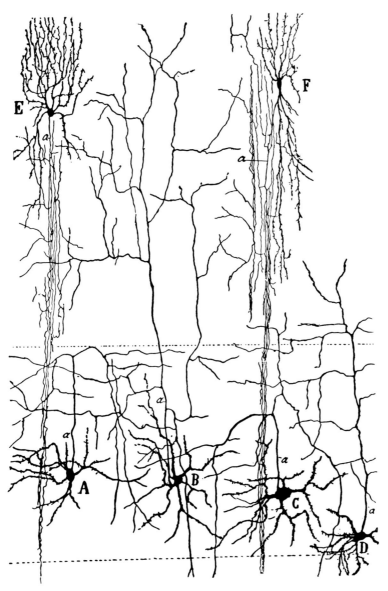

Figure 4. Reproduction of Fig. 384 from Ramón y Cajal (1911). Cells labeled A and C are interpreted as cells with relatively extended axonal arborizations (Section 3.3.4); D, as a cell with ascending axon and horizontal collaterals comparable to the ones shown in Fig. 1; cell B resembles the cell shown in Fig. 2 (Section 3.1). Cells E and F are double bouquet cells with mainly descending axonal arborizations.

dendrite of a layer V pyramid very intimately; it is most likely that similar observations prompted Ramón y Cajal (1899a) to suggest a functional relationship between the axonal arborization of his double bouquet cells and the cell bodies and apical dendrites of pyramids. It has been suggested, furthermore, that these contacts would be established onto the apical dendritic spines of pyramidal cells (Colonnier, 1966; Szentágothai, 1969, 1973), and consequently that

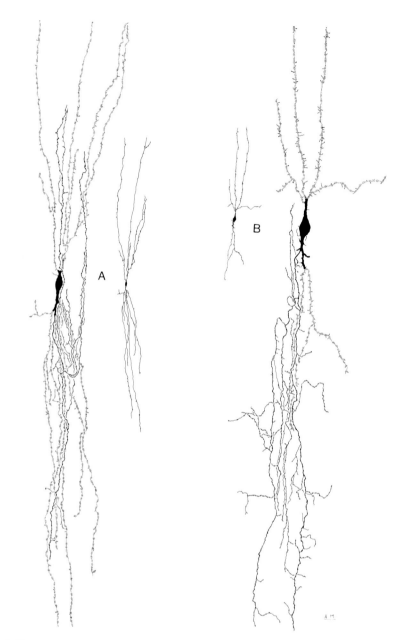

Figure 5. Two examples of double bouquet cells drawn from original Ramón y Cajal preparations of the somatosensory cortex of infants. Both have their perikarya in layer III. Insets show the total span of their dendritic arborizations. See text for details.

double bouquet cells might be excitatory. Such an assumption has recently been contested by Somogyi and Cowey (1981), who have examined double bouquet cells with vertical axonal plexuses in the visual cortices of cats and monkeys which form symmetrical synapses and, in the visual cortex of monkeys, Somogyi *et al.* (1981b) have suggested that it is these cells that can be labeled by retrograde

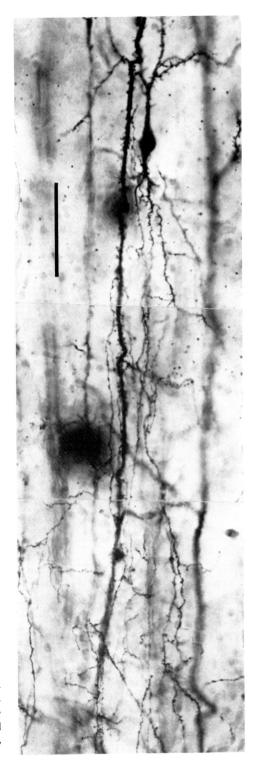

Figure 6. Photomontage of part of the cell labeled B in Fig. 5. Note the course of its descending axonal collaterals in close proximity to the apical dendrite of a layer V pyramidal cell, whose body is not shown. Calibration bar, 150 μm.

transport of [^{3}H]-GABA from deeper layers (see Chapter 5). Additionally, however, Somogyi and Cowey (1981) present a neuron in layer IV of the monkey area 17 which forms asymmetrical contacts; they interpret that neuron as being a spiny stellate cell (another neuron variety which produces columnar axonal patterns; see Section 3.5). Another interpretation is tenable, however, for Peters and Kimerer (1981) have described, in the rat visual cortex, bipolar cells which produce efferent synapses of the asymmetrical variety (see Chapter 11). Some of the bipolar cells reported by these authors have axons that form vertically oriented plexuses, as also do examples shown by Vogt and Peters (1981, their Figs. 15c, d) and McMullen and Glaser (1982, their Fig. 13), or the cell shown in Fig. 7, taken from our rabbit material. Whether bipolar cells must be considered as a distinct subgroup of double bouquet cells awaits further study, but some data seem to support the idea that two main groups of double bouquet cells must be considered.

3.2.1. Double Bouquet Cells with Ascending and Descending Axonal Collaterals

This group contains bitufted or bipolar cells with very elongate dendritic fields and perikarya located in layers II through V, but they seem to be more frequent in supragranular layers. The characteristics of the axon have been summarized above. In brief, the axon originates from the cell body or from a proximal dendrite and generates a plexus of ascending and descending collaterals. The collaterals are thin and the plexuses, as far as one can judge from the Golgi drawings, are not very dense. This description corresponds to cells A and B in Fig. 3 or to cell F in Fig. 5 of Ramón y Cajal (1900). Ramón y Cajal (1899a, 1900, 1911) stated that, in cats and dogs, these cells are less frequent than in the human cortex; he showed examples of what he considered to be their homologs in his Figs. 21G (1899c) and 347d (1911), although no comparable cells are illustrated in his study of the cat visual cortex (1921, 1922). Other examples in the literature of what we believe are similar cells are reported by O'Leary and Bishop (1938) in their Fig. 10 (rabbit visual cortex); O'Leary (1941) in his Figs. 9-11 and 10-2 (cat visual cortex); Norita and Kawamura (1981) in their Fig. 1a (Clare–Bishop area of the cat); and Lund *et al.* (1981) in their Fig. 3e (area 18 of the monkey). It is interesting to note that Jones (1975) apparently does not include similar cells in his type 3 and that they were probably not sampled by Somogyi and Cowey (1981) in their study of double bouquet cells (see Section 3.2.2).

We have chosen a few additional examples from our own material which seem to fit into this group. Besides the cell shown in Fig. 5A, which we have referred to above, there is a neuron in the cat visual cortex (Fig. 8A) with a comparable dendritic morphology but a poorly arborizing axon arising from the main descending dendritic trunk. In Figs. 9A and C, there are two neurons, also from the cat visual cortex, with more complete axonal impregnations; they are strikingly similar to cell d in Fig. 347 of Ramón y Cajal (1911). Cell B in Fig. 9 is from the rat visual cortex; though showing a similar dendritic morphology, its identity is difficult to establish since the axonal arborization is looser.

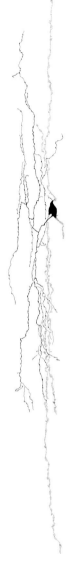

Figure 7. Bipolar cell from layer IV of the visual cortex of a rabbit. It shows an axonal plexus with vertically oriented ascending and descending axonal collaterals.

Since, as pointed out by Peters and Regidor (1981), some of the neurons considered here may be envisaged as bipolar cells, it might be of interest to know whether the synapses formed by their axons are asymmetrical, as they are in bipolar cells of the rat visual cortex (Peters and Kimerer, 1981). That this is indeed the case has been found for the cells shown in Figs. 8 and 9A. In Figs. 8B and C, two axonal boutons are presynaptic, at asymmetrical synaptic junctions (open arrows), to dendritic spines. Figure 10 shows some of the synapses formed

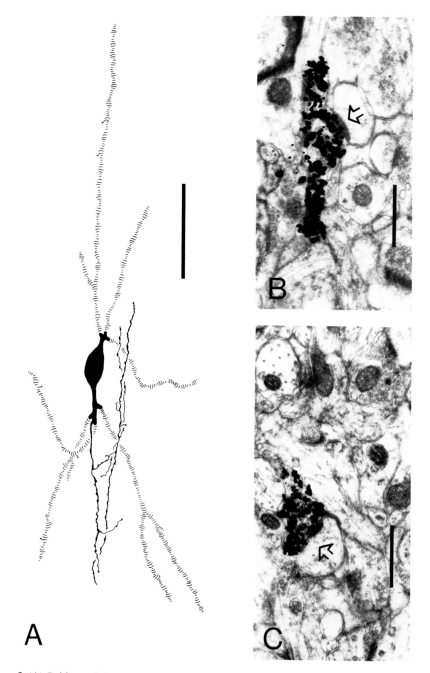

Figure 8. (A) Gold-toned fusiform neuron from deep layer III of cat area 17. Dendritic morphology suggests it could be a bipolar cell and it also resembles cell A in Fig. 5. Although impregnation was incomplete, the nature of the synapses formed by its axon could still be identified. In B and C, examples of asymmetrical synapses (open arrows) on dendritic spines are shown. Calibration bars: A, 50 μm; B and C, 0.5 μm.

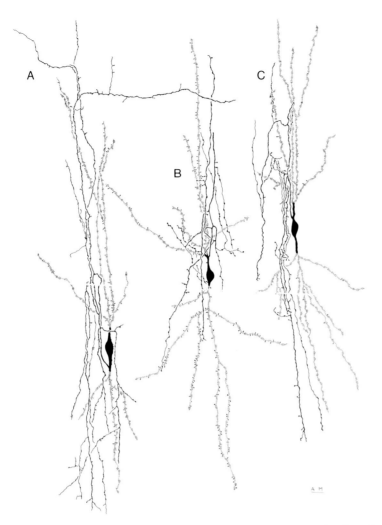

Figure 9. Examples of double bouquet cells. Cell A is from layer IV and cell C from layer III of cat area 17. Both show a columnar distribution of ascending and descending axonal collaterals, and a horizontal axonal branch in upper layer II is present in A. Cell B is from layer II–III of rat area 18a; it is comparable in dendritic morphology to cells A and C, but it differs in its axonal distribution, which is not as clearly columnar.

by axonal collaterals of the cell in Fig. 9A. In the two serial sections shown in Figs. 10A and B, two boutons are seen to contact dendritic spines; note that the postsynaptic density is not recognizable as being of an asymmetrical synapse in one of the cases (open arrow in A), whereas its nature is obvious in a serial section (B). Two more asymmetrical synapses on spines are seen in C. Since these results are preliminary, no information regarding the sources of these dendritic spines is available, and similarly, no other postsynaptic targets as reported by Peters and Kimerer (1981) for the rat bipolar neurons (shafts of apical dendrites and somata and dendrites of nonpyramidal cells) have been found in our material (see Chapter 11). The difficulty of staining the axons of bipolar

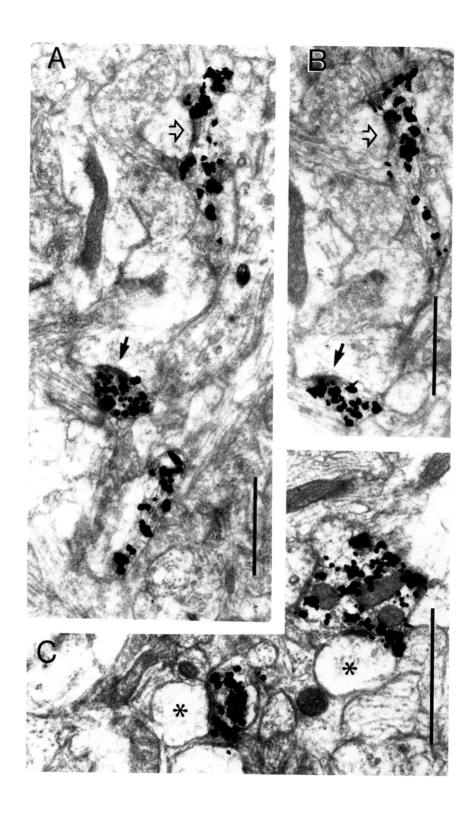

cells by the Golgi method is notorious and has made attempts at correlations between species particularly troublesome. It is hoped that further analyses of their synaptology at the electron microscope level, together with immunocytochemical studies, will help to solve the problem.

3.2.2. Double Bouquet Cells with Mainly Descending Axonal Arborizations

The cell variety is exemplified by cells E and F in Fig. 4 (taken from Ramón y Cajal, 1911, Fig. 384). As mentioned above, Ramón y Cajal did not separate these cells from his first type of double bouquet cell, but there are reasons to believe that they represent a different subtype of neurons (see, e.g., Peters and Regidor, 1981). Similar cells have frequently been shown in the literature, as they appear in rather diverging species and cortical areas: the mouse somatosensory (Lorente de Nó, 1922, his Fig. 7C) and visual (Ruiz-Marcos and Valverde, 1970, their Fig. 1e) cortices; the cat visual cortex (Peters and Regidor, 1981, Figs. 8K, L) and Clare–Bishop area (Norita and Kawamura, 1981, Figs. 1b, c); the monkey somatosensory (Jones, 1975, Fig. 8) and visual (area 18) cortices (Valverde, 1978, Fig. 3a). Besides the cell shown in Fig. 5B, drawn from preparations of Ramón y Cajal's, one example taken from our material of the cat area 17 is represented in Fig. 11A, to facilitate comparisons. It is clear that the examples listed above possess the same configurations as some of the neurons selected by Somogyi and Cowey (1981) in their Golgi–electron microscope study of double bouquet cells (e.g., their Fig. 1, from the cat, and Fig. 15, from the monkey area 17; see also Fig. 2 in Chapter 9). Excellent descriptions and illustrations of these cells are found in Jones (1975), who includes them in his type 3, and in Valverde (1978), who names them "cells with vertical axonal bundles and grape-like terminal knobs." Also, the cells with horsetail-shaped axons of Szentágothai (1973, 1975) seem to correspond to this group. The essential features of these cells are their location in superficial layers, their multipolar or bitufted dendritic trees, and their descending axonal bundles. There is, in some instances, a tendency for the superficial dendrites to form an ascending tuft which gives a peculiar appearance to some of these cells, but the ascending tufts are not exclusive to these cells. The axonal plexuses are essentially descending and clearly pass beyond the dendritic domain. Axonal collaterals become thick along their descending trajectory and intertwine together forming one or more compact fascicles of fibers, in which short-side appendages are conspicuous. Overall, these morphological characteristics are peculiar and allow them to be distinguished from the ones we have described in the preceding subsection. Some collaterals, however, take an ascending course, as in Fig. 4F.

There are, in addition, other cells which have commonly been included in this group, characterized by their being multipolar and by the distribution of their axons. Examples are shown by Lorente de Nó (1922, his Fig. 7A), Jones

---

Figure 10. Synapses formed by the axon of the gold-toned neuron shown in Fig. 9A. A and B show two serial sections in which a vertically oriented axonal branch, labeled by its content of gold particles, forms a synaptic junction on a dendritic spine (open arrows), its asymmetrical nature being evident in B; another bouton forms an asymmetrical synaptic junction on a dendritic profile of unidentified nature (arrows). C. Asymmetrical synapses on dendritic spines. Calibration bars, 1 μm.

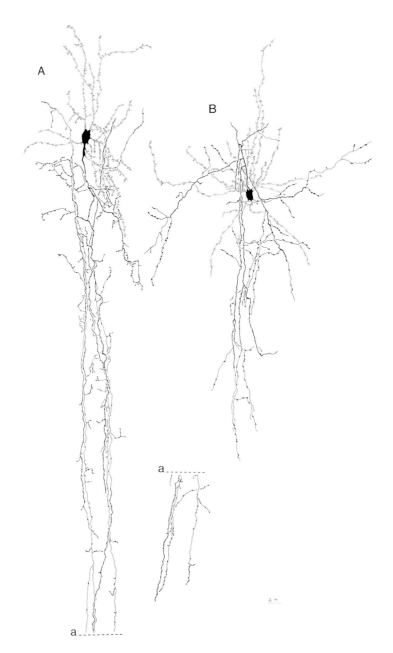

Figure 11. Double bouquet cells with descending axonal arborizations. Both have multipolar dendritic fields. A is taken from the upper tier of layer II–III of cat area 17 and shows a columnar axonal plexus in which the descending branches interlace together; inset shows the continuation of the descending axons at a. B is a similar cell from layer II–III of the visual area of a rabbit. It shows a comparable descending axonal plexus but differs in the overall distribution of the more approximal branches.

(1978, his Fig. 4c), which are similar to the cell shown by Somogyi and Cowey (1981) in their Fig. 13. Although the organization of the vertical axonal plexus is similar, there are conspicuous axonal arcades and a richer plexus within the dendritic domain which, as rightly pointed out by Jones (1975), make them reminiscent of his type 2 cells. We include an example of a cell, from the rabbit visual cortex, which is comparable (Fig. 11B; also see Fig. 2 in Chapter 13).

The forms and distribution of the synaptic boutons originating from cells with columnar, descending axons have been analyzed by Somogyi and Cowey (1981). The synapses have symmetrical membrane specializations, and these authors report more pronounced postsynaptic thickenings in the case of the cells they describe in cats than there are in monkeys. The majority of synapses are formed on dendritic shafts, which do not include the apical dendrites of pyramidal cells, but some are on dendritic spines and on perikarya of nonpyramidal neurons. Except for some differences in each of the individual cells they describe, the patterns of distribution seem consistent in all of the cases reported by these authors. This is also the case, with minor differences, for a similar cell with axonal arcades and descending axons we have analyzed in the cat visual cortex (DeFelipe and Fairén, 1981).

3.3. Cells with No Preferred Axonal Orientation

We include in this group a rather heterogeneous population of neurons, defined by a common geometrical property of their axonal fields, i.e., the lack of a preferred orientation in either the vertical (ascending or columnar) or the tangential directions. Within this group, there are some cells which can be considered as generalized (Fairén and Valverde, 1979), whereas the others are specialized. Precise differences between generalized types are difficult to establish, either on the basis of size or on the basis of subtle differences in the axonal branching patterns.

The group contains cells showing a strictly local axonal arborization (Golgi type II cells) but, also, others which display axonal aroborizations with diverse degrees of dispersion around the perikaryon or origin. For some of these cells, especially those with large perikarya and rather extended dendritic fields, the term *local* applied to their axonal trees would seem inappropriate. Depending on the size of the axonal domain, some cells may be confined to a single lamina or encompass two or more adjacent ones. A discussion of some of these cells is also presented in Chapter 13.

3.3.1. Small Multipolar Cells with Strictly Local Axonal Arborizations

These cells correspond to the "neurogliaform cells" of Ramón y Cajal (1899b,c,d, 1900, 1911, 1921, 1922; see Chapter 12). They are small cells provided with short, smooth, and finely beaded dendrites which branch at obtuse angles, not far from their points of origin; there are instances, however, in which the dendrites ramify less and are recurving. The axon is slender and is studded with dilations; it arborizes richly within the dendritic domain, in a strictly local manner. Thus, neurogliaform cells are the only *true* Golgi type II cell in the cerebral cortex. These cells have been reported in a number of species and cortical areas (Ramón y Cajal, 1911, 1921, 1922; Lorente de Nó, 1922, 1949; Ramón-Moliner, 1961; Valverde, 1971, 1978; Shkol'nik-Yarros, 1971; LeVay, 1973; Lund, 1973; Szentágothai, 1973, 1978; Jones, 1975; Lund *et al.*, 1977; Tömböl, 1978b; Fairén and Valverde, 1979; Werner *et al.* 1979; Norita and Kawamura, 1981; Peters and Regidor, 1981; see Chapter 12). In the published drawings, the morphological characteristics that define this cell group are easily recognizable, and no new details need to be added to the previous descriptions. As defined here, the essential trait is the strictly local organization of their dendritic and axonal trees. They may be more or less compact, however. It seems that in the primary sensory areas of primates, including man, neurogliaform cells are small and possess a dense axonal plexus; this makes arborization patterns difficult to analyze, as for instance in the original drawings of Ramón y Cajal. In cats and dogs (Ramón y Cajal, 1911, 1921, 1922; Fairén and Valverde, 1979; Norita and Kawamura, 1981; Peters and Regidor, 1981) or in rabbits (Tömböl, 1978b) the cells are larger and the axonal arborizations looser; they may spread out of the dendritic domain slightly. The same seems true for local cells in area 18 of monkeys (Valverde, 1978, and compare Fig. 6b in Lund *et al.*, 1981).

In the visual cortex of rodents, the presence of local neurons *sensu strictu* has been discussed, and it has been suggested (Peters and Fairén, 1978; Fairén and Valverde, 1979) that they might be represented by other nonpyramidal neurons with more extended axonal arborizations. However, this may not necessarily be the case, since Peters and Regidor (1981) report an example of a neurogliaform cell in their material of rat visual cortex. In the somatosensory cortex of mice (Lorente de Nó, 1922; Woolsey *et al.*, 1975) there is a type of smooth stellate cell which is, in its distribution, confined to a single layer IV barrel (Woolsey and Van der Loos, 1970). The cells shown in Figs. 6C and 7I of Lorente de Nó (1922) are comparable to local axon cells in other species (Valverde, 1971). In layers V and VI, Lorente de Nó (1922, 1949) represented cells with similar shapes, but less restricted in space (cf. Fig. 73, cells 24, 25, and 26, in Lorente de Nó, 1949).

Neurons with strictly local axons are present in all cortical layers (Ramón y Cajal, 1911; Ramón-Moliner, 1961; Peters and Regidor, 1981), including layer I (LeVay, 1973). Some reports, however, indicate that they are typical of layer IV in the somatosensory cortex (Jones, 1975) and in area 17 (Valverde, 1971) and 18 (Valverde, 1978; Lund *et al.*, 1981) of monkeys. It may be, however, that these layer IV cells—including those in the rodent barrel field—constitute a peculiar type, akin to Valverde's (1971) clewed cells, whereas other cells may correspond more directly, on account of their dendritic branching patterns, to the classical neurogliaform cells (cf. Szentágothai, 1973). A further account of neurogliaform cells is given in Chapter 12.

3.3.2. Chandelier Cells

These interneurons were first described by Szentágothai and Arbib (1974) in the cingulate cortex of the cat. Prior to this description, no such interneurons had been represented in any account of neurons of the cerebral cortex. This illustrates the limitations of the Golgi method for describing the distribution or the presence of a particular type of neuron in a given cortical area. There can be some debate about whether some of the interneurons described in the literature as small basket cells (e.g., Figs. 17-4 and 73 in Shkol'nik-Yarros, 1971) are chandelier cells. In any case, we have not found convincing examples after an examination of a large number of preparations from the Ramón y Cajal collection; most probably, chandelier cells were very infrequently impregnated and escaped recognition.

The name given to these cells derives from the peculiar morphology of their overall axonal distribution and of their terminal, vertical rows of axonal boutons, which Fairén and Valverde (1980) have named *specific terminal portions*. Even if there are certain differences among species and areas (e.g., Fig. 12), the basic pattern, reminiscent of a chandelier fixture, can easily be recognized (see Chapter 10).

Chandelier cells are unique among the cortical nonpyramidal cells in that they are, in absolute terms, target selective. In all Golgi–EM studies reported so far, their vertical axonal terminal portions have been found to contact only the axon initial segments of pyramidal cells, forming symmetrical synaptic specializations (Somogyi, 1977, 1979; Somogyi *et al.*, 1979, 1982, 1983; Fairén and Valverde, 1980; Fairén *et al.*, 1981; Peters *et al.*, 1982). In addition, Somogyi *et al.* (1982) have added that those individual boutons, not belonging to the specific terminal portions, also form axo-axonic synapses. This unique type of synaptic relationship has prompted the formal proposal by Somogyi *et al.* (1982) that chandelier cells should be renamed *axo-axonic cells*. While this point of view may be correct, the study of Fairén and Valverde (1980) showed that cells identical, in the Golgi picture, to the ones shown by Szentágothai (1975, 1979) behave in exactly the same way as Somogyi's axo-axonic cells. We believe that the name *chandelier cells* should be maintained because this term best describes their axonal morphology. Changing the name to reflect the synaptic target might force us to change the names of many other cells once their synaptology is accurately determined. However, most of the local axons studied so far in the cerebral cortex have postsynaptic targets that are rather diversified.

Somogyi *et al.* (1982) have questioned the identity of their axo-axonic cells to many of the chandelier cells that have been illustrated in the literature, in which electron microscope evidence of the axonal distribution has not been given. Indeed, the apical shafts of pyramidal cells, proposed by Szentágothai and Arbib (1974) and Szentágothai (1975, 1978, 1979) as the postsynaptic targets for chandelier cells, do receive multiple innervation by boutons forming symmetrical synapses (Szentágothai and Arbib, 1974; Szentágothai, 1975; Hersch and White, 1981b). The cells of origin of these boutons have not been identified. Somogyi *et al.* (1982) report preliminary data on interneurons forming multiple symmetrical synapses on this location, but they do not give any information regarding their morphology at the light microscope level. In passing, reference should also be made to the report by Müller-Paschinger *et al.* (1983) who, on the sole basis of Golgi observations, suggest that axon terminals of chandelier cells in the rabbit sensory cortices may contact virtually all portions of the pyramidal neurons.

Most of the terminal boutons of chandelier cells tend to form clusters around the most distal part of the axon initial segments of pyramidal cells, although

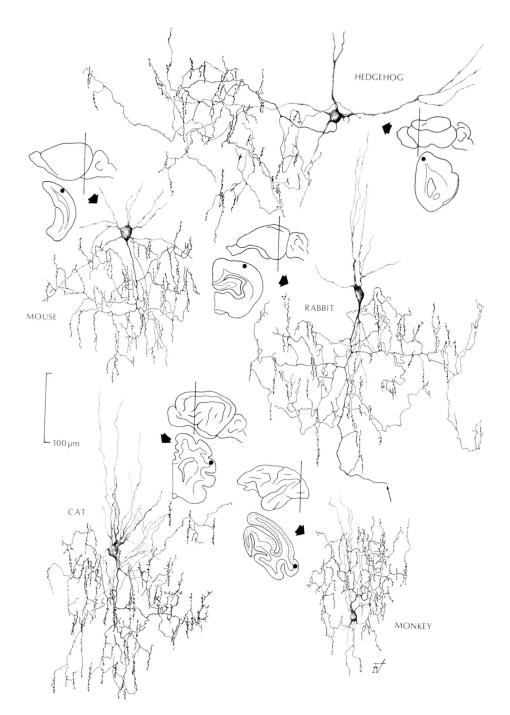

Figure 12. Examples of chandelier cells in diverse mammalian species and cortical areas. Reproduced from Valverde (1983) with permission.

some may be more proximal. There are, in addition, other interneurons whose axonal boutons occasionally contribute with similar axo-axonic synapses to the axon initial segment (Peters and Fairén, 1978; Peters and Proskauer, 1980a; DeFelipe and Fairén, 1981; Somogyi *et al.*, 1982). However, the distribution of chandelier cell axonal boutons is so typical that they can be recognized using GAD immunocytochemistry. This led Peters *et al.* (1982) to the important conclusion that they are GAD-positive and, thus, that chandelier cells are inhibitory, as had been suggested earlier (Somogyi, 1977; Fairén and Valverde, 1980) on the basis of the morphology of the synaptic contacts they produce. See Chapter 12 for additional discussion of this point.

Complexity of the specific terminal portions is variable, and some reports on the cat cerebral cortex (Szentágothai, 1975, 1979; Lund *et al.*, 1979; Fairén and Valverde, 1980; Fairén *et al.*, 1981) describe very complex ones, made occasionally by the convergence of several collaterals from the same axonal arborization into a unique terminal portion (see, e.g., Figs. 6 and 7, taken from a 3-month-old specimen, in Fairén and Valverde, 1980). Other terminal formations in the cat are simpler, formed of a single row of boutons, as in the case of chandelier cells of rats and mice. It was tentatively suggested by Fairén and Valverde (1980) and Fairén *et al.* (1981) that this might be the expression of an evolutionary trend, but reports of chandelier cells in the monkey neocortex show simple rows of terminal boutons (e.g., Jones, 1975; Somogyi *et al.*, 1982; Valverde, 1983). The alternative hypothesis that complex specific terminal portions are immature structures has been advanced by Somogyi *et al.* (1982), but Somogyi *et al.* (1983) show complex axonal terminations of similar cells in the hippocampus of adult monkeys. Clearly, the issue cannot be considered completely settled and an examination is required of terminal axonal formations of chandelier cells in immature specimens of species, such as rats or mice, where they have been reported to be simple in all cases.

Examples of chandelier cells, with or without electron microscope evidence, have been reported in different species and cortical areas, including, in the *monkey,* the visual (Tömböl, 1978a; Lund, 1981; Lund *et al.*, 1981; Somogyi *et al.*, 1982; Valverde, 1983), somatosensory (Jones, 1975; Szentágothai, 1975), and auditory cortices (Szentágothai, 1975). In the *cat,* examples have been found in the visual cortex (Tömböl, 1976, 1978b; Fairén and Valverde, 1979, 1980; Lund *et al.*, 1979; Somogyi, 1979; Peters and Regidor, 1981; Somogyi *et al.*, 1982), the Clare–Bishop area (Norita and Kawamura, 1981), the somatosensory (Tömböl, 1978b), and motor (Somogyi *et al.*, 1982) cortices, the cortex of the anterior ectosylvian sulcus (Valverde, 1983, and unpublished observations by the present authors), and the cingulate cortex (Szentágothai and Arbib, 1974; Szentágothai, 1975). In *rabbits,* they have been reported in the visual area (Valverde, 1983) and in other sensory cortices (Müller-Paschinger *et al.*, 1983). Chandelier cells in the *rat* have been encountered in the visual cortex (Somogyi, 1977; Somogyi *et al.*, 1979, 1982; Werner *et al.*, 1979; Peters *et al.*, 1982) and in the cingulate cortex (Vogt and Peters, 1981) and, in the *mouse,* in the visual cortex (Valverde, 1983), auditory cortex (Fairén *et al.*, 1981), and premotor cortex (unpublished observations). As shown in Fig. 12, taken from Valverde (1983), cells with identical terminal axonal portions are present in a primitive cortex, that of the hedgehog *Erinaceus europaeus;* Valverde has found them in the parietal region and in the interhemispheric and entorhinal cortices. Somogyi *et al.* (1982) have described chandelier cell axons in the subiculum and pyriform cortex of the rat, and, additionally, Somogyi *et al.* (1983) have provided light and electron microscope evidence that similar chandelier cells exist in the stratum pyramidale of the monkey hippocampus, which is not surprising if the synaptology of the axon initial segments of hippocampal pyramidal cells (Kosaka, 1980) is considered.

Therefore, it seems that chandelier cells occur in all mammals and are present in all cortical areas, and not exclusively in the neocortex, so that they must be regarded as an essential cellular component of the cerebral cortex.

A point of interest is whether chandelier cells distribute uniformly in the areas where they appear. In the visual cortex of cats and rats, Fairén and Valverde (1980) and Peters *et al.* (1982) have reported a greater occurrence of chandelier cells at the border of areas 17 and 18 (or 17 and 18a); while this might be due to the capriciousness of the Golgi method, it appears that certain pyramidal cells receive only a few synaptic contacts on their axon initial segments (Peters *et al.*, 1982), thus indicating that they might not be innervated by chandelier cells. An indirect approach to solve the problem of the suspected discreteness in distribution of chandelier cells may be found by reconstructing entire initial axonal segments of diverse populations of pyramidal cells identified according to their projections by using retrograde labels. Combination of HRP retrograde labeling with the Golgi staining in the same material (Somogyi *et al.*, 1979) is of interest, but it is subjected to the vagaries of the Golgi impregnation. This combined method, however, has generated the interesting observation that one of the targets of chandelier cells are callosal-projecting neurons (Somogyi *et al.*, 1979), a fact that might explain the preferential impregnation of chandelier cells at the periphery of area 17.

Similarly, new efforts are required to analyze the distribution of chandelier cells according to cortical layers. Most reports indicate that chandelier cells are more abundant in supragranular layers and there are data that indicate, at least in the monkey somatosensory and motor cortices, a richer synaptic supply to axon initial segments of pyramidal cells located in supragranular layers (Sloper and Powell, 1979). Nevertheless, chandelier cells indeed exist in the infragranular layers (Tömböl, 1976, 1978a,b; Fairén and Valverde, 1980, and unpublished results in the cat visual cortex). Occasionally, the descending axonal collaterals of superficially located chandelier cells may arborize in these layers (Lund *et al.*, 1979; Fairén and Valverde, 1980).

3.3.3. Small Basket Cells

Ramón y Cajal (1899c, 1911) described a medium-sized variety of his "cellules à double bouquet dendritique," located in the supragranular layers of the human sensory motor cortex. One such cell, taken from this last publication, is reproduced here as Fig. 13B. The peculiarity of the axon of these cells is that they form nests about the cell bodies of small-sized pyramidal cells (Fig. 13A). Comparable cells are described by O'Leary and Bishop (1938) and O'Leary (1941) in the visual cortices of rabbits and cats, respectively, but, as pointed out by Peters and Regidor (1981), the dendritic and axonal arborizations of the examples shown by O'Leary (1941) resemble those of chandelier cells. However,

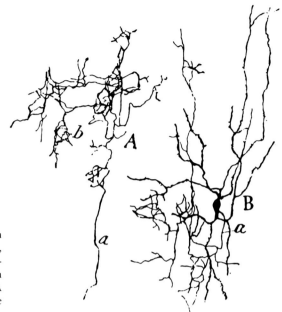

Figure 13. Reproduction of Fig. 349 from Ramón y Cajal (1911) to illustrate, in B, one of the varieties of his double bouquet cells, which in this case gives origin to pericellular axonal plexuses (b). A represents the axonal arborization of one such cell. a, Axon.

other interpretations of the drawings by Ramón y Cajal have been advanced (Marin-Padilla and Stibitz, 1974; Marin-Padilla, 1975), but it is interesting to note that this is the first formulation, in Ramón y Cajal's writings, of the concept of the neocortical basket, i.e., a cell which contributes synaptic contacts, preferentially, to cell bodies of pyramids.

There are several varieties of basket cells (Ramón y Cajal, 1911; Marin-Padilla, 1969, 1970b; Szentágothai, 1973; Jones, 1975; and see Chapter 8), and, in this section, we will refer only to what Szentágothai (1969, 1973) has named small or short-range basket cells. Golgi–EM evidence for the existence of such a variety of cells in the visual cortex of the cat has been given recently (DeFelipe and Fairén, 1982). The basic criterion for identification of small basket cells in that study was the analysis of their patterns of efferent connections, to determine whether there were signs of target selectivity (cf. Fairén and Valverde, 1979). In a preliminary evaluation of local interneurons in layer II–III of the cat area 17, using semithin sections of Golgi-stained material, some cells were found which consistently produce multiple contacts on cell bodies and proximal dendrites of pyramidal cells (Fig. 14). The synaptic nature of these contacts was demonstrated electron microscopically, but it was also found that nonpyramidal cells receive multiple synaptic contacts (DeFelipe and Fairén, 1982). In addition, multiple axosomatic autapses have recently been described in one such cell (Fairén *et al.*, 1982). In all cases, the identified synapses were of the symmetrical variety.

This type of connectivity was not evident in the preliminary light microscope evaluation of the Golgi preparations: no visible basket formations were present. Nevertheless, the cells that, according to the above criteria, proved to be basket cells show a well-defined morphology. They are multipolar cells with rather wide dendritic fields, sometimes showing a predominant dendritic tuft oriented to-

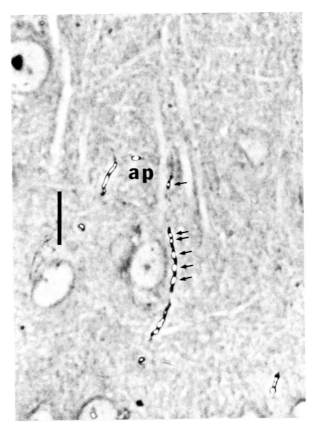

Figure 14. Phase-contrast photomicrograph of a semithin section from a Golgi preparation. Multiple axonal boutons of a common origin, traced back to a small basket cell, are seen in close apposition (arrows) to the perikaryon and apical dendrite (ap) of a pyramidal cell. Calibration bar, 20 μm.

ward the pial surface (Fairén *et al.*, 1982, and Fig. 15). In all the cases analyzed (see examples in Figs. 15 and 16), the axon is primarily descending and forms a rich local plexus through diverging, recurrent collaterals. There are some variations, however, both in the form of descending axonal branches as in Fig. 16, which resembles the cell labeled 5 in Peters and Fairén (1978), and in the presence of relatively long horizontal collaterals (Fig. 15), as in type 6 cells of Jones (1975). It may be that horizontal branches are lost, in certain cases, due to the orientation of cells in the preparations (see Section 3.3.4). Overall, the local axonal plexus is characterized by its curving preterminal axonal branches, provided with "en passant" boutons, which were later found to contact neuronal perikarya or proximal dendrites.

Cells with a similar morphology are present in the rat visual cortex (Fig. 17) and in the somatosensory cortex of the mouse. Further work is needed, however, to confirm the identity of these cells in the rodent cortex as small basket cells, and this can only be achieved by a detailed analysis of their efferent connections. It is also important to determine if small basket cells are present in different cortices. Perhaps the spherical, multipolar neurons with a local axonal

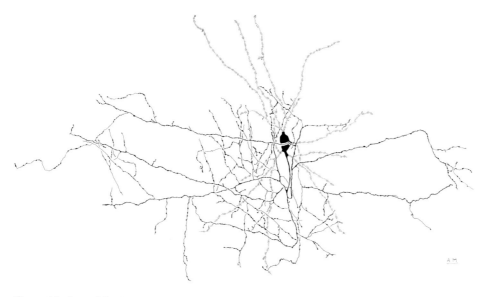

Figure 15. A small basket cell in layer II–III of kitten area 17. Note the initially descending axon, the profuse local plexus it produces, and its long horizontal collaterals.

plexus described by Peters and Regidor (1981) in the cat visual cortex and the type 6 cells of Jones (1975) in the somatosensory cortex of monkeys are neurons of this type. Other examples deserving mention include the cells shown by Lund (1973) in her Fig. 31z (monkey area 17); Szentágothai (1978) in his Fig. 5 (cat visual cortex); Norita and Kawamura (1981) in their Fig. 5 (Clare–Bishop area of the cat); McMullen and Glaser (1982) in their Fig. 5 (rabbit auditory cortex); and Lorente de Nó (1922) in his Fig. 6A (mouse barrel cortex). It seems, therefore, that small basket cells might be present in rather different cortices. Finally, it must be mentioned that there are examples in the literature of reputed small basket cells which show different appearances. See, for instance, Fig. 9 in Valverde (1983) from the hedgehog neocortex, in which bushy terminal axonal formations enter the "accentuated layer II" (Sanides and Sanides, 1974) typical of that cortex.

3.3.4. Cells with Relatively Extended, Generalized Axonal Arborizations

This group is formed of multipolar or bitufted cells with rather extended, smooth or sparsely spinous dendrites which may invade two or more contiguous layers. Their axonal plexuses are predominantly local in nature, but not as compact as in the case of neurogliaform cells, and may exceed the limits of the dendritic fields. Descending axonal branches are not uncommon and the plexuses may appear somewhat columnar (Jones, 1975; Peters and Fairén, 1978; Norita and Kawamura, 1981) but not as clearly as in the cell category reviewed in Section 3.2. Moreover, unlike cells with ascending axons (see Section 3.1) or the large basket cells (Section 3.4), their axons lack a well-defined trend to form vertically or horizontally oriented plexuses outside the dendritic domain. In

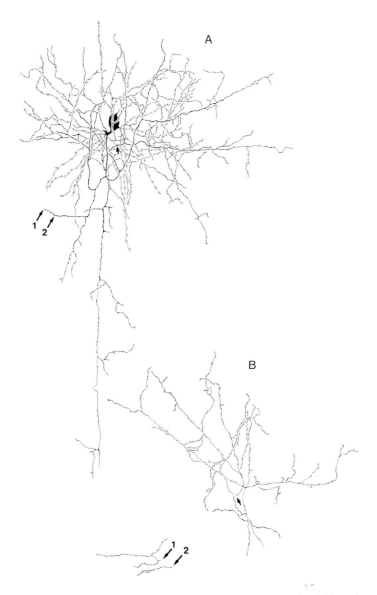

Figure 16. A small basket cell in layer II–III of cat area 17. In A, the dendritic and most of the axonal arborizations are shown. The axon emerges from the base of a dendrite and gives rise to a plexus made up of recurrent collaterals which distribute in a fanlike fashion. A vertically descending collateral is visible. B. By demounting the Golgi section and observing it from the opposite face, additional portions of the axon are resolved; they are continuous to the tracing in A at the points marked by arrows.

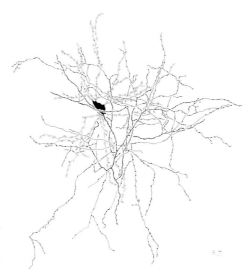

Figure 17. Multipolar neuron in upper layer II–III of rat area 17. Its axonal plexus is comparable to those of small basket cells found in the cat.

common with these cell types, the axon collaterals do not possess specialized terminal formations.

Defining this cell group is difficult, since there is a rather broad range of morphological diversity and one fears that the group as a whole might represent a common pool in which rather different types of cells are included. This is illustrated by Figs. 18 and 19. Cell A in Fig. 18 is from layer IV of the cat area 19; it shows a multipolar morphology, with sparsely spinous dendrites and somatic spines. The ascending axon forms a loose plexus in which recurving axonal arcades are visible. Cell B is a bitufted cell from layer II–III of the rat area 17 and shows a similar plexus, not strictly confined to the dendritic domain; some of the axonal branches enter layer I. Figure 19 shows a multipolar cell located in the middle layers of the cortex of the anterior ectosylvian sulcus of the cat. In this case, the perikaryon and the span of the dendrites are larger; the axon ascends and forms a plexus in which horizontal and vertical collaterals are clearly discernible. By its size and the form of its axonal arborization, this neuron resembles the ones described by Jones (1975) as type 1 cells, and it is reminiscent of a cell type reported by Valverde (1983, his Fig. 5) in the neocortex of the hedgehog. The question now arises as to whether some of the multipolar neurons with apparently generalized axonal arborizations might not be true basket cells (see Section 3.4). In fact, Marin-Padilla and Stibitz (1974), Marin-Padilla (1975), and Jones (1975) have shown that axonal patterns of basket cells vary drastically when viewed in the direction of the long horizontal collaterals, and Peters and Regidor (1981) have specifically pointed out that multipolar cells with elongated dendritic trees and horizontal axons in the cat visual cortex display recurring axonal arcades after a 90° rotation in the vertical axis. These observations clearly indicate that a bias may be introduced in previous reports of multipolar cells with generalized axonal arborizations being different from basket cells.

Clearly, the issue requires the study of the synapses formed by the axon terminals of these cells. This has been done in the rat visual cortex. Peters and

Fairén (1978) have examined, with the Golgi–EM method, smooth or sparsely spinous multipolar cells, with spherical or ovoid dendritic fields, which possess axonal arborizations similar to the examples shown in Fig. 18. The axon of these cells do not have preferred postsynaptic targets, for they contact perikarya of stellate and pyramidal neurons, shafts of apical dendrites, dendrites of smooth stellate cells, and, in one case, the axon initial segment of a pyramidal cell, always forming symmetrical synapses. On the other hand, Peters and Proskauer (1980a) have examined, also in the rat visual cortex, the synaptic relationships between the axon of a layer III multipolar cell with smooth dendrites and a Golgi-impregnated pyramidal cell, and report a substantial number of synapses formed by the stellate cell axon on the cell body and proximal dendrites of the pyramidal cell; in addition, the axon forms synapses with other pyramids, including the axon initial segment of one of them, and with cell bodies and dendrites of other aspiny nonpyramidal neurons (also see Chapter 13). As discussed in Section 3.3.3, multiplicity of the synaptic input on the same postsynaptic neuron indicates a certain degree of target selectivity; this feature differentiates small basket cells from other nonpyramidal neurons present in the superficial layers of the cat visual cortex. Whether this is also the case for the classical basket cells is not yet known, but our observation of the reality of the small basket cells and the Golgi

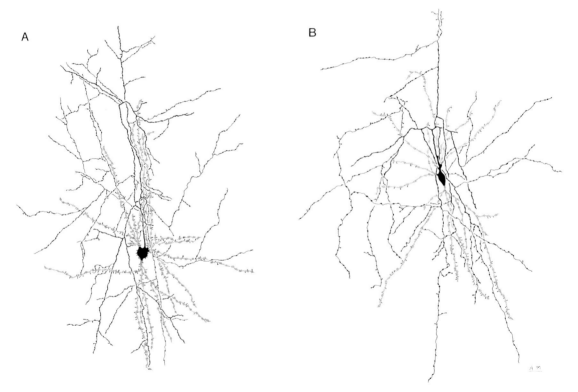

Figure 18. Nonpyramidal cells with extended axonal arborizations. A is from layer IV of cat area 19, and B from upper layer II–III of rat area 17.

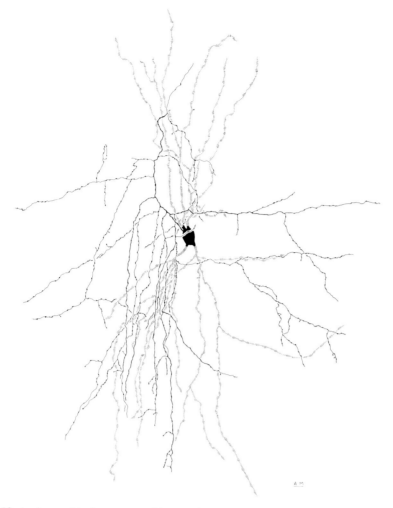

Figure 19. Aspiny multipolar neuron with extended axonal arborization from middle layers of the anterior ectosylvian sulcus of the cat.

evidence, as far as it goes (see, e.g., Fig. 17 in Jones, 1981; and Fig. 6c in Peters and Regidor, 1981), indicate that this is a most likely possibility.

It seems that a sharp distinction between the basket cells and the cells with relatively extended axonal arborizations does not exist. Several important pieces of evidence are wanting: first, a complete account of the distribution of axon terminals from basket cells, to see if they exclusively contact neuronal cell bodies and proximal dendrites; second, whether nonpyramidal cell bodies are also contacted by the axons of the large basket cells; and, third, a definition of the ratio of the axon terminals emanating from generalized multipolar neurons vs. basket cells, converging on a given postsynaptic cell. Since it has been firmly established that axosomatic synapses on pyramidal cells are GABAergic (see Chapter 8), it would be of interest to determine whether or not these terminals derive from the axonal arborizations of a uniform population of nonpyramidal neurons.

With these reservations in mind, it appears that multipolar neurons with relatively extended axonal arborizations are a common cellular component of the mammalian neocortex. They correspond to type 2 cells (Jones, 1975) or "common cells with axonal arcades" (Jones, 1981) of the monkey sensory motor cortex, but there are some doubts about their correspondence to the cells Szentágothai (1973) includes in his "category II cells with widely distributed axonal arborizations." Similar to Jones type 2 are cells which have been represented in monkey area 17 (Lund, 1973, her Figs., 24, 27, and 36) and 18 (Lund *et al.*, 1981, their Fig. 7), cat area 17 (Tömböl, 1978b, her Fig. 1e; Lund *et al.*, 1979, their Fig. 6B) and Clare–Bishop area (Norita and Kawamura, 1981, their Fig. 2),* and rat area 17 (Feldman and Peters, 1978, their Fig. 19). Examples in the human neocortex are given by Ramón y Cajal (e.g., cells A and C in Fig. 4 of the present report), and an early observation in a newborn rabbit is reported in Fig. 9 of Ramón y Cajal (1891).

Valverde and Ruiz-Marcos (1969), Valverde (1976), and Fairén and Valverde (1979) have represented similar neurons in the visual cortex of the mouse, as did Lorente de Nó (1922) in the somatosensory cortex of the same species (e.g., his Fig. 13E, but see also Fig. 73 in Lorente de Nó, 1949, where he represents diverse types of cells with intracortical axons). Valverde (1976) distinguishes two types of axonal configurations, which either distribute within a cylindrical volume of tissue, above the perikaryon of origin (type I), or are flattened and arborize both above and below the cell body (type III). The morphology of these axonal plexuses, with obvious axonal arcades, reminds one of a weeping willow tree, but as discussed in Section 3.2.2, somewhat similar cells in the monkey area 18 (Valverde, 1978), and also in other species and areas, form additional compact axonal bundles descending to lower layers and have been included by Somogyi and Cowey (1981) in the group of double bouquet cells (see Chapter 13 for an additional discussion of this point). One such interneuron, in the cat visual cortex, analyzed by DeFelipe and Fairén (1981), showed a pattern of efferent connectivity compatible with that reported by Somogyi and Cowey (1981). This implies an additional landmark to be established for the cell category we are discussing.

3.4. Cells with Horizontal Axons: The Basket Cells

As discussed in the preceding section, one of the known sources of the symmetrical, GABAergic synapses on the perikarya of pyramidal cells in the rat visual cortex are multipolar cells with smooth or sparsely spined dendrites (see Chapter 8). However, the existence of a characteristic type of nonpyramidal cell which contributes more substantially, by multiple synapses, to the afferent connectivity of pyramidal cell bodies has been postulated for higher species, and doubts arise on whether such cells do appear in more primitive cortices.

---

* As already mentioned, Peters and Regidor (1981) consider similar cells in the cat visual cortex to be basket cells seen on edge.

Ramón y Cajal (1899b,c, 1911) observed, in the human visual and motor cortices and in the visual cortex of the cat, the presence of rich axonal plexuses [nests or, according to Marin-Padilla (1969), baskets] surrounding the cell bodies of (unimpregnated) pyramidal cells, located in layers III and V. In his Fig. 361 (Ramón y Cajal, 1911) he represents a number of these plexuses, in which there is convergence of several axon collaterals originating from horizontally running axons. Later, Marin-Padilla (1969, 1970a,b, 1974) and Valverde (1983) in man, and Szentágothai (1973) and Holländer and Vanegas (1981) in cat, have represented similar plexuses and confirmed the convergence of multiple fibers into an individual pericellular plexus (see also Szentágothai, 1975, 1978). The work by Holländer and Vanegas (1981), based on the uptake of locally injected HRP, has provided electron microscope evidence that the pericellular baskets form symmetrical synapses on the pyramidal cell perikarya and proximal dendrites and, additionally, that afferent fibers may be myelinated. This agrees well, as will be shown later, with the observation by Jones (1975) of large multipolar cells of his type 1 cells which lack axonal impregnation in adult specimens.

Ramón y Cajal attributed the origin of the horizontal fibers entering the baskets to large stellate cells located in layers III and V (see Fig. 360 in Ramón y Cajal, 1911, and Fig. 20 of the present account, taken from Ramón y Cajal,

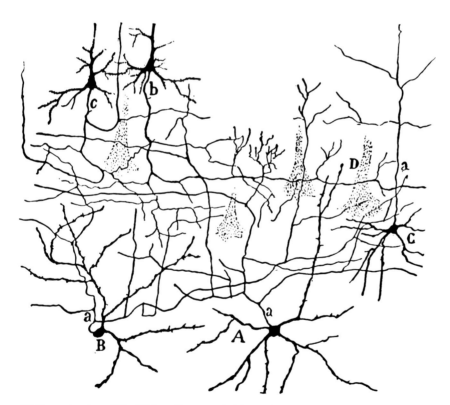

Figure 20. Reproduction of Fig. 19 from Ramón y Cajal (1899b) to illustrate cells with long horizontal axons. This is the first illustration by Ramón y Cajal of these cells which were presumed to contribute to the pericellular plexuses about pyramidal cell somata.

1899b). That the origin of perisomatic axonal boutons must be local was shown by Szentágothai (1965), since they persist in isolated cortical slabs. Convincing Golgi evidence was given, in the human motor cortex, by Marin-Padilla (1969, 1970a,b). Thus, basket cells are large multipolar cells which, in immature specimens, show a sparse population of dendritic spines (also see Chapter 8). The poorly arborizing dendrites radiate in all directions but the vertical ones predominate. The axons are either ascending or descending and soon form long branches coursing horizontally over distances of up to 1–2 mm, but additional long oblique branches are present. Besides these general characteristics, a conspicuous feature is the component of short vertical collaterals which, in Marin-Padilla's drawings, are seen to join Golgi-stained, pericellular baskets. Perhaps, the failure to simultaneously impregnate these plexuses and the axons of individual basket cells has somewhat jeopardized the interpretation of the short, vertically oriented collaterals of these cells, for these structures are not easily recognizable as specialized terminal formations in the absence of impregnation of the axonal plexuses to what they contribute, and, also, because the contribution of an individual basket cell to a given pyramidal cell perikaryon is likely to be less dense, as pointed out by Jones (1981; see, for instance, his Fig. 17), than in the case of the cerebellar basket cells. Consequently, many reports of Golgi-impregnated cells with long horizontal axons in diverse species fail to recognize them as true basket cells. One interesting point, already noted by Ramón y Cajal, is that each basket cell contributes to the pericellular plexuses of a number of pyramidal cells.

Two examples, drawn from preparations of the Ramón y Cajal collection, are presented in Fig. 21, mainly to compare the dimensions of the cells reported by Ramón y Cajal (1899b,c, 1911) with those of more recent accounts. Cell A is from deep layer III of the visual cortex of a 27-day-old infant, and B from layer III of the motor cortex of a newborn. Both of them fit well with the description given above, both in their dendritic morphology and in that their axons form long horizontal or oblique collaterals, with short-side appendages.

In the sensory motor cortex of monkeys, Jones (1975) has described, as type 1 cells, similar large multipolar neurons with long horizontal axons. In adult specimens, the axons are myelinated, but the cells can still be recognized on the basis of somal size and dendritic distribution. Type 1 cells vary in their dimensions according to their locations, the ones in area 2 and in area 4 being the largest. There is also a size segregation according to layers, the deeper cells being larger than the superficial ones, as also pointed out by Ramón y Cajal (1911) and Marin-Padilla (1969, 1970b). In spite of the fact that the smallest ones, such as the "short-range basket cells" (Szentágothai, 1969, 1973), similar to type 6 cells of Jones (1975), must be considered as a variety of basket cells, we have chosen to consider them separately (see Section 3.3.3).

Whether basket cells are present in all mammalian species has not been definitely settled. In the following selection of examples published by different authors, their identification of the neurons as putative basket cells is based on the presence of the basic morphological patterns just discussed; but it must be pointed out that, in certain cases, the identification is based on the present authors' concepts. In the *monkey*, such cells are illustrated in area 17 by Lund (1973, her Fig. 29), and by Lund *et al.* (1981, their Fig. 10i) in area 18. There are no doubts that the neocortex of *carnivores* contains basket cells (e.g., in cat area 17, Tömböl, 1978b, her Fig. 7; Lund *et al.*, 1979, their Fig. 8A; Peters and Regidor, 1981, their Figs. 5F, H; Gilbert and Wiesel, 1979, their Fig. 2b; in Clare–Bishop area of the cat, Norita and Kawamura, 1981, their Figs. 4a and 5a; in area 17 of the dog, Shkol'nik-Yarros, 1971, her Figs. 36 and 37; in cat auditory cortex, Sousa-Pinto, 1973, his Figs. 17F, H). Examples drawn from our own material of cats are shown in Figs. 19 and 22A. The cell in Fig. 19 could be considered to be a basket cell by virtue of its similarity to a drawing by Jones (1975) of a type 1 cell in the monkey somatosensory cortex (his Fig. 2), but their vertical axonal branches are striking. Figure 22A represents a more typical example, even if the long axonal collaterals are oblique. In *rabbits,* reports include the visual (O'Leary and Bishop, 1938, their Figs. 14-4 and 14-11; Tömböl, 1978b, her Fig. 8) and auditory cortices (McMullen and Glaser, 1982, their Fig. 12). As pointed out by Peters and Regidor (1981), the possibility must be considered that some of the examples we have included in our review of cells with relatively extended axonal arborizations (see Section 3.3.4) might in fact be basket cells, but this must await further studies.

Whether basket cells are present in rodents is an unsettled question. It has been suggested earlier (Peters and Fairén, 1978; Peters and Proskauer, 1980a;

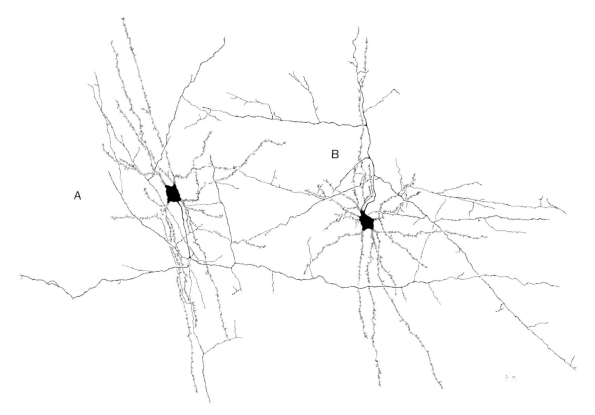

Figure 21. Two large multipolar neurons with long horizontal axons (presumably large basket cells) drawn from original preparations of Ramón y Cajal. See text for details.

Peters and Regidor, 1981) that in these species, they could be represented by the smooth or sparsely spinous multipolar neurons. In fact, the axons of certain of these cells are myelinated (Peters and Proskauer, 1980b), a characteristic common to basket cells of higher species, but these cells with myelinated axons may well represent a heterogeneous population. Looking for nonpyramidal cells with long horizontal axons, we have examined preparations of the rat visual cortex. In Fig. 22B is a multipolar neuron, located in layer II–III of area 18a. The axon stems from the side of the perikaryon and tends to form horizontally oriented collaterals. However, there are certain differences with respect to the typical cases found in other species by other authors. A case in point is the cell labeled H in Fig. 7 by Lorente de Nó (1922), as are some interneurons present in phylogenetically older cortices, such as the interhemispheric cortex (Iwahori and Mizuno, 1981, their Figs. 3F and 5). On the other hand, Lorente de Nó (1933) in the mouse entorhinal cortex has represented multipolar cells with horizontal axons having vertical collaterals, which may resemble basket cells. Finally, some doubts on the interpretation of the cell shown in Fig. 5 by Valverde (1983) have been commented upon in the preceding section.

Axonal geometry is an interesting feature of basket cells. Marin-Padilla (1969, 1970b) and Jones (1975) have found that the axons distribute within narrow slabs of tissue, precisely oriented in a plane perpendicular to the long axis of the pre- and postcentral gyri. The possible correlation between this spatial

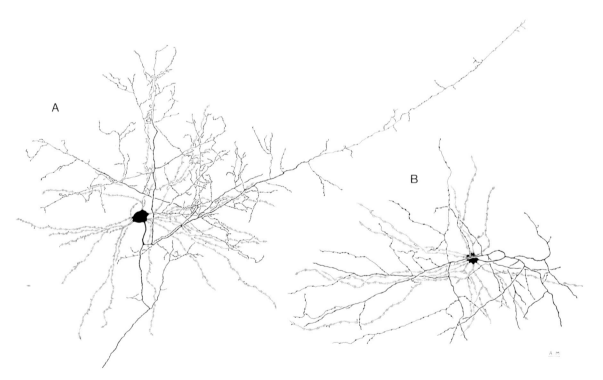

Figure 22. A is a spiny multipolar cell, considered a putative basket cell, from layer III of cat area 17. Within the axonal plexus, long horizontal or oblique branches predominate. B is a smaller neuron from layer II–III of rat area 18a. The axon stems from the lateral aspect of the perikaryon and tends to form horizontal branches.

arrangement and certain properties of the functional columns has been suggested by Marin-Padilla (1970b) and stressed by Jones (1975, 1981) and Peters
and Regidor (1981) (see Chapter 8). Thus, in the sensory motor cortex, the
basket cells may mediate the inhibition of the columns adjacent to the one which
is excited by a peripheral stimulus (Powell and Mountcastle, 1959). In the visual
cortex, a similar flattened distribution in tissue slabs has been recognized (Peters
and Regidor, 1981), but their precise spatial orientation is not yet known in that
cortex. However, as discussed by Jones (1975, 1981), Peters and Regidor (1981),
and in Chapter 8, basket cells in that cortex might play a role in the determination
of orientation columns (Hubel and Wiesel, 1974; Hubel *et al.*, 1978).

3.5. Spiny Stellate Cells

Several types of nonpyramidal cells from immature specimens are more or
less richly endowed with dendritic spines; especially in the old literature, many
types of nonpyramidal cells which are recognized today as smooth or sparsely
spined are represented with conspicuous spiny dendrites. It is customary, however, to reserve the term *spiny stellate cells* (LeVay, 1973; Lund, 1973) to a type
of nonpyramidal cell specifically located in layer IV (or in any of its subdivisions)
of the primary sensory areas (see Chapter 7). Jones (1975) reports them, however,
in the motor cortex. Spiny stellate cells do not seem to constitute a uniform
population, for substantial differences have been reported to exist between species, the cortical area or even the sublayer in which they are located. Nevertheless,
it is useful to consider these cells as a group. In general, they are defined as
multipolar neurons with spinous dendrites comparable to those of pyramidal
cells, but they lack a typical apical dendrite. The density of spines, however, is
less than that of pyramidal cells (Jones, 1975; see Chapter 4), and visible differences exist in this respect among the subtypes present in layer IV of the
monkey visual cortex (see, e.g., Figs. 3 and 5A in Fairén and Valverde, 1979).
It may be that some of the cells reported as spiny stellate cells are in fact true
pyramidal cells in which the apical dendrite failed to impregnate or was not
included in the Golgi section during tissue processing. In some instances, some
of the dendrites are not confined to layer IV, but instead enter suprajacent
layers, as in the case of *star pyramids,* a term coined by Lorente de Nó (1949).
Perhaps, the distinction Lorente de Nó (1949) made between star pyramids and
star cells is mose evident in the barrel field of rodents, i.e., the cortical representation of the mystacial vibrissae of the animal's snout. In his initial account
of this cortex (Lorente de Nó, 1922), both differences and similarities between
the two types are obvious (see his Figs. 5 and 9), for there are identical patterns
of local dendrite distribution clearly related to the presence of "glomérulos"
(barrels: Woolsey and Van der Loos, 1970) and perhaps to the termination of
thalamocortical fibers in discrete territories (Lorente de Nó, 1922; Killackey,
1973; Steffen, 1976; White, 1979). The patterns vary according to whether the
cells are located in the periphery of a "glomerulo" (barrel wall or septum) or in
its center (barrel hollow). Thus, the patterns of distribution of the dendrites are
"context-dependent characteristics" (Woolsey *et al.*, 1975) that allow for a
straightforward differentiation between star pyramids and true pyramidal cells.

On the other hand, star pyramids differ from star cells in that they possess a thin and poorly arborizing ramifying ascending dendrite which may reach layer I.

Lorente de Nó (1922) considers his star cells to be equivalent to the long-axoned star cells that Ramón y Cajal (1911) described in the human visual cortex and in the visual cortex of the cat (Ramón y Cajal, 1911, 1921, 1922). Ramón y Cajal gave the first description of these large cells in 1899 (Ramón y Cajal, 1899a,b), insisting that their axons project out of the cortex, a fact that has been confirmed for some such neurons in the visual cortex of the cat (Innocenti and Fiore, 1976; Shatz, 1977; Sanides and Donate-Oliver, 1978; Innocenti, 1979; Sanides, 1979; Hornung and Garey, 1980, 1981a; Meyer and Albus, 1981), as well as in layer IVb of the visual cortex of the monkey (Lund et al., 1975; Lund, 1981). However, the distant target areas are not the same for the cat as for the primate (see Lund et al., 1979; Lund, 1981; and see Chapter 16).

Spiny stellate cells in layer IV of the cat visual cortex are Ramón y Cajal's star cells (Ramón y Cajal, 1899b, 1911, 1921, 1922; O'Leary, 1941; Shkol'nik-Yarros, 1971; LeVay, 1973; Szentágothai, 1973; Lund et al., 1979; Fairén and Valverde, 1979; Peters and Regidor, 1981). They are large cells with long dendrites richly supplied with spines; cells located in the lower tier of layer IV are smaller (Garey, 1971; Lund et al., 1979; Hornung and Garey, 1981b; Peters and Regidor, 1981).

The axon originates from the lower pole of the perikaryon, initially descends and gives off horizontal or recurrent collaterals. Although an idea of the axonal distribution can be obtained with the Golgi method, it is apparent that impregnations are not complete (see Lund et al., 1979): the intracellular HRP injection by Gilbert and Wiesel (1979, 1981) of one such cell in layer IVab shows a very extensive arborization through layers IVab and II–III, not restricted to the dendritic tree. The axonal arborization of layer IVc spiny stellate cells seems to be much more restricted (Lund et al., 1979; Gilbert and Wiesel, 1979, 1981).

In the monkey area 17, several varieties of spiny stellate cells are present (Valverde, 1971; Lund, 1973; Lund and Boothe, 1975; Fairén and Valverde, 1979; Lund, 1981), but they have been reported to be absent of area 18 (Valverde, 1978; Lund et al., 1981). In area 17, morphology varies according to the sublayer in which the cells are located. First, there is a type of long-projecting, spiny stellate cell in layer IVb (Lund et al., 1975; Lund, 1981) which seems to be the homolog of the large star cell of Ramón y Cajal, which is also present in human visual cortex (Ramón y Cajal, 1899a,b, 1911). On the other hand, in layers IVa and IVc there are distinct populations of spiny stellate cells which have a lesser spine density (see Fig. 3 in Fairén and Valverde, 1979) and possess intracortical axons (Valverde, 1971; Lund, 1973; Lund and Boothe, 1975; Fairén and Valverde, 1979; Lund, 1981). The most conspicuous type, apparently absent from the visual cortex in nonprimates, is located in the lower part of layer IVc; the axon first descends but soon forms recurrent branches which ascend in a strictly columnar fashion. An interesting, additional feature of spiny stellate cells in the primate visual cortex is the existence of quite specific, differential patterns of axonal projections to the suprajacent layers, depending on the position of parent cells at the different levels of layer IV (see Lund, 1981, and Chapter 7 for a review). Given, however, that this is based solely on Golgi studies, where there are no guarantees of complete axonal staining, complementary evidence must be sought to fully substantiate the reality of these differential projections.

Unlike the situation in the rodent barrelfield, in the visual cortex of primates (and also in cats) there are no indications of dendritic asymmetries which could reflect a spatial relationship between the distribution of thalamocortical axons and that of spiny dendrites (Lund, 1981, and Chapter 7). The application of a recently developed technique (Botteri *et al.*, 1982) might shed some light on this issue.

An interesting discussion on spiny stellate cells in the monkey somatosensory cortex is given by Jones (1975). It seems that the majority of these cells possess dendrites entering layer III and, thus, they may be classified as star pyramids; their axons are not dissimilar to those of spiny stellate cells in layer IVc of the monkey visual cortex in that their strongly recurrent collaterals distribute in a columnar fashion. Spiny stellate cells with dendrites confined to layer IV (more commonly impregnated in area 3) have axons with a relatively wider distribution through their recurrent ascent. In addition, a descending branch of the axon may be present in both subtypes.

In the rodent visual cortex, Golgi studies usually refer to the apparent scarcity of spiny stellate cells; this is somewhat surprising, since such cells are an outstanding component of the somatosensory cortex in such species. Typical examples are shown by Valverde (1968) in his Fig. 7 and by Feldman and Peters (1978) but, clearly, the problem of identification of these cells in the visual cortex of rodents is not settled yet (cf. Parnavelas *et al.*, 1977b; Somogyi, 1978).

4. Concluding Remarks

The present account attempts to describe the different sets of nonpyramidal neurons present in the neocortex of a variety of mammalian species. Basically, morphological criteria have been employed, but data on synaptology and cytochemistry have been useful in defining characteristics within this rather diversified group of neurons. We offer a general overview which may serve as a body of reference for more specific studies dealing with the neuronal composition of particular cortical areas. An additional step has been to explore whether the differences between cortical areas in diverse mammalian species can be based on differences in the types of neuronal units they contain. After completing this overview, our conclusion is that, along the evolutionary scale, each one of the well-defined nonpyramidal cell classes is basically stable: similarities between the neuronal components of the various areas in the diverse species are more evident than their dissimilarities. Of course, exceptions exist and these have been discussed in the preceding sections.

Is there a basic uniformity in the cellular composition of the cerebral neocortex? The answer must await futher analyses. It must be emphasized that we have deliberately looked for basic structural patterns which would permit comparisons to be made, and we have intentionally underestimated certain morphological details, when comparing cells in different species. It is uncertain whether we have succeeded in selecting the essential features which define nonpyramidal cell groups. It is discouraging to realize that even after more than a century of possessing suitable methods to reveal the forms of neurons, morphological criteria to define neuronal groups are not established. There are many examples of neurons, both in our preparations and in the literature, whose interpretation largely evades us. Moreover, it is an everyday experience of many Golgi workers that *new* types appear each time a successful preparation is examined; this has prompted the common trend to consider higher brains as more diversified in cell types than the most primitive ones are. The conclusion is clear: glimpses at neuronal geometry now need to be complemented by other approaches if valid criteria are to emerge. In addition, the fact must be seriously considered that Golgi observations have covered but minute parts of the neocortical mantle. Very little has been said about the association cortices.

The question of the basic uniformity in the composition of the cerebral cortex has been the subject of countless discussions; it was already embroidered in the early efforts by Ramón y Cajal to disclose the structural basis of the cortical parcellations made by the cytoarchitectonic schools, and it still pervades much of the contemporary Golgi-based literature. It is our hope that by studying the particularities of organization of nonpyramidal cells in the different cortical fields, the nature and fundamental significance of cytoarchitectonic distinctions will become clearer.

The idea that nonpyramidal neurons or, in general terms, local circuit neurons increase in number and diversity in phylogeny was advanced by Ramón y Cajal (1911) (see Rakic, 1975, for a review). Modern concepts on the modular organization of the cerebral cortex (Mountcastle, 1957, 1979; Hubel and Wiesel, 1962, 1977; Szentágothai, 1975, 1978; Jones, 1981) suggest that the cellular components of the modules are basically unvaried; what makes for differences are the number of modules and their connections (Rockel *et al.*, 1980).

Two converging lines of evidence support the idea of uniformity. First, neuron counting (Rockel *et al.*, 1974, 1980; Powell, 1981; Powell and Hendrickson, 1981) reveals that the total number of neurons in narrow columns of uniform width through the full depth of the cortex, in diverse species and areas, is remarkably constant. There is an exception, however, in both the monocular and the binocular segments of the area 17 of monkeys, in which the number of cells is more that twice that in other cortical areas.* The second line of evidence comes from the comparison of the ratio between pyramidal and nonpyramidal neurons, identified according to conventional electron microscope criteria. The ratio is remarkably constant in monkeys (Sloper, 1973; Tömböl, 1974; Sloper *et al.*, 1979) and in rats and cats (Winfield *et al.*, 1980).

Within the modules, elaboration of the neuropil differs in the various species (e.g., Mountcastle, 1979). The idea that cells with specialized axonal arborizations are more abundant in higher species (Fairén and Valverde, 1979) could only reflect an elaboration of dendritic and axonal processes. Uniformity of the basic types of nonpyramidal cells along the evolutionary scale has been suggested by various authors using the Golgi methods (e.g., Szentágothai, 1979), and the

---

* Besides the possibility that certain nonpyramidal neurons only appear in area 17 of primates (e.g., some varieties of stellate cells; see Section 3.5), there are histochemical indications of a unique organization of that cortex (Hendrickson *et al.*, 1981; Horton and Hubel, 1981; Livingstone and Hubel, 1982; Hunt, 1982).

present reexamination of the problem strongly favors this point of view. The most noticeable fact is that most of the nonpyramidal cell varieties have been found in all species of mammals which so far have been examined by the present authors or by others, and little variation has been found even for certain of the cell types previously considered as specialized (Fairén and Valverde, 1979). A reevaluation of what is meant by specialized axonal arborizations is needed. Our proposal is that the qualification of *specialized* must be reserved for those cells whose axonal arborizations are selective for their postsynaptic partners (see Fairén and Valverde, 1980, and DeFelipe and Fairén, 1982, for additional discussion). An outstanding example of specialized cell is the chandelier cell, and this cell type is present all along the evolutionary scale, from insectivores to primates. Perhaps, another strong candidate is the basket cell, but data about its constancy in phylogeny are still scarce.

ACKNOWLEDGMENTS. We wish to express our sincere gratitude to Ms. Alicia Mimbrera for her patience and skill in preparing the figures in their final form, to Ms. Rosa Martínez-Ruiz for technical assistance during the initial phases of the present work, and to Ms. Christine Verven for secretarial help. Ms. M. Angustias Pérez de Tudela has helped us with the references. We are indebted to Dr. F. Valverde for allowing us to examine his Golgi preparations of hedgehogs and monkeys and to Dr. P. J. Berbel for putting his Golgi preparations of rats at our disposal. Dr. A. Carrato, Director of the Instituto Cajal, offered us the unique opportunity to study preparations from the Cajal collection. We thank both the Instituto Cajal and Elsevier Biomedical Press for permission to reproduce published illustrations.

During the final preparation of the manuscript, A.F. was on leave at the Laboratoire de Neuromorphologie, INSERM U. 106, Suresnes, France. He wishes to thank Dr. C. Sotelo for all the facilities offered. Original work reported has been supported by grants from Fundacion E. Rodriguez Pascual and CAICYT.

5. References

Botteri, C., Nguyen-Legros, J., and Hauw, J.-J., 1982, Radioautographic assessment of ocular dominance columns in Golgi-impregnated sections of the primary visual cortex in monocularly deprived monkeys, *Neurosci. Lett.* **31**:111–115.

Chronwall, B. M., and Wolff, J. R., 1978, Classification and location of neurons taking up ^{3}H-GABA in the visual cortex of rats, in: *Amino Acids as Chemical Transmitters* (F. Fonnum, ed.), pp. 297–303, Plenum Press, New York.

Chronwall, B., and Wolff, J. R., 1980, Prenatal and postnatal development of GABA-accumulating cells in the occipital neocortex of rat, *J. Comp. Neurol.* **190**:187–208.

Colonnier, M., 1964, The tangential organization of the visual cortex, *J. Anat.* **98**:327–344.

Colonnier, M., 1966, The structural design of the neocortex, in: *Brain and Conscious Experience* (J. C. Eccles, ed.), pp. 1–23, Springer-Verlag, Berlin.

Colonnier, M., 1968, Synaptic patterns on different cell types in the different laminae of the cat visual cortex: An electron microscope study, *Brain Res.* **9**:268–287.

Davis, T. L., and Sterling, P., 1979, Microcircuitry of cat visual cortex: Classification of neurons in Layer IV of area 17, and identification of the patterns of lateral geniculate input, *J. Comp. Neurol.* **188**:599–628.

DeFelipe, J., and Fairén, A., 1981, Interneurones with axonal arcades in the cat visual cortex: A Golgi–EM study, *Neurosci. Lett. Suppl.* **7:**S399.

DeFelipe, J., and Fairén, A., 1982, A type of basket cell in superficial layers of the cat visual cortex: A Golgi–electron microscope study, *Brain Res.* **244:**9–16.

Emson, P. C., and Hunt, S. P., 1981, Anatomical chemistry of the cerebral cortex, in: *The Organization of the Cerebral Cortex* (F. O. Schmitt, F. G. Worden, G. Adelman, and S. G. Dennis, eds.), pp. 325–345, MIT Press, Cambridge, Mass.

Fahrenkrug, J., 1980, Vasoactive intestinal polypeptide, *Trends Neurosci.* **3:**1–2.

Fairén, A., and Valverde, F., 1979, Specific thalamo-cortical afferents and their presumptive targets in the visual cortex: A Golgi study, in: *Development and Chemical Specificity of Neurons, Progress in Brain Research*, Vol. 51 (M. Cuénod, G. W. Kreutzberg, and F. E. Bloom, eds.), pp. 419–438, Elsevier, Amsterdam.

Fairén, A., and Valverde, F., 1980, A specialized type of neuron in the visual cortex of cat: A Golgi and electron microscope study of chandelier cells, *J. Comp. Neurol.* **194:**761–779.

Fairén, A., DeFelipe, J., and Martínez-Ruiz, R., 1981, The Golgi–EM procedure: A tool to study neocortical interneurons, in: *Eleventh International Congress of Anatomy: Glial and Neuronal Cell Biology*, pp. 291–301, Liss, New York.

Fairén, A., DeFelipe, J., and Van der Loos, H., 1982, Autapses in a neocortical basket cell, *Neurosci. Lett. Suppl.* **10:**S169–S170.

Feldman, M. L., and Peters, A., 1978, The forms of non-pyramidal neurons in the visual cortex of the rat, *J. Comp. Neurol.* **179:**761–794.

Garey, L. J., 1971, A Light and electron microscopic study of the visual cortex of the cat and monkey, *Proc. R. Soc. London Ser. B* **179:**21–40.

Garvey, C. F., Young, J. H., Jr., Coleman, P. D., and Simon, W., 1973, Automated three-dimensional dendrite tracking system, *Electroencephalogr. Clin. Neurophysiol.* **35:**199–204.

Gilbert, C. D., and Wiesel, T. N., 1979, Morphology and intracortical projections of functionally characterised neurones in the cat visual cortex, *Nature (London)* **280:**120–125.

Gilbert, C. D., and Wiesel, T. N., 1981, Laminar specialization and intracortical connections in cat primary visual cortex, in: *The Organization of the Cerebral Cortex* (F. O. Schmitt, F. G. Worden, G. Adelman, and S. G. Dennis, eds.), pp. 163–191, MIT Press, Cambridge, Mass.

Glaser, E. M., and Van der Loos, H., 1965, A semi-automatic computer microscope for the analysis of neuronal morphology, *IEEE Trans. Biomed. Eng.* **12:**22–31.

Glaser, E. M., Van der Loos, H., and Gissler, M., 1979, Tangential orientation and spatial order of cat auditory cortex: A computer microscope study of Golgi-impregnated material, *Exp. Brain Res.* **36:**411–431.

Gray, E. G., 1959, Axosomatic and axodendritic synapses of the cerebral cortex: An electron microscopy study, *J. Anat.* **93:**420–433.

Hendrickson, A. E., 1982, The orthograde axoplasmic transport autoradiographic technique and its implications for additional neuroanatomical analysis of the striate cortex, in: *Cytochemical Methods in Neuroanatomy* (V. Chan-Palay and S. L. Palay, eds.), pp. 1–16, Liss, New York.

Hendrickson, A. E., Hunt, S. P., and Wu, J.-Y., 1981, Immunocytochemical localization of glutamic acid decarboxylase in monkey striate cortex, *Nature (London)* **292:**605–607.

Hendry, S. H. C., and Jones, E. G., 1981, Sizes and distributions of intrinsic neurons incorporating tritiated GABA in monkey sensory-motor cortex, *J. Neurosci.* **1:**390–408.

Hendry, S. H. C., Houser, C. R., Jones, E. G., and Vaughn, J. E., 1983a, Synaptic organization of immunocytochemically identified GABA neurons in the monkey sensory-motor cortex, *J. Neurocytol.* **12:**639–660.

Hendry, S. H. C., Jones, E. G., and Beinfeld, M. C., 1983b, Cholecystokinin-immunoreactive neurons in rat and monkey cerebral cortex make symmetric synapses and have intimate associations with blood vessels, *Proc. Natl. Acad. Sci. U.S.A.* **80:**2400–2404.

Hersch, S. M., and White, E. L., 1981a, Thalamocortical synapses involving identified neurons in mouse primary somatosensory cortex: A terminal degeneration and Golgi/EM study, *J. Comp. Neurol.* **195:**253–263.

Hersch, S. M., and White, E. L., 1981b, Quantification of synapses formed with apical dendrites of Golgi-impregnated pyramidal cells: Variability in thalamocortical inputs, but consistency in the ratios of asymmetrical to symmetrical synapses, *Neuroscience* **6:**1043–1051.

Hökfelt, T., and Ljungdahl, A., 1972, Autoradiographic identification of cerebral and cerebellar cortical neurons accumulating labeled gamma-aminobutyric acid (^{3}H-GABA), *Exp. Brain Res.* **14:**354–362.

Holländer, H., and Vanegas, H., 1981, Identification of pericellular baskets in the cat striate cortex: Light and electron microscopic observations after uptake of horseradish peroxidase, *J. Neurocytol.* **10:**577–587.

Hornung, J. P., and Garey, L. J., 1980, A direct pathway from thalamus to visual callosal neurons in cat, *Exp. Brain Res.* **38:**121–123.

Hornung, J. P., and Garey, L. J., 1981a, Ultrastructure of visual callosal neurons in cat identified by retrograde axonal transport of horseradish peroxidase, *J. Neurocytol.* **10:**297–314.

Hornung, J. P., and Garey, L. J., 1981b, The thalamic projection to cat visual cortex: Ultrastructure of neurons identified by Golgi impregnation or retrograde horseradish peroxidase transport, *Neuroscience* **6:**1053–1068.

Horton, J. C., and Hubel, D. H., 1981, Regular patchy distribution of cytochrome oxidase staining in primary visual cortex of macaque monkey, *Nature (London)* **292:**762–764.

Houser, C. R., Hendry, S. H. C., Jones, E. G., and Vaughn, J. E., 1983, Morphological diversity of immunocytochemically identified GABA neurons in the monkey sensory-motor cortex, *J. Neurocytol.* **12:**617–638.

Hubel, D. H., and Wiesel, T. N., 1962, Receptive fields, binocular interactions and functional architecture in the cat's visual cortex, *J. Physiol. (London)* **160:**106–154.

Hubel, D. H., and Wiesel, T. N., 1974, Sequence regularity and geometry of orientation columns in the monkey striate cortex, *J. Comp. Neurol.* **158:**267–294.

Hubel, D. H., and Wiesel, T. N., 1977, Functional architecture of macaque monkey visual cortex, *Proc. R. Soc. London Ser. B* **198:**1–59.

Hubel, D. H. Wiesel, T. N., and Stryker, M. P., 1978, Anatomical demonstration of orientation columns in macaque monkey, *J. Comp. Neurol.* **177:**361–380.

Hunt, S. P., 1982, GABA produces excitement in the visual cortex, *Trends Neurosci.* **5:**101–102.

Innocenti, G. M., 1979, Adult and neonatal characteristics of the callosal zone at the boundary between areas 17 and 18 in the cat, in: *Structure and Function of Cerebral Commissures* (I. Steele Russell, M. W. Van Hof, and G. Berlucchi, eds.), pp. 244–258, Macmillan & Co., London.

Innocenti, G. M., and Fiore, L., 1976, Morphological correlates of visual field transformation in the corpus callosum, *Neurosci. Lett.* **2:**245–252.

Iwahori, N., and Mizuno, N., 1981, A Golgi study on the neuronal organization of the interhemispheric cortex in the mouse. II. Intrinsic neurons, *Anat. Embryol.* **161:**483–498.

Jones, E. G., 1975, Varieties and distribution of non-pyramidal cells in the somatic sensory cortex of the squirrel monkey, *J. Comp. Neurol.* **160:**205–268.

Jones, E. G., 1981, Anatomy of cerebral cortex: Columnar input–output organization, in: *The Organization of the Cerebral Cortex* (F. O. Schmitt, F. G. Worden, G. Adelman, and S. G. Dennis, eds.), pp. 199–235, MIT Press, Cambridge, Mass.

Jones, E. G., and Hartman, B. K., 1978, Recent advances in neuroanatomical methodology, *Annu. Rev. Neurosci.* **1:**215–296.

Killackey, H. P., 1973, Anatomical evidence for cortical subdivisions based on vertically discrete thalamic projections from the ventral posterior nucleus to cortical barrels in the rat, *Brain Res.* **51:**326–331.

Kosaka, T., 1980, The axon initial segment as a synaptic site: Ultrastructure and synaptology of the initial segment of the pyramidal cell in the rat hippocampus (CA3 region), *J. Neurocytol.* **9:**861–882.

LeVay, S., 1973, Synaptic patterns in the visual cortex of the cat and monkey: Electron microscopy of Golgi preparations, *J. Comp. Neurol.* **150:**53–86.

Livingstone, M. S., and Hubel, D. H., 1982, Thalamic inputs to cytochrome oxidase-rich regions in monkey visual cortex, *Proc. Natl. Acad. Sci. USA* **79:**6098–6101.

Llinás, R., and Hillman, D. E., 1975, A multipurpose tridimensional reconstruction computer system for neuroanatomy, in: *Golgi Centennial Symposium: Perspectives in Neurobiology* (M. Santini, ed.), pp. 71–79, Raven Press, New York.

Lorén, I., Emson, P. C., Fahrenkrug, J., Björklund, A., Alumets, J., Håkanson, R., and Sundler, F., 1979, Distribution of vasoactive intestinal polypeptide in the rat and mouse brain, *Neuroscience* **4:**1953–1976.

Lorente de Nó, R., 1922, La corteza cerebral del ratón. (Primera contribución-La corteza acústica), *Trab. Lab. Invest. Biol. Madrid* **20:**41–78.

Lorente de Nó, R., 1933, Studies on the structure of the cerebral cortex. I. The area entorhinalis, *J. Psychol. Neurol.* **45:**381–438.

Lorente de Nó, R., 1934, Studies on the structure of the cerebral cortex. II. Continuation of the study of the ammonic system, *J. Psychol. Neurol.* **46:**113–177.

Lorente de Nó, R., 1949, Cerebral cortex: Architecture, intracortical connections, motor projections, in: *Physiology of the Nervous System* (J. F. Fulton, ed.), 3rd ed., pp. 288–313, Oxford University Press, London.

Lund, J. S., 1973, Organization of neurons in the visual cortex, area 17, of the monkey *(Macaca mulatta), J. Comp. Neurol.* **147:**455–496.

Lund, J. S., 1981, Intrinsic organization of the primate visual cortex, area 17, as seen in Golgi preparations, in: *The Organization of the Cerebral Cortex* (F. O. Schmitt, F. G. Worden, G. Adelman, and S. G. Dennis, eds.), pp. 105–124, MIT Press, Cambridge, Mass.

Lund, J. S., and Boothe, R. G., 1975, Interlaminar connections and pyramidal neuron organisation in the visual cortex, area 17, of the macaque monkey, *J. Comp. Neurol.* **159:**305–334.

Lund, J. S., Lund, R. D., Hendrickson, A. E., Bunt, A. H., and Fuchs, A. F., 1975, The origin of efferent pathways from the primary visual cortex, area 17, of the macaque monkey as shown by retrograde transport of horseradish peroxidase, *J. Comp. Neurol.* **164:**287–304.

Lund, J. S., Boothe, R. G., and Lund, R. D., 1977, Development of neurons in the visual cortex (area 17) of the monkey *(Macaca nemestrina)*: A Golgi study from fetal day 127 to postnatal maturity, *J. Comp. Neurol.* **176:**149–188.

Lund, J. S., Henry, G. H., MacQueen, C. L., and Harvey, A. R., 1979, Anatomical organization of the primary visual cortex (area 17) of the cat: A comparison with area 17 of macaque monkey, *J. Comp. Neurol.* **184:**599–618.

Lund, J. S., Hendrickson, A. E., Ogren, M. P., and Tobin, E. A., 1981, Anatomical organization of primate visual cortex area VII, *J. Comp. Neurol.* **202:**19–45.

McDonald, J. K., Parnavelas, J. G., Karamanlidis, A. N., and Brecha, N., 1982a, The morphology and distribution of peptide-containing neurons in the adult and developing visual cortex of the rat. II. Vasoactive intestinal polypeptide, *J. Neurocytol.***11:**825–837.

McDonald, J. K., Parnavelas, J. G., Karamanlidis, A. N., Rosenquist, G., and Brecha, N., 1982b, The morphology and distribution of peptide-containing neurons in the adult and developing visual cortex of the rat. III. Cholecystokinin, *J. Neurocytol.* **11:**881–895.

McMullen, N. T., and Glaser, E. M., 1982, Morphology and laminar distribution of nonpyramidal neurons in the auditory cortex of the rabbit, *J. Comp. Neurol.* **208:**85–106.

Mann, M. D., 1979, Sets of neurons in somatic cerebral cortex of the cat and their ontogeny, *Brain Res. Rev.* **1:**3–45.

Marin-Padilla, M., 1969, Origin of the pericellular baskets of the pyramidal cells of the human motor cortex: A Golgi study, *Brain Res.* **14:**633–646.

Marin-Padilla, M., 1970a, Prenatal and early postnatal ontogenesis of the human motor cortex: A Golgi study. I. The sequential development of the cortical layers, *Brain Res.* **23:**167–183.

Marin-Padilla, M., 1970b, Prenatal and early postnatal ontogenesis of the human motor cortex: A Golgi study. II. The basket–pyramidal system, *Brain Res.* **23:**185–191.

Marin-Padilla, M., 1972, Prenatal ontogenetic history of the principal neurons of the neocortex of the cat *(Felis domestica)*: A Golgi study. II. Developmental differences and their significances, *Z. Anat. Entwicklungsgesch.* **136:**125–142.

Marin-Padilla, M., 1974, Three-dimensional reconstruction of the pericellular nests (baskets) of the motor (area 4) and visual (area 17) areas of the human cerebral cortex: A Golgi study, *Z. Anat. Entwicklungsgesch.* **144:**123–135.

Marin-Padilla, M., 1975, LCN's in the neocortex, in: *Local Circuit Neurons, Neurosci. Res. Program Bull.* Vol. 13 (P. Rakic, ed.), pp. 385–392.

Marin-Padilla, M., and Marin-Padilla, T., 1982, Origin, prenatal development and structural organization of layer I of the human cerebral (motor) cortex: A Golgi study, *Anat. Embryol.* **164:**161–206.

Marin-Padilla, M., and Stibitz, G. R., 1974, Three-dimensional reconstruction of the basket cell of the human motor cortex, *Brain Res.* **70:**511–514.

Martinotti, C., 1889, Contributo allo studio della corteccia cerebrale, ed all'origine centrale dei nervi, *Ann. Freniatr. Sci. Affini* **1**:314–381.

Martinotti, C., 1890, Beitrag zum Studium der Hirnrinde und dem Centralursprung der Nerven, *Int. Monatschr. Anat. Physiol.* **7**:69–90.

Meyer, G., and Albus, K., 1981, Spiny stellates as cells of origin of association fibers from area 17 to area 18 in the cat's neocortex, *Brain Res.* **210**:335–341.

Morrison, J. H., 1982, Principles of organization of neurotransmitter systems in neocortex, *Anat. Rec.* **204**:24A–25A.

Mountcastle, V. B., 1957, Modality and topographic properties of single neurons of cat's somatic sensory cortex, *J. Neurophysiol.* **20**:408–434.

Mountcastle, V. B., 1979, An organizing principle for cerebral function: The unit module and the distributed system, in: *The Neurosciences: Fourth Study Program* (F. O. Schmitt and F. G. Worden, eds.), pp. 21–42, MIT Press, Cambridge, Mass.

Müller-Paschinger, I.-B., Tömböl, T., and Petsche, H., 1983, Chandelier neurons within the rabbits' cerebral cortex: A Golgi study, *Anat. Embryol.* **166**:149–154.

Norita, M., and Kawamura, K., 1981, Non-pyramidal neurons in the medial bank (Clare–Bishop area) of the middle suprasylvian sulcus: A Golgi study in the cat, *J. Hirnforsch.* **22**:9–28.

O'Leary, J. L., 1941, Structure of the area striata of the cat, *J. Comp. Neurol.* **75**:131–164.

O'Leary, J. L., and Bishop, G. H., 1938, The optically excitable cortex of the rabbit, *J. Comp. Neurol.* **68**:423–478.

Parnavelas, J. G., Lieberman, A. R., and Webster, K. E., 1977a, Organization of neurons in the visual cortex, area 17, of the rat, *J. Anat.* **124**:305–322.

Parnavelas, J. G., Sullivan, K., Lieberman, A. R., and Webster, K. E., 1977b, Neurons and their synaptic organization in the visual cortex of the rat: Electron microscopy of Golgi preparations, *Cell Tissue Res.* **183**:499–517.

Pasternak, J., and Woolsey, T. A., 1975, On the "selectivity" of the Golgi–Cox method, *J. Comp. Neurol.* **160**:307–312.

Peters, A., and Fairén, A., 1978, Smooth and sparsely-spined stellate cells in the visual cortex of the rat: A study using a combined Golgi–electron microscope technique, *J. Comp. Neurol.* **181**:129–172.

Peters, A., and Kimerer, L. M., 1981, Bipolar neurons in rat visual cortex: A combined Golgi–electron microscope study, *J. Neurocytol.* **10**:921–946.

Peters, A., Miller, M., and Kimerer, L. M., 1983, Cholecystokinin-like immunoreactive neurons in rat cerebral cortex, *Neuroscience* **8**:431–448.

Peters, A., and Proskauer, C. C., 1980a, Synaptic relationships between a multipolar stellate cell and a pyramidal neuron in the rat visual cortex. A combined Golgi–electron microscope study, *J. Neurocytol.* **9**:163–183.

Peters, A., and Proskauer, C. C., 1980b, Smooth or sparsely spined cells with myelinated axons in rat visual cortex, *Neuroscience* **5**:2079–2092.

Peters, A., and Regidor, J., 1981, A reassessment of the forms of nonpyramidal neurons in area 17 of cat visual cortex, *J. Comp. Neurol.* **203**:685–716.

Peters, A., Proskauer, C. C., and Ribak, C. E., 1982, Chandelier cells in rat visual cortex, *J. Comp. Neurol.* **206**:397–416.

Powell, T. P. S., 1981, Certain aspects of the intrinsic organisation of the cerebral cortex, in: *Brain Mechanisms and Perceptual Awareness* (O. Pompeiano and C. Ajmone-Marsan, eds.), pp. 1–19, Raven Press, New York.

Powell, T. P. S., and Hendrickson, A. E., 1981, Similarity in number of neurons through the depth of the cortex in the binocular and monocular parts of area 17 of the monkey, *Brain Res.* **216**:409–413.

Powell, T. P. S., and Mountcastle, V. B., 1959, Some aspects of the functional organization of the cortex of the postcentral gyrus of the monkey: a correlation of findings obtained in a single unit analysis with cytoarchitecture, *Bull. Johns Hopkins Hosp.* **105**:133–162.

Rakic, P., 1975, *Local Circuit Neurons, Neurosci. Res. Program Bull.* **13**:291–446.

Ramón-Moliner, E., 1961, The histology of the postcruciate gyrus in the cat. III. Further observations, *J. Comp. Neurol.* **117**:229–249.

Ramón y Cajal, S., 1891, Sur la structure de l'écorce cérébrale de quelques mammifères, *Cellule* **7**:3–54.

Ramón y Cajal, S., 1899a, Apuntes para el estudio estructural de la corteza visual del cerebro humano, *Rev. Ibero-Am. Cie. Med. (Madrid)* **1899:**1–14.

Ramón y Cajal, S., 1899b, Estudios sobre la corteza cerebral humana: Corteza visual, *Rev. Trimest. Microgr.* **4:**1–63.

Ramón y Cajal, S., 1899c, Estudios sobre la corteza cerebral humana: Estructura de la corteza motriz del hombre y mamíferos superiores, *Rev. Trimest. Microgr.* **4:**117–200.

Ramón y Cajal, S., 1899d, Comparative study of the sensory areas of the human cortex, in: *Clark University, Decennial Celebration* (W. E. Story and L. N. Wilson, eds.), pp. 311–382, Norwood Press, Norwood, Mass.

Ramón y Cajal, S., 1900, Estudios sobre la corteza cerebral humana. III. Estructura de la corteza acústica, *Rev. Trimest. Microgr.* **5:**129–183.

Ramón y Cajal, S., 1911, *Histologie du Système Nerveux de L'Homme et des Vertébrés* (translated by L. Azoulay) Vol. II, Maloine, Paris.

Ramón y Cajal, S., 1921, Textura de la corteza visual del gato, *Trab. Lab. Invest. Biol. Madrid* **19:**113–144.

Ramón y Cajal, S., 1922, Studien über die Sehrinde der Katze, *J. Psychol. Neurol.* **29:**161–181.

Ribak, C. E., 1978, Aspinous and sparsely-spinous stellate neurons in the visual cortex of rats contain glutamic acid decarboxylase, *J. Neurocytol.* **7:**461–478.

Ribak, C. E., Harris, A. B., Vaughn, J. E., and Roberts, E., 1979, Inhibitory, GABAergic nerve terminals decrease at sites of focal epilepsy, *Science* **205:**211–214.

Ribak, C. E., Bradburne, R. M., and Harris, A. B., 1982, A preferential loss of GABAergic, symmetric synapses in epileptic foci: A quantitative ultrastructural analysis of monkey neocortex, *J. Neurosci.* **2:**1725–1735.

Rockel, A. J., Hiorns, R. W., and Powell, T. P. S., 1974, Numbers of neurons through full depth of neocortex, *J. Anat.* **118:**371.

Rockel, A. J., Hiorns, R. W., and Powell, T. P. S., 1980, The basic uniformity in structure of the neocortex, *Brain* **103:**221–244.

Rowe, M. H., and Stone, J., 1977, Naming of neurones: Classification and naming of cat retinal ganglion cells, *Brain Behav. Evol.* **14:**185–216.

Rowe, M. H., and Stone, J., 1980, The interpretation of variation in the classification of nerve cells, *Brain Behav. Evol.* **17:**123–151.

Ruiz-Marcos, A., and Valverde, F., 1970, Dynamic architecture of the visual cortex, *Brain Res.* **19:**25–39.

Sanides, D., 1979, Commissural connections of the visual cortex of the cat, in: *Structure and Function of Cerebral Commissures* (I. Steele Russell, M. W. Van Hof, and G. Berlucchi, eds.), pp. 236–243, Macmillan & Co., London.

Sanides, D., and Donate-Oliver, F., 1978, Identification and localisation of some relay cells in cat visual cortex, in: *Architectonics of the Cerebral Cortex* (M. A. B. Brazier and H. Petsche, eds.), pp. 227–234, Raven Press, New York.

Sanides, D., and Sanides, F., 1974, A comparative Golgi study of the neocortex in insectivores and rodents, *Z. Mikrosk. Anat. Forsch.* **88:**957–977.

Scheibel, M. E., and Scheibel, A. B., 1970, The rapid Golgi method: Indian summer or renaissance?, in: *Contemporary Research Methods in Neuroanatomy* (W. J. H. Nauta and S. O. E. Ebbesson, eds.), pp. 1–11, Springer-Verlag, Berlin.

Scheibel, M. E., and Scheibel, A. B., 1978, The methods of Golgi, in: *Neuroanatomical Research Techniques* (R. T. Robertson, ed.), pp. 89–114, Academic Press, New York.

Shatz, C., 1977, Anatomy of interhemispheric connections in the visual system of Boston Siamese and ordinary cats, *J. Comp. Neurol.* **173:**497–518.

Shkol'nik-Yarros, E. G., 1971, *Neurons and Interneuronal Connections of the Central Visual System*, Plenum Press, New York.

Sholl, D. A., 1956, *The Organization of the Cerebral Cortex*, Methuen, London.

Sims, K. B., Hoffman, D. L., Said, S. I., and Zimmerman, E. A., 1980, Vasoactive intestinal polypeptide (VIP) in mouse and rat brain: An immunocytochemical study, *Brain Res.* **186:**165–183.

Sloper, J. J., 1973, An electron microscope study of the neurons of the primate motor and somatic sensory cortices, *J. Neurocytol.* **2:**351–359.

Sloper, J. J., and Powell, T. P. S., 1979, A study of the axon initial segment and proximal axon of neurons in the primate motor and somatic sensory cortices, *Philos. Trans. R. Soc. London Ser. B* **285:**173–197.

Sloper, J. J., Hiorns, R. W., and Powell, T. P. S., 1979, A qualitative and quantitative electron microscopic study of the neurons in the primate motor and somatic sensory cortices, *Philos. Trans. R. Soc. London Ser. B* **285**:141–171.

Smit, G. J., and Colon, E. J., 1969, Quantitative analysis of the cerebral cortex. I. A selectivity of the Golgi–Cox staining technique, *Brain Res.* **13**:485–510.

Somogyi, P., 1977, A specific 'axo-axonal' interneuron in the visual cortex of the rat, *Brain Res.* **136**:345–350.

Somogyi, P., 1978, The study of Golgi stained cells and of experimental degeneration under the electron microscope: A direct method for the identification in the visual cortex of three successive links in a neuron chain, *Neuroscience* **3**:167–180.

Somogyi, P., 1979, An interneurone making synapses specifically on the axon initial segment of pyramidal cells in the cerebral cortex of the cat, *J. Physiol. (London)* **296**:18–19P.

Somogyi, P., and Cowey, A., 1981, Combined Golgi and electron microscopic study on the synapses formed by double bouquet cells in the visual cortex of the cat and monkey, *J. Comp. Neurol.* **195**:547–566.

Somogyi, P., Hodgson, A. J., and Smith, A. D., 1979, An approach to tracing neuron networks in the cerebral cortex and basal ganglia: Combination of Golgi staining, retrograde transport of horseradish peroxidase and anterograde degeneration of synaptic boutons in the same material, *Neuroscience* **4**:1805–1852.

Somogyi, P., Freund, T. F., Halász, N., and Kisvárday, Z. F., 1981a, Selectivity of neuronal [^{3}H]-GABA accumulation in the visual cortex as revealed by Golgi staining of the labeled neurons, *Brain Res.* **225**:431–436.

Somogyi, P., Cowey, A., Halász, N., and Freund, T. F., 1981b, Vertical organization of neurones accumulating ^{3}H-GABA in visual cortex of rhesus monkey, *Nature (London)* **294**:761–763.

Somogyi, P., Freund, T. F., and Cowey, A., 1982, The axo-axonic interneuron in the cerebral cortex of the rat, cat and monkey, *Neuroscience* **7**:2577–2607.

Somogyi, P., Nunzi, M. G., Gorio, A., and Smith, A. D., 1983, A new type of specific interneuron in the monkey hippocampus forming synapses exclusively with the axon initial segments of pyramidal cells, *Brain Res.* **259**:137–142.

Sousa-Pinto, A., 1973, The structure of the first auditory cortex (A I) in the cat. I. Light microscopic observations on its organization, *Arch. Ital. Biol.* **111**:112–137.

Steffen, H. 1976, Golgi-stained barrel-neurons in the somatosensory region of the mouse cerebral cortex, *Neurosci. Lett.* **2**:57–59.

Steffen, H., and Van der Loos, H., 1980, Early lesions of mouse vibrissal follicles: Their influence on dendrite orientation in the cortical barrelfield, *Exp. Brain Res.* **40**:419–431.

Szentágothai, J., 1965, The use of degeneration methods in the investigation of short neuronal connexions, in: *Degeneration Patterns in the Nervous System, Progress in Brain Research*, Vol. 14 (M. Singer and J. P. Schadé, eds.), pp. 1–32, Elsevier, Amsterdam.

Szentágothai, J., 1969, Architecture of the cerebral cortex, in: *Basic Mechanisms of the Epilepsies* (H. H. Jasper, A. A. Ward, and A. Pope, eds.), pp. 13–28, Little, Brown, Boston.

Szentágothai, J., 1973, Synaptology of the visual cortex, in: *Handbook of Sensory Physiology*, Vol. VII/3, *Central Visual Information*, Part B (R. Jung, ed.), pp. 269–324, Springer-Verlag, Berlin.

Szentágothai, J., 1975, The "module-concept" in cerebral cortex architecture, *Brain Res.* **95**:475–496.

Szentágothai, J., 1978, The neuron network of the cerebral cortex: A functional interpretation, *Proc. R. Soc. London Ser. B* **201**:219–248.

Szentágothai, J., 1979, Local neuron circuits of the neocortex, in: *The Neurosciences: Fourth Study Program* (F. O. Schmitt and F. G. Worden, eds.), pp. 399–415, MIT Press, Cambridge, Mass.

Szentágothai, J., and Arbib, M. A., 1974, *Conceptual Models of Neural Organization, Neurosci. Res. Program Bull.* **12**:307–510.

Tömböl, T., 1974, An electron microscopic study of the neurons of the visual cortex, *J. Neurocytol.* **3**:525–531.

Tömböl, T., 1976, Golgi analysis of the internal layers (V–VI) of the cat visual cortex, *Exp. Brain Res. Suppl.* **1**:292–295.

Tömböl, T., 1978a, Some Golgi data on visual cortex of the rhesus monkey, *Acta Morphol. Acad. Sci. Hung.* **26**:115–138.

Tömböl, T., 1978b, Comparative data on the Golgi architecture of interneurons of different cortical areas in cat and rabbit, in: *Architectonics of the Cerebral Cortex* (M. A. B. Brazier and H. Petsche, eds.), pp. 59–76, Raven Press, New York.

Tyner, C. F., 1975, The naming of neurons: Applications of taxonomic theory to the study of cellular populations, *Brain Behav. Evol.* **12:**75–96.

Uylings, H. B. M., Parnavelas, J. G., and Walg, H. L., 1981, Morphometry of cortical dendrites, in: *Eleventh International Congress of Anatomy: Advances in the Morphology of Cells and Tissues,* pp. 185–192, Liss, New York.

Valverde, F., 1968, Structural changes in the area striata of the mouse after enucleation, *Exp. Brain Res.* **5:**274–292.

Valverde, F., 1970, The Golgi method: A tool for comparative structural analyses, in: *Contemporary Research Methods in Neuroanatomy* (W. J. H. Nauta and S. O. E. Ebbesson, eds.), pp. 12–31, Springer-Verlag, Berlin.

Valverde, F., 1971, Short axon neuronal subsystems in the visual cortex of the monkey, *Int. J. Neurosci.* **1:**181–197.

Valverde, F., 1976, Aspects of cortical organization related to the geometry of neurons with intra-cortical axons, *J. Neurocytol.* **5:**509–529.

Valverde, F., 1978, The organization of area 18 in the monkey: A Golgi study, *Anat. Embryol.* **154:**305–334.

Valverde, F., 1983, A comparative approach to neocortical organization based on the study of the brain of the hedgehog *(Erinaceus europaeus),* in: *Ramón y Cajal's Contribution to the Neurosciences* (S. Grisolía, C. Guerri, F. Samson, S. Norton, and F. Reinoso-Suárez, eds.), pp. 149–170, Elsevier, Amsterdam.

Valverde, F,. and Ruiz-Marcos, A., 1969, Dendritic spines in the visual cortex of the mouse: Introduction to a mathematical model, *Exp. Brain Res.* **8:**269–283.

Van der Loos, H., 1976, Neuronal circuitry and its development, in: *Perspectives in Brain Research, Progress in Brain Research,* Vol. 45 (M. A. Corner and D. S. Swaab, eds.), pp. 259–278, Elsevier, Amsterdam.

Vincent, S. R., Johansson, O., Hökfelt, T., Meyerson, B., Sachs, C., Elde, R. P., Terenius, L., and Kimmel, J., 1982a, Neuropeptide coexistence in human cortical neurones, *Nature (London)* **298:**65–67.

Vincent, S. R., Skirboll, L., Hökfelt, T., Johansson, O., Lundberg, J. M., Elde R. P., Terenius, L., and Kimmel, J., 1982b, Coexistence of somatostatin- and avian pancreatic polypeptide (APP)-like immunoreactivity in some forebrain neurons, *Neuroscience* **7:**439–446.

Vogt, B. A., and Peters, A., 1981, Form and distribution of neurons in rat cingulate cortex: Areas 32, 24 and 29, *J. Comp. Neurol.* **195:**603–625.

Wann, D. F., Woolsey, T. A., Dierker, M. L., and Cowan, W. M., 1973, An on-line digital-computer system for the semiautomatic analysis of Golgi-impregnated neurons, *IEEE Trans. Biomed. Eng.* **20:**233–247.

Werner, L., Hedlich, A., Winkelmann, E., and Brauer, R., 1979, Versuch einer Identifizierung von Nervenzellen des visuellen Kortex der Ratte nach Nissl- und Golgi-Kopsch-Darstellung, *J. Hirnforsch.* **20:**121–139.

White, E. L., 1979, Thalamocortical synaptic relations: A review with emphasis on the projections of specific thalamic nuclei to the primary sensory areas of the neocortex, *Brain Res. Rev.* **1:**275–311.

White, E. L., and Rock, M. P., 1980, Three-dimensional aspects and synaptic relationships of a Golgi-impregnated spiny stellate cell reconstructed from serial thin sections, *J. Neurocytol.* **9:**615–636.

White, E. L., and Rock, M. P., 1981, A comparison of thalamocortical and other synaptic inputs to dendrites of two non-spiny neurons in a single barrel of mouse SmI cortex, *J. Comp. Neurol.* **195:**265–277.

Winfield, D. A., Gatter, K. C., and Powell, T. P. S., 1980, An electron microscopic study of the types and proportions of neurons in the cortex of the motor and visual areas of the cat and rat, *Brain* **103:**245–258.

Wolff, J. R., and Chronwall, B. M., 1982, Axosomatic synapses in the visual cortex of adult rat: A comparison between GABA-accumulating and other neurons, *J. Neurocytol.* **11:**409–425.

Wong, W. C., 1967, The tangential organization of dendrites and axons in three auditory areas of the cat's cerebral cortex, *J. Anat.* **101:**419–433.

Woolsey, T. A., and Dierker, M. L., 1982, Morphometric approaches to neuroanatomy with emphasis on computer-assisted techniques, in: *Cytochemical Methods in Neuroanatomy* (V. Chan-Palay and S. L. Palay, eds.), pp. 69–91, Liss, New York.

Woolsey, T. A., and Van der Loos, H., 1970, The structural organization of layer IV in the somatosensory region (S I) of mouse cerebral cortex, *Brain Res.* **17**:205–242.

Woolsey, T. A., Dierker, M. L., and Wann, D. F., 1975, Mouse SmI cortex: Qualitative and quantitative classification of Golgi-impregnated barrel neurons, *Proc. Natl, Acad. Sci. USA* **72**:2165–2169.

7

Spiny Stellate Neurons

JENNIFER S. LUND

1. Introduction

The spiny stellate neuron occupies a special position in the neuropil of the mammalian cerebral cortex. It is often the principal target of thalamic axons, appearing in considerable numbers in a specialized stratum in middle depth between pia and white matter in primary sensory regions of the cortex. The synthesis of incoming information achieved by these neurons is a crucial initial step in the cortical processing of afferent activity and it is therefore of interest to consider their organization in some detail. Since most study has been made of the visual cortical areas and this is the particular interest of this author, many points will be illustrated in terms of the visual cortex. There is no reason to believe, however, that once more is known of other sensory regions of cortex that similar features of organization will not be found there also.

2. Morphology and Synaptic Relations of the Spiny Stellate Neuron

This class of neurons resembles the cortical pyramidal neuron morphologically in having dendrites with synapse bearing spiny projections (see Figs. 1–3). They are distinguished from pyramidal neurons by the absence of the extended apical dendrite characteristic of the pyramidal neuron (Lund, 1973; see for

JENNIFER S. LUND • Departments of Psychiatry, Neurology, and Ophthalmology, University of Pittsburgh School of Medicine, Pittsburgh, Pennsylvania 15261.

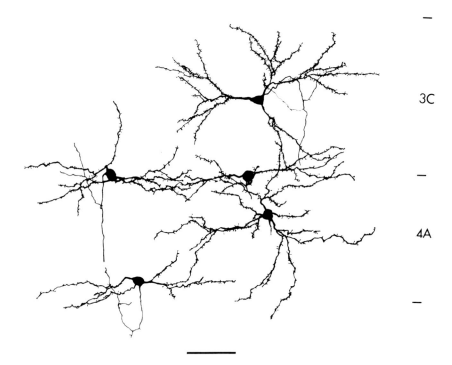

3C

4A

Figure 1. Drawing of Golgi-impregnated spiny stellate neurons from tree shrew visual cortex. Note the differences in horizontal stratification of the dendrites of the individual neurons. This stratification is believed to relate to the distribution of different populations of thalamocortical axons. Scale bar = 50 μm.

comparison the pyramidal neurons of Fig. 18). The spiny stellate neuron is distinguished from other classes of stellate cells in the cortex by its prominent dendritic spine population in the adult animal. The dendrites of other stellate neurons of the cortex become spine-free or only very sparsely spined at maturity, although most bear spines or spicules during early development (Lund *et al.*, 1977). The spiny stellate neurons share many characteristics with pyramidal neurons, despite the absence of an apical dendrite. Where they occur, they can comprise the majority of the neurons in the layer, in contrast to the relatively low density of smooth or sparsely spined neurons in the population. They share this characteristic with the pyramidal neurons which also numerically predominate over the nonspiny stellate neurons (Mates and Lund, 1983a). The spiny stellate neuron and pyramidal neuron also share a common anatomical polarity, in that their axons almost always leave the soma from the side facing the white matter. Their axons travel toward the white matter for a short distance, even if their final destination lies on the pial side of the cell. This differs from smooth or sparsely spined stellate neurons whose axons either have no predictable polarity to their origin or, more often, arise on the pial aspect of the soma (Lund, 1973).

As one studies the variety of forms that are found in both pyramidal and spiny stellate neuron classes, a suspicion arises that in fact there may be a con-

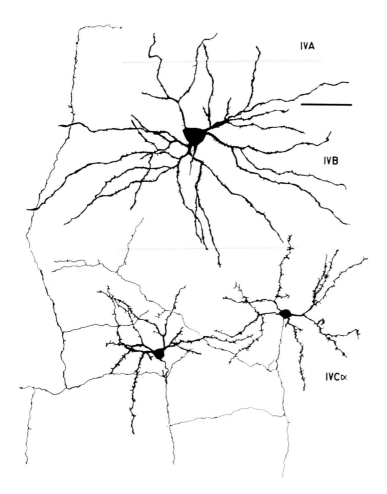

Figure 2. Drawing of Golgi-impregnated spiny stellate neurons from macaque monkey striate visual cortex. Scale bar = 50 μm. Reproduced from Lund (1973) with permission.

tinuum of form between the two groups. For instance, in primate VI visual cortex there is a class of small pyramidal neurons lying at the top of lamina 5 that, at first glance, appears to be a spiny stellate population (Fig. 4B). However, these neurons have a fine, aspinous process, quite unlike the rest of their dendrites, resembling a vestigial apical dendrite emerging from the pial side of the neuron. For this reason these neurons have been classified as pyramidal rather than spinous stellate (Lund, 1973). Another example of an apparently intermediary form is found in the cat visual cortex where large spinous stellate neurons in upper lamina 4 (Fig. 4A) have a short "apical" dendrite that divides into a bunch of lateral branches, actually no longer than the basal dendrites (Lund *et al.*, 1979). It would be possible to consider these neurons as pyramidal cells with truncated apical dendrites. Lorente de Nó (1938) was evidently struck by the possibility of intermediary forms since he called some groups of neurons *star pyramids,* apparently on the grounds that their basal dendrites in the middle cortical layers formed a radiate field, like true spiny stellate neurons in the same lamina, whereas the possession of an apical dendrite (albeit with few collateral branches) extending into more superficial laminae required recognition as characteristic of a pyramidal neuron. Star pyramids and other intermediary forms between spiny stellate and pyramidal morphology are typical of the primate somatosensory cortex (Jones, 1975) (see Figs. 5–7).

The majority of spiny stellate neurons apparently resemble pyramidal neurons in the type of synaptic segregation seen on their somal and dendritic surfaces (Colonnier, 1968; Lund and Lund, 1970; LeVay, 1973; Mates, 1981). Both forms of spiny neuron have been found to have relatively few synaptic contacts on their somata, all of type 2 morphology [i.e., making symmetric contact apposition (Gray, 1959) and containing pleomorphic vesicles (Colonnier, 1968); see Figs. 8–10]. Type 2 contacts are also present on their dendritic shafts, in gradually diminishing numbers toward the distal tips of the dendrites, and occasionally found on spine stalks or tips. The spine tips are occupied by type 1 synapses [asymmetric contact site and round synaptic vesicles (Gray, 1959; Colonnier, 1968); see Figs. 8–10], usually only one per spine tip and occasionally sharing the spine with a type 2 contact. Very occasional type 1 contacts have been described on the dendritic shafts, but as we shall see later this may be a sign of immaturity. This type of synaptology is in general not found on the smooth dendritic or sparsely spined stellate neurons where the dendritic and somal surface are well covered with both type 1 and type 2 contacts. However, apparent

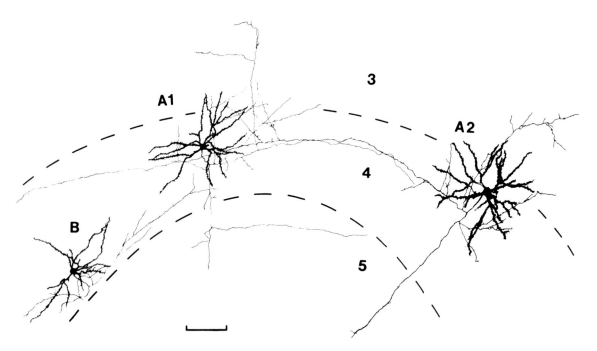

Figure 3. Drawing of Golgi-impregnated spiny stellate neurons from cat striate visual cortex. Scale bar = 100 μm. Reproduced from Lund *et al.* (1979) with permission.

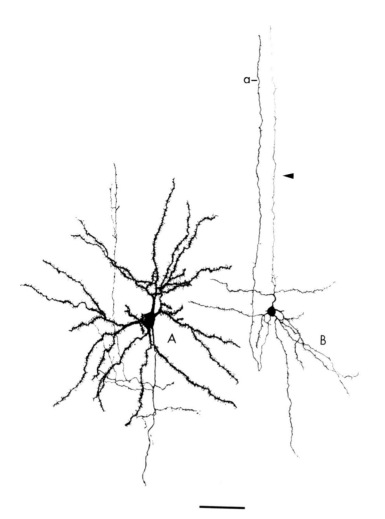

Figure 4. Spiny neurons that could be considered intermediary in form between pyramidal and spiny stellate neurons. (A) Drawing of large spiny stellate neuron from cat striate visual cortex with short apical dendrite (arrow). (B) Small pyramidal neuron with poorly developed apical dendrite (arrow) from layer 5A of macaque monkey striate cortex. The rising axon (a) of this cell is larger in diameter than the apical dendrite. Scale bar = 50 μm. (A) From Lund *et al.* (1979); (B) reproduced from Lund (1973) with permission.

exceptions have been described to these broad patterns of synaptology in spiny vs. nonspiny neuron groups: for instance, in the cat, large spiny stellate neurons which project across the corpus callosum have been described as having both type 1 and type 2 contacts on their cell bodies (Hornung and Garey, 1981), and further work correlating the light microscopic morphology with electron microscopy of synaptology is needed.

The axons of the spiny stellate neurons are found to form synapses of type 1 morphology (LeVay, 1973; see Fig. 10H), in this respect again resembling the pyramidal neuron rather than the majority of the smooth dendritic neuron class

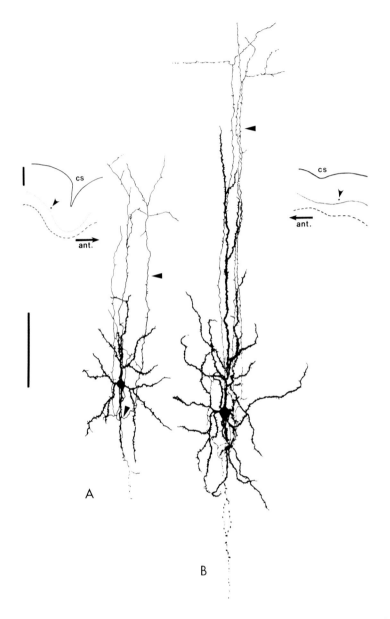

Figure 5. Drawings of spiny stellate (A) and star pyramid (B) neurons from lamina 4 of squirrel monkey somatosensory cortex, area 3. The dendritic spines and pronounced ascending dendritic system give such cells a superficial resemblance to pyramidal neurons. Note also the strongly recurrent axon branches (arrows). Golgi rapid preparations. Scale bar against cells = 100 μm. Scale bar in cortex diagram = 1 mm. Reproduced from Jones (1975) with permission.

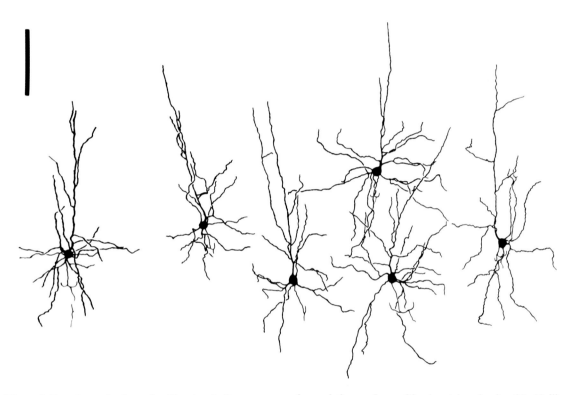

Figure 6. Drawings of spiny cells of lamina 4 of somatosensory cortex, area 3, in squirrel monkey. Dendritic spines and distal portions of the axons are not drawn. In every case there is a strong ascending dendritic system which extends beyond the confines of lamina 4 into lamina 3B. Unlike a pyramidal neuron, however, the soma is always round and there is no pronounced basal dendritic spray. Scale bar = 100 μm. Reproduced from Jones (1975) with permission.

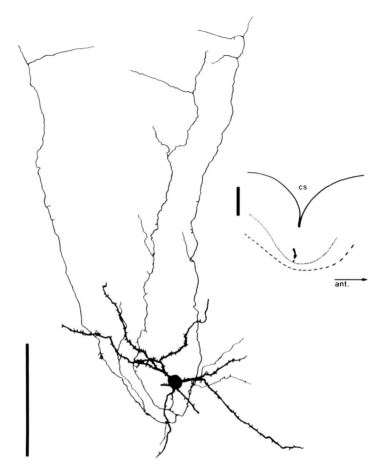

Figure 7. Drawing of a spiny stellate neuron from somatosensory cortex, area 3, in squirrel monkey, lying in layer 4 of the floor of the central sulcus. Scale bar with cell = 100 μm; scale bar in cortex diagram = 1 mm. Reproduced from Jones (1975) with permission.

which make type 2 contacts in most cases (exceptions do exist—see Peters and Kimerer, 1981). It must also be remembered that the morphological descriptions, type 1 or type 2, for presynaptic axonal processes and their apposition sites are extremely broad. Type 1 contacts are derived from both extrinsic afferents and neurons intrinsic to the cortex, and therefore the broad class of type 1 contact includes many different varieties of terminal within it; we urgently need some techniques for recognizing subgroups within the class. The same is true for type 2 contacts, although most, if not all, of these terminals derive from intrinsic cortical neurons (see Chapter 13). The only biochemical correlate known for type 2 terminals is the finding that many are rich in glutamic acid decarboxylase (GAD), or accumulate tritiated GABA (Somogyi *et al.*, 1981a,b), suggestive of an inhibitory function. In this respect, spiny stellate neurons may differ from pyramidal neurons in lacking a marked population of type 2 synaptic contacts on their initial axon segments (Somogyi, 1977; Mates, 1981). These contacts are

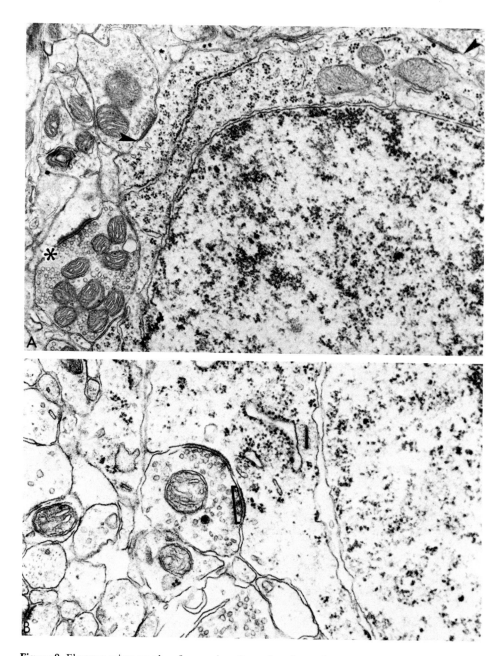

Figure 8. Electron micrographs of examples of type 1 and type 2 synapses in layer 4C of macaque monkey visual cortex. (A) Type 2 contacts onto spiny stellate neuron soma. Asterisk marks type 1 synapse typical of those contacting spine tips on the spiny stellate neuron dendrites. (B) One type 2 contact site is bracketed, another is unmarked, from an axon terminal contacting a spiny stellate neuron soma. Magnification approximately × 35,000 (A) and × 40,000 (B). From Mates and Lund (1983a) with permission.

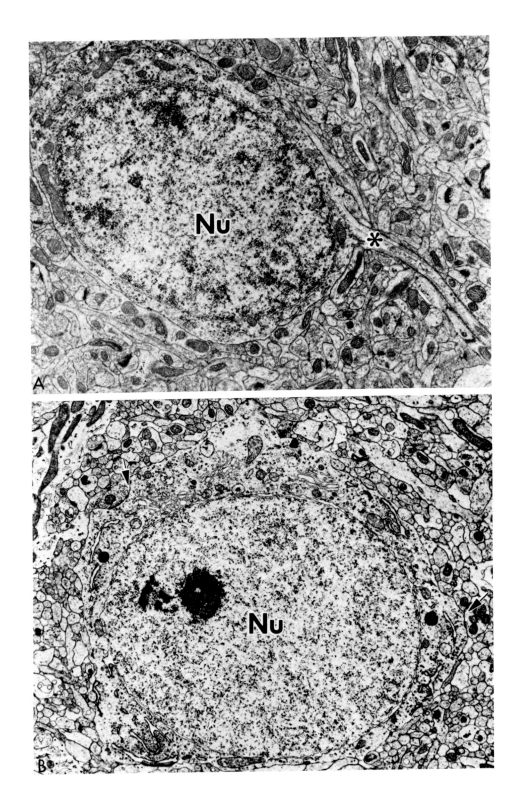

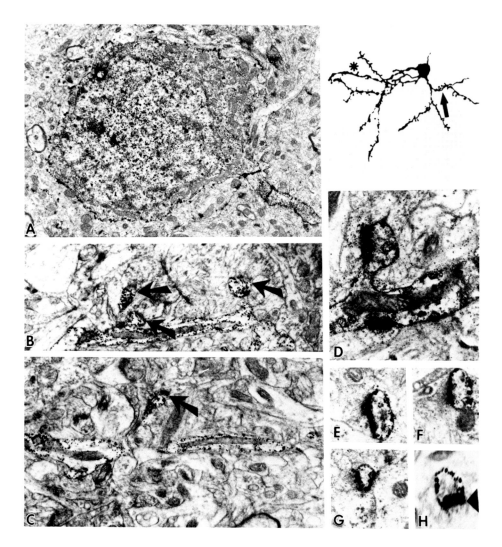

Figure 10. Light and electron micrographs of a Golgi-impregnated spiny stellate neuron, gold-toned for electron microscopy, from lamina 4Cβ of macaque visual cortex. (A) Gold-toned thin section of cell body of neuron. (Inset) Drawing of the spiny stellate neuron seen by light microscopy prior to thin sectioning. (B, C) Arrows point to spines. (D–G) A spine (aserisk in inset) receiving a synapse. Every fourth section of a row of serial sections is shown. (H) Axon terminal of the same spiny stellate neuron making a type 1 synapse. Magnification × 7000 (A), approximately × 18,000 (B, C), approximately × 22,000 (D–H). Reproduced from Mates and Lund (1983a) with permission.

←

Figure 9. Electron micrographs of spiny stellate neuron cells in macaque monkey visual cortex. Nu, nucleus; asterisk marks axon initial segment. Arrows indicate type 2 synapses. Magnification × 10,960. From Mates and Lund (1983a) with permission.

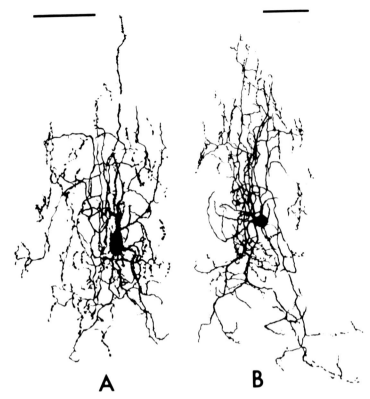

Figure 11. Drawings of two examples of "chandelier" stellate neurons found in granular layer 4 of visual area VII in macaque monkey visual cortex. Golgi impregnations in 3-month-old infant monkey. Scale bars = 50 μm. Reproduced from Lund *et al.* (1981) with permission.

often prominent on the axon initial segment of pyramidal neurons and have been shown (Somogyi, 1977) to derive from a particular variety of smooth dendritic neuron, the chandelier cell (Fig. 11 and Chapter 10). The chandelier cell is generally not evident in regions of spiny stellate neurons lacking pyramidal neurons but can be found if pyramidal neurons form part of the population as well [for instance, in layer 4 of the cat cortex (Fairén and Valverde, 1980)]. It may be that the spiny stellate neuron differs from pyramidal neurons in the manner in which inhibitory control is exerted on the cell, inhibitory contacts on cell body and dendrites evidently being of different origin, and probably functionally different in this situation from those on the axon initial segment.

3. Distribution and Axonal Projections of Spiny Stellate Neurons

The spiny stellate neuron population is sharply confined within a middle stratum of particular regions of sensory cerebral cortex. Their presence has been recognized in primary visual cortex (Lund, 1973; Lund *et al.*, 1979), in somatosensory cortex (Jones, 1975; Woolsey *et al.*, 1975a,b), and in auditory cortex (Winer, 1982). In at least part of the stratum these cells may be particularly small and extremely densely packed; this "granular" layer, so-called by early neuroanatomists on the basis of the fine grain appearance of the cytoarchitecture in stains for Nissl substance (see Figs. 12–15), is generally designated as all, or part, of lamina 4. The presence of a zone of small, closely packed neurons in Nissl-stained material in midcortical depth, even in a sensory area of cortex, should not, however, be taken as a sure indication of the presence of spiny stellate neurons. For instance, in the visual association area, V2 or area 18, of the macaque monkey cortex there is a well-developed "granular" layer 4 (Fig. 16). However, in contrast to adjacent V1 (area 17), this layer is composed of closely packed small pyramidal neurons (Fig. 16) with a small proportion of smooth dendritic or sparsely spined stellate cells (including chandelier neurons such as those shown in Fig. 11), but no spiny stellate neurons are to be found (Lund *et al.*, 1981). The transition from several laminae containing spiny stellate neuron populations in V1 to their absence in V2 occurs abruptly at the junction of the two regions. It is clear in somatosensory cortex that neighboring areas

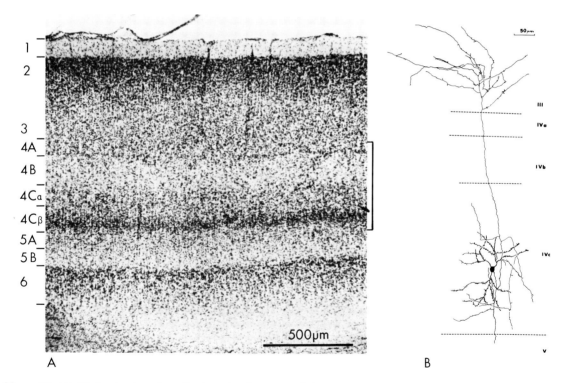

Figure 12. (A) Nissl-stained section of striate visual cortex of macaque monkey. Bracket indicates stratum of spiny stellate neurons. Note the different cell packing densities at different depths within the stratum and the laminar subdivisions 4A, 4B, 4Cα, and 4Cβ that have been recognized within the stratum by virtue of the distribution of different thalamic axon populations (to laminae 4Cα, 4Cβ, and 4A), and reciprocal relationship to extrastriate visual area MT (lamina 4B). (B) Drawing of a Golgi-impregnated spiny stellate neuron of lamina 4Cβ from macaque striate cortex with rising axon arborizing in laminae 4A–lower 3. (B) reproduced from Lund (1973) with permission.

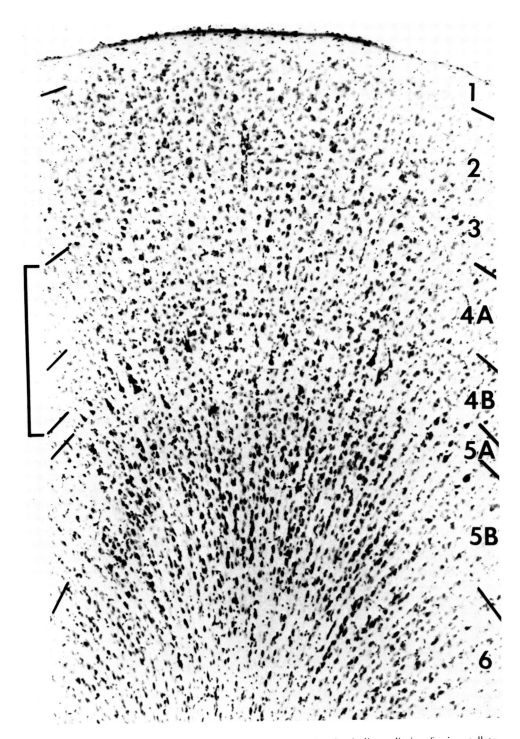

Figure 13. Nissl-stained section of cat striate visual cortex. Bracket indicates limits of spiny stellate stratum which has two subdivisions, 4A and 4B, which receive input from different populations of thalamic axons. Magnification approximately × 100. Reproduced from Lund *et al.* (1979) with permission.

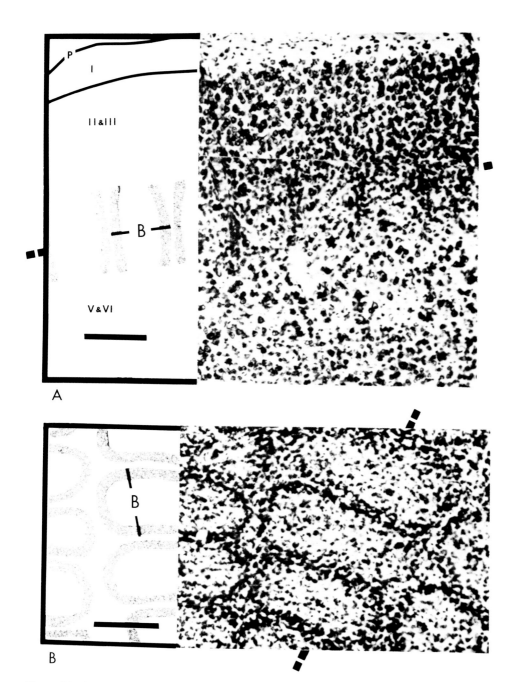

Figure 14. Photomicrographs of methylene blue-stained sections through the posteromedial barrel subfield of mouse somatosensory cortex. In coronal section (A), layer IV is characterized by "columns" of closely packed cells with less densely packed regions between. The hatched line at the edges idicates the level at which the tangential section shown in (B) was taken. Line B in both figures indicates the same dimension of the barrel-shaped arrays of cells seen in the two planes of section. Further tangential sections of this region of cortex are shown in Fig. 15. Each vibrissa on the animal's nuzzle is represented within a single barrel array. Scale bars = 100 μm. Reproduced from Woolsey and Van der Loos (1970) with permission.

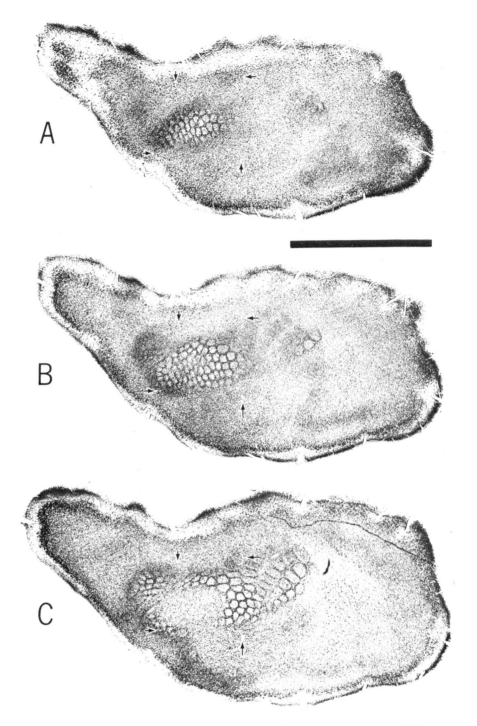

Figure 15. Photomicrographs of tangential sections from the somatosensory cortex of the mouse showing the barrel field (vibrissa-l representation). The ring-shaped concentrations of neurons occur within layer IV, the spiny stellate stratum, of this region of cortex (see Fig. 14). 50-μm sections; scale bar = 2 mm. Reproduced from Woolsey and Van der Loos (1970) with permission.

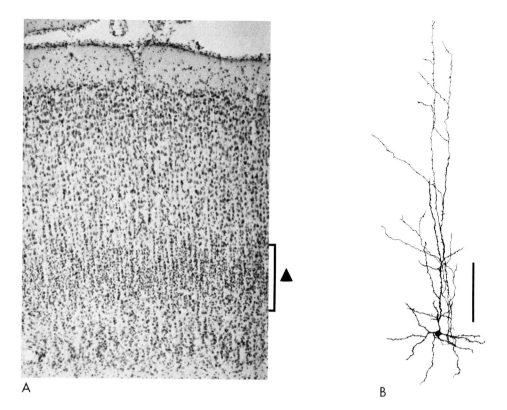

Figure 16. (A) Nissl section through visual cortical area VII of macaque monkey (magnification × 97). The bracketed zone, lamina 4, is a densely packed small-cell granular layer. However, unlike area VI (striate cortex), the cells in this zone are pyramidal neurons [example shown in (B)] with recurrent rising axon trunks. No spiny stellate neurons are to be found in this region of the neocortex. (B) Scale bar = 100 μm; from Lund *et al.* (1981) with permission.

(S1, S2, S3) contain different proportions of spiny stellate neurons (Jones, 1975) and that in those animals with well-developed vibrissae the cortical whisker area has a particularly rich and well-organized stratum of spiny stellate neurons (Figs. 14, 15) (Woolsey *et al.*, 1975a). This curiously parcellated distribution suggests that the spiny stellate neuron must fulfill a rather special role in cerebral cortex function.

While all the dendrites of a particular spiny stellate neuron are of similar length, they may be strongly stratified horizontally within individual laminae, or they may be radiate or even vertically elongate in distribution (Lund, 1973; Winer, 1982). Their dendrites may also obey the boundaries of structural feature within a lamina, such as in the vibrissal barrel fields of somatosensory cortex (Woolsey *et al.*, 1975a; Steffan, 1976). The strata containing spiny stellate neurons may have laminar subdivisions distinguished in part by their different cell packing densities and cell size, and in part by the proportion of pyramidal neurons present in addition to spinous stellate neurons (Lund, 1973; Lund and Boothe, 1975; Humphrey and Lund, 1979, and unpublished observations). Figure 17i shows, in diagrammatic form, laminar subdivisions distinguishable in the spiny stellate neuron strata in visual cortex of monkey, cat, and tree shrew. However, the laminar subdivisions can generally be most clearly distinguished on the basis of the distribution—often segregated with sharp boundaries—of different populations of afferent axon terminal fields, particularly the thalamic axon populations (Hubel and Wiesel, 1972; Harting *et al.*, 1973; LeVay and Gilbert, 1976; Ferster and LeVay, 1978; Fitzpatrick *et al.*, 1982; Blasdel and Lund, 1982, 1983). This multiple layering of the afferents to the spiny stellate neuron population can reach considerable complexity and has been most clearly demonstrated in the primary visual cortex (see Fig. 17ii). It is clear, however, that the laminar distribution of the thalamic afferents is not always a simple replication of the segregation of neuron populations seen in the thalamic nuclei of origin. While some afferent axon segregation clearly reflects thalamic and even sensory receptor segregation patterns (as in the vibrissal representation of somatosensory cortex—see Fig. 15), other cortical segregation patterns in spiny stellate laminae seem to reflect a new order peculiar to the needs of cortical processing of afferent activity.

The stratum of spiny stellate neurons in sensory cortex occupies a position just external to a band of pyramidal neurons (termed *lamina 5* efferent to the superior or inferior colliculi and pulvinar complex (Gilbert and Kelly, 1975; Lund *et al.*, 1975). Lamina 5 in turn lies external to a second band of pyramidal neurons just above the white matter—lamina 6—which are efferent to those thalamic nuclei giving rise to the afferents to the spiny stellate stratum (Gilbert and Kelly, 1975; Lund *et al.*, 1975; LeVay and Sherk, 1981). The lamina 6 pyramidal neurons also project intrinsically via rising axon collaterals to the spiny stellate stratum above, often with a stratified axonal distribution reflecting the divisions of the stratum created by thalamic inputs, but also creating new linkages between these laminar subdivisions (Lund and Boothe, 1975; Lund *et al.*, 1979; Gilbert and Wiesel, 1979). Their apical dendrites may also enter into the divisions of the spiny stellate neuropil with arborizations again reflecting its laminar subdivisions. This is illustrated in more detail in Figs. 18 and 19B in relation to the visual cortex. The spiny stellate stratum therefore is intimately connected with lamina 6 neurons in a feedback relationship at both cortical and thalamic levels.

The axons of spiny stellate neurons are largely (but not exclusively) intrinsic in their projections. In the visual cortex, where their relays have been best explored, they travel relatively short distances from the cells of origin to laminae above and below and also establish connections within the lamina of origin (Lund, 1973; Lund and Boothe, 1975; Lund *et al.*, 1979; Gilbert and Wiesel, 1979). The emphasis in the projections is on ascending (pial-ward) projection to other laminae within the spiny neuron stratum and to pyramidal neuron populations with accompanying nonspiny stellate neurons external to the stratum (divisions of laminae 3, 2, and 1). The lamina subdivisions outlined by the afferent axon populations are also often reflected in differential relays of the spiny stellate neurons lying postsynaptic to each input, each projecting to different destinations; this is illustrated in Fig. 19A for monkey visual cortex. Some populations of spiny stellate neurons do, however, send their axons long distances, to other cortical areas. For instance, in the primary visual cortex of the primate, one

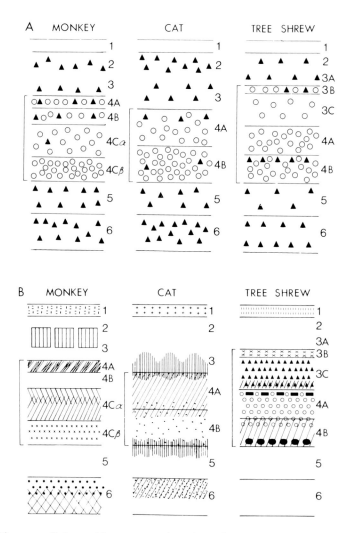

Figure 17. Diagrams of pia to white matter sections through primary visual cortex of monkey, cat, and tree shrew. (A) Comparison of the distribution of spiny stellate neurons (○) and pyramidal neurons (▲). It can be seen that the spiny stellate neurons occupy a stratum in middle depth in each animal. The degree to which pyramidal neuron somata and basal dendritic fields occur within the stratum depends on the species and the laminar subdivisions within the stratum. Data from Lund (1973), Lund *et al.* (1979), and Lund and Humphrey (unpublished observations). (B) Diagrams illustrating the complex patterns of distribution of thalamic axon populations from the dorsal lateral geniculate nucleus in macaque monkey, cat, and tree shrew, primary visual cortex. The brackets indicate the stratum of spiny stellate neurons. No attempt has been made here to identify the origins of each axon population but different populations are marked by different hatching patterns. It can be seen that some populations terminate outside the stratum of spiny stellate neurons although the stratum does serve as a principal recipient zone for many inputs. Data derived from many sources including Hubel and Wiesel (1972), LeVay and Gilbert (1976), Fitzpatrick *et al.* (1982), Blasdel and Lund (1983), and Conley *et al.* (1984).

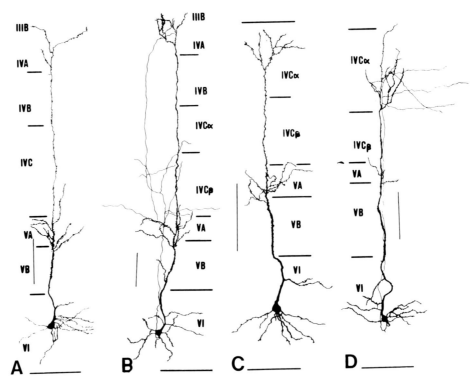

Figure 18. Drawing of Golgi-impregnated layer 6 pyramidal neurons from infant macaque monkey visual cortex. The apical dendrites and recurrent axon collaterals of these neurons relate to specific laminar subdivisions of the spiny stellate neuron stratum. These same neurons may also send an axon projection back to the dorsal lateral geniculate nucleus which provides the main input to the spiny stellate neuron stratum. Scale bars (vertical line beside each neuron) measure 100 μm. Reproduced from Lund and Boothe (1975) with permission.

subdivision of the spiny stellate neuron population (in lamina 4B) sends axons to a distant visual association area MT in the middle temporal sulcus (Lund *et al.*, 1975; Spatz, 1977; Tigges *et al.*, 1981). In the cat, large spiny stellate neurons (in lamina 4A) send axons to the contralateral homotypic area via the corpus callosum (Hornung and Garey, 1981) and small ones (again in 4A) project to ipsilateral area 18 (Meyer and Albus, 1981). Spiny stellate neurons have not, however, been found to project subcortically. In contrast, the great majority of efferent neurons of the cortex are pyramidal neurons, forming both cortico-cortical and cortico-thalamic connections. However, within the pyramidal neuron population there are varieties that are entirely intrinsically projecting, much as the majority of spiny stellate neurons. These include pyramidal neurons that occur in the spiny stellate stratum, where they seem to mimic the stellate neuron axon intrinsic distribution patterns, and most notably, a population of small pyramidal neurons at the junction of lamina 5 and the spiny stellate stratum which receive input from the spiny stellate neurons and which project via recurrent collaterals to the overlying layers superficial to the spiny stellate stratum (Lund, 1973; Lund and Boothe, 1975).

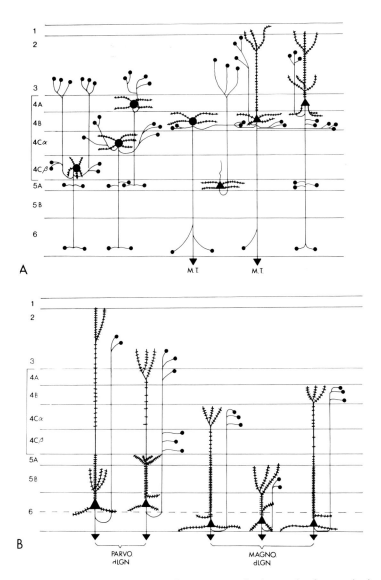

Figure 19. Diagram of projections of spiny stellate neurons of primary visual cortex in the macaque monkey. The projections of the spiny stellate neurons within each subdivision of the stratum are specific for that subdivision and represent the relay of different kinds of thalamic information to different locations within primary visual cortex. Note that lamina 4B, which does not receive direct thalamic visual input, contains pyramidal as well as spiny stellate neurons which are efferent to cortical area MT. In contrast, the other populations of spiny stellate neurons are entirely intrinsic in their projections. Data from Lund (1973), Lund and Boothe (1975), and Lund *et al.* (1975). (B) Diagram of relationships of axons and dendrites of layer 6 pyramidal neurons to the overlying laminae of the primary visual cortex in macaque monkey. These dendritic and axonal projections relate both to thalamic axon laminar distribution patterns and to the organization of axon relays of the spiny stellate neurons [see (A) above]. Drawings of Golgi-impregnated neurons showing these projections are shown in Fig. 18.

4. Comparison of Stratum of Spiny Stellate Neurons in Visual Cortex of Several Different Mammals

It is of interest to explore the organization of a spiny stellate stratum in some detail for one of the mammalian sensory cortical areas and examine in different species how this stratum may change its substructure. The primary visual cortex serves well for such a comparison and the diagrams of Fig. 17 summarize what is known of the organization of this stratum in cat, macaque monkey, and tree shrew from published and unpublished work. The reader is advised to study these diagrams as we discuss the organizational features of the stratum (the reader should be aware that different laminar numbering schemes apply to the different species and do not denote homologies). There is a considerable diversity of relationship between the neurons of the stratum and thalamic inputs in different mammalian groups, principal differences being seen in the degree of lamination of thalamic axon populations, the admixture of pyramidal neurons to some laminae and not others, and the entry of afferent axons from sources other than the thalamus into divisions of the stratum. The claustrum has been shown to specifically emphasize a projection to the thalamic receiving layers of striate cortex in cat and tree shrew, which therefore includes the spiny stellate stratum in both. However, the claustral input has not been shown to obey the narrower subdivisions observed for thalamic inputs from the lateral geniculate nucleus (Carey et al., 1980; LeVay and Sherk, 1981). In the primate it is found that anterior visual cortex projects back to one division, 4B, of the spiny stellate stratum.

Spiny stellate neurons appear in some lamina subdivisions of their stratum to exclude pyramidal neuron cell bodies and their basal dendrites almost entirely from the population (Fig. 17i). Lamina 4C of the macaque striate cortex (Lund and Boothe, 1975) is an example of such a population where only extremely rare examples of pyramidal neurons are to be found [even these few have very poorly developed apical dendrites and for division 4C even the apical dendritic trunks of lower pyramidal neurons passing through the layer become spine poor (Fig. 19B)]. A similar exclusion of pyramidal neurons is seen in tree shrew laminae 4A and 3C (Humphrey and Lund, 1979, and unpublished observations). Other laminae of the stratum in tree shrew and monkey are occupied by both pyramidal and spiny stellate neurons. The lower division of lamina 4 (4B) of the tree shrew has a population of small pyramidal neurons mixed with spiny stellate neurons. These pyramidal neurons are particularly numerous at the upper border of 4B and show a marked horizontal stratification of their basal dendrites. Their apical dendrites and recurrent axon trunks pass upward to arborize in lamina 3B, the same destination as the axon trunks of the spiny stellate neurons of the same subdivision. In the cat, pyramidal neurons are found throughout the stratum of spiny stellate neurons, though decreasing in number at the base (O'Leary, 1941; Lund et al., 1979). The macaque monkey has one subdivision (4B) which also has a prominent population of pyramidal neurons, although the largest neurons of the lamina are spiny stellate cells. As yet, the functional significance of these different proportions of spiny stellate and pyramidal neurons within single laminae is obscure; it is evidently not related to the presence or absence of direct thalamic input to the sublamina. However, two particular anatomical features may be of functional importance. First, the apical dendrite of the pyramidal neuron allows these cells to sample activity in laminae otherwise out of range of the rest of the cell's dendrites. This may be of particular importance, in the visual cortex at least, where there is little or no descending axon arborization within the spiny stellate stratum from pyramidal neurons lying superficial to it (Fisken *et al.*, 1975; Lund and Boothe, 1975). Correspondingly, if the lamina contains no pyramidal neurons, it is effectively isolated from much of the activity ongoing within the cortex, having access only to those afferent axons terminating in the lamina. A study of Fig. 17i will show examples of laminae that are isolated in this fashion, while others have access via pyramidal neuron dendritic extensions to more superficial laminar environments.

The spiny stellate stratum serves as the main terminal zone for thalamic afferents in primary visual cortex. Some thalamic axon populations terminate exclusively within the stratum and occupy clearly defined lamina territories (Fig. 17ii). Examples of such axons are a population originating from parvocellular laminae of the lateral geniculate nucleus of the macaque monkey which establish highly ordered, restricted fields within lamina 4Cβ (Fig. 20), a lamina which apparently does not receive afferents from other cell groups of the geniculate (Hubel and Wiesel, 1972; Blasdel and Lund, 1983). In the tree shrew there is an extremely complex ordering of thalamic axon territories (Fig. 17ii) within the spiny stellate zone, with projections occupying zones that can occupy extremely narrow subdivisions within the depth of the stratum, and with complex patterns of partial overlap of the terminal fields of different axon populations (Harting *et al.*, 1973; Casagrande and Harting, 1975; Hubel, 1975; Conley *et al.*, 1984). This finely ordered axonal distribution is accompanied by markedly stratified dendritic fields of the stellate neurons (Fig. 21) and, when they occur, of the basal dendritic fields of admixed pyramidal neuron groups, suggesting a concomitant restriction of the postsynaptic neurons to input only from similarly

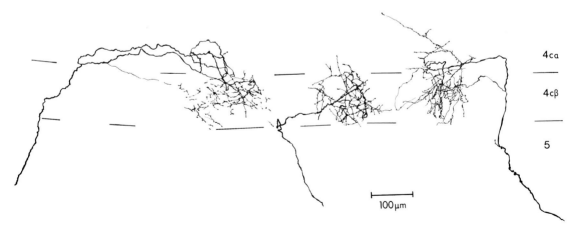

4cα

4cβ

5

100μm

Figure 20. Drawing of thalamic axon arbors (arising from the parvocellular laminae of the lateral geniculate nucleus) in lamina 4Cβ of macaque monkey primary visual cortex. These axons were filled with HRP from large injections of this substance into the underlying white matter. Each arbor is extremely dense and confined to a single small region of this subdivision of the spiny stellate neuron stratum. Compare with the axon of Fig. 22 derived from magnocellular LGN. Reproduced from Blasdel and Lund (1983) with permission.

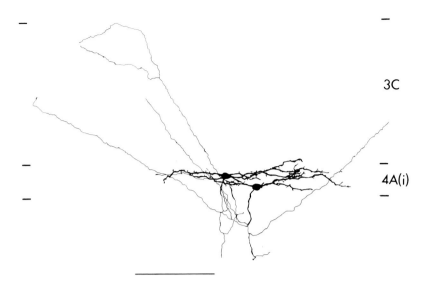

3C

4A(i)

Figure 21. Highly stratified spiny stellate neurons from tree shrew visual cortex. These neurons lie at the top of lamina 4 and form the postsynaptic surface for a narrow tier of thalamocortical input from a particular component of the LGN (Conley *et al.*, 1984). Scale bar = 100 μm. See also Fig. 1 which illustrates further examples of these neurons (Humphrey and Lund, unpublished observations).

laminated afferent axon terminal fields (Humphrey and Lund, 1979). As mentioned earlier, the laminar distribution of thalamic axons in the cortical neuropil does not always replicate that shown in the segregation of the neurons of origin in the geniculate laminae. This feature, of new kinds of order being established in the cortex compared to the thalamic nucleus of origin, is seen in primate (Fitzpatrick *et al.*, 1982; Blasdel and Lund, 1983), cat (LeVay and Gilbert, 1976), and tree shrew (Conley *et al.*, 1984). In cat, for instance, neurons contained within single laminae of the lateral geniculate nucleus—e.g., lamina A—project to separate laminae of the cortex, neurons of so-called Y type projecting to cortical lamina 4A and neurons of X type projecting to lamina 4B (LeVay and Gilbert, 1976).

   While the stratum of spiny stellate neurons provides a major target for thalamic axon terminals, it is also true that some populations of thalamic axons terminate outside such strata (see Fig. 17ii), or have one set of collaterals, generally the more prominent, within the stratum and one set outside. In the primate and cat primary visual cortex, thalamic axons from large cells of the lateral geniculate nucleus have their major distribution to lamina 4 (4A in the cat, 4Cα in the primate) but these axons also send fine collaterals to lamina 6 (Fig. 22) where spiny stellate neurons are not part of the neuron population (Ferster and LeVay, 1978; Blasdel and Lund, 1983). Other axon populations arising from the lateral geniculate nucleus of these same animals, but taking origin from different cell groups, terminate in cortical laminae apparently entirely lacking spiny stellate neurons; for example, the small-cell c laminae of the cat geniculate project to bands immediately above and below the stratum of spiny stellate neurons (Ferster and LeVay, 1978) and the intercalated, small-cell zones in the

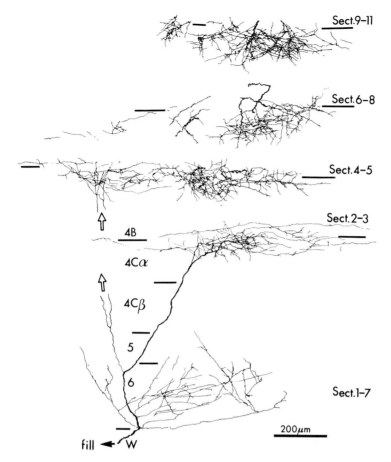

Sect.9–11

Sect.6–8

Sect.4–5

Sect.2–3

4B

4Cα

4Cβ

5

6

Sect.1–7

200 μm

fill ← W

Figure 22. A thalamic axon terminal arbor in the primary visual cortex of macaque monkey. This axon was identified physiologically by extra- and intracellular recording and then filled with HRP by intracellular iontophoresis. Compare the dimensions of this axon arbor in lamina 4Cα of the spiny stellate stratum to those shown in Fig. 20 in the immediately subjacent lamina 4Cβ. The terminal field in 4Cβ has been drawn separately for several groups of 90-μm sections so as to avoid overcomplexity in the reconstruction. The axon also has collaterals in lamina 6. It was identified as arising from the magnocellular division of the LGN by its physiological characterisitics. Reproduced from Blasdel and Lund (1983) with permission.

monkey geniculate project to patches in laminae 2–3, also lacking spiny stellate neurons (Fitzpatrick *et al.*, 1982).

5. Patterned Substructure within Strata of Spiny Stellate Neurons

The varied relationships between thalamic axon and spiny stellate neuron populations suggest that such an association is conditional on the type of thalamic axon, or at least on the type of information it carries to the cortex. At present,

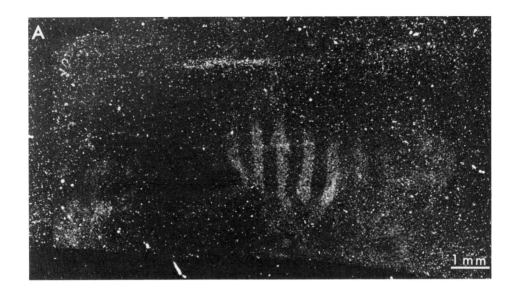

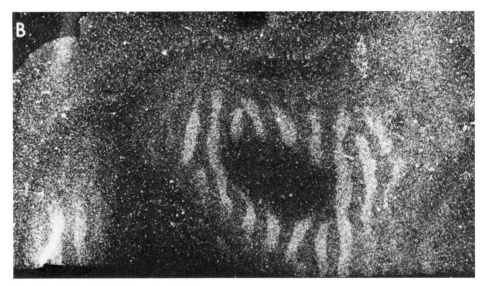

Figure 23. Normal macaque monkey visual cortex. The right eye was injected 14 days prior to sacrifice with 2.0 mCi of tritiated proline and fucose. The radioactive material has been transported transneuronally from the eye, through the LGN to the visual cortex. These autoradiograms, taken darkfield, are of tangential sections through the dome-shaped operculum of the right occipital lobe, ipsilateral to the injected eye. (A) Section with center region through layer 4C of the spiny stellate stratum. The light stripes represent the terminal fields of relays from the right eye with gaps of equal width which contain the unlabeled relays from the left eye. (B) 169 μm deeper than (A). (C) Reconstruction of a series of sections including those in (A) and (B) to show the striped segregation of the thalamic input in lamina 4C. Anterior—up, medial to left. Reproduced from Hubel *et al.* (1977) with permission.

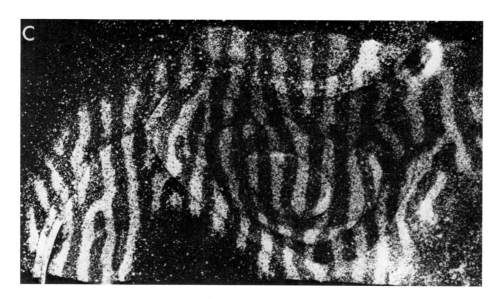

Figure 23. *(continued)*

however, it is unclear what functions are carried out in the stratum of spiny stellate neurons that would help clarify their role in any region of sensory cortex. In this respect, interesting functional parcellation of the neuropil within single laminae of the spiny neuron population can occur in a variety of ways. In the macaque visual cortex, regularly alternating bandlike zones (Fig. 23) are established within layer 4C by the thalamic axons served by the left and right eye (Wiesel *et al.*, 1974; Hubel and Wiesel, 1977). This lateral alternating segregation according to ocularity is determined by a competitive interaction (Fig. 24) during development between the thalamic axons of each ocularity (Hubel *et al.*, 1977). Despite the sharply segregated territories established by the afferent axons, there is no indication of the boundaries of these regions in terms of the distribution of the spiny neuron populations or their dendritic orientation (Lund, 1973). This differs from the striking parcellation of territory shown by both neurons and afferents in the somatosensory cortex of animals with prominent vibrissal follicle representation (Woolsey *et al.*, 1975a) (see Fig. 15).

A fine-scale honeycomb pattern of axon terminal distribution (Fig. 25) seen in lamina 4A of macaque primary visual cortex (Hendrickson *et al.*, 1978; Blasdel and Lund, 1983) is another example of the parcellation of territory within spiny stellate domains—as yet without functional explanation. These patterned relationships of afferent to spiny stellate neuron populations have been identified usually because of the accessibility of the thalamic axons to anatomical labels distant from their cortical terminal zones. However, even when thalamic axons are not involved, it has been found that the axons of the spiny stellate neurons themselves may form patterned connections within the lamina they occupy in the cortex. Such patterning of the spiny stellate neuron intrinsic connections has been identified in lamina 4B (Fig. 26) of macaque and squirrel monkey visual

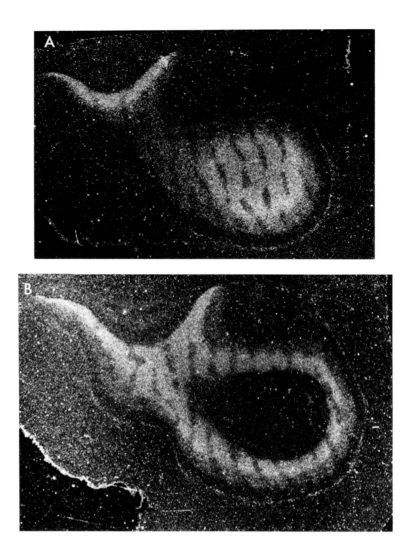

Figure 24. Macaque monkey whose right eyelids were sutured closed from age 2 weeks to 18 months. The left, normal eye was injected with tritiated proline–fucose mixture 14 days prior to sacrifice. The autoradiograms were prepared as described in Fig. 23 and are from the operculum of the left hemisphere. (A) Center region of section is a tangential cut through lamina 4C of the spiny stellate stratum. (B) 200 μm deeper than (A). (C) Result of reconstruction of nine such sections with total depth of 900 μm. Label in (C) representing the input from the normal eye is in the form of swollen bands which in places coalesce, obliterating the narrow gaps which represent the territory connected to the closed eye. The thin, almost continuous belt of label in (A) (also part of the spiny stellate stratum) is seen in all three sections. The six dots in (C) represent lesions made during physiological recording and mark the changes in ocular dominance and are clearly at or close to the stripe boundaries. Reproduced from Hubel *et al.* (1977) with permission.

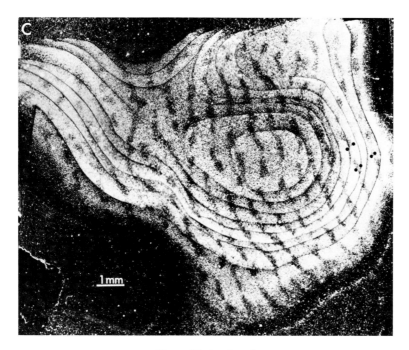

Figure 24. *(continued)*

cortex (Rockland and Lund, 1982, 1983). This laminar subdivision of the spiny stellate neuron stratum is of particular interest in that it apparently does not receive thalamic input but instead is both the source of efferents to, and the recipient of afferents from, a visual association area in the middle temporal gyrus (Lund *et al.,* 1975; Spatz, 1977; Tigges *et al.,* 1981). This lamina also receives a prominent input from the zone of spiny stellate neurons immediately internal to it, 4Cα, which in turn receives its input from the magnocellular division of the lateral geniculate nucleus (Hubel and Wiesel, 1972; Lund, 1973). The internal patterned relays within lamina 4B have been shown using transport of the tracer substance HRP injected into the layer. Both spiny stellate neurons and pyramidal neurons of the layer contribute long horizontal axon collaterals which terminate in a latticelike pattern within the lamina. Interestingly, these latticelike, periodic connections are aligned with a similar set of connections made within layers 2–3 by pyramidal neurons (Rockland and Lund, 1983). The scale and overall patterning of these connections resemble aspects of the patterns seen in experiments using the metabolic marker 2-deoxyglucose to label zones of neuropil active under particular conditions of visual stimulation (Hubel *et al.,* 1978; Hendrickson and Wilson, 1979; Horton and Hubel, 1981; Humphrey and Hendrickson, 1983). The patterns seen in laminae 2–3 also include periodic zones of thalamic input (Hubel and Livingston, 1981; Fitzpatrick *et al.,* 1982); it is possible, therefore, that these connections may be part of the anatomical substrate serving the specialization of cortical neuron response properties for particular stimulus characteristics.

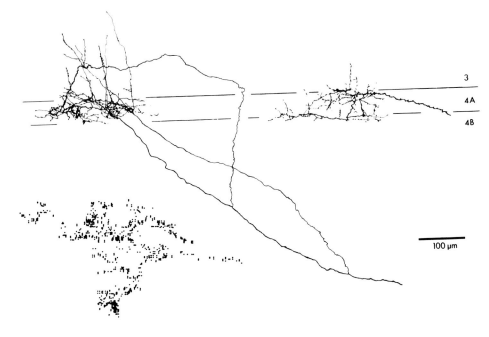

Rotated 90 Degrees About X Axis

Figure 25. Thalamic axon arborization in lamina 4A of the macaque visual cortex identified following filling with HRP by white matter injection. The terminal fields of these axons in the spiny stellate neuron stratum have a curious honeycomb distribution, here illustrated in the computer-derived rotation of the terminal boutons so that the lamina is viewed from above. Such axon patterns indicate an elaborate substructure within this layer. Reproduced from Blasdel and Lund (1983) with permission. See also autoradiographic data of Hendrickson *et al.* (1978).

6. Relationships between Smooth Dendritic and Spiny Stellate Neurons

The spiny stellate neuron stratum contains a population of smooth or sparsely spined neurons which are far less numerous than the population of spine-bearing neurons (Mates, 1981). In the visual cortex of the primate, they have been estimated at no more than 5% of the neuron population of lamina 4C on the basis of quantitative electron microscope analysis (Mates, 1981; Mates and Lund, 1983a). This is probably comparable to their proportion in other layers outside the stratum where pyramidal neurons replace the spiny stellate neuron population. Lamina 6 of the macaque for instance has again about 4–5% smooth dendritic stellate neurons in its neuron population (Mates and Lund, 1983c). While more work is needed in defining the morphology of these relatively infrequent neurons, in the visual cortex, at least, there appear to be particular varieties which accompany the spiny stellate cells (Fig. 27). It is also noticeable that there are relatively few varieties of these neurons in the spiny stellate stratum of tree shrew and primate compared to the large number of different forms of smooth or sparsely spined neurons to be found in layers 2–3 (Lund, 1973;

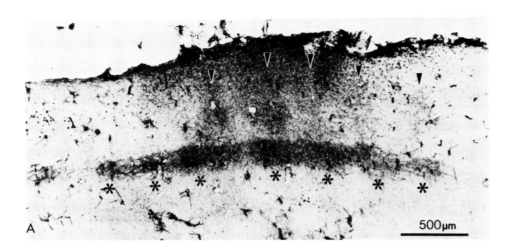

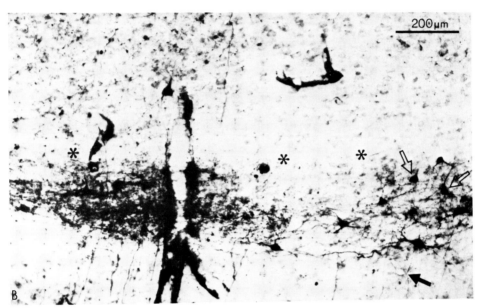

Figure 26. Photomicrographs of periodic (asterisked below each patch) distribution of HRP transported anterogradely and retrogradely by the neurons of lamina 4B in squirrel monkey primary striate cortex. This periodic label following small injections of HRP is believed to result from long-distance, regularly arranged periodic axon projections from neurons within the layer [both spiny stellate and pyramidal neurons appear to participate, see (B); open arrow indicates a pyramidal neuron, filled arrow indicates a spiny stellate neuron recurrent axon collateral]. Reproduced from Rockland and Lund (1983) with permission.

Humphrey and Lund, 1979, and work in progress; also see Chapters 6 and 13). Within the spiny stellate neuron stratum, these neurons provide the main source of type 2 (presumed inhibitory) synaptic contacts on the cell bodies and dendritic shafts of the spiny cells (LeVay, 1973; Mates and Lund, 1983a). The degree to which smooth dendritic neurons located in other laminae contribute synapses to the stratum may depend on the species. In the cat, there appear to be reciprocal

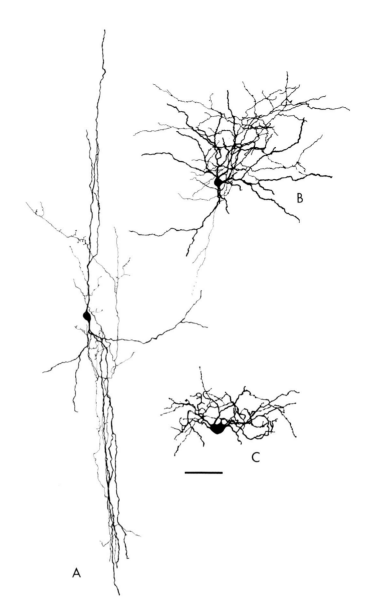

Figure 27. Smooth dendritic stellate neurons (drawn from Golgi impregnations) characteristic of the stratum of spiny stellate neurons in the tree shrew. Similar varieties occur in the primate. Cell A has vertically oriented dendrites and axon which freely cross the laminar boundaries within the cortex. Cell B can encompass several, but not all, subdivisions of the spiny stellate stratum, appearing to affect a partial link between several subdivisions. Cell C lies within the borders of single subdivision of the spiny stellate stratum apparently interacting only with the spiny neurons of that narrow subdivision (see also Fig. 28). Scale bar = 50 μm. From Lund and Humphrey (unpublished observations).

projections between layers 2–3 and the spiny stellate stratum of lamina 4 by the smooth dendritic neurons of each division (Lund *et al.*, 1979). In the tree shrew and macaque monkey, however, the stratum appears much more self-contained and isolated from input from smooth dendritic neurons of deeper or more superficial layers (Lund, 1973).

In the tree shrew and macaque visual cortex, one class of smooth dendritic neuron appears particularly frequent in the stratum. Its axon and dendrites are restricted to single lamina subdivisions (as defined by thalamic axon relays) within the stratum. The neuron class (Figs. 27C, 28) is characterized by having heavily beaded axons which in part at least contribute to the population of type 2 somatic synapses on the spiny stellate neurons (Mates and Lund, 1983a). Figure 29 shows this correlation in Golgi–EM material. Another class of smooth dendritic neuron spreads dendrites and axon across more than one laminar subdivision of the stratum as defined by geniculate inputs, affecting some kind of functional bridge between these subdivisions, but not bridging the whole stratum (Fig. 27B). For instance, such neurons encompass either the upper or the lower division of lamina 4 in the tree shrew within their axonal and dendritic tree but extend very little into the other division. Only one class of sparsely spined neurons found quite widely distributed in mammalian cortex seems indifferent to the laminar subdivisions of the stratum. These neurons form narrow, vertically oriented dendritic and axonal arrays (Fig. 27A) extending beyond the limits of the stratum. This is perhaps the neuron class described by Peters and Kimerer (1981) in the rat visual cortex as an exception to the general rule of smooth dendritic neurons making type 2 contacts. This neuron variety appears to make type 1 contacts and may contain the vasointestinal polypeptide (VIP) (Emson and Lindvall, 1979; Loren *et al.*, 1979; Sims *et al.*, 1980). The cell body, however, resembles the other classes of smooth dendritic neurons in bearing both type 1 and type 2 contacts (see Chapter 11).

The activity of the interneurons with axons making type 2 contacts on the spiny stellate neurons is likely to be a crucial element in the overall activity of the stratum. These neurons, as well as the spiny stellate neurons, have been shown to be a target of thalamic axon synapses (Peters *et al.*, 1979; White, 1980); their relative infrequency in the stratum means that, even with some degree of overlap of their axons, each such neuron exerts control over a group of spiny stellate neurons, effectively dividing the population of spiny neurons into small subgroups.

7. Development of Spiny Stellate Neurons

The developmental origin of the spiny stellate neurons has so far only been defined in terms of their place in a gradient of generation time of cerebral cortex neurons. As shown by thymidine labeling studies (Angevine and Sidman, 1961; Rakic, 1975), the first generated cortical neurons lie deepest in the neuropil of the cortical gray matter in the adult, and successively later-generated neurons, which migrate through them, lie more and more superficial, until the last gen-

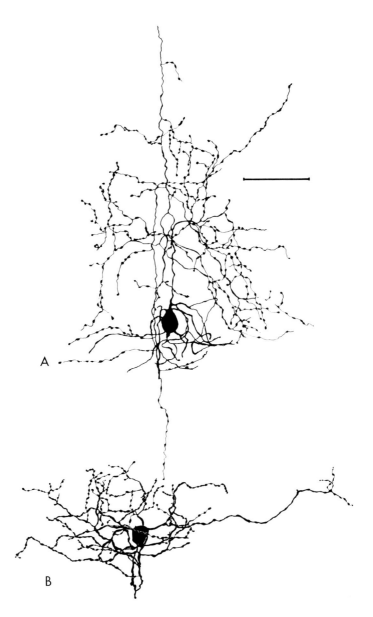

Figure 28. Examples of a particularly abundant smooth dendritic cell type seen in macaque (cell A) and tree shrew (cell B). These neurons obey the laminar boundaries of single subdivisions of the spiny stellate stratum and appear to provide much of the inhibitory control for the spiny stellate neurons. They comprise less than 5% of the neuron population whereas the spiny stellate neurons comprise at least 90% of the neurons of the layer. Scale bar = 50 μm. (A) reproduced from Lund (1973) with permission.

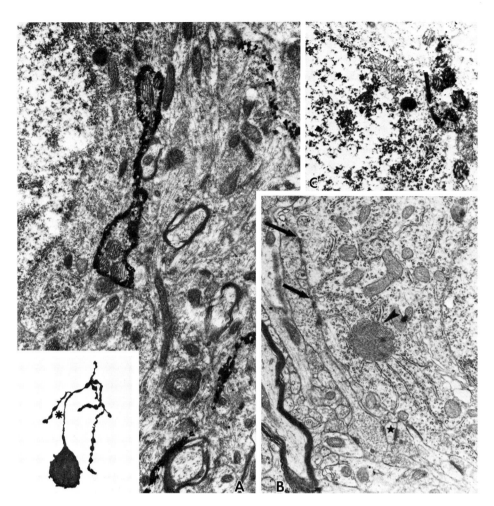

Figure 29. (A) Electron micrograph of a gold-toned Golgi-impregnated neuron (inset: initial portion of axon and soma) of the variety shown in Fig. 28A, from macaque monkey visual cortex, lamina 4C. This variety of neuron contributes type 2, probably inhibitory, synaptic contacts to the cell bodies and dendritic shafts of the spinous stellate neurons of the lamina. Magnification × 16,400. (B) Arrow points to symmetric, type 2, synapse between gold-toned bouton and spinous stellate neuron soma of neuron shown in (A). (C) Conventional EM material from lamina 4Cβ. Arrows point to type 2 synapses. Star: spine receiving both type 1 and type 2 synapses. Arrow: cytoplasmic inclusion body. Magnification × 21,000. Reproduced from Mates and Lund (1983) with permission.

erated neurons are found in lamina 2 closest to the pia (layer I has few cells and is present as the marginal zone at the earliest stages of development; see Chapter 14). The precursors of the spiny stellate neurons therefore undergo their final division in the middle period of this generative sequence [Rakic (1975) provides information on the timing of last divisions and migration of the neuron populations of the macaque monkey striate cortex]. It is unknown if these cells are derived from a particular stem population of generative cells, if they represent a particular stage in the sequence of division of generative cells, or whether their

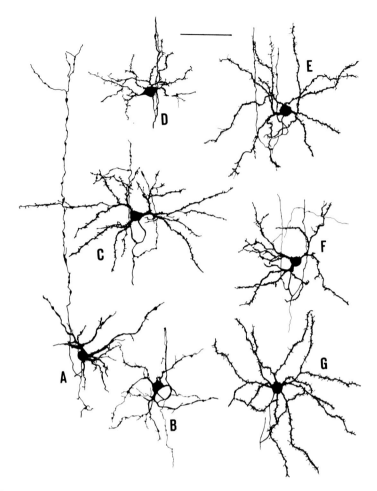

Figures 30–31. Developmental sequence of spiny stellate neurons in lamina 4Cβ of macaque monkey visual cortex. Drawings from Golgi preparations of visual cortex from a series of pre- and postnatal ages: (A, B) E127; (C, D) E145; (E) E156; (F, G) birth; (H) 3 months; (I, J) 9 months; (K, L) adult. A gradual sequence of acquisition of dendritic spines can be seen to occur, particularly postnatally (H–J), but the adult neuron (K, L) is clearly much spine poorer than the infant. See Fig. 34 for a quantitative assessment of this change in spine populations. Scale bars = 50 μm. Reproduced from Lund *et al.* (1977) with permission.

final characteristics are determined during migration or on arrival in final position in midcortical depth. Interaction with the cortical environment may well determine their morphology, but their stellate form and other characteristics are evident in their earliest growth phase following migration (Lund and Boothe, 1975). It is clear in at least the primate that the boundaries of their stratum of occurrence are much more sharply defined than the distribution of neurons according to generation time, suggesting cortical environment may play a decisive role in their final pattern of distribution (see Lund, 1973; Rakic, 1975).

The relative numbers of spiny stellate neurons and smooth dendritic neu-

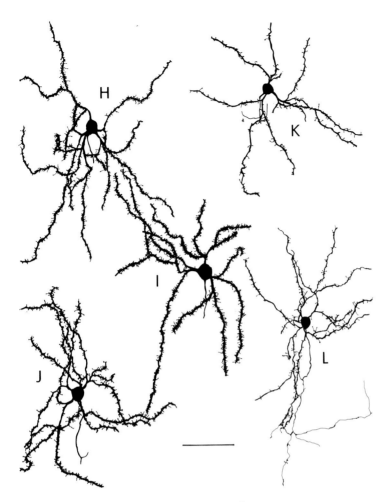

Figure 31. *(continued)*

rons seems to be determined early in development, probably during generation, and these two groups can be distinguished as soon as synaptic development gets under way by the different patterns of synaptic contacts on their somata (Mates, 1981; Mates and Lund, 1983a). As mentioned earlier, the spiny stellate neuron has only type 2 contacts in relatively low numbers on its cell body, while the smooth dendritic neuron has both type 1 and type 2 contacts in large numbers on the soma. The dendritic surface of the spiny stellate neuron develops its population of spines as a gradual process (Figs. 30–32), which can include both pre- and postnatal periods depending on the relative developmental rate of the species considered (Morest, 1969; Lund *et al.*, 1977). Particularly marked phases of rapid addition of spines occur postnatally, or when the eyes open to visual stimulation in the case of the visual cortex (Valverde, 1968; Lund *et al.*, 1977;

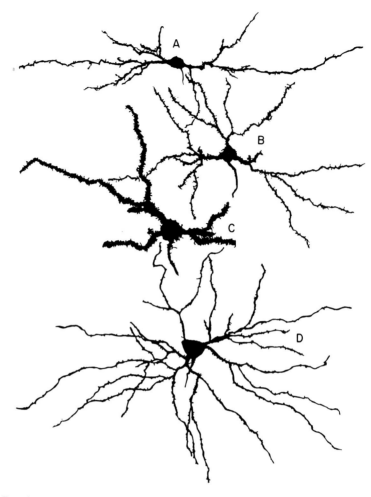

Figure 32. Drawings of Golgi-impregnated neurons during maturation from lamina 4B of macaque monkey visual cortex. A dramatic increase in dendritic spine populations occurs in the young postnatal animal, but many of these synapse-bearing processes are lost as the neuron matures. Ages of animals: (A) E145; (B) E156; (C) 3 months postnatal (incompletely drawn); (D) adult. Scale bar = 50 μm. Reproduced from Lund *et al.* (1977) with permission.

Figure 33. Electron micrographs illustrating the suggested sequence of spine formation on spiny stellate neurons of lamina 4C of macaque monkey primary visual cortex. (A) Type 1 synaptic contact onto dendrite (asterisk); animal 1 week old. (B) Type 1 synapses surrounding "bulge" on dendrite (asterisk). This portion of the dendrite now contains flocculent material characteristic of mature spine cytoplasm; animal 1 week old. (C) Continuation of spine (asterisk) development; animal 1 week old. (D) Mature spine (asterisk) receiving a type 1 synapse. Magnification × 22,000. Reproduced from Mates and Lund (1983) with permission.

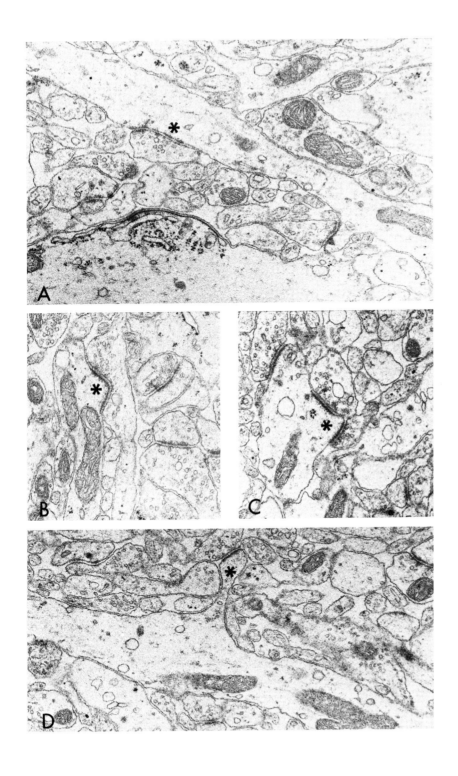

Boothe *et al.*, 1979). Following this phase of spine acquisition, even in normal development, dendritic development is then characterized by a loss of some proportion of these spines, particularly during the later postnatal developmental period, to reach a more stable adult spine population.

It appears that the outgrowth of the dendritic spine is triggered by the formation of a type 1 synaptic contact directly onto the dendritic shaft of the young neuron (Mates, 1981; Mates and Lund, 1983b). The dendritic membrane responds to the contact by an outgrowth from the region contacted and the type 1 synapse is carried out with the region which then forms the spine process (Fig. 33). It is unclear why the type 2 contacts on the same dendritic shafts do not elicit a similar spine outgrowth. Some of the type 2 contacts appear to get caught up in the outgrowth and are carried out along the spine membrane, for they are occasionally found on the spine tip, shaft, or base, always accompanied by a type 1 contact on the spine tip. However, they commonly remain on the main dendritic shaft and soma. In the macaque monkey visual cortex, where the development of these neurons has been studied in detail (Boothe *et al.*, 1979), the formation of spines (and therefore of type 1 synapses) accelerates after birth and a peak population of spines is seen on these neurons by 5–12 weeks of age. The rate of addition of new spines and the total population generated varies in the spiny stellate neuron population and seems to depend on the laminar subdivision of the stratum in which the neurons are found (Fig. 34). The different rates probably reflect the relative rate of maturation and synapse formation of

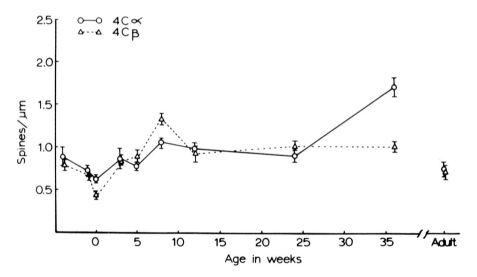

Figure 34. Changes in the average number of spines per micrometer on the dendrites of spiny stellate neurons in laminae 4Cα and 4Cβ of the macaque monkey striate visual cortex in a series of immature animals and in the adult. It is clear that a rapid increase in spine numbers occurs on these neurons between birth and 8 weeks of age. There is also a marked decrease in number of spines by the time the animal is mature. The progression of spine acquisition and loss also seems to differ between different subdivisions (here 4Cα and 4Cβ) of the spiny stellate neuron stratum. Reproduced from Boothe *et al.* (1979) with permission.

different populations of thalamic axon synapses, as well as input from maturing axon collaterals from pyramidal neurons in lamina 6 and intrinsic projections of the axons of the spiny neurons themselves. As noted earlier, a certain proportion of these spine synapses do not survive; both pre- and postsynaptic elements may detach from one another and undergo apparent atrophy and loss (Mates, 1981; Mates and Lund, 1983b). Figure 35 shows examples of this phenomenon from the macaque primary visual cortex, lamina 4C. The attrition of these contacts is seen by light microscopy as a gradually diminishing population of spines on the dendrites of the spiny stellate neurons. It is possible that this loss of synaptic contacts during development represents a refinement of the synaptic inputs to the neuron and is reflected in the sensitivity of the visual cortex to interruption of visual input during the early postnatal period (Wiesel and Hubel, 1965; Baker *et al.*, 1974; Crawford *et al.*, 1975; Hubel *et al.*, 1977). A sequence of acquisition and loss of spines is seen also in the pyramidal neuron populations of other laminae. The different time course of spine acquisition and loss seen on the spiny stellate neurons in the α and β subdivisions of lamina 4C of the monkey is reflected in similarly differing time courses of this same process occurring on pyramidal neurons of lamina 6 (Fig. 36). These neurons are differentially associated with the α and β divisions via both apical dendritic extensions and recurrent axons abors (see Figs. 18, 19B). The process of overproduction of synaptic contacts and subsequent loss of a certain proportion of synapses during maturation of the spiny stellate neuron is reminiscent of the process of synapse formation and loss at the neuromuscular junction during maturation (e.g., Brown *et al.*, 1976; Diamond, 1982). This also seems to reflect a refinement of functional links influenced by the early afferent activity of the system affecting both pre- and postsynaptic processes.

In the same maturational period that spines and their synapses are undergoing marked changes in number, there is also an increase and subsequent decrease in the population of type 2 contacts on the spiny stellate neuron cell bodies (Mates, 1981; Mates and Lund, 1983c). However, no sign of death or atrophy of these contacts has been detected to explain their decrease in number. After calculating the effects of the various changing volumetric relationships of the developing neuropil (expanding distance between cell bodies, changes in size and number of contact sites over time, and changes in size of the postsynaptic cell bodies), it is concluded that the apparent reduction in number of type 2 contacts (Fig. 37) on the spiny neuron cell bodies is due to redistribution of the contacts, probably to dendritic surfaces, rather than loss. The type 2 axon arbors of the smooth dendritic neurons retain a more or less constant volume in this postnatal period while the distance between neuron somata increases as the neuropil expands. It appears therefore that the spiny neuron cell bodies are drawn out of range of a certain proportion of type 2 axon arbors and these displaced contacts are either drawn out along the dendritic shafts or shift their contact site to other elements in the neuropil. It is concluded that the type 2 contacts increase in number to their final adult population in the postnatal period. Changes may then occur in their locus but probably not in overall numbers. The physiological consequences of these maturational changes in locus of type 2 synaptic populations on the spiny neurons have not been investigated.

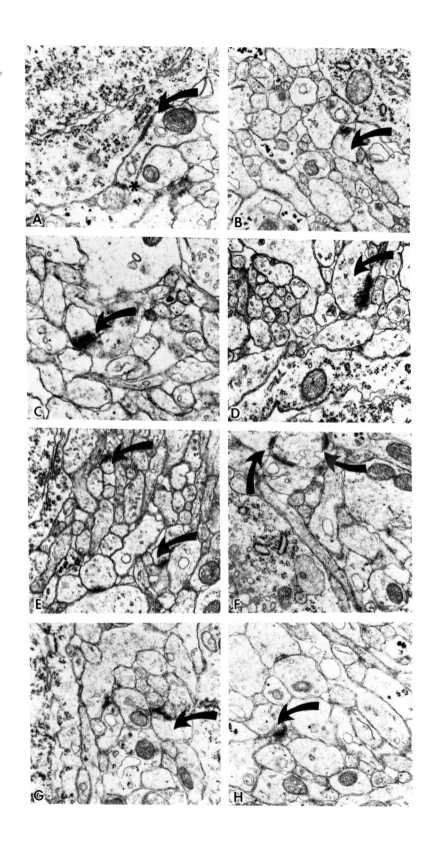

Disturbance of the sensory input during this critical postnatal phase of development reveals the importance of afferent information to the subsequent organization of the stratum of spiny stellate neurons. In the somatosensory cortex rodent vibrissal representation, it is found that the striking barrellike arrays of these neurons seen in the adult cortex develop postnatally (Rice and Van der Loos, 1977). Following removal of certain of the vibrissal skin follicles at birth, the "barrels" in the cortex representing the damaged vibrissae fail to develop and, instead, a small area of uniformly distributed neurons is seen (Van der Loos and Woolsey, 1973). As the counterpart to this is the finding that if the animal develops with an aberrant extra vibrissa, a new "barrel" develops to accommodate it at a cortical level. These findings imply that the afferents to the spiny stellate stratum govern the development of laterally parcellated organization within the stratum. As was mentioned earlier in the chapter, a similar phenomenon occurs in the visual cortex of Old World primates. Here, thalamic afferents relaying information from the right and left eye form an alternating, segregated, stripelike distribution (Wiesel *et al.*, 1974; Hubel and Wiesel, 1977). These axon territories are not apparently reflected in striking patterns of cell distribution or dendritic arbors of the postsynaptic neurons to the degree seen in the vibrissal representation of somatosensory cortex. However, it can be concluded from the results of physiological investigations (Hubel and Wiesel, 1977; Poggio and Fischer, 1977) that this afferent parcellation must be reflected functionally in the later relays of the axons of the postsynaptic spiny stellate neurons to create binocular neurons and disparity-sensitive cells. This parcellation of thalamic axons has been shown to derive from a competitive interaction between the thalamic axons, which initially overlap their territories, for acquisition of synaptic sites within the spiny stellate stratum (Hubel, 1975; LeVay *et al.*, 1981). Afferents deprived of normal visual input (e.g., by monocular eyelid closure) are at a competitive disadvantage and occupy narrow territorial stripes compared to the expanded territorial stripes of axons served by the normal undeprived eye (Fig. 38). The influence of the afferent activity is believed to be not only responsible for the maintenance of a juvenile, widely spreading, distribution of thalamic axons in these monocular deprivation experiments but it can also allow an active reacquisition of territory by axons that have already apparently completed segregation (LeVay *et al.*, 1981) amongst the spiny stellate neurons. This has been shown by examining the thalamic axon distribution after reversal of monocular suture, opening the sutured eye and closing the experienced eye.

←

Figure 35. Electron micrographs illustrating loss of type 1 synapses and dendritic spines as part of the normal process of spiny stellate neuron maturation. (A) Asterisk marks a dendrite receiving a type 1 synapse; the arrow points to an asymmetric postsynaptic thickening where the presynaptic axonal process has been replaced by a cell body. (B, C, E, H) Spines with glia or debris on the presynaptic side. (D, F) Presynaptic axons with debris on the postsynaptic side. (G) Two axon terminals sharing a single postsynaptic thickening. (Magnification × 20,000.) Age of animal: (A) 8 week of age; (B, D, E, F) 5 weeks of age; (C, G, H) 3 weeks of age. Reproduced from Mates and Lund (1982b) with permission.

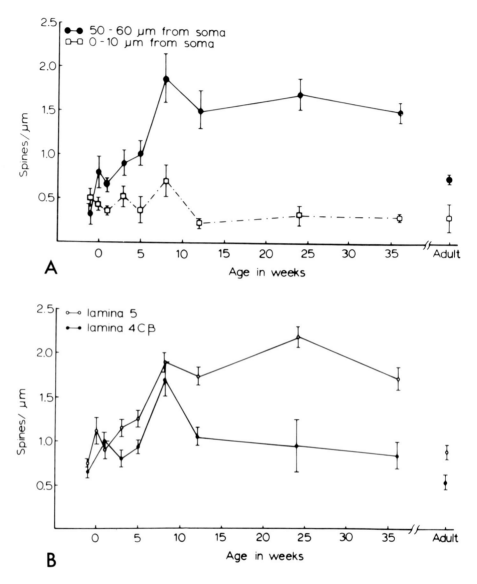

Figure 36. Spine acquisition and loss during maturation on the dendrites of pyramidal neurons in upper lamina 6 of macaque monkey striate cortex. (A) Spine frequency on the basal dendrites within lamina 6 as a function of age. Two separate curves are shown, one for counts on segments 0–10 μm from the soma and the other for counts on segments 50–60 μm from the soma. Error bars are ± 1 S.E.M. computed across individual neurons. (B) Spine frequency on the apical dendrites as a function of the lamina in which the dendritic segment is found (here laminae 5 and 4Cβ). Error bars as in (A). It is noticeable that spine acquisition and loss follows a different sequence depending on laminar environment and that the sequence within the stratum of spiny stellate neurons (4Cβ) differs from either basal dendrites or the lamina 5 apical dendritic segment. Reproduced from Boothe *et al.* (1979) with permission.

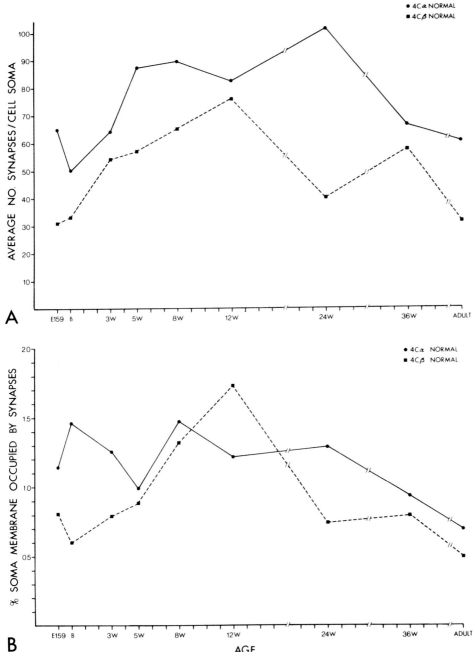

Figure 37. Changes in number of type 2 synaptic contacts on the cell bodies of spiny stellate neurons in laminae 4Cα and 4Cβ in the macaque monkey striate cortex during maturation. (A) The average number of type 2 synaptic contacts on each soma from embryonic day 159 to postnatal maturity. (B) The percentage of the total surface area of somal membrane occupied by type 2 contacts during maturation. While marked increase and decrease is seen in the numbers of these contacts during maturation, it is believed that the later reduction in number to the adult is due to a redistribution of these contacts, probably to the dendrites of the same neurons. Reproduced from Mates and Lund (1983c) with permission.

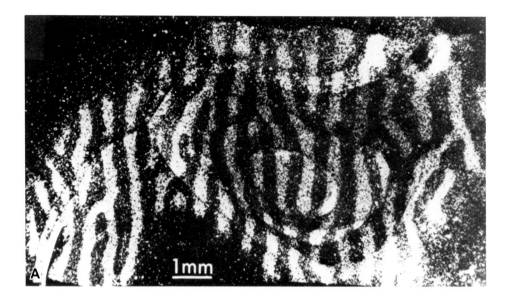

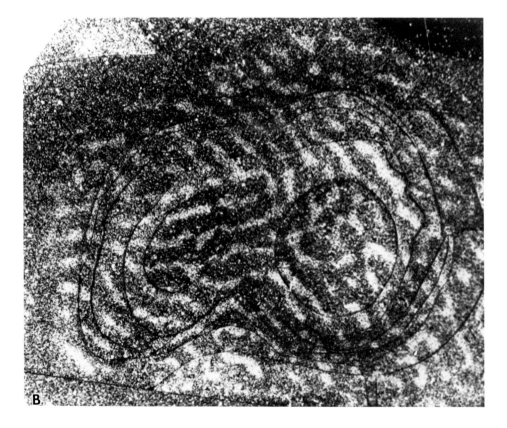

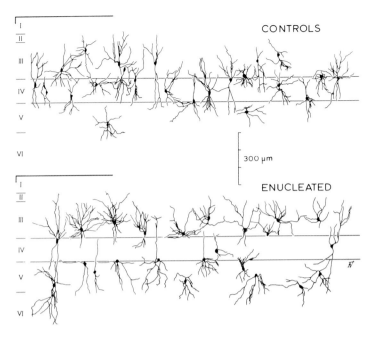

CONTROLS

300 μm

ENUCLEATED

Figure 39. Composite drawing of spiny stellate neurons with ascending axons in the area striata from mice aged 48 days. Stellate neurons in normal mice appear with bodies and dendrites distributed randomly through layers V, IV, and III (controls). In mice enucleated at birth, the orientation of dendrites outside layer IV is evident (enucleated). The axons were not traced. Golgi method. Reproduced from Valverde (1968) with permission.

While the thalamic fibers have considerable influence on the structural organization of the stratum, the spiny stellate neurons continue to occupy the same stratum of cortex even if all afferents are removed by lesions early in development (Valverde, 1968; Van der Loos and Dörfl, 1978). They may, however, reflect deafferentation or deprivation of input in a variety of ways including a reorientation of their dendrites into neighboring laminae (Fig. 39), apparently seeking new afferents (Valverde, 1968), a dispersion of ribosomes or granular endoplasmic reticulum in their cytoplasm (LeVay, 1977; Haseltine *et al.*, 1979), and changes in spine populations on their dendrites (Boothe *et al.*, 1979).

←—————————————————————————————

Figure 38. (A) Reconstruction of serial tangential radioautograms illustrating stripelike pattern of the relays from a single eye into layer 4C of the normal macaque monkey visual cortex. (For further details see Fig. 23.) (B) Reconstruction of serial tangential radioautograms from layer 4C of the visual cortex in a macaque monkey with its right eyelids sutured closed from age 3 weeks to 7 months. The right, deprived, eye was injected with tritiated proline–fucose mixture. The reconstruction is made up from seven serial sections with total depth of 640 μm. The labeled, bright, stripelike territories of the relays from the closed eye are markedly shrunken compared to the normal (A). Reproduced from Hubel *et al.* (1977) with permission.

9. Function of the Spiny Stellate Neuron

The function of the spiny stellate neuron population in the various sensory areas of the neocortex is poorly understood. This function is not simply a direct relationship to thalamic inputs, since only certain of the thalamic fiber populations terminate amongst them, while other populations are excluded, terminating in other laminae. They must therefore be concerned with processing particular kinds of input, and the physiological transformation of this information and its subsequent relay to other elements of the cortical neuropil becomes of great interest. It has been proposed both in somatosensory cortex and in visual cortex that the numerical relationships between the afferent fibers and the postsynaptic stellate neuron populations may have important functional consequences (Kerwin and Woolsey, 1975; Barlow, 1979). Certainly in both these areas the more numerous the afferent fiber population, the more numerous the postsynaptic neuron population in the lamina of termination. The densely packed cells of the granular layer, 4Cβ, of the macaque spiny stellate stratum, which is postsynaptic to axons with very small arbors arising from the parvocellular laminae of the lateral geniculate nucleus (Hubel and Wiesel, 1972; Blasdel and Lund, 1983), appear to outnumber their afferent neuron population by at least 30 to 1 (see Barlow, 1981). Barlow (1979, 1981) has suggested that this is a device restoring a fine-grain version of the visual image sufficient to provide the basis for vernier acuity observed behaviorally, but not achieved at the level of the opic fiber input. However, the representation of sensory surfaces in the cortical neuropil at the level of the spiny stellate neuron stratum certainly presents other puzzles. The dimensions of the spread of single afferent terminal fields (compare Figs. 20 and 22) and their frequency against the packing density and dendritic spread of the postsynaptic neurons may well be extremely important in this transformation, but much further work is needed before we can define the nature of the change and the anatomical substrate for it.

The correlation of lamination and morphology of cortical neurons with physiological properties in the visual cortex has indicated that the spiny stellate neuron often reflects many of the properties of the thalamic inputs impinging on them (Hubel and Wiesel, 1962, 1968). However, in some instances a major transformation of properties can occur even within the spiny stellate stratum. This is shown in primary visual cortex where some such neurons in the cat have been identified as "simple" cells (Gilbert and Wiesel, 1979). For these cells (Figs. 40, 41), specific line orientation becomes a crucial element in the visual stimulus eliciting a response from the neuron. This differs sharply from the thalamic input neurons for which line orientation is immaterial. However, the properties of the "simple" cell are not found uniquely in the spiny stellate stratum or in this cell type. Pyramidal and smooth dendritic neurons of layers 3 and 6 have been shown to have simple cell properties (Kelly and Van Essen, 1974; Gilbert and Wiesel, 1979) and, moreover, populations of pyramidal neurons in layers 2–3 have been shown to have nonoriented circular receptive fields like those of the spiny stellate neurons of layer 4 in macaque (Hubel and Livingston, 1981). It must be concluded, therefore, that the properties of the postsynaptic cells so far described correlate more with their relationship to direct thalamic input than to stellate or pyramidal morphology. Physiological properties that seem to re-

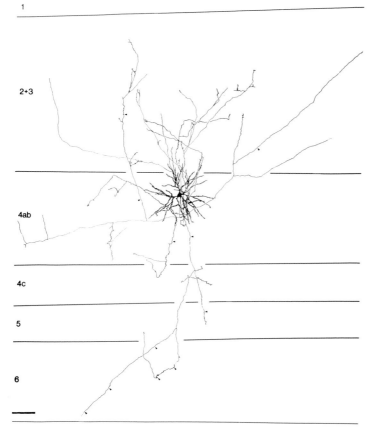

Figure 40. A spiny stellate neuron from layer 4ab of cat striate cortex. The cell was identified and characterized physiologically and then intracellularly filled with HRP. The drawing is made from the cell after the brain was sectioned and prepared histologically. The neuron had a "simple" receptive field with on-center and off-flanks. The arrows indicate the position of nodes of Ranvier. Scale bar = 100 μm. Reproduced from Gilbert and Wiesel (1979) with permission.

quire greater correlation of different thalamic inputs, such as are seen in the complex cell type of the visual cortex, have not been correlated with spiny stellate neuron morphology, but have been identified as a property of cells in laminae rich in pyramidal neurons deep and superficial to the spiny stellate stratum (Hubel and Wiesel, 1962, 1968; Gilbert and Wiesel, 1979).

10. Summary

This survey of the organization of the spiny stellate neuron strata points out the key position occupied by these neurons at the interface between major components of thalamic input and cerebral cortex. The elaborate structuring of this relationship between particular thalamic axon populations and cortical neu-

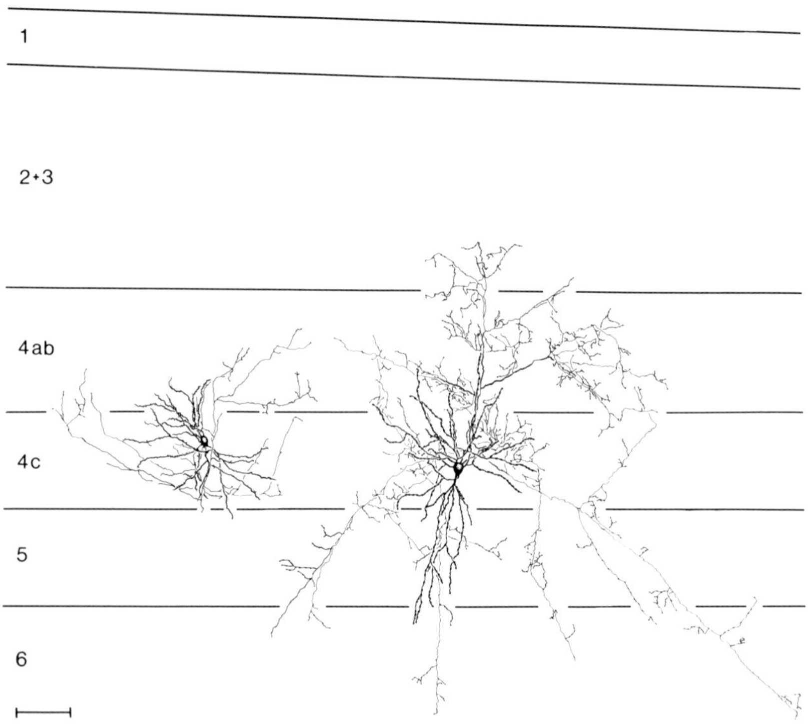

Figure 41. A spiny stellate cell (left) and a smooth dendritic stellate cell (right) in layer 4c of cat striate cortex. Preparation as in Fig. 40. Both neurons had "simple" receptive fields with on-center and off-flanks. Scale bar = 100 μm. Reproduced from Gilbert and Wiesel (1979) with permission.

ropil, and the sensitivity of this relationship to early afferent activity is particularly striking. It is clear that not only does a new synthesis of sensory information occur within the stratum but, in turn, the subdivisions of the stratum each pass on this information in orderly and discrete fashion as a series of relays to the adjoining cortical neuropil superficial and deep to the stratum. It is these relays that must lay the basis for many of the amazing functional capabilities of the cortex.

11. References

Angevine, J. B., Jr., and Sidman, R. L., 1961, Autoradiographic study of cell migration during histogenesis of cerebral cortex in the mouse, *Nature (London)* **192:**766–768.

Baker, F. H., Gregg, P., and Von Noorden, G. K., 1974, Effects of visual deprivation and strabismus on the response of neurons in the visual cortex of the monkey, including studies on the striate and prestriate cortex in the normal animal, *Brain Res.* **66:**185–208.

Barlow, H. B., 1979, Reconstructing the visual image in space and time, *Nature (London)* **279:**189–190.

Barlow, H. B., 1981, Critical limiting factors in the design of the eye and visual cortex, *Proc. R. Soc. London Ser. B* **212:**1–34.

Blasdel, G. G., and Lund, J. S., 1982, Physiological and morphological analysis of afferent axons in thalamo-recipient laminae of macaque striate cortex, *Soc. Neurosci. Abstr.* **8:**705.

Blasdel, G. G., and Lund, J. S., 1983, Termination of afferent axons in macaque striate cortex, *J. Neurosci.* **3:**1389–1413.

Boothe, R. G., Greenough, W. T., Lund, J. S., and Wrege, K., 1979, A quantitative investigation of spine and dendrite development of neurons in visual cortex (area 17) of *Macaca nemestrina* monkeys, *J. Comp. Neurol.* **186:**473–490.

Brown, M. C., Jansen, K. S., and Van Essen, D., 1976, Polyneuronal innervation of skeletal muscle in newborn rats and its elimination during maturation, *J. Physiol. (London)* **261:**387–422.

Carey, R. G., Bear, M. F., and Diamond, I. T., 1980, The laminar organization of the reciprocal projections between the claustrum and striate cortex in the tree shrew, *Tupaia glis, Brain Res.* **184:**193–198.

Casagrande, V. A., and Harting, J. K., 1975, Transneuronal transport of tritiated fucose and proline in the visual pathway of the tree shrew *Tupaia glis, Brain Res.* **96:**367–372.

Colonnier, M., 1968, Synaptic patterns on different cell types in the different laminae of the cat visual cortex: An electron microscope study, *Brain Res.* **9:**268–287.

Conley, M., Fitzpatrick, D., and Diamond, I. T., 1984, The projection of individual layers of the lateral geniculate nucleus to striate cortex in the tree shrew, *J. Neurosci.* **4** (in press).

Crawford, M. L., Blake, J. R., Cool, S. J., and Von Noorden, G. K., 1975, Physiological consequences of unilateral and bilateral eyelid closure in macaque monkeys: Some further observations, *Brain Res.* **84:**150–154.

Diamond, J., 1982, The patterning of neuronal connections, *Am. Zool.* **22:**154–172.

Emson, P. C., and Lindvall, O., 1979, Distribution of putative neuro-transmitters in the neocortex, *Neuroscience* **4:**1–30.

Fairén, A., and Valverde, F., 1980, A specialized type of neuron in the visual cortex of the cat: A Golgi and electron microscope study of chandelier cells, *J. Comp. Neurol.* **194:**761–779.

Ferster, D., and LeVay, S., 1978, The axonal arborizations of lateral geniculate neurons in the striate cortex of the cat, *J. Comp. Neurol.* **182:**923–944.

Fisken, R. A., Garey, L. J., and Powell, T. P. S., 1975, The intrinsic association and commissural connections of area 17 of the visual cortex, *Philos. Trans. R. Soc. London Ser. B* **272:**487–536.

Fitzpatrick, D., Itoh, K., and Diamond, I. T., 1982, The laminar organization of the lateral geniculate body and the striate cortex in the squirrel monkey *(Saimiri sciureus)*, *J. Neurosci.* **3:**673–702.

Gilbert, C. D., and Kelly, J. P., 1975, The projections of cells in different layers of the cat's visual cortex, *J. Comp. Neurol.* **163:**81–106.

Gilbert, C. D., and Wiesel, T. N., 1979, Morphology and intracortical projections of functionally characterized neurons in the cat visual cortex, *Nature (London)* **280:**120–125.

Gray, E. G., 1959, Axosomatic and axodendritic synapses of the cerebral cortex, *J. Anat.* **93:**420–433.

Harting, J. K., Diamond, I. T., and Hall, W. C., 1973, Anterograde degeneration study of the cortical projections of the lateral geniculate and pulvinar nuclei in the tree shrew *(Tupaia glis)*, *J. Comp. Neurol.* **150:**393–440.

Haseltine, E. C., DeBruyn, E. J., and Casagrande, V. A., 1979, Demonstration of ocular dominance columns in Nissl-stained sections of monkey visual cortex following enucleation, *Brain Res.* **176:**153–158.

Hendrickson, A. E., and Wilson, J. R., 1979, A difference in ^{14}C deoxyglucose autoradiographic patterns in striate cortex between *Macaca* and *Saimiri* monkeys following monocular stimulation, *Brain Res.* **170:**353–358.

Hendrickson, A. E., Wilson, J. R., and Ogren, M. P., 1978, The neuroanatomical organization of pathways between dorsal lateral geniculate nucleus and visual cortex in Old and New World primates, *J. Comp. Neurol.* **182:**123–136.

Hornung, J. P., and Garey, L. J., 1981, Ultrastructure of visual callosal neurons in cat identified by retrograde axonal transport of horseradish peroxidase, *J. Neurocytol.* **10:**297–314.

Horton, J. C., and Hubel, D. H., 1981, Regular patchy distribution of cytochrome-oxidase staining in primary visual cortex of macaque monkey, *Nature (London)* **292:**762–764.

Hubel, D. H., 1975, An autoradiographic study of the retino-cortical projections in the tree shrew, *(Tupaia glis), Brain Res.* **96:**41–50.

Hubel, D. H., and Livingston, M. S., 1981, Regions of poor orientation tuning coincide with patches of cytochrome oxidase staining in monkey striate cortex, *Soc. Neurosci. Abstr.* **7:**357.

Hubel, D. H., and Wiesel, T. N., 1962, Receptive fields, binocular interaction, and functional architecture in the cat's visual cortex, *J. Physiol (London)* **160:**106–154.

Hubel, D. H., and Wiesel, T. N., 1968, Receptive fields and functional architecture of monkey striate cortex, *J. Physiol. (London)* **196:**215–243.

Hubel, D. H., and Wiesel, T. N., 1972, Laminar and columnar distribution of geniculo-cortical fibers in the macaque monkey, *J. Comp. Neurol.* **146:**421–450.

Hubel, D. H., and Wiesel, T. N., 1977, Functional architecture of macaque monkey visual cortex, *Proc. R. Soc. London Ser. B* **198:**1–59.

Hubel, D. H., Wiesel, T. N., and LeVay, S., 1977, Plasticity of ocular dominance columns in monkey striate cortex. *Philos. Trans. R. Soc. London Ser. B* **278:**377–410.

Hubel, D. H., Wiesel, T. N., and Stryker, M. P., 1978, Anatomical demonstration of orientation columns in macaque monkey, *J. Comp. Neurol.* **177:**361–379.

Humphrey, A. L., and Hendrickson, A. E., 1983, Background and stimulus-induced patterns of high metabolic activity in the visual cortex (area 17) of the squirrel and macaque monkey, *J. Neurosci.* **3:**345–358.

Humphrey, A. L., and Lund, J. S., 1979, Anatomical organization of layer IV in tree shrew striate cortex (area 17): Evidence for two sublaminae, *Soc. Neurosci. Abstr.* **5:**789.

Jones, E. G., 1975, Varieties and distribution of non-pyramidal cells in the somatic sensory cortex of the squirrel monkey, *J. Comp. Neurol.* **160:**205–268.

Kelly, J. P., and Van Essen, D. C., 1974, Cell structure and function in the visual cortex of the cat, *J. Physiol. (London)* **238:**515–547.

Kerwin, J. L., and Woolsey, T. A., 1975, A proportional relationship between peripheral innervation density and cortical neuron number in the somatosensory cortex of the mouse, *Brain Res.* **99:**349–353.

LeVay, S., 1973, Synaptic patterns in the visual cortex of the cat and monkey: Electron microscopy of Golgi preparations, *J. Comp. Neurol.* **150:**53–86.

LeVay, S., 1977, Effects of visual deprivation on polyribosome aggregation in visual cortex of the cat, *Brain Res.* **119:**73–86.

LeVay, S., and Gilbert, C. D., 1976, Laminar patterns of geniculocortical projection in the cat, *Brain Res.* **113:**1–19.

LeVay, S., and Sherk, H., 1981, The visual claustrum of the cat. I. Structure and connections, *J. Neurosci.* **1:**956–980.

LeVay, S., Wiesel, T. N., and Hubel, D. H., 1981, The development of ocular dominance columns in normal and visually deprived monkeys, *J. Comp. Neurol.* **191:**1–51.

Loren, I., Emson, P. C., Fahrenkrug, J., Björklund, A., Alumets, J., Håkanson, R. P., and Sundler, F., 1979, Distribution of vasoactive intestinal polypeptide in rat and mouse brain, *Neuroscience* **4:**1953–1976.

Lorente de Nó, R., 1938, Cerebral cortex: Architecture, intracortical connections, motor projections, in: *Physiology of the Nervous System* (J. F. Fulton, ed.), 2nd ed., pp. 288–313, Oxford University Press, London.

Lund, J. S., 1973, Organization of neurons in the visual cortex, area 17, of the monkey *(Macaca mulatta)*, *J. Comp. Neurol.* **147:**455–496.

Lund, J. S., and Boothe, R., 1975, Interlaminar connections and pyramidal neuron organization in the visual cortex, area 17, of the macaque monkey, *J. Comp. Neurol.* **159:**305–334.

Lund, J. S., and Lund, R. D., 1970, The termination of callosal fibers in the paravisual cortex of the rat, *Brain Res.* **17:**25–45.

Lund, J. S., Lund, R. D., Hendrickson, A. E., Bunt, A. H., and Fuchs, A. F., 1975, The origin of efferent pathways from the primary visual cortex, area 17, of the macaque monkey, *J. Comp. Neurol.* **164:**287–304.

Lund, J. S., Boothe, R. G., and Lund, R. D., 1977, Development of neurons in the visual cortex of the monkey *(Macaca nemestrina)*: A Golgi study from fetal day 127 to postnatal maturity, *J. Comp. Neurol.* **176:**149–188.

Lund, J. S., Henry, G. H., MacQueen, C. L., and Harvey, A. R., 1979, Anatomical organization of the visual cortex of the cat: A comparison with area 17 of the macaque monkey, *J. Comp. Neurol.* **184:**559–618.

Lund, J. S., Hendrickson, A. E., Ogren, M. P., and Tobin, E. A., 1981, Anatomical organization of primate visual cortex, area VII, *J. Comp. Neurol.* **202:**19–45.

Mates, S., 1981, Neuronal maturation and synapse formation in layer 4 of macaque striate cortex, Ph.D. thesis, University of Washington, Seattle.

Mates, S. L., and Lund, J. S., 1983a, Neuronal composition and development in lamina 4C of monkey striate cortex, *J. Comp. Neurol.* **221**:60–90.

Mates, S. L., and Lund, J. S., 1983b, Developmental changes in the relationship between type 1 synapses and spiny neurons in the monkey visual cortex, *J. Comp. Neurol.* **221**:91–97.

Mates, S. L., and Lund, J. S., 1983c, Developmental changes in the relationship between type 2 synapses and spiny neurons in the monkey visual cortex, *J. Comp. Neurol.* **221**:98–105.

Meyer, G., and Albus, K., 1981, Spiny stellates as cells of origin of association fibers from area 17 to area 18 in the cat's neocortex, *Brain Res.* **210**:335–341.

Morest, D. K., 1969, The growth of dendrites in the mammalian brain, *Z. Anat. Entwicklungsgesch.* **138**:290–317.

O'Leary, J. L., 1941, Structure of the area striata of the cat, *J. Comp. Neurol.* **75**:131–161.

Peters, A., and Kimerer, L. M., 1981, Bipolar neurons in rat visual cortex: A combined Golgi–electron microscope study, *J. Neurocytol.* **10**:921–946.

Peters, A., Proskauer, C. C., Feldman, M. L., and Kimerer, L., 1979, The projection of the lateral geniculate nucleus to area 17 of the rat cerebral cortex. V. Degenerating axon terminals synapsing with Golgi impregnated neurons, *J. Neurocytol.* **8**:331–357.

Poggio, G. F., and Fischer, B., 1977, Binocular interaction and depth sensitivity in striate and prestriate cortex of behaving rhesus monkey, *J. Neurophysiol.* **40**:1392–1406.

Rakic, P., 1975, Timing of major autogenetic events in the visual cortex of the rhesus money, in: *Brain Mechanisms in Mental Retardation* (N. A. Buchwald and M. Brazier, eds.), pp. 3–40, Academic Press, New York.

Rice, F. L., and Van der Loos, H., 1977, Development of the barrels and barrel field in the somatosensory cortex of the mouse, *J. Comp. Neurol.* **171**:545–560.

Rockland, K. S., and Lund, J. S., 1982, Lattice-like intrinsic neural connections in primate striate visual cortex, *Soc. Neurosci. Abstr.* **8**:706.

Rockland, K. S., and Lund, J. S., 1983, Intrinsic laminar lattice connections in primate visual cortex, *J. Comp. Neurol.* **216**:303–318.

Sims, K. B., Hoffman, D. L., Said, S. I., and Zimmerman, E. A., 1980, Vasoactive intestinal polypeptide (VIP) in mouse and rat brain: A immunocytological study, *Brain Res.* **186**:165–183.

Somogyi, P., 1977, A specific axo-axonal neuron in the visual cortex of the rat, *Brain Res.* **136**:345–350.

Somogyi, P., Freund, T. F., Halasz, N., and Kisvarday, Z. F., 1981a, Selectivity of neuronal [³H]-GABA accumulation in the visual cortex as revealed by Golgi staining of the labelled neurons, *Brain Res.* **225**:431–436.

Somogyi, P., Cowey, A., Halasz, N., and Freund, T. F., 1981b, Vertical organization of neurones accumulating [³H]-GABA in visual cortex of rhesus monkey, *Nature (London)* **294**:761–763.

Spatz, W. B., 1977, Topographically organized reciprocal connections between areas 17 and MT (visual area of superior temporal sulcus) in the marmoset *Callithrix jacchus*, *Exp. Brain Res.* **27**:559–572.

Steffan, H., 1976, Golgi stained barrel-neurons in the somatosensory region of the mouse cerebral cortex, *Neurosci. Lett.* **2**:57–59.

Tigges, J., Tigges, M., Anschel, S., Cross, N. A., Ledbetter, W. D., and McBride, R. L., 1981, Areal and laminar distribution of neurons interconnecting the central visual cortical areas 17, 18, 19 and MT in squirrel monkey *(Saimiri)*, *J. Comp. Neurol.* **202**:539–560.

Valverde, F., 1968, Structural changes in the area striata of the mouse after enucleation, *Exp. Brain Res.* **5**:274–292.

Van der Loos, H., and Dörfl, J., 1978, Does the skin tell the somatosensory cortex how to construct a map of the periphery?, *Neurosci. Lett.* **7**:23–30.

Van der Loos, H., and Woolsey, T. A., 1973, Structural alterations following early injury to sense organs, *Science* **179**:395–398.

White, E. L., 1980, Thalamocortical synaptic relations: A review with emphasis on the projections of specific thalamic nuclei to the primary sensory areas of the neocortex, *Brain Res. Rev.* **1**:275–311.

Wiesel, T. N., and Hubel, D. H., 1965, Comparison of the effects of unilateral and bilateral eye closure on cortical unit responses in kittens, *J. Neurophysiol.* **28**:1029–1040.

Wiesel, T. N., Hubel, D. H., and Lam, D. M., 1974, Autoradiographic demonstration of ocular-dominance columns in the monkey striate cortex by means of transneuronal transport, *Brain Res.* **79**:273–279.

Winer, J. A., 1982, The stellate neurons in layer IV of primary auditory cortex (AI) of the cat: A study of columnar organization, *Soc. Neurosci. Abstr.* **8:**1020.

Woolsey, T. A., and Van der Loos, H., 1970, The structural organization of the mouse cerebral cortex: The description of a cortical field composed of discrete cytoarchitectonic units, *Brain Res.* **17:**205–242.

Woolsey, T. A., Dierker, M. L., and Wann, D. F., 1975a, Mouse SmI cortex: Qualitative and quantitative classification of Golgi-impregnated barrel neurons, *Proc. Natl. Acad. Sci. USA* **72:**2165–2169.

Woolsey, T. A., Welker, C., and Schwartz, R. H., 1975b, Comparative anatomical studies of the SmI face cortex with special reference to the occurrence of "barrels" in layer IV, *J. Comp. Neurol.* **164:**79–94.

8

Basket Cells

EDWARD G. JONES and STEWART H. C. HENDRY

1. Background

1.1. Ramón y Cajal

In his general account of the cerebral cortex, Ramón y Cajal (1911) remarked (p. 556) that he had discovered first in the visual cortex and later in the motor cortex some particularly abundant large cells with long horizontal axon collaterals in layer III. These he thought probably ended in pericellular nests of terminal branches ("nids pericellulaires") around the somata of pyramidal cells in layers II and IV.

The cells (Fig. 1) belonged to his category of "cellules a cylindre-axe court" and, along with his double bouquet cells, dominated layer III. As described by him they were star-shaped and voluminous, with extremely long, diverging dendrites having few or no spines. The axon initially ascended and though it might then arc downwards for a short distance, it quickly gave rise to many very long horizontal or oblique branches. Then, "après un trajet fort compliqué, ces longues branches se résolvent en arborisations qui embarassent étroitement le corps des cellules pyramidales et la racine de leurs grosses expansions protoplasmiques" (p. 557). These pericellular nests about the somata and proximal dendrites of layer III pyramidal cells, received branches of many horizontal axons and a single axon could contribute terminal branches to many nests. Each pericellular nest was comprised of many short varicose ramifications, the vari-

EDWARD G. JONES and STEWART H. C. HENDRY • James L. O'Leary Division of Experimental Neurology and Neurological Surgery and McDonnell Center for Studies of Higher Brain Function, Washington University School of Medicine, Saint Louis, Missouri 63110.

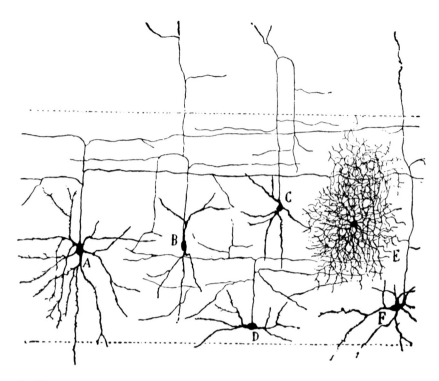

Figure 1. Figure 368 of Ramón y Cajal (1911) showing drawings of Golgi-impregnated cells from the motor cortex of a human infant. The cell somata are in what would now be called the deep part of layer III. Five of the cells (A–D, F) have ascending axons and horizontal axon collaterals though Ramón y Cajal chose to emphasize this feature only in regard to cells A and D.

cosities being directly applied to the membranes of the pyramidal cell soma (Fig. 2). Though invariably referring to the terminations as nests (nids), Ramón y Cajal repeatedly remarked on their similarity to the terminations of basket cells ("cellules à corbeilles") in the cerebellum. His failure to call the cerebral cortical cells *basket cells* may stem from his use of the term *basket* (corbeille) for the dense plexuses of terminations made by the axons of one form of double bouquet cell about other somata. Even here, however, his usage is not consistent and in the legend to his Fig. 395 he refers to a cell with an axon like that of the double bouquet cell as giving rise to pericellular nests.

Allowing for this not atypical inconsistency, we can assume that Ramón y Cajal observed a particularly large, multipolar cell in the middle layers of the cortex. It possessed long horizontal axon collaterals that he believed terminated on pyramidal cell somata in a manner resembling that of basket cell axons on the Purkinje cells of the cerebellum.

When we look further into his writings, we find that Ramón y Cajal was rarely, if at all, able to trace the horizontal parent axons of the pericellular nests to their cells of origin, so that his relating the nests to the large multipolar cells, though these certainly had horizontal axons, was somewhat conjectural. Indeed, in one figure (his 362), not apparently described in his text, he shows what he labels as an extrinsic afferent fiber contributing terminals to a typical nest around

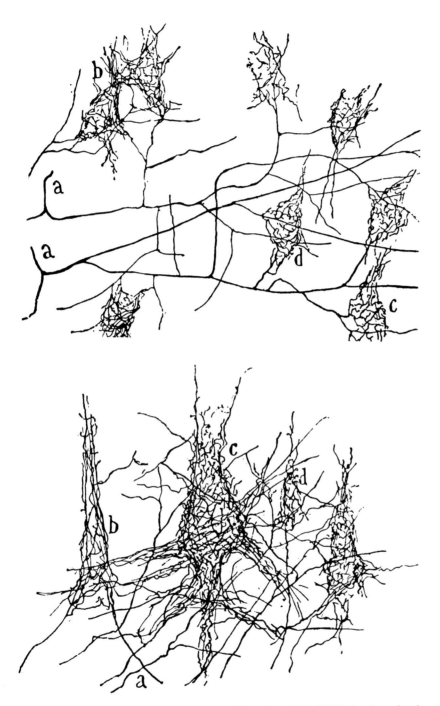

Figure 2. Figures 361 (upper) and 362 (lower) of Ramón y Cajal (1911) showing what he called pericellular nests about the somata of pyramidal neurons in the deep part of layer III of a human infant. In the lower figure, "a" is identified as "afferent fibers."

a pyramidal cell body. Furthermore, although he later illustrates and describes large multipolar cells with ascending axons and long horizontal collaterals in deeper layers of the cortex (our layers IV to VI) and in many cortical areas (Fig. 3), he makes no comment about whether they, too, contribute to pericellular nests or whether such nests exist around pyramidal cells in layers other than layer III. In his account of the visual cortex of the cat, published late in his career (1922), he does not seem to mention pericellular nests of the type described earlier.

1.2. Other Studies

In ensuing years, large multipolar cells with ascending axons, sometimes giving rise to horizontal collaterals, were mentioned at intervals (Lorente de Nó, 1922, 1949; O'Leary, 1941), but no worker seems to have related these to the pericellular nest of Ramón y Cajal and its seems doubtful that the nests, though mentioned, were ever clearly observed in those years. It is to Marin-Padilla (1969, 1972, 1974) that we owe the first modern description of the cells, the recognition of the connection of their axons with the pericellular nests of Ramón y Cajal, and the use of the word *baskets* for these and, thus, *basket cell* for the parent cell (Fig. 4). Marin-Padilla's studies were carried out with the rapid Golgi method on the motor cortex and visual cortex of fetal and early postnatal human brains. His more complete descriptions are from the motor area. In blocks from the postnatal specimens, he was able to demonstrate elaborate pericellular baskets encompassing the somata of pyramidal cells in layers III and V (Fig. 5). Each of the baskets arose from one or more horizontal axons, each up to 1 mm in length, which were in turn derived from what he termed *medium-sized stellate cells* with somata mainly in layers III and V (Fig. 4). Marin-Padilla described the cells as basically multipolar in shape but with longer vertical than horizontal dendrites. The vertical dendrites could extend from layers II to VI. All dendrites possessed a moderate number of dendritic spines. The axons ascended or descended before giving off its horizontal collaterals, exactly as described by Ramón y Cajal. In a later paper (1974), Marin-Padilla noted that the dendritic field tended to be flattened so that the basket cells formed a slablike dendritic field, approximately 0.2 mm thick, mainly at right angles to the long axis of the precentral gyrus but extending throughout all layers. He also noted (1972) that certain small cells of layer II had many similarities to the large basket cells of deeper layers but was unable to trace their axons to fully developed pericellular baskets. He felt that this was because they had not fully matured at the ages he was studying. Finally, he suggested that axons contributing to the pericellular baskets might arise from sources other than the basket cells since in a 2½-day-old infant brain he was able to trace large ascending axons from layer VI into the baskets around pyramidal cells of layer V. These axons he took to be derived from the ventral lateral complex of the thalamus, though this now seems unlikely.

Basket cells comparable to those described by Marin-Padilla were later mentioned by Szentágothai (1969, 1970, 1973) in somatic sensory, motor, and visual areas of the cat cortex, though he did not describe basketlike terminations as

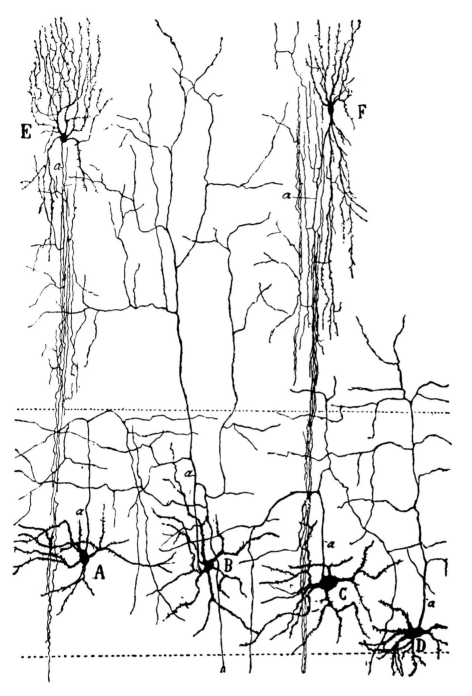

Figure 3. Figure 384 of Ramón y Cajal (1911) showing four multipolar cells (A–D) with ascending axons and horizontal collaterals in supervening layers. The cell somata are in layer IV of the human visual cortex. Cells E and F in layer III are double bouquet cells.

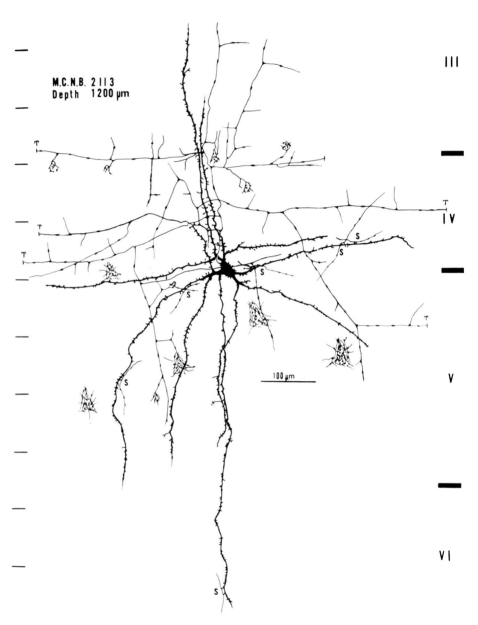

Figure 4. Camera lucida drawing of a basket cell from the junction of layers IV and V in the motor cortex of a human infant. Courtesy of Marin-Padilla (1969).

elaborate as those illustrated by Ramón y Cajal and Marin-Padilla. The basket cell Szentágothai assumed could operate in an inhibitory manner akin to that of its namesake in the cerebellar cortex, and it has for some years formed a central element in his thinking on the functional organization of the neocortex (Szentágothai, 1973, 1975, 1978).

Large multipolar cells with ascending axons were mentioned in other Golgi studies of several cortical areas in a number of studies but, probably because of the difficulty of impregnating the axons or the pericellular baskets, a "basket cell" was either not specifically identified or its existence denied (O'Leary, 1941; Lorente de Nó, 1949; Ramón-Moliner, 1961; Lund, 1973). See Chapter 6 for another account.

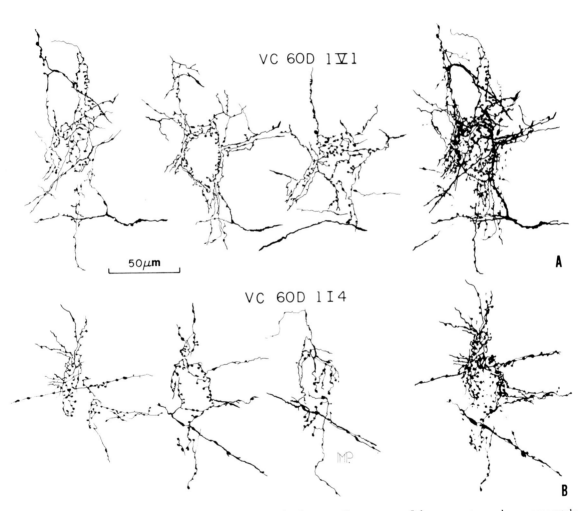

Figure 5. Two pericellular nests (A, B) from the human visual cortex. Components of the two nests are drawn separately on the left. Courtesy of Marin-Padilla (1972).

2. Golgi Morphology

In 1975 in a Golgi study of the pre- and postcentral gyri of monkeys, Jones again drew attention to the basket cells as one of the more common and easily recognized varieties of intrinsic neuron in these areas. The identification depends in the first instance on the large size of the soma. For cells in layer V, this approaches in diameter that of the largest pyramidal cell (15–30 μm) (Figs. 6, 7). From this large soma, 4–10 thick dendrites, 50 to 10 μm in diameter, radiate outwards, mostly vertically upwards and downwards. The dendrites are sinuous,

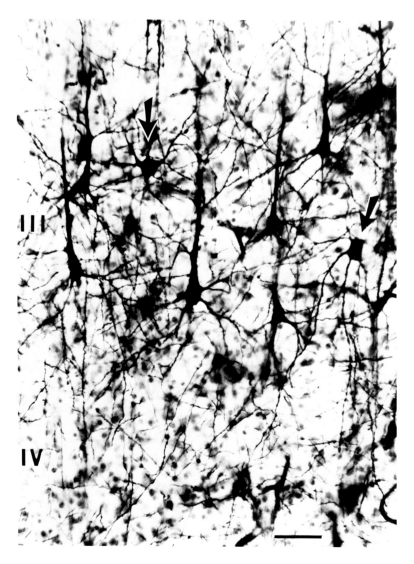

Figure 6. Large multipolar or basket cells (arrows) from layer III of the somatic sensory cortex of a cynomolgus monkey. Counterstained Golgi–Cox preparation. In size the somata of the basket cells approach those of the large pyramidal cells. Bar represents 50 μm.

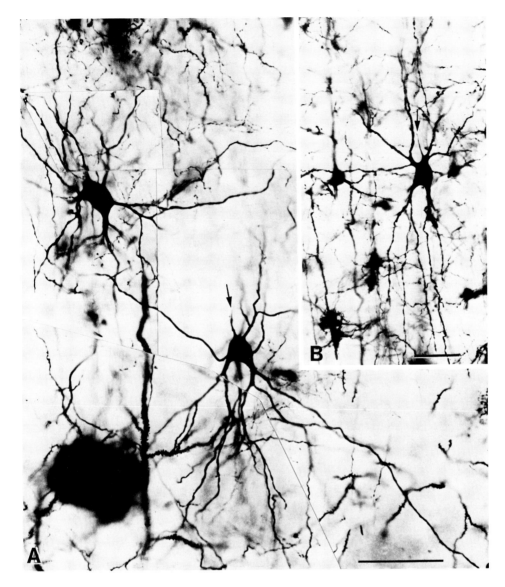

Figure 7. (A) Golgi–Kopsch and (B) Golgi–Cox preparations from the somatic sensory cortex of a squirrel monkey showing large multipolar cells. (B) shows the more common, elongated form of the basket cell. Arrows indicate the typical ascending initial segments of the axons in (A) and (B). Bars represent 50 μm.

branch only once or twice, and bear few or no spines in mature animals. In immature animals, the spine population is somewhat higher, though never particularly dense. The vertical dendrites are particularly long, and collectively, can extend through all layers of the cortex irrespective of the layer in which the soma lies.

The thick axon almost invariably ascends from an elongated hillock on the upper end of the soma or from the base of an ascending dendrite. In adult animals, the axons is rarely impregnated beyond the initial segment. It was suggested that this was because it quickly became myelinated, a prediction that has subsequently been confirmed (Peters and Proskauer, 1980b; Hendry *et al.*, 1983) (see Fig. 15). In immature monkeys, however, it was possible to impregnate the axons of several of these large multipolar cells over much of their extent (Fig. 8). In these cases, the initial segment is seen to rise vertically for a variable distance, commonly reaching into two or more cortical layers above the layer containing the soma. As it ascends, it gives off at several levels four or more horizontal collaterals that can extend for 1 mm or more in either direction. Instead of continuing upwards, the initial axons of some cells arch vertically downwards into subjacent layers, again giving off long horizontal collaterals at all levels as they do so. A single basket cell can, therefore, have horizontal axon collaterals running through several cortical layers.

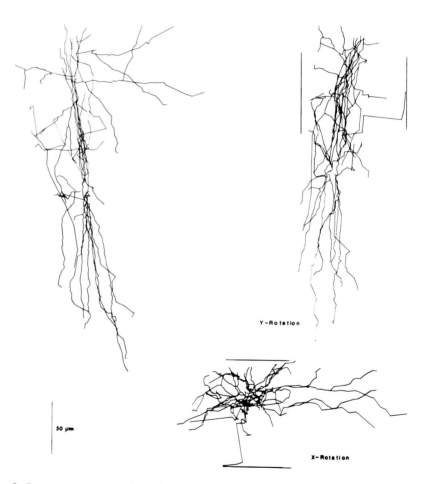

Figure 8. Computer reconstructions of a basket cell with impregnated axon collaterals from the postcentral gyrus of an infant squirrel monkey, seen en face (left), from the side (top right), and from the surface of the brain (bottom right). Surfaces of the (sagittal) section are indicated by short lines. Figure at bottom right shows typical anteroposterior orientation of axon collaterals in pre- and postcentral gyri. From Jones (1975).

The horizontal axon collaterals give off short ascending or descending terminal branches at intervals. These branches run over the surfaces of pyramidal cell bodies and the proximal portions of their dendrites, commonly reaching the axon hillock (Fig. 9). As they do so, they form chains of boutonlike dilations in intimate contact with the pyramidal cell. In the study of Jones (1975), no baskets composed of multiple axon branches of this type were observed, but the indi-

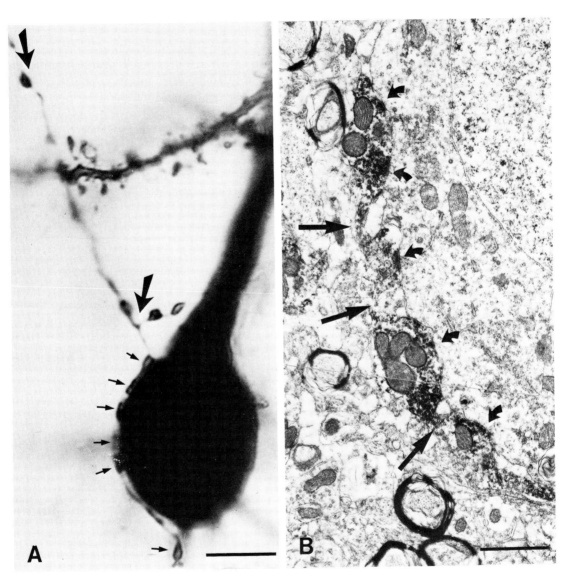

Figure 9. (A) Golgi–Kopsch-impregnated axon of a basket cell descending toward a pyramidal cell soma and branching (large arrows). One branch forms boutonlike terminations on the soma and appears to continue onto the axon hillock (small arrows). Postcentral gyrus of an infant squirrel monkey. From Jones (1975). (B) Immunocytochemical staining of basketlike axon terminations (arrows) on surface of a pyramidal cell soma in layer V of somatic sensory cortex of a cynomolgus monkey. Antiserum to GABA-synthetic enzyme, GAD. From Hendry *et al.* (1983). Bars represent 5 μm in (A) and 1 μm in (B).

vidual terminal branches shown in Fig. 9 have all the characteristics of the components of the pericellular baskets described by Ramón y Cajal and Marin-Padilla. Jones referred to the parent cells as *type I cells*, though recognizing their similarity to basket cells. It now seems appropriate to refer to them by this latter name.

A characteristic feature of the large basket cells of the sensory motor cortex is the orientation, not only of their dendritic fields, but also of their horizontal axon collaterals (Fig. 8). The dendritic field is flattened into a parasagittal slab, as noted by Marin-Padilla in the human motor cortex. But the axon collaterals, too, are aligned in the same plane so that they run in a preferred orientation, anteroposteriorly, orthogonal to the long axes of the pre- and postcentral gyri. The collaterals are long and even in infant squirrel monkeys may be as long as 1 mm. Such observations, made in Golgi preparations, received support from the experimental results of Gatter and Powell (1978). After placing extremely narrow needle lesions through the depth of the monkey precentral cortex, they noted that the ensuing axonal degeneration, spreading out 1–2 mm beyond the lesion particularly in layers III and V, was more extensive sagittally than mediolaterally. This they attributed to involvement of the basket cell axons. In a concurrent electron microscopic study, Gatter *et al.* (1978) noted that the majority of the degenerating axon terminals detected 0.5–2.5 mm beyond the damage in layer V were on the somata and proximal dendrites of large pyramidal cells. Such terminals had symmetrical membrane thickenings. Though degenerating terminals formed a high proportion of the axosomatic populations, others were normal, perhaps implying their origin from basket cells unaffected by the lesion.

The basket cells of the monkey sensory motor cortex have their somata concentrated in layers III and V. Moderate numbers of somata are found in layers IV and VI. In layer VI, they can be extended into a more horizontal form as the cortex folds in the floor of a sulcus. Whether any basket cells are present in layer II is at the moment debatable. In this layer, there are many aspiny or sparsely spiny nonpyramidal cells (type 6 of Jones, 1975) that resemble the basket cells of deeper layers in all except size. The somata are rarely greater than 12 μm in diameter. They have horizontal axons, mainly in layers I and II but, unfortunately, these have never been traced to pericellular terminations (but see Chapter 6).

3. Distribution

Ramón y Cajal based his description of what we have come to call basket cells on material taken from layer III of the human motor cortex but he shows large, relatively spine-free, multipolar cells with their somata situated in several deeper layers of the human motor (e.g., his Figs. 360, 368), somatic sensory (e.g., his Fig. 375), and temporal (e.g., his Figs. 358, 395, 399) areas and giving off ascending axons with long horizontal collaterals in supra- and subjacent layers. In the visual cortex, comparable cells, as illustrated, are smaller, appear to have more dendritic spines, and the horizontal axon branches seem less long (e.g., his Fig. 384). Though demonstrating a pericellular nest around a pyramidal cell in the cerebral cortex of a dog (his Fig. 363), he makes no mention of the putative basket cells in other species.

The most complete descriptions of basket cells therefore still derive from accounts of the somatic sensory and motor cortex of primates (Marin-Padilla, 1969, 1972, 1974; Jones, 1975). In these areas in monkeys and man, the cells are particularly large and, thus, readily identified, at least in layers III–VI (Fig. 10). In other areas of the cortex and in other species such as the cat (Peters and Regidor, 1981), there are reasons for believing that comparable cells are present but full details remain to be elucidated. The lack of data probably derives mostly from failure to completely impregnate the axons and pericellular baskets in Golgi preparations but the less obvious difference in size between possible basket cells and other intrinsic neurons in the rather thin but densely populated visual cortex of monkeys and throughout the cortex of other species has also made identification difficult.

In Valverde's (1976, 1978) drawings of Golgi-impregnated cells from the visual and paravisual cortex of mice and monkeys, a few cells having some similarities to basket cells can be identified. The cells are multipolar, of medium to large size, lack dendritic spines, and have ascending axons commonly arising from the base of an ascending dendrite. Where drawn, only some of the branches of the axons are horizontally oriented and no pericellular baskets are mentioned but a few short varicose collaterals are shown ramifying over the surfaces of pyramidal somata in layers III or V. Feldman and Peters (1978) have identified medium to large, aspiny multipolar cells in layers III–VI of the rat visual cortex. These cells have ascending or descending axons that do not impregnate well beyond their initial segments (Peters and Proskauer, 1980b). Another Golgi-impregnated cell examined electron microscopically by Peters and Proskauer (1980a) had an ascending axon with short horizontal and some descending branches ending in part on the soma and proximal dendrites of a pyramidal cell in layer III of the rat visual cortex. Shkol'nik-Yarros (1971) in her description of the visual cortex of the dog shows (her Fig. 36) what may be part of a horizontal axon system sectioned tangentially, the smaller branches of which she says terminate in pericellular nests. Tömböl (1978) mentions Golgi-impregnated basket cells in the striate area of the rhesus monkey. Though not describing their axonal ramifications in detail, she mentions small forms in layers II and III and large forms in deeper layers.

In the cat striate cortex after injections of horseradish peroxidase, Holländer and Vanegas (1981) described anterogradely labeled axon terminals arising from myelinated axons and ending around the soma of a layer V pyramidal cell near the injection site. The nest, though possibly less complicated, is similar to the pericellular nests described in the neonatal human visual cortex by Marin-Padilla (1974).

Apart from these observations, and the statements made by Szentágothai in his several review articles regarding the ubiquity of basket cells, we still do not have a strong body of evidence for their existence in cortical areas outside the sensory motor regions of primates. It would be surprising, however, if a type of cell were to be found represented in only two cortical areas of a single order. It seems logical to assume that something akin to the basket cell of the sensory motor regions will ultimately be demonstrated in its entirety in other neocortical areas (see chapter by Martin and Whitteridge in Volume 2).

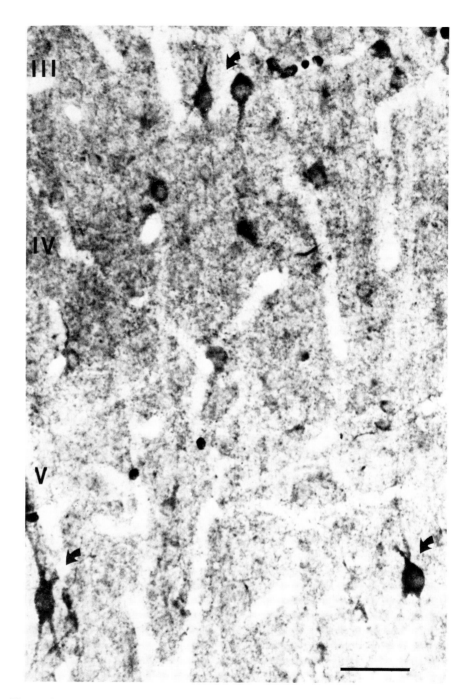

Figure 10. Immunocytochemical staining of large multipolar, presumed basket neurons (arrows) in layers III–IV of area 3b of a cynomolgus monkey. Antiserum to GAD. Note high concentration of GAD-positive axon terminals in layer IV. Bar represents 75 μm. From Houser *et al.* (1983).

If we can provisionally accept that the largest nonpyramidal cells in the sensory motor cortex are basket cells, it is possible to provide a few details of their fine structure. Colonnier (1968) and Jones and Powell (1970a; Peters, 1971) first noted that nonpyramidal cells in the visual and somatic sensory cortex of cats could usually be distinguished from pyramidal cells, even in isolated thin sections, by virtue of their high complement of cytoplasmic organelles, beaded or undulating dendrites, and a high concentration of asymmetric and symmetric synapses on both somata and dendritic shafts.

Later in the monkey sensory motor areas, Sloper and Powell (1979a,b) made a further distinction between large nonpyramidal cells (which they regarded as basket cells) and small nonpyramidal cells. As described by them, the somata and dendrites of the large cells had an abundant cytoplasm, full of organelles, especially stacks of rough-surfaced endoplasmic reticulum and mitochondria (Fig. 11). Axons ascended and in two cases were observed to become myelinated. The dendrites were moderately varicose and, together with the soma, received a particularly high density of both symmetric and asymmetric synapses. By contrast, the small nonpyramidal cells had sparser cytoplasm and fewer organelles and received a lower density of axosomatic synapses. The larger cell type was concentrated in layers III–V and formed 5–7% of the total cell population, versus 72% for pyramidal cells and 21–23% for small nonpyramidal cells. A concurrent study showed that the majority of dendritic shafts and somata contacted by degenerating thalamic or commissural axon terminals were of the large nonpyramidal type (Fig. 11). This implies that, along with dendritic spine-bearing cells, basket cells are major recipients of extrinsic afferent inputs. A similar conclusion has been arrived at by White (1978) in his studies of nonspiny multipolar cells in the somatic sensory cortex of the mouse.

5. Labeling by [³H]-GABA and by Immunocytochemistry

The large basket cells of the sensory motor cortex appear to synthesize the transmitter substance GABA. The evidence for this is twofold: (1) If [³H]-GABA is injected into the monkey sensory motor cortex, preferably after administration of a GABA transaminase inhibitor, only nonpyramidal neurons concentrate the injected GABA and a substantial proportion of these, especially in layers III–V, have somata with diameters approaching those of the largest pyramidal cells (in monkeys in excess of 15 μm) (Fig. 12; Hendry and Jones, 1981). A second population has somal diameters in the range of 6–15 μm (2) Immunocytochemical staining of the monkey sensory motor cortex with antiserum against the GABA-synthetic enzyme, GAD, also shows staining of two populations of nonpyramidal cells, one of which has very large somata, is concentrated in layers III–V (Fig. 10), receives many synapses, and is rich in organelles (see Figs. 14, 17) (Houser *et al.*, 1983). If animals are pretreated with colchicine in order to block somatofugal axoplasmic transport, and thus, cause GAD to accumulate in

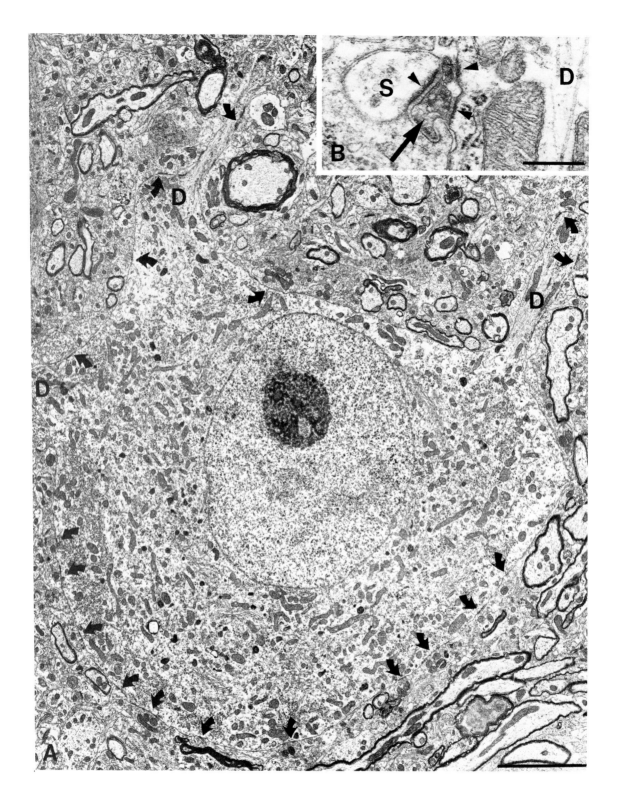

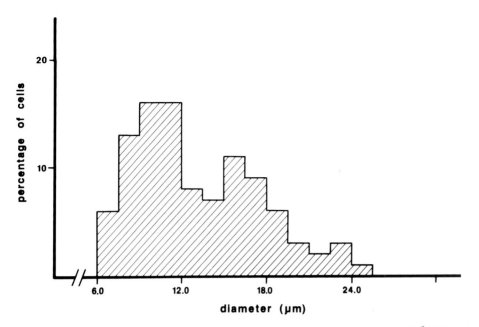

Figure 12. Bimodal size spectrum of neuronal somata showing selective uptake of [³H]-GABA injected into area 3b of a cynomolgus monkey. Large somata, above 12 μm, are thought to represent basket cells. From Hendry and Jones (1981).

somata and dendrites, it is not only possible to show that the large stained cells are multipolar in form but also that they have ascending axon initial segments that give rise to long horizontal collaterals (Fig. 13). Electron microscopy shows that many or all of these collaterals are myelinated and 3 to 5 μm in diameter (Figs. 15–17; Hendry *et al.*, 1983).

The size and morphology of these immunocytochemically stained cells alone seem to point to their identification as basket cells which we, therefore, conclude are probably GABAergic in function. This conclusion is strengthened by the evidence that many, perhaps all, synapses on the somata of pyramidal cells are also GAD positive (Fig. 16). Colonnier (1968) first noted and Jones and Powell (1970a) and Peters and Kaiserman-Abramof (1970) confirmed that all synaptic terminals on the somata of pyramidal cell neurons form symmetric membrane contacts and possess synaptic vesicles that flatten in aldehyde-fixed material. This raised the possibility of an inhibitory function for the basket cells. Later, in the first detailed immunocytochemical study of GAD localization in the cerebral

←

Figure 11. (A) Electron micrograph of a large multipolar, presumed basket neuron from layer IV of somatic sensory cortex of a cynomolgus monkey. Dendrites indicated by D. Note high concentration of cytoplasmic organelles and large numbers of axosomatic synapses (arrows). (B) Degenerating thalamocortical axon terminal (arrow) making synaptic contact (arrowheads) with a dendrite (D) of cell A and with an unidentified dendritic spine (S). Bars represent 3 μm in (A) and 1 μm in (B).

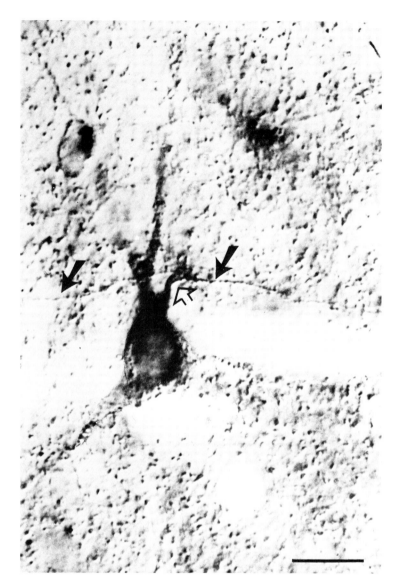

Figure 13. Large multipolar neuron immunocytochemically stained for GAD in layer V of motor cortex of a cynomolgus monkey. Large size, multipolar form, ascending axon (open arrow), and horizontal collaterals (closed arrows) indicate it to be a probable basket cell. Nomarski photomicrograph. Bar represents 25 μm. From Houser *et al.* (1983).

cortex, Ribak (1978) noted that pyramidal cell somata in the visual cortex of the rat were commonly surrounded by numerous GAD-positive axon terminals. Subsequent examination of the monkey cerebral cortex has revealed a similar staining pattern in the visual (Hendrickson *et al.*, 1981) and sensory motor areas (Fig. 16) (Houser *et al.*, 1983; Hendry *et al.*, 1983). In the sensory motor cortex, all axon terminals in a section through a pyramidal cell soma can be GAD positive. Commonly, several are joined by thin unmyelinated axon segments and arise from a single myelinated parent axon (Figs. 9, 16). It is easy to see in these appearances the fine structural correlate of the terminal axonal elements of the pericellular nest or baskets described in Golgi preparations (cf. Figs. 9A and B).

These last observations raise two points for discussion. First, it seems from the observations on the visual cortex that a population of GABAergic intrinsic neurons with basket-type terminations is probably present in that area as in the sensory motor areas. Second, the possibility, raised by Ramón y Cajal and Marin-Padilla, that extrinsic afferent fibers may also contribute to the pericellular baskets around pyramidal cell somata seems ruled out. All extrinsic afferents to the cortex appear to terminate in asymmetrical synaptic complexes, contain spherical vesicles in aldehyde-fixed material, and have rarely, if ever, been demonstrated to end on pyramidal cell somata (Jones, 1968; Jones and Powell, 1970b; Colonnier and Rossignol, 1969). Furthermore, GABA and GAD levels in the cerebral

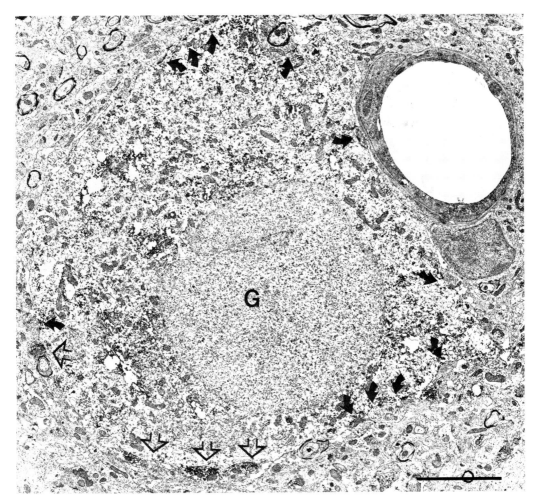

Figure 14. Electron micrograph showing soma of a large, organelle-filled neuron (G) immunocytochemically stained for GAD in layer IV of somatic sensory cortex of a cyno- molgus monkey. Filled arrows indicate unstained synapses, open arrows GAD-positive synapses on the soma. Bar represents 7 μm.

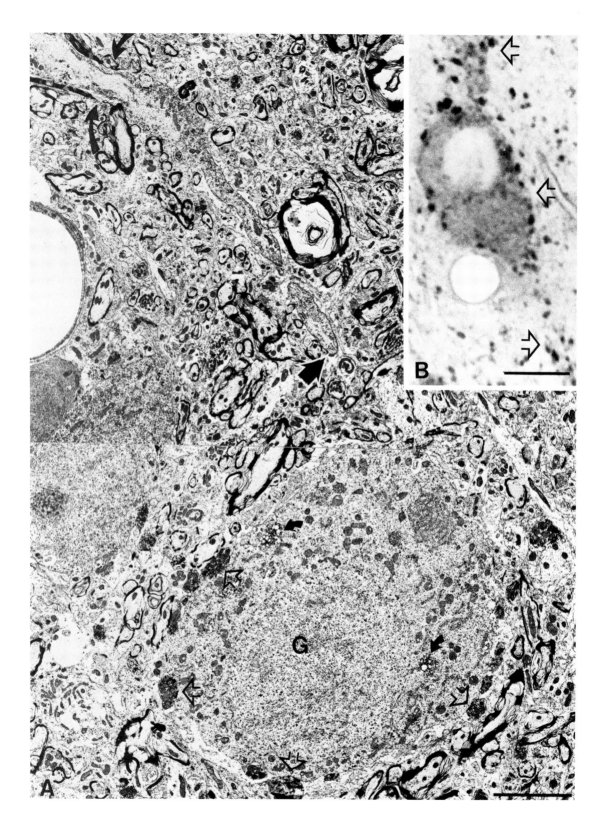

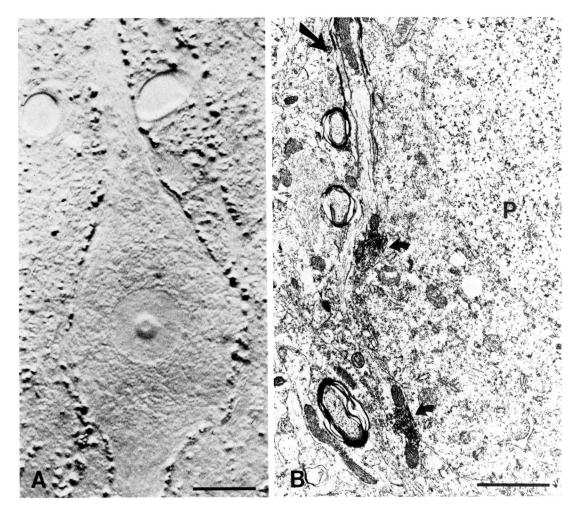

Figure 16. (A) Nomarski photomicrograph showing GAD-positive axon terminals on the soma and dendrites of a pyramidal cell in the motor cortex of a cynomolgus monkey. From Houser *et al.* (1983). (B) Electron micrograph of a myelinated GAD-positive axon (large arrow) making syn-aptic contacts (small arrows) on soma of a pyramidal neuron (P) in layer III of area 3a of a cynomolgus monkey. Bars represent 12 μm in (A) and 7 μm in (B). From Hendry *et al.* (1983).

←

Figure 15. (A) Edge of a large GAD-positive neuronal soma in layer V of somatic sensory cortex of a cynomolgus monkey. Small arrows indicate reaction product in soma and GAD-positive axon terminals ending on it. Large arrows indicate ascending axon that arose from this cell. Axon be-comes myelinated at upper left. From Hendry *et al.* (1983). (B) Plastic section of a large GAD-positive multipolar neuron from area 3b of a cynomolgus monkey. Arrows indicate GAD-positive axon terminals on its soma and dendrites. Bars represent 2 μm in (A) and 25 μm in (B).

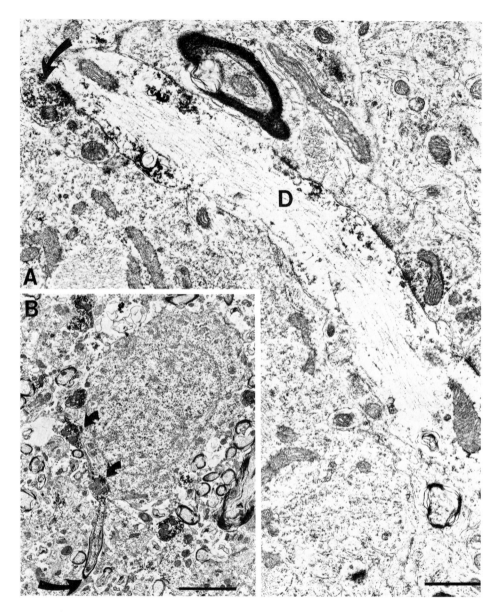

Figure 17. (A) Large GAD-positive dendrite (D) of a putative basket cell receiving multiple axon terminals, one of which (arrow) is also GAD positive—layer III of area 1 of a cynomolgus monkey. From Hendry *et al.* (1983). (B) Small, unlabeled, nonpyramidal soma in layer IV of area 3b of a cynomolgus monkey receiving axon terminals from a GAD-positive myelinated axon (arrows). From Hendry *et al.* (1983). Bars represent 2 μm in (A) and 10 μm in (B).

cortex are only transiently altered after the destruction of seemingly all extrinsic afferents (Iversen *et al.,* 1971; Ulmar, 1975; Ulmar *et al.,* 1976; Emson and Lindvall, 1979). Ramón y Cajal and Marin-Padilla did not trace the fibers that they thought were afferents back into the white matter but only down to layer V or VI. Hence, it is possible that they were visualizing large myelinated axons ascending from deeply placed basket cells to pyramidal somata in more superficial layers.

We do not yet know whether all GAD-containing axon terminals ending on pyramidal cell somata arise from basket cells. There is an extremely large population of small GABAergic cortical interneurons in which are included several of the types defined in morphological studies (Hendry and Jones, 1981; Houser *et al.,* 1982; Hendry *et al.,* 1983). The axons of some of these appear to have selective terminations on axon initial segments, and other sites (Peters *et al.,* 1982; Fairén and Valverde, 1980; Somogyi, 1977; Hendry *et al.,* 1983), but terminations on pyramidal cell somata have also been described (Peters and Fairén, 1978; Somogyi and Cowey, 1981). This raises the semantic question as to whether all axosomatic terminations on pyramidal cells should be considered parts of the pericellular basket or nest and whether their parent cells, by extrapolation, should all be called basket cells. This approach has little to commend it, for the classical basket cell, by its large size, horizontal myelinated axon, and dense pericellular terminations on pyramidal cell somata, clearly stands apart from the other intrinsic cell types, most of which have a stereotyped axonal morphology of their own. Such considerations might become relevant, however, if some cortical areas, such as the visual or some layers such as layer II in which classical pericellular baskets have not been demonstrated, were to be shown to lack the typical basket cell.

The extent to which basket cell axons form terminations on synaptic targets other than the somata of pyramidal cells is incompletely known. Electron microscopic immunocytochemical studies reveal GAD-positive terminals arising from myelinated axons terminating on certain nonpyramidal cells but it is not certain if all these myelinated axons arise from basket cells (Fig. 17). Myelinated, GAD-positive axons also terminate on the somata of large GAD-positive neurons, presumably basket cells (Figs. 14, 15, 17). The large GAD-positive somata can receive as many GAD-positive terminals as pyramidal cell somata. This arrangement forces us to think of GABA-mediated disinhibition as a feature of cortical function.

6. Functions of Basket Cells

There had been no confirmed single-unit recordings from basket cells in any area of cortex at the time of writing (but see chapter by Martin and Whitteridge in Volume 2). Stimulation of extrinsic afferents, however, invariably results in short-latency, monosynaptic EPSPs in a significant proportion of cortical neurons. This is commonly succeeded by di- or polysynaptic IPSPs (Toyama *et al.,* 1974). From this we may assume that the inhibitory effect is mediated by intrinsic cortical neurons that are excited by an afferent volley. Because of the extremely high concentration of GABAergic neurons demonstrated by auto-radiography or immunocytochemistry in the cortex, it also seems justifiable to assume that many of these will be involved in the inhibitory effect.

When considering how the large basket cells of the sensory motor cortex could fit into a scheme of intracortical processing, three features stand out: (1) The dendrites of the cells are particularly concentrated in the layers in which all extrinsic afferents to the cortex (thalamic, associational, callosal) terminate. In this position, some at least receive thalamic axon terminals (Fig. 11) (Sloper and Powell, 1979b) and according to White (1978), in the mouse somatic sensory cortex, cells that may be comparable to the basket cells are among those receiving the highest density of thalamic synapses. (2) The basket cells and especially their axons are preferentially oriented anteroposteriorly in the sensory motor cortex and a single cell can have axon terminals on pyramidal cell somata in several layers. (3) The axons are long, thick, myelinated, and presumably rapidly conducting.

All of these features suggest an organization in which the GABAergic basket cell can be driven monosynaptically by extrinsic afferents and rapidly transmit a powerful inhibitory influence over relatively long distances, in a preferred orientation to pyramidal cells throughout much of the vertical depth of the cortex in an adjacent zone. If we postulate that basket cells in a vertical column of cortex are excited along with other cells as part of the early cortical response to an external stimulus, then these cells could provide for the near-simultaneous inhibition of cells in neighboring vertical columns (Fig. 18). In the somatic sensory cortex of monkeys, a phenomenon of this kind has in fact been observed: activation of one column of cells with common receptive field and submodality properties, is usually accompanied by inhibition of neighboring columns (Mountcastle and Powell, 1959). Similar phenomena have not been reported in other cortical areas though it is not difficult to make conjectures about how basket cells with axons oriented in preferred directions could participate in the molding of columns or other modular units with particular kinds of receptive field properties, such as are seen, for example, in the visual cortex (Blakemore and Tobin, 1972; Schiller *et al.*, 1976; Hubel and Wiesel, 1977; Hammond, 1978; Orban *et al.*, 1980). Many of these receptive field properties appear to be influenced by GABA (Sillito, 1975, 1977a,b, 1979; Sillito and Versiani, 1977; Tsumoto *et al.*, 1979).

7. Summary

The basket cell has become recognized as an entity mainly in the sensory motor areas of primates, including man. There is reason to believe, however, that comparable cells may be present in other areas and in other species.

In the sensory motor regions, the basket cell is a large, nonspiny multipolar neuron with a soma approaching in size that of the larger pyramidal cells. Though basket cell somata are concentrated in layers III–V, their dendrites are long and often can span virtually the whole thickness of the cortex. The axon usually ascends from the soma, becomes myelinated, and gives off numerous

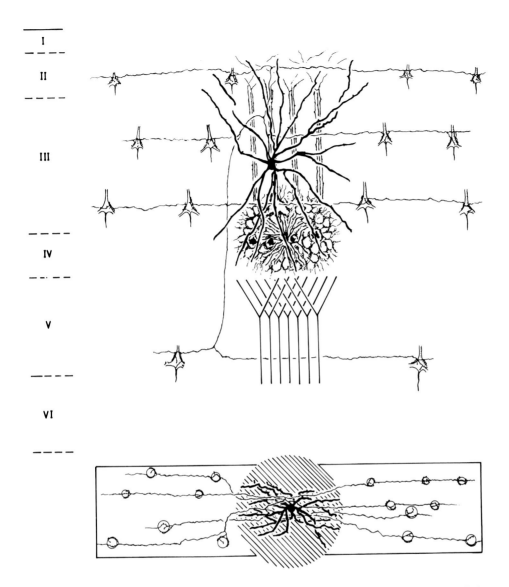

Figure 18. Schematic figure from Jones (1981) suggesting one mode of action of basket cells in monkey somatic sensory cortex. Bundle of incoming thalamocortical axons carrying place- and modality-specific information sets up with local interneurons, a focus of excitation in layer IV. This serves as a basis for excitation of a narrow vertical column of cortical cells. Thalamic axon terminations on inhibitory basket cells would lead, via the long collaterals of the latter, to inhibition of cells in neighboring columns. Because of orientation of basket cells (below), such inhibition might operate in a preferred anteroposterior direction.

horizontally disposed axon collaterals extending for 1–2 mm, mainly in an anteroposterior direction, through all cortical layers. Smaller side branches terminate in pericellular baskets around the somata and proximal dendrites of pyramidal cells.

The basket cell appears to be one of several forms of GABAergic intrinsic cortical neuron. It is presumably inhibitory to the pyramidal cells. As well as receiving a substantial number of extrinsic, thalamic, and commissural axon terminals, the basket cell itself is contacted by numerous GABAergic terminals.

ACKNOWLEDGMENTS. This work was supported by Grant NS10526 from the National Institutes of Health, United States Public Health Service, and by the Washington University McDonnell Center for Studies of Higher Brain Function. We are grateful for the collaboration of Dr. Carolyn Houser and Dr. James E. Vaughn, City of Hope Medical Center, Duarte, California, whose work is supported by Grant NS18858.

8. References

Blakemore, C., and Tobin, E. A., 1972, Lateral inhibition between orientation detectors in the cat's visual cortex, *Exp. Brain Res.* **15:**439–440.

Colonnier, M., 1968, Synaptic patterns on different cell types in the different laminae of the cat visual cortex: An electron microscope study, *Brain Res.* **9:**268–287.

Colonnier, M., and Rossignol, S., 1969, Discussion. Heterogeneity of the cerebral cortex, in: *Basic Mechanisms of the Epilepsies* (H. H. Jasper, A. A. Ward, and A. Pope, eds.), pp. 29–40, Little Brown, Boston.

Emson, P.C., and Lindvall, O., 1979, Distribution of putative neurotransmitters in the neocortex, *Neuroscience* **4:**1407–1439.

Fairén, A., and Valverde, F., 1980, A specialized type of neuron in the visual cortex of cat: A Golgi and electron microscope study of chandelier cells, *J. Comp. Neurol.* **194:**761–780.

Feldman, M., and Peters, A., 1978, The forms of non-pyramidal neurons in the visual cortex of the rat, *J. Comp. Neurol.* **179:**761–794.

Gatter, K.C., and Powell, T. P. S., 1978, Intrinsic connections of the cortex of area 4 of the monkey, *Brain* **101:**513–541.

Gatter, K. C., Sloper, J. J., and Powell, T. P. S., 1978, An electron microscopic study of the termination of intracortical axons upon Betz cells in area 4 of the monkey, *Brain* **101:**543–553.

Hammond, P., 1978, Directional tuning of complex cells in area 17 of the feline visual cortex, *J. Physiol. (London)* **285:**479–491.

Hendrickson, A., Hunt, S. P., and Wu, J.-Y., 1981, Immunocytochemical localization of glutamic acid decarboxylase in monkey striate cortex, *Nature (London)* **292:**605–607.

Hendry, S. H. C., and Jones, E. G., 1981, Sizes and distributions of intrinsic neurons incorporating tritiated GABA in monkey sensory-motor cortex, *J. Neurosci.* **1:**390–408.

Hendry, S. H. C., Houser, C. R., Jones, E. G., and Vaughn, J. E., 1983, Synaptic organization of immunocytochemically characterized GABAergic neurons in the monkey sensory-motor cortex, *J. Neurocytol.* **12:**639–660.

Holländer, H., and Vanegas, H., 1981, Identification of pericellular baskets in the cat striate cortex: Light and electron microscopic observations after uptake of horseradish peroxidase, *J. Neurocytol.* **10:**577–587.

Houser, C. R., Hendry, S. H. C., Jones, E. G., and Vaughn, J. E., 1983, Morphological diversity of GABAergic neurons characterized immunocytochemically in monkey sensory-motor cortex, *J. Neurocytol.* **12:**617–638.

Hubel, D. H., and Wiesel, T. N., 1977, Functional architecture of macaque monkey visual cortex, *Proc. R. London Ser. Soc. B* **198:**1–59.

Iversen, L. L., Mitchell, J. F., and Srinivarsan, V., 1971, The release of gamma-aminobutyric acid during inhibition in the cat visual cortex, *J. Physiol. (London)* **212:**519–534.

Jones, E. G., 1968, An electron microscopic study of the termination of afferent fibre systems within the somatic sensory cortex of the cat, *J. Anat.* **103:**595–597.

Jones, E. G., 1975a, Varieties and distribution of non-pyramidal cells in the somatic sensory cortex of the squirrel monkey, *J. Comp. Neurol.* **160:**205–268.

Jones. E. G., 1981, Anatomy of cerebral cortex: Columnar input–output relations, in: *The Cerebral Cortex* (F. O. Schmitt, F. G. Worden, G. Adelman, and S. G. Dennis, eds.), pp. 199–235, MIT Press, Cambridge, Mass.

Jones, E. G., and Powell T. P. S., 1970a, Electron microscopy of the somatic sensory cortex of the cat. I. Cell types and synaptic organization, *Phils. Trans. R. Soc. London Ser. B* **257**:1–11.

Jones, E. G., and Powell, T. P. S., 1970b, An electron microscopic study of the laminar pattern and mode of termination of the afferent fibre pathways to the somatic sensory cortex, *Phils. Trans. R. Soc. London Ser. B* **257**:45–62.

Lorente de Nó, R., 1922, La corteza cerebral del ratón (Primera contribucion-La corteza acustica), *Trab. Lab. Invest. Biol Madrid* **20**:41–78.

Lorente de Nó, R., 1949, Cerebral cortex: Architecture, intracortical connections, motor projections, in: *Physiology of the Nervous System* (J. F. Fulton, ed.), 3rd ed., pp. 288–313, Oxford University Press, London.

Lund, J. S., 1973, Organization of neurons in the visual cortex, area 17, of the monkey *(Macaca mulatta,) J. Comp. Neurol.* **147**:455–496.

Marin-Padilla, M., 1969, Origin of the pericellular baskets of the pyramidal cells of the human motor cortex, *Brain Res.* **14**:633–646.

Marin-Padilla, M., 1972, Double origin of the pericellular baskets of the pyramidal cells of the human motor cortex: A Golgi study, *Brain Res.* **38**:1–12.

Marin-Padilla, M., 1974, Three-dimensional reconstruction of the pericellular nests (baskets) of the motor (area 4) and visual (area 17) areas of the human cerebral cortex: A Golgi study, *Z. Anat. Entwicklungsgesch.* **144**:123–135.

Mountcastle, V. B., and Powell, T. P. S., 1959, Neural mechanisms subserving cutaneous sensibility, with special reference to the role of afferent inhibition in sensory perception and discrimination, *Bull. Johns Hopkins Hosp.* **105**:201–232.

O'Leary, J. L., 1941, Structure of the area striata of the cat, *J. Comp. Neurol.* **75**:131–164.

Orban, G. A., Kato, H., and Bishop, P. O., 1980, End-zone region in receptive fields of hypercomplex and other striate neurons in the cat, *J. Neurophysiol.* **42**:818–832.

Peters, A., 1971, Stellate cells of the rat parietal cortex, *J. Comp. Neurol.* **141**:345–373.

Peters, A., and Fairén, A., 1978, Smooth and sparsely-spined stellate cells in the visual cortex of the rat: A study using a combined Golgi–electron microscope technique. *J. Comp. Neurol.* **181**:129–172.

Peters, A., and Kaiserman-Abramof, I. R., 1970, The small pyramidal neuron of the rat cerebral cortex: The perikaryon, dendrites and spines, *Am. J. Anat.* **127**:321–355.

Peters, A., and Proskauer, C. C., 1980a, Synaptic relationships between a multipolar stellate cell and a pyramidal neuron in the rat visual cortex—A combined Golgi–electron microscope study, *J. Neurocytol.* **9**:163–184.

Peters, A., and Proskauer, C. C., 1980b, Smooth or sparsely spined cells with myelinated axons in rat visual cortex, *Neuroscience* **5**:2079–2092.

Peters, A., and Regidor, J., 1981, A reassessment of the forms of non-pyramidal neurons in area 17 of the cat visual cortex, *J. Comp. Neurol.* **203**:685–716.

Peters, A., Feldman, M., and Saldanha, J., 1976, The projection of the lateral geniculate nucleus of area 17 of the rat cerebral cortex. II. Terminations upon neuronal perikarya and dendritic shafts, *J. Neurocytol.* **5**:85–107.

Peters, A., Proskauer, C. C., and Ribak, C. E., 1982, Chandelier cells in rat visual cortex, *J. Comp. Neurol.* **206**:397–416.

Ramón-Moliner, E., 1961, The histology of the postcruciate gyrus of the cat. III. Further observations, *J. Comp. Neurol.* **117**:229–249.

Ramón y Cajal, S., 1911, *Histologie due Système Nerveux de l'Homme et des Vertébrés* (translated by L. Azoulay), Vol. II, Maloine, Paris.

Ramón y Cajal, S., 1922, Studien über die Sehrinde der Katze, *J. Psychol. Neurol.* **29**:161–181.

Ribak, C. E., 1978, Aspinous and sparsely -spinous stellate neurons in the visual cortex of rats contain glutamic acid decarboxylase, *J. Neurocytol.* **7**:461–478.

Schiller, P. H., Finlay, B. L., and Volman, S. F., 1976, Quantitative studies of single-cell properties in monkey striate cortex. V. Multivariate statistical analyses and models, *J. Neurophysiol.* **39**:1362–1374.

Shkol'nik-Yarros, E. G., 1971, *Neurons and Interneuronal Connections of the Central Visual System*, Plenum Press, New York.

Sillito, A. M., 1975, The contribution of inhibitory mechanisms to the receptive field properties of neurones in the striate cortex of the cat, *J. Physiol. (London)* **250**:305–329.

Sillito, A. M., 1977a, The spatial extent of excitatory and inhibitory zones in the receptive field of superficial layer hypercomplex cells, *J. Physiol. (London)* **273**:791–803.

Sillito, A. M., 1977b, Inhibitory processes underlying the directional specificity of simple, complex and hypercomplex cells in the cat's visual cortex, *J. Physiol. (London)* **271**:699–720.

Sillito, A. M., 1979, Inhibitory mechanisms influencing complex cell orientation selectivity and their modification at high resting discharge levels, *J. Physiol. (London)* **289**:33–53.

Sillito, A. M., and Versiani, V., 1977, The contribution of excitatory and inhibitory inputs to the length preference of hypercomplex cells in layers II and III of the cat's striate cortex, *J. Physiol. (London)* **273**:775–790.

Sloper, J. J., and Powell, T. P. S., 1979a, Ultrastructural features of the sensorimotor cortex of the primate, *Philos. Trans. R. Soc. London Ser. B* **285**:123–139.

Sloper, J. J., and Powell, T. P. S., 1979b, An experimental electron microscopic study of afferent connections to the primate motor and somatic sensory cortices, *Philos. Trans. R. Soc. London Ser. B* **285**:199–226.

Somogyi, P., 1977, A specific axo-axonal interneuron in the visual cortex of the rat, *Brain Res.* **136**:345–350.

Somogyi, P., and Cowey, A., 1981, Combined Golgi and electron microscopic study on the synapses formed by double bouquet cells in the visual cortex of the cat and monkey, *J. Comp. Neurol.* **195**:547–566.

Szentágothai, J., 1969, Architecture of the cerebral cortex, in: *Basic Mechanisms of the Epilepsies* (H. H. Jasper, A. A. Ward, and A. Pope, eds.), pp. 13–28, Little, Brown, Boston.

Szentágothai, J., 1970, Les circuits neuronaux de l'écorce cérébrale, *Bull. Acad. R. Med. Belg.* **10**:475–492.

Szentágothai, J., 1973, Synaptology of the visual cortex, in: *Handbook of Sensory Physiology*, Vol. VII/3 *Central Processing of Visual Information*, Part B *Visual Centers of the Brain* (R. Jung, ed.), pp. 269–324, Springer, Berlin.

Szentágothai, J., 1975, The "module-concept" in cerebral cortex architecture, *Brain Res.* **95**:475–496.

Szentágothai, J., 1978, The neuron network of the cerebral cortex: A functional interpretation, *Proc. R. Soc. London Ser. B* **201**:219–248.

Tömböl, T., 1978, Some Golgi data on the visual cortex of the rhesus monkey, *Acta Morphol. Acad. Sci. Hung.* **26**:115–138.

Toyama, K., Matsunami, K., Ohno, T., and Tokashiki, S., 1974, An intracellular study of neuronal organization in the visual cortex, *Brain Res.* **14**:518–520.

Tsumoto, T., Eckart, W., and Creutzfeldt, O. D., 1979, Modification of orientation sensitivity of cat visual cortex neurons by removal of GABA-mediated inhibitory, *Exp. Brain Res.* **34**:351–363.

Ulmar, G., 1975, Some biochemical changes in the isolated cortex of the rat, *Exp. Brain Res.* **1**:337–342.

Ulmar, G., Ljüngdahl, A., and Hökfelt, T., 1976, Enzyme changes after undercutting of cerebral cortex in the rat, *Neurology* **46**:199–208.

Valverde, F., 1976, Aspects of cortical organization related to the geometry of neurons with intra-cortical axons, *J. Neurocytol.* **5**:509–529.

Valverde, F., 1978, The organization of area 18 in the monkey, *Anat. Embryol.* **154**:305–334.

White, E. L., 1978, Identified neurons in mouse SmI cortex which are post-synaptic to thalamocortical axon terminals: A combined Golgi–electron microscopic and degeneration study, *J. Comp. Neurol.* **181**:627–662.

9

Double Bouquet Cells

PETER SOMOGYI and ALAN COWEY

1. Introduction

The name *double bouquet cell* has been used for certain cortical neurons since Ramón y Cajal's vivid description of the "cellule à double bouquet dendritique" in diverse cortical areas of man (Ramón y Cajal, 1911). The term originally embraced several forms of neurons with somewhat different features but which had in common a characteristic bitufted dendritic arborization with its long axis oriented radially, i.e., at right angles to the pia. After being overlooked for several decades, interest in these neurons was rekindled by Colonnier (1966) and Szentágothai (1969, 1971) who called particular attention to the bundles of radially oriented axon collaterals apparent in Ramón y Cajal's drawings.

These neurons deserve attention because their bundles of radially oriented, translaminar axon collaterals are well suited to distributing information in the vertical direction through layers II–V, and such an arrangement could be related to the results of physiological studies which demonstrate a columnar organization of the visual (Hubel and Wiesel, 1977) as well as other cortical areas (Mountcastle, 1957; Asanuma, 1975).

Following Colonnier's investigation (1966), double bouquet cells were reported in many species and in various cortical areas (see below), but the term *double bouquet cell* or *bitufted cell* has been used of neurons which had only the dendritic arborization *or* the axon resembling the neurons in the original de-

PETER SOMOGYI • First Department of Anatomy, Semmelweis University Medical School, Budapest 1450, Hungary. *Present address:* Department of Human Physiology, The Flinders Medical Centre, Bedford Park, Australia 5042.   ALAN COWEY • Department of Experimental Psychology, University of Oxford, Oxford OX1 3UD, England.

scription. First of all, therefore, we should attempt to define more precisely the characteristics of neurons we call *double bouquet cells*, especially as the original description may have included several types of neuron (Ramón y Cajal, 1899, 1900, 1911), as pointed out recently (Peters and Regidor, 1981).

2. Characteristics Defining Double Bouquet Cells

The term *double bouquet cell* will be applied to neurons with their perikarya in layers II and III and which have an axon traversing layers II–V, usually in a tight bundle consisting of varicose, radially oriented collaterals. Some of these main collaterals may run outside the bundle and sometimes the bundle is not compact. As the position of the perikaryon may vary considerably within layers II–III, only the axons of deeper double bouquet cells give a prominent ascending plexus reaching layer II to match the descending plexus to layer V. The branching of the main axon into ascending and descending collaterals always takes place within a 50- to 80-μm stratum about 50–100 μm from the perikaryon. These axons often but not invariably arise from neurons which have a radially elongated soma and a lower and upper dendritic spray, originating from two or three main shafts as depicted in Ramón y Cajal's drawings (1899, 1900). However, qualitatively similar dendritic features may be possessed by neurons which have a very different type of axon, e.g., the axo-axonic or chandelier cells (Somogyi, 1977; Szentágothai, 1978; Fairén and Valverde, 1980; Somogyi *et al.*, 1982; Peters *et al.*, 1982).

Therefore, in the present chapter we use the axon as a primary identifying feature of double bouquet cells and deal with previously reported cells only briefly if the axon was not sufficiently documented or was clearly of a different type.

Double bouquet cells are also different from bipolar neurons which have sparser, longer dendrites, smaller perikarya, and establish different synaptic contacts (Peters and Kimerer, 1981; also see Chapters 6 and 11).

3. Double Bouquet Cells in Different Species

3.1. Man

It is the historical importance of Ramón y Cajal's description (1899, 1900, 1911) of double bouquet cells in the human cortex which prompts a survey in descending evolutionary order. He illustrated the presence of these neurons in various areas of the very young infant's cortex. The neurons presented in his figures (1899, Figs. 8, 11 E, F; 1900, Fig. 5F) fulfill the criteria proposed above because the axons have a radial course. The axonal features are particularly clear in his Fig. 8, but the vertical bundles are wider than those of neurons described later. He also described the vertical axons as traversing the entire cortex, which is not so in other species, e.g., "Ces filaments sont si longs qu'ils

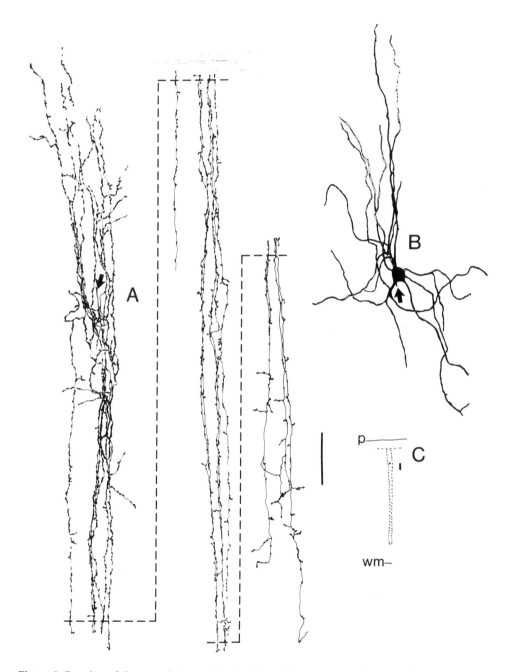

Figure 1. Drawing of the axonal (A) and the dendritic (B) arborization of a double bouquet cell in the striate cortex of the rhesus monkey. Arrows indicate the same axon initial segment. The descending axon plexus is continuous along the dashed line. (C) The position of the perikaryon (dot) and the axon bundle (broken outline) is indicated between the pia (p) and the white matter (wm). Scales: (A, B) 50 μm; (C) 100 μm. Modified from Somogyi and Cowey (1981) with permission.

peuvent s'étendre à toute la hauteur de l'écorce" (1911, p. 541). But without further studies on specimens from adults, it is not possible to establish whether the differences are due to the young age of the subjects or other factors. However, age differences will not easily explain why they are so much commoner in man, e.g., "Le nombre des corpuscules à double bouquet dendritique est extraordinairement grand chez l'homme" (1911, p. 539).

3.2. Other Primates

Compared with the number of papers dealing with the morphology of neurons in the cortex of monkeys studied by Golgi methods, descriptions of double bouquet cells with radially disposed axons are rare. They have been described in the striate and prestriate visual cortex (Szentágothai, 1971, 1973, 1978; Valverde, 1978; Tömböl, 1978; Somogyi and Cowey, 1981), in areas 1, 2, and 3 of the somatosensory cortex (Jones, 1975), and in area 5 of the parietal cortex (Jones, 1975). The most detailed acount of the axon has been given by Jones (1975) whose description can be applied to these neurons wherever they have been reported. The axon usually emerges from the base of the perikaryon (Fig. 1) or from the lower main dendritic shaft (Fig. 2A), and takes a descending course. Rarely it ascends immediately (Valverde, 1978). At 30–50 μm from its origin, it divides into thin smooth collaterals which themselves branch to form a spray of 3 to 10 main radial branches (Figs. 1, 2A). A distinct features of the axon is that "the thin stem branch which forms each ascending or descending arcade suddenly becomes very much thicker" (Jones, 1975). The thick radial branches are crowded with bulbous enlargements and terminal boutons on the end of thin stalks (Figs. 1, 2B). The radial branches together form tight fasciculi 20–50 μm in diameter (Fig. 2B) resembling a horse tail (Szentágothai, 1973, 1978), but wider axonal fasciculi have also been reported (Valverde, 1978). The main branches give rise to short collaterals in layers III and II, especially in the region of the dendritic arborization, and sometimes a few collaterals in layer V (Figs. 1, 2A).

The soma is 10–18 μm in diameter, round or ovid, and bears smooth or sparsely thorny dendrites which are also predominantly oriented in a radial direction (Figs. 1, 2A) but which may occasionally take a lateral course. The bitufted character of the dendritic arborization is not always prominent in the monkey (Fig. 1) and more or less round dendritic fields have also been described (Jones, 1975; Valverde, 1978).

Figure 2. (A) Drawing of a double bouquet cell in the striate cortex of the rhesus monkey. The perikaryon and the dendrites are in layer III but the axon bundle covers layers II–V. (B) Photomontage of the axon bundle (ab) of a similar cell in layer III of monkey striate cortex. (C–E) Electron micrographs of symmetrical synaptic contacts (solid arrows) established by Golgi-impregnated boutons of the double bouquet cell shown in (B), with spines (s) and a dendritic shaft (d). The spines receive asymmetrical synaptic contacts (open arrows) from boutons containing round synaptic vesicles. Scales: (A) 100 μm; (B) 20 μm; (C–E) 0.2 μm. Drawing courtesy of T. F. Freund. (B), (C), and (E) modified from Somogyi and Cowey (1981) with permission.

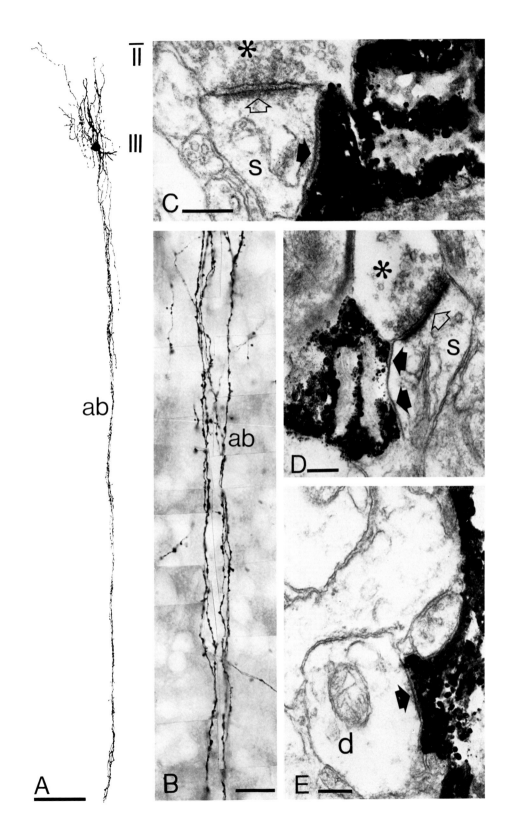

3.3. Cat

Few studies describe cells with long radial axons in this species. Colonnier (1966) mentions them, and although Szentágothai (1973) describes some similar cells in the somatosensory and visual cortex of the cat, his neurons with perikarya in layer IV may be of different types. Double bouquet cells with vertical axons have been described in the suprasylvian gyrus of young cats (Norita and Kawamura, 1981). In a previous study, we provided a detailed description of double bouquet cells in the striate (area 17) and peristriate (area 18) cortex of the cat (Somogyi and Cowey, 1981). The axonal features are similar to those in the monkey, described above, but with some differences. Thus, the main radial branches have fewer bulbous swellings and give out short collaterals especially in layer III and to a lesser extent in layer V (Figs. 3, 6A; see also Figs. 1 and 2 in Somogyi and Cowey, 1981). The radial axon plexus is usually less tightly arranged than in the monkey and may be 50–150 μm in diameter.

In the cat, the perikarya and dendrites are invariably of the characteristic bitufted type (Figs. 3B, E, 4B, 6A) and the main orientation of the dendrites is unambiguously radial. Although some proximal dendrites initially follow a lateral course, they soon bifurcate and divide into ascending and descending branches (Figs. 3, 4B, 6A). In cross-section, the radially disposed dendritic array rarely exceeds 100 μm.

On the basis of dendritic features, similar cells have recently been described in the visual cortex (Peters and Regidor, 1981), but the axons of these neurons seem somewhat different perhaps because of the young ages of the animals.

3.4. Rodents

With regard to axonal features, similar cells have not been described in rodents, despite numerous morphological investigations. However, there are several reports of neurons which in either their dendritic features or to a lesser extent their axonal characteristics, may be the forerunners of double bouquet cells in cat and primates. Lorente de Nó (1922) provided drawings of neurons from the parietal cortex of the rat which have their perikarya in layers III or IV and their axon running from layers I to V, with several main vertical collaterals and profuse arborizations in layers III and V (his Figs. 7A, B). The main dendrites are also radially oriented, but both the dendritic and the axonal arborizations are more diffuse than described above in the cat and monkey. In other studies on the visual cortex of mouse (Valverde, 1976) and rat (Peters and

$\longrightarrow$

Figure 3. Drawings of Golgi-impregnated double bouquet cells in the striate cortex of cat. The axon drawn in (A) belongs to the perikaryon and dendrites drawn separately in (B). Arrows indicate the axon initial segment. (C) and (F) show the position of the neurons in the cortex, with the territory of the axon outlined. The position of the cortical area in which they are located is shown in the lateral gyrus in (D). The dendritic arborization of a second neuron is shown in (E). Scales: (A, B, E) 50 μm; (C, F) 200 μm; (D) 2 mm.

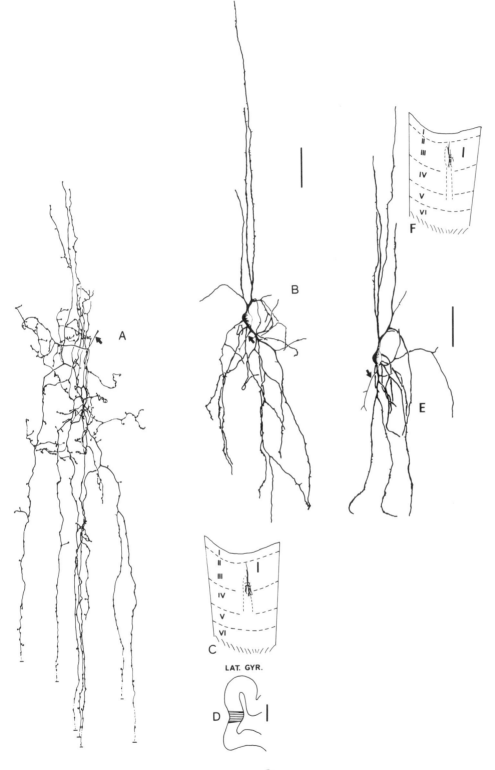

LAT. GYR.

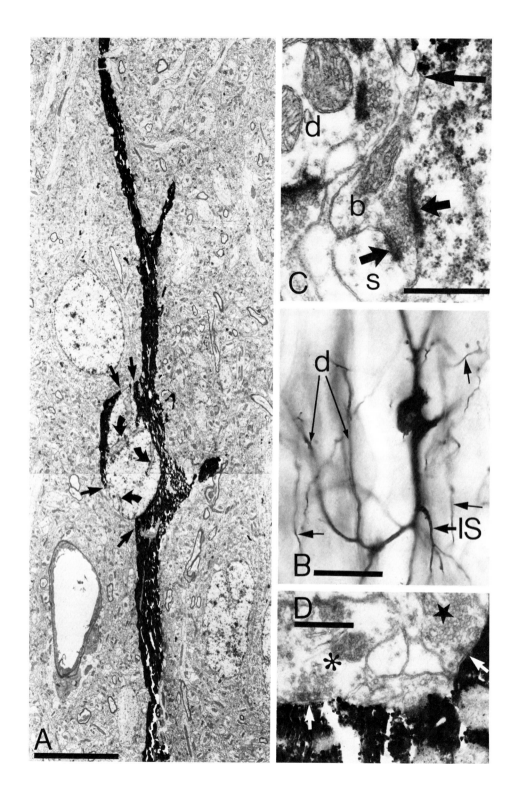

Fairén, 1978), smooth and sparsely spined stellate cells in layer III were shown to send a long vertical axon collateral to layer V, but no axon fascicles have been described (see Chapter 13). The efferent synaptic connections of the neurons in the rat show both similarities and differences to the double bouquet cells of the cat and monkey (Peters and Fairén, 1978; Somogyi and Cowey, 1981).

Bitufted cells have been described in the rat on the basis of dendritic features (Feldman and Peters, 1978) but the majority are outside layers II–III. Thus, they probably belong to other classes of neurons.

In conclusion, the double bouquet cells of cats and monkeys, which have radial axon bundles, most closely resemble and may be related to certain smooth and sparsely spiny stellate (multipolar or nonpyramidial) neurons which are present in rodents in layers II–III and have descending axons. From rodent to primate, there is a clear but still unquantified progression to a tighter axonal plexus, with less branching and more boutons concentrated on the main radial collaterals. There is suggestive but incomplete evidence that the axonal branches traverse all layers in man.

4. The Fine Structure of Double Bouquet Cells

A qualitative description of gross characteristics detectable with the light microscope is a necessary first step in identifying neurons and speculating on their function, but such descriptions have limitations when used to compare neurons in different species or to develop our ideas about their function. Until we can study the physiological and pharmacological properties of individual neurons that are marked and subsequently studied structurally [e.g., the basket cells studied by Martin *et al.* (1983) and Kisvárday *et al.* (1983)], the best procedure is to analyze the ultrastructure, and in particular the synaptic connections, of Golgi-impregnated cells first identified in the light microscope. This was the procedure adopted for double bouquet cells in the cat and monkey by Somogyi and Cowey (1981), with the following results.

Figure 4. (A) Electron micrograph of a Golgi-impregnated double bouquet cell in layer III of the striate cortex of the cat, also shown in light micrographs (B) and Fig. 6A. The perikaryon is partially impregnated. Precipitate is not present between straight arrows and is also absent from the deep nuclear invaginations (curved arrows) and from the nucleus. (B) Light micrograph of the same neuron as in (A). Note the fusiform perikaryon with a lower and upper dendritic trunk, the axon initial segment (IS), recurving dendrites (d), and varicose axons (arrows) which ascend toward layer II. (C) Electron micrograph of the perikaryon at the border of the impregnated and nonimpregnated parts (long arrow). The perikaryon receives an asymmetrical synaptic contact (thick arrow) from a bouton (b) containing round vesicles and also making a synapse (thick arrow) with a spine (s). An adjacent dendrite (d) receives similar synaptic contacts. Note the large number of free polysomes in the cytoplasm. (D) Branching point of the dendrite of the same neuron, receiving synapses (arrows) from a bouton with round vesicles (star) and another with small pleomorphic vesicles (asterisk). Scales: (A) 10 μm; (B) 25 μm; (C, D) 0.5 μm.

4.1. Characteristics of the Perikarya and Dendrites in the Cat

For the present account, one neuron was examined in the striate cortex of the cat (Fig. 4) using methods described earlier (Somogyi, 1978). The neuron was not densely or uniformly impregnated, which provided an opportunity to study some of the internal detail. The eccentrically placed nucleus had deep invaginations of the nuclear membrane so that it formed several separated profiles (Fig. 4A). Free polysomes were present in conspicuously high density in the thin rim of the cytoplasm (Fig. 4C). Mitochondria were present in moderate numbers, and the Golgi apparatus was located in the perikaryon and proximal dendrites. These are common features of cortical neurons and we have detected nothing unique about the internal features of the perikaryon of the double bouquet cell.

The perikaryon received few synaptic contacts, and mostly from boutons containing flattened, pleomorphic vesicles. But occasionally boutons containing round synaptic vesicles and making asymmetrical synaptic contacts were also found (Fig. 4C). These two basic types of bouton also contacted the dendritic shafts and thorny appendages (Fig. 4D), but on the dendrites more boutons with round vesicles were seen.

The axon initial segment was also studied in this and another neuron of the same type but afferent synaptic contacts on this position of the neuron were never observed.

The above features are similar to those of some other types of identified nonpyramidal neurons with smooth or sparsely spiny dendrites (Peters and Fairén, 1978; Peters et al., 1982; Peters and Kimerer, 1981; Somogyi et al., 1982), and so far no qualitative feature has been found which would make it possible to recognize double bouquet neurons without Golgi impregnation.

Since there are indications that different types of cortical interneurons differ in their postsynaptic targets, we analyzed the synaptic connections made by axon terminals of double bouquet cells (Somogyi and Cowey, 1981).

4.2. Efferent Synaptic Connections in Cat and Monkey

4.2.1. Characteristics of Double Bouquet Cell Boutons and Synapses

In our previous study (Somogyi and Cowey, 1981), identified Golgi-impregnated axon collaterals were followed in serial sections. In electron micrographs, the synapses formed by the impregnated boutons were compared to

Figure 5. Electron micrographs of Golgi-impregnated synaptic boutons originating from double bouquet cells in cat striate cortex. The boutons shown in (A), (C), and (D) belong to the neuron shown in Figs. 4 and 6A, while the one shown in (B) belongs to the neuron in Figs. 3A and B. (A) A smooth dendrite (d) containing a lamellar body (lb) receives a symmetrical synaptic contact (arrow) from the impregnated bouton and an asymmetrical contact from a bouton containing round vesicles (star). (B) After partial removal of the Golgi precipitate, flattened, pleomorphic vesicles (white arrows) are seen in a bouton making symmetrical synaptic contact (arrow) with a dendrite. (C) Multiple synaptic contacts (arrows) established by a collateral with the same dendrite which also receives numerous asymmetrical synaptic contacts from boutons with round vesicles (asterisk). (D) Symmetrical axosomatic synapse established on the perikaryon of a nonpyramidal neuron. Scales: (A–D) 0.25 μm. Modified from Somogyi and Cowey (1981) with permission.

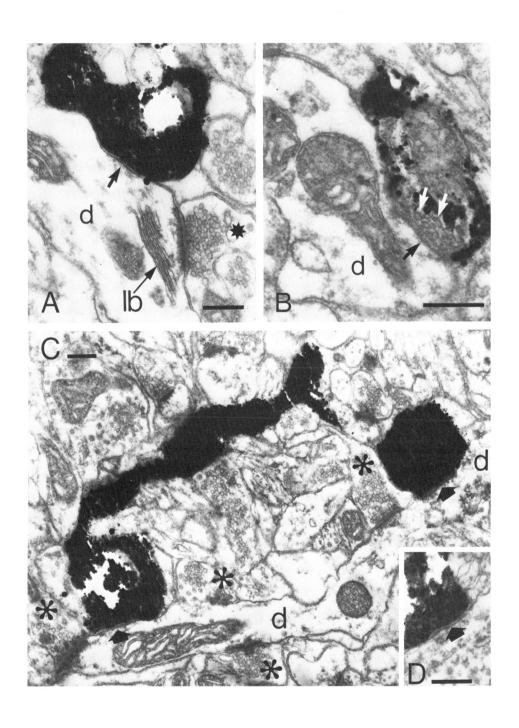

synapses established by unstained boutons with the same postsynaptic target (Figs. 2C, D, 5A, C) as well as to adjacent synapses in the same section.

In the cat, double bouquet cells form symmetrical, type II (Gray, 1959), synaptic contacts (Fig. 5). As compared to symmetrical axosomatic synapses received by pyramidal cells, the postsynaptic membrane thickening appears more pronounced in some cases (Fig. 5C). The thickness of the membrane specialization naturally depends on the plane of the section, but it never equaled the thickness of asymmetrical axospinous or axodendritic postsynaptic specializations (Fig. 5). Apart from the criterion of postsynaptic membrane density, synapses were also identified by the electron-dense cleft material which occasionally contained an additional electron-dense line.

In the monkey, one double bouquet cell was stained in a similar way. Seventeen synapses were identified and all were typical symmetrical, type II synapses (Figs. 2C–E).

The silver chromate precipitate had been partially removed from the boutons of two cells in the cat, enabling us to study the synaptic vesicles (Somogyi and Cowey, 1981). The vesicles were flattened or pleomorphic (Fig. 5B). Occasionally, large dense core vesicles were also present. This pattern of vesicles corresponded closely to that found in unstained boutons in the same material, where symmetrical membrane specialization and pleomorphic vesicles occurred together.

4.2.2. Electron Microscopy of Postsynaptic Structures

The form and distribution of postsynaptic structures are summarized in Table I which shows a difference between cat and monkey and also between areas 17 and 18 in the cat. However, it is not clear whether the differences represent anything other than sampling artifacts. Of 66 boutons studied in area 17 of the cat, 57 terminated on small or medium-sized dendritic shafts (Figs. 5A–C) which had no particular orientation. Some of these dendrites were traced in serial sections and they were never found to give rise to spines. In more than half of the sections showing an impregnated bouton from a double bouquet cell, the dendrite also received one or more unimpregnated synaptic boutons (Figs. 5A, C), the majority of which established asymmetrical contacts. Six impregnated axosomatic synapses (Figs. 5D) were identified on four nonpyramidal neurons, three of which were fusiform and had dendrites extending from the upper and lower pole of the perikaryon. These neurons were identified as nonpyramidal since their perikarya received both asymmetrical and symmetrical synapses from unstained boutons (Colonnier, 1968; Parnavelas et al., 1977). The perikarya, axon initial segments, or main dendritic shafts of pyramidal cells were never encountered among the postsynaptic structures. Unfortunately, it was not possible to identify the parent cell of the three spines postsynaptic to double bouquet cells in area 17 of the cat.

One neuron was studied from area 18 of the cat. Although spines postsynaptic to the axon were more frequent (26%), the majority of the synapses were still established with dendritic shafts. One of these shafts was about 2 μm thick and followed a radial course, both characteristics of an apical dendrite. The shaft itself received only symmetrical synapses but two spines bearing asymmetrical synapses emerged from its surface. A further shaft in synaptic contact with an

Table I. Type and Distribution of Structures Postsynaptic to Double Bouquet Cells

Animal	Cortical region	Cell No.	Layers examined by electron microscopy	Number of identified boutons contacting:			
				Spines	Dendritic shafts	Perikarya of nonpyramidal neurons	Total
Monkey	Area 17	1 (Figs. 1, 2B–E)	III–IV	14 (40%)	21 (60%)		35 (100%)
Cat	Area 17	2 (Figs. 4, 5A, C, D, 6A)	III–IV–V	1	47	5	53
		3 (Figs. 3, 5B)	III	1	7	1	9
		4	III	1	3	—	4
	Total			3 (4.6%)	57 (86.4%)	6 (9%)	66 (100%)
	Area 18	5	III	5 (26%)	14 (74%)	—	19 (100%)

impregnated bouton gave rise to two spines bearing asymmetrical synapses. The remaining dendrites were all small or medium size and had no particular orientation. They received remarkably few unstained boutons, suggesting that some or all of them are different from those described in area 17.

One double bouquet neuron from layer III of the striate cortex of the monkey was reprocessed for electron microscopy. Its boutons innervated many more spines than the boutons in the cat (Table I), and more of the spines were in layer III than in layer IV. Each of these spines received one asymmetrical synapse from an unstained bouton containing round synaptic vesicles (Figs. 2C, D) in addition to the symmetrical synapse established by the impregnated bouton. The spines had long thin stalks which made it impossible to identify their parent dendrites with certainty. As in the cat, the postsynaptic dendritic shafts (Fig. 2E) had no particular orientation, were of small or medium diameter, and about one in five made asymmetrical synaptic contacts with nonimpregnated boutons.

We were particularly interested to see whether one postsynaptic element receives many synapses from one double bouquet cell or whether the innervation is much more frugal. In both cat and monkey, two reconstructions were made from serial sections. It was clear that even the most closely adjacent boutons usually innervate different structures. Neighboring synapses on the same dendrite were rarely observed (Fig. 5C). However, two of the postsynaptic perikarya received two adjacent synapses from the same double bouquet cell.

4.2.3. Discussion of Efferent Synaptic Connections

It has been suggested that the vertical axon bundles of layer III double bouquet cells terminate mainly on the apical dendrites of pyramidal cells (Ramón y Cajal, 1911; Colonnier, 1966; Szentágothai, 1973, 1975, 1978; Jones, 1975). This proposal could not be substantiated by our electron microscopic study (Somogyi and Cowey, 1981), and from an examination of Golgi material Valverde (1978) had previously questioned whether the apical dendrites were the predominant postsynaptic targets.

In our material, many of the postsynaptic dendritic shafts in area 17 of the cat probably belong to nonpyramidal neurons as shown by the fine structural characteristics and synaptic input of the dendrites. All four postsynaptic perikarya also belonged to nonpyramidal cells. However, some of the dendritic shafts postsynaptic to layer III double bouquet cells could be basal dendrites of pyramidal cells or side branches of apical dendrites. In area 18 of the cat, two spiny dendrites were the postsynaptic target. In layer III, the spines probably belonged to pyramidal cells and they may be a significant postsynaptic target in area 18. In the monkey, the proportion of spines receiving input from double bouquet cells was greater than in the cat and there were fewer in layer IV than in layer III, where the majority can belong only to pyramidal cells. So, as well as the nonpyramidal neurons demonstrated in area 17 of the cat, certain parts of pyramidal cells also seem to receive synapses from the descending axons of double bouquet cells.

The idea that apical dendrites are the principal postsynaptic target of double bouquet cells was attractive, since it seemed to explain the narrow, strictly radial course of the axonal branches and suggested a climbing type of interaction. This could not be confirmed in our investigation, since the radial beaded axons appear not to follow any particular postsynaptic structure. Several synapses on the same dendrite were rarely observed. However, since the double bouquet cell has a dense vertical axon plexus and high bouton density, its axon is likely to encounter different dendrites of the same postsynaptic neuron.

It is probably unwise to stress the differences in the nature of the postsynaptic targets in monkey and cat and the differences between areas 17 and 18 in the cat. Nevertheless, the dissimilarities between cat and monkey for the most extensively studied neurons in area 17 are sufficiently great to suggest that real differences may exist.

5. Possible Transmitters Used by Double Bouquet Cells

5.1. Comparison of Double Bouquet Cells with Neurons Containing Glutamic Acid Decarboxylase

In our analysis of double bouquet cells from the monkey, all identified synapses were unquestionably symmetrical, i.e., type II. Although the postsynaptic membrane specialization was more pronounced in the cat, it fell far short of the thickening seen at asymmetrical synapses. Consequently, even in the cat too the contacts made by double bouquet cells are also most reasonably classified as type II. Furthermore, the presence of pleomorphic vesicles in the boutons indicates that these boutons form type II synapses. Glutamic acid decarboxylase (GAD), the enzyme synthesizing γ-aminobutyric acid (GABA), has been localized in boutons which form symmetrical synaptic contacts in the cortex of monkey (Ribak *et al.*, 1979) and cat (Somogyi *et al.*, 1983b). Thus, it is possible that the boutons of double bouquet cells also contain GAD and that they therefore use GABA as their transmitter.

It is even more pertinent that neurons of similar size and shape to double bouquet cells in layers II and III of cat visual cortex contain GAD (Somogyi *et al.*, 1983b). Some of these neurons were also Golgi impregnated, which revealed their dendritic arborization (Somogyi *et al.*, 1983b). At least one cell in layer II had very similar features to those of double bouquet cells. Unfortunately, few of the neurons containing GAD have had a Golgi-impregnated axon, and none of those successfully impregnated had axons characteristic of double bouquet cells.

The comparisons described above are necessarily limited and we have therefore used other approaches in an attempt to determine the transmitters used by double bouquet cells and other interneurons. In one line of experiments, using immunocytochemical methods, we have characterized neurons containing putative transmitters, including various peptides. In another approach, we have been studying the selective uptake and transport of [^{3}H]-GABA in combination with Golgi impregnation. Both procedures have provided information which, although indirect, can help to elucidate the function of these neurons.

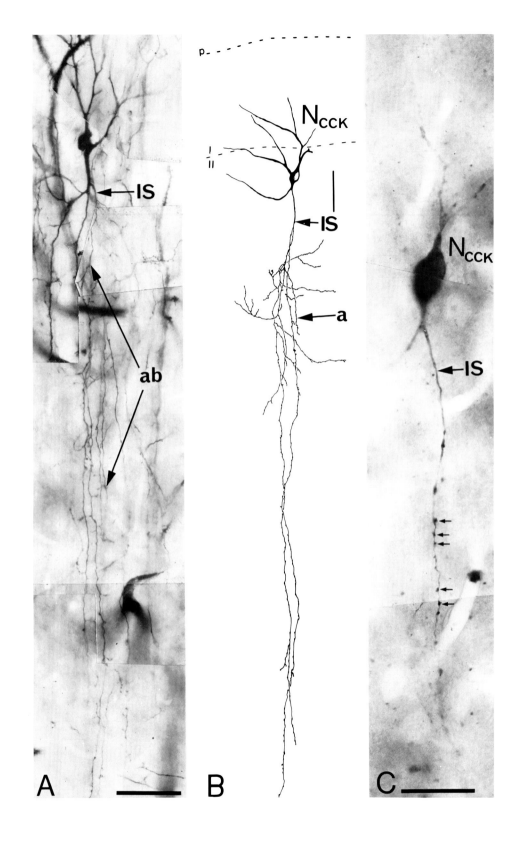

5.2. Some Cholecystokinin Immunoreactive Neurons Are Similar to Double Bouquet Cells

Following pilot experiments which indicated that some nonpyramidal cells in layers II–III contain cholecystokinin (CCK)-immunoreactive material, we studied the striate cortex of cats using the unlabeled antibody enzyme method (Sternberger *et al.*, 1970). An antiserum specific for the COOH terminus of CCK8 (Dockray, 1980) was applied to colchicine-injected striate cortex in a procedure which allows detailed visualization of immunoreactive neurons (Somogyi and Takagi, 1982). In some fortunate examples, the neurons were revealed almost in their entirety, and one such cell is shown in Figs. 6B and C. The shape of the perikaryon, the disposition of the dendrites, and the origin and course of the axon are similar to those of Golgi-impregnated double bouquet cells described above. The axon descends from layer II to layer V. Although it is far more difficult to follow immunoreactive axon collaterals than Golgi-impregnated ones, two long descending radial branches (Fig. 6B) exhibiting bulbous enlargements (Fig. 6C) and boutons on short stalks could be identified.

These findings raise the possibility that some double bouquet cells contain CCK. Earlier immunocytochemical studies also showed vertically arranged CCK-immunoreactive dots in the cortex (Emson and Hunt, 1981). However, it is already clear that many CCK-immunoreactive neurons in cat visual cortex are not double bouquet cells. For example, neurons with different axons have been encountered and many CCK-immunoreactive perikarya can be found in layers V–VI, which do not contain double bouquet cells.

Clearly, further studies are necessary to determine the afferent and efferent synaptic relations of CCK-immunoreactive neurons, which appear morphologically similar to double bouquet cells. In addition, more detailed visualization of CCK neurons is necessary using the recently developed combined Golgi impregnation–immunocytochemical staining of the same neuron (Freund and Somogyi, 1983; Somogyi *et al.*, 1983b) before it can be established that some or all double bouquet cells contain CCK.

5.3. [³H]-GABA-Accumulating Neurons in Layers II and Upper III Project to Deeper Layers

From another line of experiments in which we studied the distribution of selectively labeled neuronal perikarya following [³H]-GABA injections into different layers of the visual cortex (Cowey *et al.*, 1981; Somogyi *et al.*, 1981, 1983a), evidence was obtained that GABA may be a transmitter used by double bouquet

---

Figure 6. (A) Photomontage of a Golgi-impregnated double bouquet cell in the striate cortex of cat, also shown in Fig. 4. The axon initial segment (is) originates from the lower dendritic trunk and gives a descending axon bundle (ab). (B) Drawing of CCK-immunoreactive neuron (N_{CCK}) with a descending axon plexus (a) in the striate cortex of cat. The axon initial segment originates from the lower dendritic trunk. The perikaryon is at the border of layers I and II. (C) Light micrograph of the same neuron as in (B). Note the varicose (small arrows) descending axon. Scales: (A, B) 50 μm; (C) 25 μm.

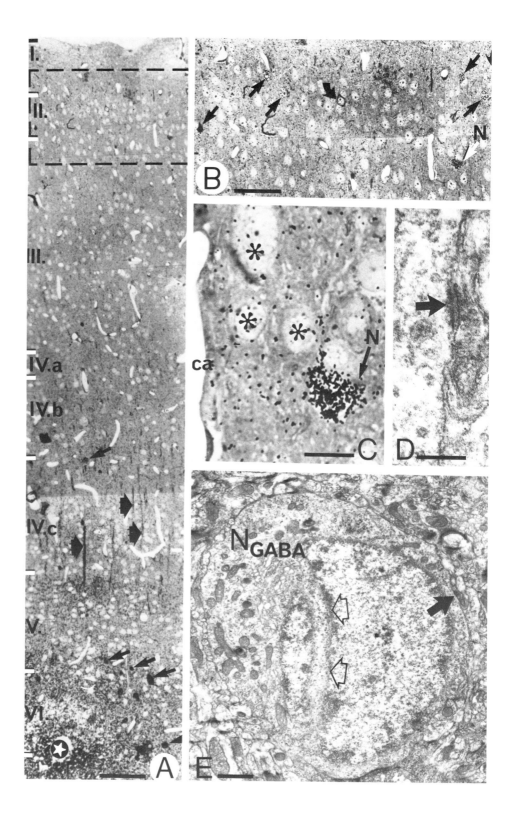

cells. It was noticed in the monkey that when the injection site was in the deep layers (V and VI), in addition to the labeled neurons always present around the injection track, another group of neurons appeared in layers II and upper III (Figs. 7A, B). These neurons lay directly above the injection site but could not have been labeled by local uptake of [^{3}H]-GABA in the region of their perikarya because there were few or no [^{3}H]-GABA accumulating neurons below them in layers IV ab and lower III, even though these layers contain numerous labeled neurons when [^{3}H]-GABA is directly injected into them. The only simple explanation for the heavy labeling of these neurons in layers II and upper III is that they accumulated the labeled substance by retrograde axonal transport from their terminals within the injection site in the deeper layers. This is supported by the simultaneous presence of strongly labeled fiber bundles (Fig. 7A) passing radially through layer IV. The neurons were small to medium in size, and fusiform or elongated (Figs. 7B, C). We studied the fine structural characteristics of these [^{3}H]-GABA-accumulating neurons (Somogyi *et al.*, 1981) and found that they have an eccentric nucleus with clumps of chromatin, and invaginations of the nuclear membrane (Fig. 7E). The neurons had large numbers of free polysomes and received asymmetrical synapses on the soma (Fig. 7D). These features are characteristic of nonpyramidal cells.

The identity of the [^{3}H]-GABA-accumulating neurons becomes apparent when they are Golgi impregnated. An example is shown in Fig. 8. We have few examples of such neurons, but all were nonpyramidal cells with smooth dendrites, very similar in dendritic and somatic features to double bouquet cells. Unfortunately, we have still not succeeded in impregnating the axons of the neurons that are Golgi-stained and have accumulated [^{3}H]-GABA, so that there is not unequivocal evidence that these neurons are double bouquet cells. Nevertheless, the results show that there is a population of aspiny neurons in layers II and upper III, where double bouquet cells occur, which selectively accumulate [^{3}H]-GABA through their descending axons and which are therefore likely to be GABAergic. The labeled axon bundles suggest that they could be the double bouquet cells. Interestingly, such a population of GABA-accumulating neurons which can be labeled in the upper layers following injections in layer V and VI, has been found in the rat (Cowey *et al.*, 1981), cat (unpublished observation),

---

Figure 7. (A–C) Light micrographs of semithin sections (1 μm) processed for autoradiography and cut from a Golgi-impregnated, gold-toned thick section of the striate cortex of the monkey. (A) The cortex was injected with [^{3}H]-GABA through a capillary nearly perpendicular to the plane of the section. Labeled neurons selectively accumulating [^{3}H]-GABA (small arrows) are present around the injection track (star) which is at the border of the white matter and layer VI. The framed area in layers II and upper III contains another group of labeled neurons and is shown in (B). Thick arrows indicate strongly labeled fiber bundles passing through layer IV. (B) High magnification of framed area in (A) showing neurons that have accumulated [^{3}H]-GABA (small arrows) and unlabeled gold-toned pyramidal neurons (curved arrows) in layers II and upper III. One labeled neuron (N) is shown at even higher magnification in (C) among unlabeled neurons (asterisk). A capillary (ca) is indicated. (D, E) Electron micrographs of a neuron (N$_{GABA}$) in layer II from the area shown in (A) and (B), and which was shown by light microscopic autoradiography to accumulate [^{3}H]-GABA from the deeper layers. The neuron has a deeply indented nucleus (open arrows) and receives an asymmetric synaptic contact (solid arrows) on the perikaryon. Scales: (A) 100 μm; (B) 50 μm; (C) 10 μm; (D) 0.2 μm; (E) 1 μm.

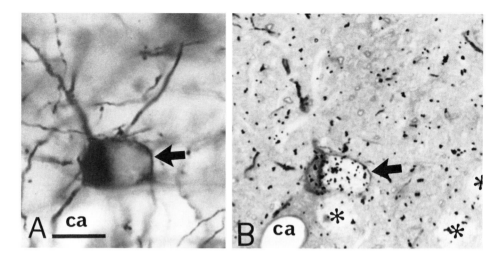

Figure 8. (A) Light micrograph of a Golgi-impregnated gold-toned neuron with smooth dendrites in layer II of monkey prestriate cortex (area 18, V II). This neuron was situated directly above an [³H]-GABA injection track in layer VI. (B) Semithin section (1 μm) cut from the perikaryon (arrow) of the same neuron and processed for autoradiography. This neuron selectively accumulated [³H]-GABA when compared to neighboring unlabeled neurons (asterisk). A capillary (ca) serves as reference in the two micrographs. Scales: 10 μm. Courtesy of Z. F. Kisvárday.

and monkey (Somogyi *et al.*, 1981), so they probably form a basic feature of cortical circuitry.

5.4. Conclusions on the Possible Transmitter(s) of Double Bouquet Cells

The types of synapses formed by double bouquet cells and their other morphological features suggest that they use GABA as a transmitter (Somogyi and Cowey, 1981; Somogyi *et al.*, 1981). This idea is compatible with results obtained from the immunocytochemical demonstration of GAD and from the autoradiographic demonstration of [³H]-GABA following its selective uptake (see Sections 5.1 and 5.3). GABA is an inhibitory neurotransmitter in the cerebral cortex (Krnjevic and Schwartz, 1967; Krnjevic, 1974), which would mean that double bouquet cells with vertical axon bundles are inhibitory. In addition, CCK may be present in some double bouquet cells, either alone or together with other transmitter candidates (see Section 5.2).

6. Functional Implications

Earlier light microscopic studies led to the suggestion (Colonnier, 1966; Szentágothai, 1973) that the vertical disposition of axons of double bouquet cells mediated excitation, and the similarly oriented apical dendrites were considered as the primary postsynaptic targets. In our electron microscopic studies, we could not find a preferential association between apical dendrites of pyramidal neurons and the axons of double bouquet cells, although more work is necessary especially in the monkey. The idea that apical dendrites receive input from double bouquet cells was attractive, for it seemed to explain the narrow and strictly radial course of the axon, and it suggested a climbing type of interaction. However, the small diameter of the axon cylinder may be the basis of other types of neuronal interaction, and we consider some of them.

It was suggested (Somogyi and Cowey, 1981) that perhaps one should think of not one neuron, but assemblies of double bouquet cells with vertical axons forming dense "curtains" from layer II down to layer V. Viewed from the surface of the cortex, these curtains could be long and narrow, with sharp edges caused by the small lateral spread of the axon. Such axonal assemblies could contribute to differences in the activity of neighboring neuron populations contained within slablike pieces of cortex.

Unfortunately, there is still no evidence about the lateral distribution of double bouquet cells in the cortex, largely because only a small proportion of neurons are impregnated by the Golgi method. Only when it is possible to selectively reveal all or most of the double bouquet cells in a particular region will it be possible to relate them with any confidence to functional groups of neurons such as those contained within the ocular dominance slabs. And even then, an apparently uniform anatomical distribution may conceal physiological specialization that depends on their inputs.

Another likely consequence of the tight radial axon plexus of double bouquet cells is that their action on any particular postsynaptic neuron will be localized to a particular region of that neuron. Thus, while one double bouquet cell may have negligible effect on the postsynaptic neuron as a whole its local effect on a dendrite or spine may be powerful and may interact significantly with other inputs to the same region. It was a striking feature of the postsynaptic spines in the monkey that the type II symmetrical synapse formed by the bouton of a double bouquet cell was invariably accompanied by a type I, asymmetrical synapse from a different bouton, as if the two types of inputs were competing for the same spine.

Another type of interaction was suggested on the basis of results obtained in cat striate cortex (Somogyi and Cowey, 1981), in which a substantial proportion of the elements postsynaptic to double bouquet cells belong to nonpyramidal cells. Many of the latter are GABAergic, as revealed by the presence of GAD immunoreactivity in their perikarya (Somogyi *et al.*, 1983b). If double bouquet cells are also GABAergic and inhibitory, as we suggest, it means that any synaptic interaction between them and other GABAergic neurons would produce disinhibition at the synapses of the latter. In fact, in the striate cortex of the cat, GAD-immunoreactive neurons receive numerous GAD-positive synaptic contacts both on their perikarya and dendrites as revealed by simultaneous Golgi impregnation (Somogyi *et al.*, 1983b), and some of these boutons may originate from double bouquet cells. Disinhibitory interactions have been proposed to explain some of the discharge characteristics of visual cortical neurons excited by retinal stimulation (Toyama *et al.*, 1977). Thus, it has been reported that the initial excitation in all cells is followed by a depression, apparently mediated by IPSPs, which was in turn rapidly succeeded by a rebound excitation possibly as a result of inhibition of the first-order inhibitory interneuron. To a first approximation, the double bouquet cell described in area 17 of the cat ideally fits the role of the putative second-order inhibitory neuron because (1) its synaptic structure suggests that it is inhibitory; (2) it frequently makes synapses with perikarya and dendrites of other nonpyramidal cells, which may also be inhibitory; (3) its soma and dendrites reside primarily in upper layer III, and are thus unlikely to receive input from specific afferents which could cause the first-order inhibition; (4) it provides the highest bouton density of any cortical interneuron yet described, so that its local effect is probably very powerful.

Finally, it is worth comparing the geometrically specific axon of the double bouquet cell with that of another local-circuit interneuron, the axoaxonic cell, which is now known to make synapses exclusively with the axon initial segments of pyramidal cells in the rat, cat, and monkey (Somogyi, 1977, 1979; Somogyi et al., 1979, 1982; Fairén and Valverde, 1980; Peters et al., 1982). The axo-axonic cell (also known as the chandelier cell, although the two may not always be identical) has a much more dispersed axonal arborization but extraordinary specificity with respect to target structure. This contrasts with the spatial specificty of layer III double bouquet cells, whose radially oriented tightly confined axonal terminal field is unique among known cortical local-circuit interneurons. Their postsynaptic targets are more diverse than those of axo-axonic cells, but nevertheless they appear to exclude the perikarya, axon initial segments, and even the apical dendrites (one possible example found) of pyramidal cells. When contrasted in this way with the different, but still highly specific pattern of connections made by other types of neurons those of the double bouquet cell illustrate the extraordinary specificity and intricacy of the local circuitry of the cerebral cortex.

ACKNOWLEDGMENTS. The authors are grateful to Mrs. K. Boczko, Miss K. Szigeti, Miss S. Thomas, and Dr. S. Totterdel for their excellent assistance at various stages of experiments reported here. The gift of CCK antiserum from Dr. G. Dockray is gratefully acknowledged, as is unpublished material and comment on the manuscript from T. F. Freund and Z. F. Kisvárday. This work was supported by the MRC, the E.P. Abraham Cephalosporin Trust, the Wellcome Trust, the International Cultural Institute (Budapest), and the Hungarian Academy of Sciences. P. S. was supported at the Department of Pharmacology, Oxford University, by the Wellcome Trust during part of this work.

7. References

Asanuma, H., 1975, Recent developments in the study of the columnar arrangement of neurons within the motor cortex, *Physiol. Rev.* **55:**143–156.

Colonnier, M. L., 1966, The structural design of the neocortex, in: *Brain and Conscious Experience* (J. C. Eccles, ed.), pp. 1–23, Springer, Berlin.

Colonnier, M. L., 1968, Synaptic patterns on different cell types in the different laminae of the cat visual cortex. An electron microscope study, *Brain Res.* **9:**268–287.

Cowey, A., Freund, T. F., and Somogyi, P., 1981, Organization of [³H]GABA-accumulating neurones in the visual cortex of the rat and the rhesus monkey, *J. Physiol. (London)* **320:**15–16P.

Dockray, G. J., 1980, Cholecystokinins in rat cerebral cortex: Identification, purification and characterization by immunochemical methods, *Brain Res.* **188:** 155–165.

Emson, P. C., and Hunt, S. P., 1981, Anatomical chemistry of the cerebral cortex, in: *The Organization of the Cerebral Cortex* (F. O. Schmitt, F. G. Worden, G. Adelman, and S. G. Dennis, eds.), pp. 325–345, MIT Press, Cambridge, Mass.

Fairén A., and Valverde, F., 1980, A specialized type of neuron in the visual cortex of cat: A Golgi and electron microscope study of chandelier cells, *J. Comp. Neurol.* **194**:761–780.

Feldman, M. L., and Peters, A., 1978, The forms of non-pyramidal neurons in the visual cortex of the rat, *J. Comp. Neurol.* **179**:761–793.

Freund, T. F., and Somogyi, P., 1983, The section–Golgi impregnation procedure. I. Description of the method and its combination with histochemistry after intracellular iontophoresis or retrograde transport of horseradish peroxidase, *Neuroscience* **9**:463–474.

Gray, E. G., 1959, Axo-somatic and axo-dendritic synapses of the cerebral cortex: An electron microscope study, *J. Anat.* **93**:420–433.

Hubel, D. H., and Wiesel, T. N., 1977, Functional architecture of the macaque monkey visual cortex, Ferrier Lecture, *Proc. R. Soc. London Ser. B* **198**:1–59.

Jones, E. G., 1975, Varieties and distribution of non-pyramidal cells in the somatic sensory cortex of the squirrel monkey, *J. Comp. Neurol.* **160**:205–268.

Kisvárday, Z. F., Martin, K. A. C., Somogyi, P., and Whitteridge, D., 1983, The physiology, morphology and synaptology of basket cells in the cat's visual cortex, *J. Physiol. (London)* **334**:33P.

Krnjevic, K., 1974, Chemical nature of synaptic transmission in vertebrates, *Physiol. Rev.* **54**:318–450.

Krnjevic, K., and Schwartz, S., 1967, The action of γ-aminobutyric acid on cortical neurones, *Exp. Brain Res.* **3**:320–336.

Lorente de Nó, R., 1922, La corteza cerebral del ratón, *Trab. Lab. Invest. Biol. Madrid* **20**:41–78.

Martin, K. A. C., Somogyi, P., and Whitteridge, D., 1983, Physiological and morphological properties of identified basket cells in the cat's visual cortex. *Exp. Brain Res.* **50**:193–200.

Mountcastle, V. B., 1957, Modality and topographic properties of single neurons of cat's somatic sensory cortex, *J. Neurophysiol.* **20**:408–434.

Norita, M., and Kawamura, K., 1981, Non-pyramidal neurons in the medial bank (Clare–Bishop area) of the middle suprasylvian sulcus: A Golgi study in the cat, *J. Hirnforsch.* **22**:9–28.

Parnavelas, J. G., Sullivan, K., Lieberman, A. R., and Webster, K. E., 1977, Neurons and their synaptic organization in the visual cortex of the rat, *Cell Tissue Res.* **183**:499–517.

Peters, A., and Fairén, A., 1978, Smooth and sparsely-spined stellate cells in the visual cortex of the rat: A study using a combined Golgi–electron microscope technique, *J. Comp. Neurol.* **181**:129–172.

Peters, A., and Kimerer, L. M., 1981, Bipolar neurons in rat visual cortex—A combined Golgi–electron microscope study, *J. Neurocytol.* **10**:921–946.

Peters, A., and Regidor, J., 1981, A reassessment of the forms of nonpyramidal neurons in area 17 of cat visual cortex, *J. Comp. Neurol.* **203**:685–716.

Ramón y Cajal S., 1899, Estudios sobre la corteza cerebral humana: Corteza visual, *Rev. Trimest. Microsc.* **4**:1–63.

Ramón y Cajal, S., 1900, Estudios sobre la corteza cerebral humana. III. Estructura de la corteza acústica, *Rev. Trimest. Microsc.* **5**:129–183.

Ramón y Cajal, S., 1911, *Histologie du Système Nerveux de l'Homme et des Vertébrés* (translated by L. Azoulay), Vol. II, Maloine, Paris.

Ribak, C. E., Harris, A. B., Vaughn, J. E., and Roberts, E., 1979, Inhibitory, GABAergic nerve terminals decrease at sites of focal epilepsy, *Science* **205**:211–213.

Somogyi, P., 1977, A specific axo-axonal interneuron in the visual cortex of the rat, *Brain Res.* **136**:345–350.

Somogyi, P., 1978, The study of Golgi stained cells and of experimental degeneration under the electron microscope: A direct method for the identification in the visual cortex of three successive links in a neuron chain, *Neuroscience* **3**:167–180.

Somogyi, P., 1979, An interneuron making synapses specifically on the axon initial segment (AIS) of pyramidal cells in the cerebral cortex of the cat, *J. Physiol. (London)* **296**:18–19P.

Somogyi, P., and Cowey, A., 1981, Combined Golgi and electron microscopic study on the synapses formed by double bouquet cells in the visual cortex of the cat and monkey, *J. Comp. Neurol.* **195**:547–566.

Somogyi, P., and Takagi, H., 1982, A note on the use of picric acid–paraformaldehyde–glutaraldehyde fixative for correlated light and electron microscopic immunocytochemistry, *Neuroscience* **7**:1779–1783.

Somogyi, P., Hodgson, A. J., and Smith, A. D., 1979, An approach to tracing neuron networks in the cerebral cortex and basal ganglia: Combination of Golgi-staining, retrograde transport of horseradish peroxidase and anterograde degeneration of synaptic boutons in the same material, *Neuroscience* **4**:1804–1852.

Somogyi, P., Cowey, A., Halasz, N., and Freund, T. F., 1981, Vertical organization of neurons accumulating ³H-GABA in the visual cortex of the rhesus monkey, *Nature (London)* **294**:761–763.

Somogyi, P., Freund, T. F., and Cowey, A., 1982, The axo-axonic interneuron in the cerebral cortex of the rat, cat and monkey, *Neuroscience* **7**:2577–2609.

Somogyi, P., Cowey, A., Kisvárday, Z. F., Freund, T. F., and Szentágothai, J., 1983a, Retrograde transport of ³H-GABA reveals specific interlaminar connections in the striate cortex of monkey, *Proc. Natl. Acad. Sci. USA* **80**:2385–2389.

Somogyi, P., Freund, T. F., Wu, J.-Y., and Smith, A. D., 1983b, The section Golgi impregnation procedure. II. Immunocytochemical demonstration of glutamate decarboxylase in Golgi-impregnated neurons and in their afferent synaptic boutons in the visual cortex of the cat, *Neuroscience* **9**:475–490.

Sternberger, L. A., Hardy, P. H., Curculis, J. J., and Meyer, H. G., 1970, The unlabelled antibody-enzyme method of immunohistochemistry: Preparation and properties of soluble antigen–antibody complex (horseradish peroxidase–antihorseradish peroxidase) and its use in identification of spirochetes, *J. Histochem. Cytochem.* **18**:315–333.

Szentágothai, J., 1969, Architecture of the cerebral cortex, in: *Basic Mechanisms of the Epilepsies* (H. H. Jasper, A. A. Ward, and A. Pope, eds.), pp. 13–28, Little, Brown, Boston.

Szentágothai, J., 1971, Some geometrical aspects of the neocortical neuropil, *Acta Biol. Acad. Sci. Hung.* **22**:107–124.

Szentágothai, J., 1973, Synaptology of the visual cortex, in: *Handbook of Sensory Physiology*, Vol. VII/3B, *Central Processing of Visual Information* (R. Jung, ed.), pp. 269–324, Springer, Berlin.

Szentgothai, J., 1975, The "module-concept" in cerebral cortex architecture, *Brain Res.* **95**:475–496.

Szentgothai, J., 1978, The neuron network of the cerebral cortex: A functional interpretation, Ferrier Lecture, *Proc. R. Soc. London Ser. B* **201**:219–248.

Tömböl, T., 1978, Some Golgi data on visual cortex of the rhesus monkey, *Acta Morphol. Acad. Sci. Hung.* **26**:115–138.

Toyama, K., Maekawa, K., and Takeda, T., 1977, Convergence of retinal inputs onto visual cortical cells. I. A study of the cells monosynaptically excited from the lateral geniculate body, *Brain Res.* **137**:207–220.

Valverde, F., 1976, Aspects of cortical organization related to the geometry of neurons with intracortical axons, *J. Neurocytol.* **5**:509–529.

Valverde, F., 1978, The organization of area 18 in the monkey: A Golgi study, *Anat. Embryol.* **154**:305–334.

10

Chandelier Cells

ALAN PETERS

1. Introduction

In Golgi preparations, chandelier cells are recognized by the form of their axons, which terminate in vertically oriented "candles," each one consisting of a series of axonal boutons or swellings linked together by thin connecting pieces. Surprisingly, chandelier cells were not recognized until 1974, when Szentágothai and Arbib encountered them in the cingulate gyrus of cat. In the following year, Szentágothai (1975) enlarged upon the description of these neurons in his discussion of the modules of neurons in the visual cortex, and at the same time Jones (1975) described similar neurons in monkey somatosensory cortex, referring to them as type 4 cells.

Szentágothai (1975) considered the axonal candles of the chandelier cells to be arranged along the apical dendrites of pyramidal cells, but in 1977 Somogyi corrected this interpretation, when he examined similar neurons in rat visual cortex. Using a Golgi–EM technique, in which impregnated cells were first identified in the light microscope and subsequently studied in the electron microscope, Somogyi (1977, 1979) was able to show that the axon terminals comprising the candles are not arranged around apical dendrites but synapse with the axon initial segments of pyramidal cells. Because of the sites where their synapses are formed, Somogyi (1977) referred to these presynaptic cells as specific axo-axonal interneurons, but it is now apparent that these axo-axonal interneurons and Szentágothai's chandelier cells are similar.

ALAN PETERS • Department of Anatomy, Boston University School of Medicine, Boston, Massachusetts 02118.

2. Distribution of Chandelier Cells

Most attention has been paid to the chandelier cells in the visual cortex, in which they have now been identified in the rat (Somogyi, 1977; Somogyi *et al.*, 1979, 1982; Peters *et al.*, 1982), cat (Tömböl, 1978; Fairén and Valverde, 1980; Lund *et al.*, 1979; Peters and Regidor, 1981), and monkey (Lund *et al.*, 1981). It is apparent, however, that chandelier cells are by no means confined to the visual cortex, for they occur in the somatosensory cortex of the monkey (Jones, 1975), as well as in the auditory cortex of the monkey (Szentágothai, 1975), cat (Szentágothai, 1975), and rat (Peters, unpublished results), in the suprasylvian sulcus, or Clare–Bishop area, of the cat (Norita and Kawamura, 1981), and in the cingulate cortex (Vogt and Peters, 1981) and subiculum and pyriform cortex of the rat (Somogyi *et al.*, 1982). In addition, chandelier cells have even been encountered in the neocortex of the hedgehog (Valverde and Lopez-Mascaraque, 1981) (see also Chapter 6). In many of these studies, the chandelier cells have been described as being most prominent in the supragranular layers. For example, in rat visual cortex, Somogyi (1977) states that they are most common in layers II and III, and Peters *et al.* (1982) report a similar result. Similarly, Fairén and Valverde (1980) and Peters and Regidor (1981) find chandelier cells to be prominent in supragranular layers in cat visual cortex. In this cortex, other chandelier cells have been encountered in layers IV and V, and Jones (1975) also describes them to be present in all layers in monkey somatosensory cortex, although he comments that chandelier cells are most prominent in layer III. The distribution of chandelier cells may vary in different cortical areas, however, for Lund *et al.* (1981) have recently shown that one of the main differences between the primary and secondary visual areas of monkey cortex is the presence of chandelier cells in layer IV of the secondary visual area (see Fig. 4) and their absence from this layer in the primary visual area. Lund *et al.* (1981) consider that this difference can be attributed to the fact that layer IV of the secondary visual area contains many small pyramidal neurons, which they believe to be the targets of the layer IV chandelier cell axons.

3. Cell Bodies and Dendrites

It is fortunate that the axons of the chandelier cells form such charactertistic terminals, for the cell bodies and dendritic arbors seem to be quite variable (Figs. 1–4). Thus, although the cell bodies of most chandelier cells have been described as being ovoid, or fusiform in shape, with dendrites extending from the upper and lower poles of the cell body to produce a bitufted dendritic tree (Fig. 1); other chandelier cells are more multipolar with the dendrites emerging more

Figure 1. Golgi–Kopsch-impregnated chandelier cell in layer II of area 17 of rat visual cortex. The cell has dendrites which emerge preferentially from the upper and lower surfaces of the cell body, and some of the dendrites in the upper tuft reach the pial surface. The axon emerges from the lower surface of the cell body to form axonal candles (arrows). Bar equals 25 μm.

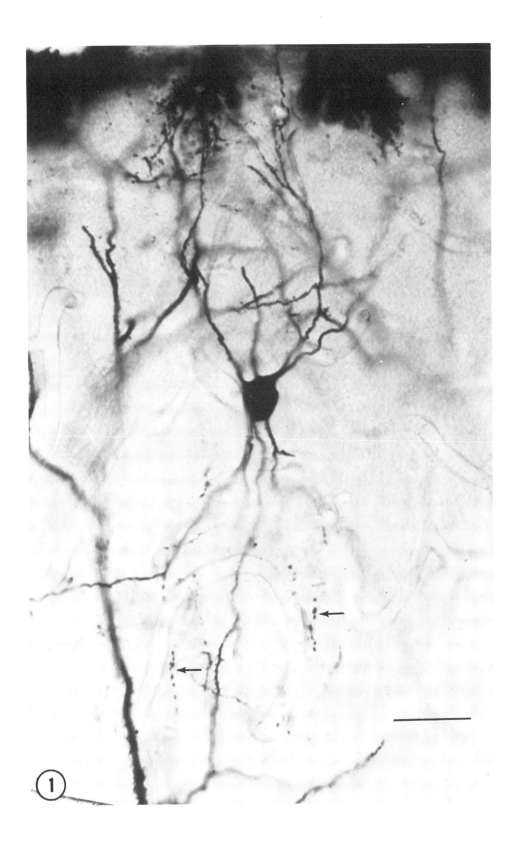

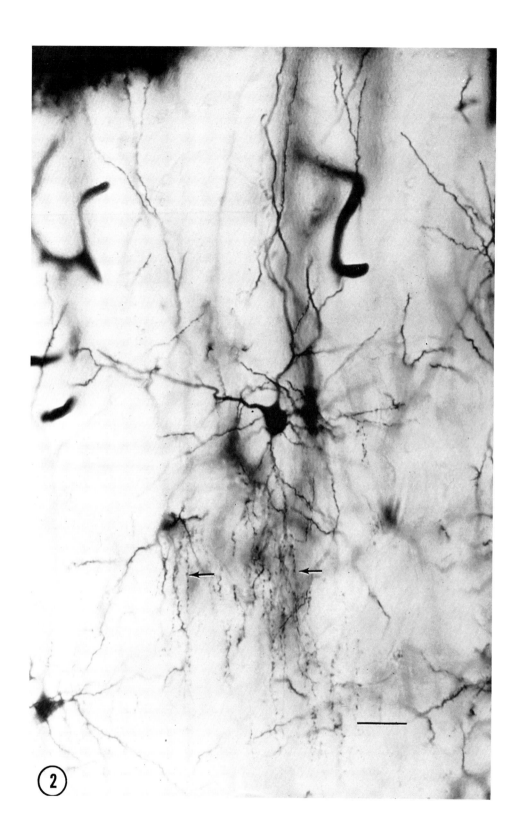

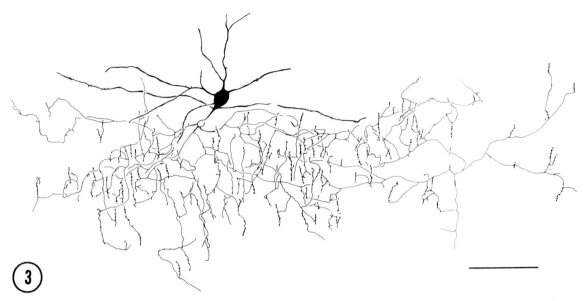

③

Figure 3. Camera lucida drawing of a rapid Golgi-impregnated chandelier cell from layer II of area 41 of rat cerebral cortex. The cell is multipolar and the long, thin dendrites possess few spines. The axon arises from the base of the cell body and branches extensively to form a widely spread plexus which terminates in numerous axonal candles. Bar equals 25 μm.

randomly from the surface of the rounded cell body (Figs. 2–4). Not uncommonly, the dendrites of the chandelier cells in supragranular layers can reach as far as the outer portion of layer I (Figs. 1 and 2), where they may pass tangentially, parallel to the pial surface, while the dendrites of the lower tuft may reach as far as layer IV (e.g., Somogyi, 1977; Peters *et al.*, 1982). Further, as mentioned by Fairén and Valverde (1980), the ascending tuft of dendrites is frequently more profuse than the descending one, and this bias may be so pronounced that it can result in a morphology reminiscent of a "flame-shaped" cell described by Szentágothai (1975, his Fig. 18).

In all cases, the dendrites of chandelier cells seem to have relatively even diameters, although they are gradually tapering toward their ends. Most of the primary dendrites branch close to the cell body, and while additional branching may occur more distally, the dendritic tree is never profuse, and the dendrites bear only few spines (Figs. 1–3).

The only account of the fine structure of the cell body and dendrites of chandelier cells is that given by Peters *et al.* (1982) in their account of these cells in rat visual cortex. Using a Golgi–EM technique, these authors show that the

Figure 2. Golgi–Kopsch-impregnated chandelier cell in layer II of rat visual cortex. This cell is located at the area 17/18a border. The dendrites have a multipolar configuration, and some of the long ascending dendrites reach the pial surface. The axon arises from the base of a descending dendrite and produces a prolific plexus in which the terminals form vertical strings of axonal terminals (arrows). Bar equals 25 μm.

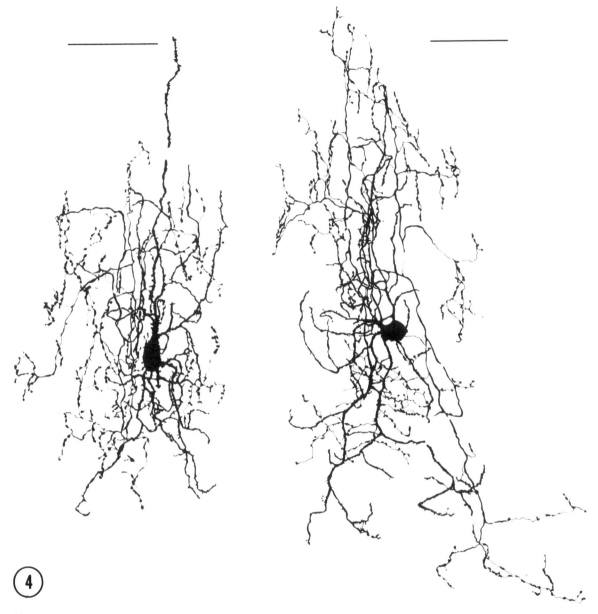

④

Figure 4. Drawings of two examples of chandelier cells present in layer IV of visual cortex area VII of a 3-month-old macaque monkey. Scale bars equal 50 μm. From Lund *et al.* (1981).

Figure 5. Electron micrograph of the cell body of a Golgi-impregnated and gold-toned chandelier cell. The nucleus (N) is pale and has a folded nuclear envelope. The perikaryon contains many ribosomes, some of which are attached to the parallel arrays of cisternae of rough endoplasmic reticulum (ER). The axon (Ax) extends from the hillock at the base of the cell body. Axosomatic synapses are indicated by arrows. Bar equals 2.5 μm.

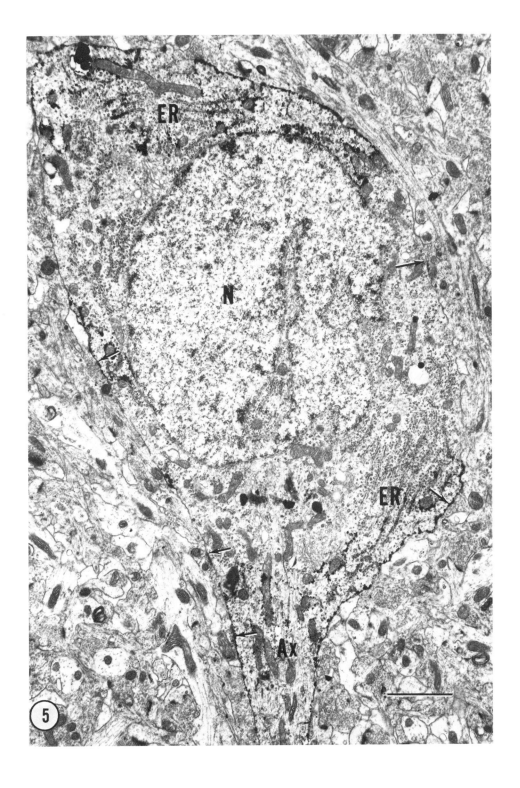

pale nuclei of these neurons are often rounded, although the nuclear envelope may sometimes display some infolding and ruffling (Fig. 5). In contrast to the pale nuclei, the perikaryal cytoplasm is darkened by the presence of many ribosomes, both attached to the outer surfaces of the cisternae forming the well-developed stacks of rough endoplasmic reticulum (RER) and free in the cytoplasm. The RER also extends into the rather thick bases of the primary dendrites but is not prominent in the more distal lengths of dendrites, for there the cytoplasm is dominated by microtubules and cisternae of various sizes. Such cytological features are common to most nonpyramidal cells, so that in thin sections the cell bodies and dendrites of chandelier cells possess no characteristics which would allow them to be easily distinguished from other types of nonpyramidal cells. Further, in common with other nonpyramidal cells in rat cerebral cortex examined by electron microscopy, for example other smooth and sparsely spinous multipolar and bitufted neurons (Peters and Fairén, 1978; Peters and Proskauer, 1980a,b) and bipolar cells (Peters and Kimerer, 1981), the cell bodies and dendrites of chandelier cells receive axon terminals which form asymmetric and symmetric axosomatic synapses (Fig. 5, arrows). At present, the origins of the axon terminals synapsing with the dendrites and cell bodies of chandelier cells are not known, although it is likely that in rat visual cortex the axon terminals forming the symmetric synapses are derived from the smooth and sparsely spinous cells described by Peters and Fairén (1978), since the axons of these neurons appear to be the source of the majority of the symmetric axosomatic and axodendritic synapses present in that cortex (also see Peters and Proskauer, 1980b).

4. Axons

The axons of chandelier cells in rat cortex emerge directly from the cell body, or from one of the descending primary dendrites close to the cell body. The rather thick axonal trunk then descends, giving off collateral branches which extend at right angles from the main trunk, and branches many times to produce a profuse plexus in the vicinity of the parent cell body (Fig. 3). In monkey somatosensory cortex (Jones, 1975), the disposition of the axonal plexus depends on the location of the parent cell body. Thus, chandelier cells with somata in deep layer III and in layer IV tend to have ascending axons, while those with cell bodies in layer II and the superficial one-third of layer III tend to have descending axons, and cells in the middle of layer III have axons which both descend and ascend. This latter disposition of the axon is also similar to that

Figure 6. A portion of the Golgi-impregnated axonal plexus of a chandelier cell in area 17 of rat visual cortex. The characteristic vertically oriented strings of axonal boutons (arrows) are apparent. Rapid Golgi impregnation. Bar equals 25 μm.

Figure 7. A portion of the Golgi-impregnated axonal plexus of a chandelier cell from area 18a of rat visual cortex. The axonal plexus gives off many vertically oriented candles consisting of strings of axonal boutons (arrows). Photograph made by multiple exposures. Golgi–Kopsch impregnation. Bar equals 25 μm.

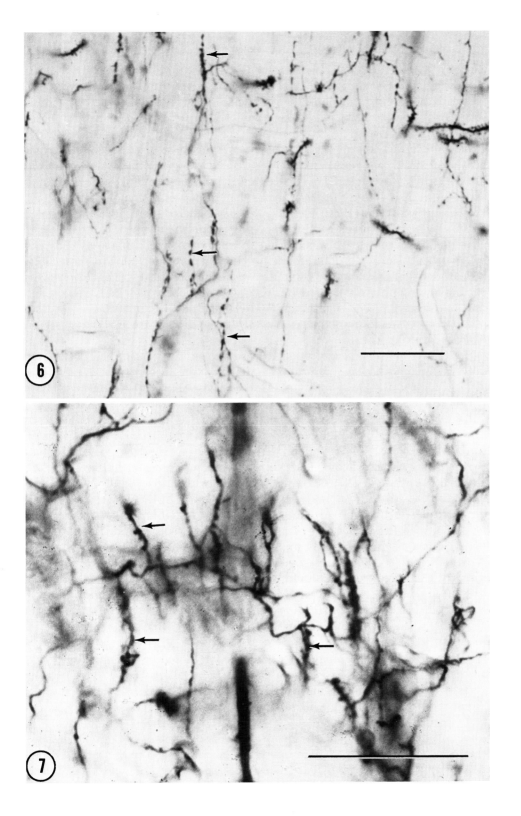

shown by chandelier cells in layer IV of the secondary visual area of monkey cortex, for these cells have their plexuses all around the cell body (Fig. 4). In all cases, however, the axonal plexus gives rise to numerous, vertically oriented strings of axonal swellings, which are the "candles" of the chandelier and are so typical of the chandelier cell. In the rat, each candle consists of a relatively simple string of axonal boutons joined together by thin strands, so that the boutons resemble beads strung along a necklace (Figs. 6 and 7). Some of these strings of boutons can be 30 µm long and the intervals between successive boutons vary between 2 and 5 µm (Peters *et al.*, 1982), with an average of five to seven boutons in each string (Somogyi, 1977). The axonal candles in the monkey have a similar appearance (Fig. 4), but in the cat the axonal candles may be more complex, for Fairén and Valverde (1980) have shown that some of them have the form of "braids," which are produced by branching within the terminal complex.

The axonal plexus formed within the vicinity of the parent cell body can be up to 200 µm wide. The depth it occupies may vary, and in most Golgi preparations it appears to be contained within a cylindrical space. However, by examining computer-generated reconstructions of chandelier cell axonal plexuses in cat visual cortex, Fairén and Valverde (1980) conclude that rather than occupying a cylinder-shaped territory, the axonal candles are aggregated within narrow slabs of cortical tissue.

In rat visual cortex, impregnated axonal plexuses of chandelier cells have only been seen within layer II/III, in the vicinity of the parent cell body (Somogyi, 1977; Peters *et al.*, 1982), although a descending branch of the primary axon may descend beyond the level of this plexus. In cat visual cortex, however, Fairén and Valverde (1980) have shown that in addition to the local plexus, the axons of some chandelier cells may produce a second plexus in a deeper cortical layer. In this same cortex, Tömböl (1978) depicts a layer IV chandelier cell with a local plexus in the vicinity of the cell body and a second plexus within layers V and VI, while Lund *et al.* (1979) have also shown a chandelier cell in layer III of cat visual cortex with a secondary axonal plexus in layer VI. In all cases, this second plexus seems less extensive than the one in the vicinity of the cell body, and having formed its plexuses the chandelier cell axon may continue into the white matter, for a destination as yet unknown.

Finally, in describing the light microscopic appearance of Golgi-impregnated axons of chandelier cells, it should be stated that not all of the axonal swellings, or boutons, of the axons are contained within the vertically oriented candles. Some branches of the axon are more obliquely oriented, do not appear to form candles, and have boutons en passant arranged at infrequent intervals along their courses (Fig. 3).

As first shown by Somogyi (1977), when Golgi-impregnated chandelier cells are examined in the electron microscope, the axonal candles produced by the vertical strings of terminals are found to be arranged alongside the axon initial segments of pyramidal neurons. This has recently been confirmed by Fairén and Valverde (1980) and Peters *et al.* (1982) and such an arrangement can sometimes even be seen in Golgi preparations examined by light microscopy (Fig. 8). In Somogyi's study, the axon terminals were still filled with the Golgi deposit, but in the studies by Fairén and Valverde (1980) and Peters *et al.* (1982) in which the material was gold-toned (Fairén *et al.*, 1977; Peters, 1981) so that

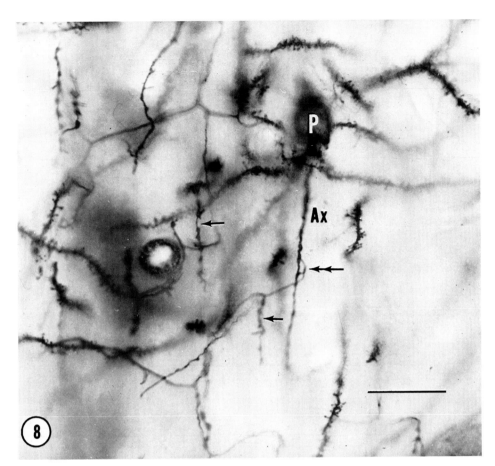

Figure 8. A rapid Golgi impregnation showing the axon (Ax) of a layer II pyramidal neuron, the cell body (P) of which is visible. On the left is a portion of the axonal plexus of a chandelier cell from which arise a number of axonal candles (arrows). A branch of the chandelier cell axon extends toward the axon of the pyramidal cell and branches (double arrow) to wrap around the pyramidal cell axon. Bar equals 25 μm.

the cytoplasmic details are revealed, it is apparent that the irregularly shaped chandelier cell axon terminals are filled by pleomorphic synaptic vesicles (see Fig. 11). The axon terminals are flattened against the surfaces of pyramidal axon initial segments (Figs. 9 and 10), which are recognized as axon initial segments by the presence of a dense undercoating of the axolemma and the occurrence of fascicles of microtubules in the axoplasm (e.g., Palay *et al.*, 1968; Peters *et al.*, 1968). That the postsynaptic axon initial segments belong to pyramidal cells is evident in those examples in which the axon initial segment can be seen to extend from the parent cell body. The identity of the postsynaptic cell has also been demonstrated rather nicely by Somogyi *et al.* (1979) in an experiment in which the axon terminals of a Golgi-impregnated chandelier cell have been shown to synapse with the axon initial segments of pyramidal neurons caused to be filled

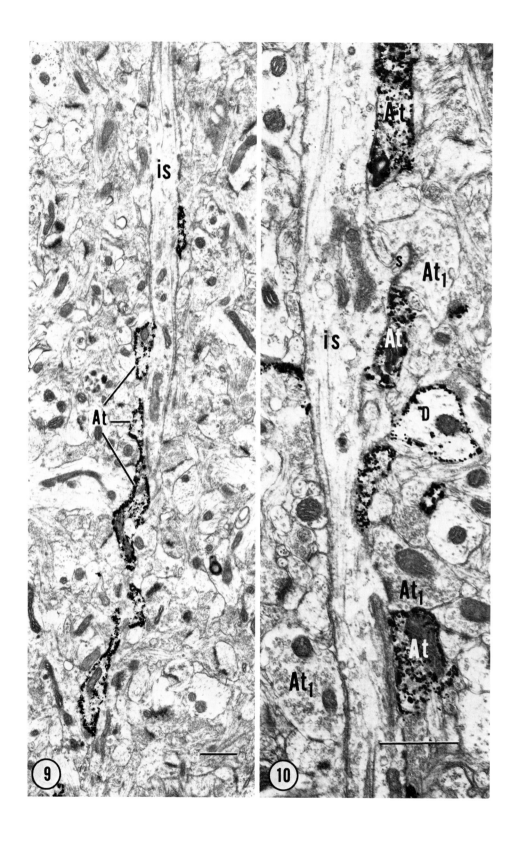

with HRP by an injection of HRP into areas 17 and 18a of the contralateral hemisphere.

The synapses formed between chandelier cell axon terminals and the axon initial segments of pyramidal neurons are of the symmetric variety (Fig. 11). Sometimes the synaptic vesicles are accumulated next to one or two small junctional zones, at which the cleft between the pre- and the postsynaptic membranes is about 20 nm wide and there is a slight accumulation of dense material associated with the cytoplasmic faces of both synapsing membranes. At other junctions, however, the synaptic complexes are more extensive, so that one or two complexes can occupy much of the length of the interface between the pre- and the postsynaptic membranes. Thus, there is some variability in the form of the axo-axonal synapses formed by the chandelier cell axon terminals.

In summary then, the chandelier cell axon terminals have rather irregular shapes, are filled by synaptic vesicles, and form symmetric synaptic junctions with the axon initial segments of pyramidal cells. In gold-toned preparations of Golgi-impregnated chandelier cells, other, and unimpregnated axon terminals with the same features as those listed above may also synapse with the pyramidal cell axon initial segments (Figs. 10 and 13). The conclusion reached by Somogyi (1977), Fairén and Valverde (1980), and Peters *et al.* (1982) is that these unimpregnated axon terminals also belong to chandelier cells, so that an initial axon segment of a pyramidal cell can receive axon terminals from more than one chandelier cell (see Somogyi *et al.*, 1982). This arrangement is not ubiquitous, however, for it is evident in gold-toned preparations that some supragranular pyramidal cells appear to receive terminals from only a single chandelier cell, while a survey of normally prepared material shows that yet others receive no chandelier cell axon terminals. At present, the significance of these different arrangements is not known.

It should be emphasized that these observations on Golgi-impregnated chandelier cells examined with the electron microscope are confined to the supragranular layers of cat and rat visual cortex. Examination of thin sections of normally prepared rat visual cortex, however, suggests that irregularly shaped axon terminals resembling those of chandelier cells are at least uncommon on the axon initial segments of layer V pyramidal neurons (Peters *et al.*, 1982), and this observation is compatible with that of Sloper and Powell (1979) in monkey motor somatosensory cortex, for they find that there are about three times as many axo-axonal synapses along the initial segments of pyramidal cells in supragranular as compared with those in infragranular layers. These observations taken in conjunction with those on Golgi-impregnated material suggest, then,

---

Figure 9. Electron micrograph of gold-labeled chandelier cell terminals (At) aligned alongside the axon initial segment (is) of a layer III pyramidal cell. The most proximal terminal of the chandelier cell candle is 12 μm distant from the axon hillock of the pyramidal cell. Area 18 of rat cortex. Bar equals 1 μm.

Figure 10. Electron micrograph of gold-toned chandelier cell axon terminals (At) lying alongside the axon initial segment (is) of a layer III pyramidal cell. In addition to the gold-labeled axon terminals, unlabeled axon terminals (At$_1$) are also synapsing with the axon initial segment and one of them is synapsing with a spine (S). The field also contains a gold-labeled profile of a chandelier cell dendrite (D). Rat visual cortex. Bar equals 1 μm.

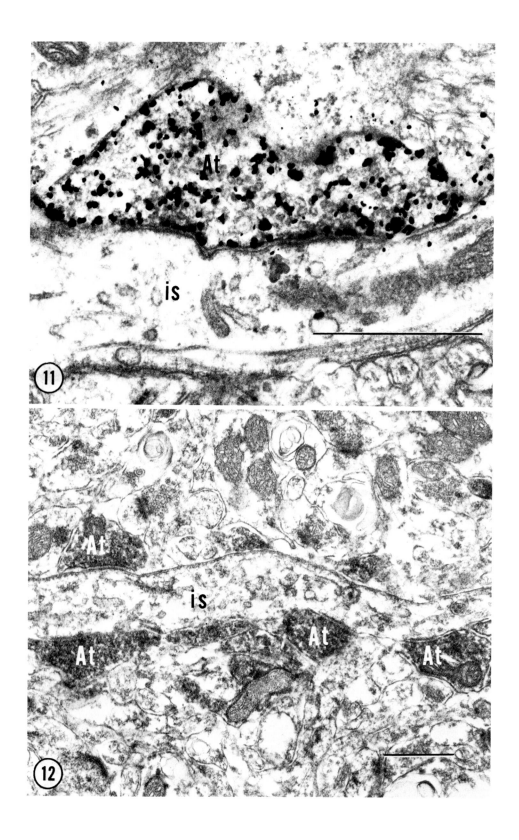

that infragranular pyramidal cells receive many fewer chandelier cell axon terminals than the pyramidal cells in supragranular layers. Interestingly, however, as pointed out above, some granular layers may contain chandelier cell axon terminals, as for example the secondary visual area of the macaque, in which Lund *et al.* (1981) describe the axon initial segments of the small pyramidal neurons in layer IV to be coated with axon terminals forming symmetric synapses.

The question arises as to whether neurons other than pyramidal cells receive the axon terminals of chandelier cells. Chandelier cell terminals have not been seen in Golgi–EM preparations to synapse with the axon initial segments of nonpyramidal cells, and in rat visual cortex at least, the smooth and sparsely spinous cells which occur throughout layers II through V, and can have either unmyelinated (Peters and Fairén, 1978) or myelinated (Peters and Proskauer, 1980a) axons, have only one or two rounded axon terminals synapsing with their axon initial segments. The same is also true of the bipolar cells in this cortex (Peters and Kimerer, 1981), and the nonpyramidal cells of monkey somatosensory cortex are similar in having few axo-axonal synapses (Sloper and Powell, 1979). It would appear then that at least the strings of axon terminals contained in the candles formed by the chandelier cell synapse specifically with the axon initial segments of pyramidal cells. It should be recalled, however, that a few branches of the axonal plexus of the chandelier cell appear not to form vertical strings of axon terminals (Fig. 3). Instead, these branches pass in an oblique direction and have swellings arranged along their lengths at infrequent intervals, but so far these particular axonal branches have not been traced.

If the chandelier cell axon terminals do indeed synapse only with the axon initial segments of pyramidal cells, then the chandelier cells are probably unique among cortical neurons, for the other types of cortical neurons which form symmetric synapses and have so far been examined in Golgi–EM preparations, have various elements postsynaptic to them. Thus, the smooth or sparsely spinous stellate cells of rat visual cortex form symmetric synapses with the cell bodies and dendrites of both nonpyramidal and pyramidal neurons, as well as axon hillocks and the proximal portions of axon initial segments (see Peters and Fairén, 1978; Peters and Proskauer, 1980b; Parnavelas *et al.*, 1977). Similarly, the double bouquet cells which also form symmetric synapses have a variety of postsynaptic targets. These neurons have vertically arranged axonal bundles which traverse layers II through V, and in examining such neurons from cat and monkey cortex, Somogyi and Cowey (1981) have shown that although their axons synapse predominantly with dendritic shafts, they also synapse with neuronal cell bodies and dendritic spines. In addition, DeFelipe and Fairén (personal communication) have shown that neurons which they regard as being basket cells in the supra-

←

Figure 11. Electron micrograph of a gold-labeled chandelier cell axon terminal (At) which contains pleomorphic vesicles forming a symmetric axo-axonal synapse with the axon initial segment (is) of a layer III pyramidal cell. Rat visual cortex. Bar equals 1 μm.

Figure 12. Electron micrograph of rat visual cortex treated with GAD antiserum. A length of axon initial segment (is) is surrounded by GAD-labeled axon terminals (At) which are forming symmetric synaptic junctions. Bar equals 1 μm.

granular layers of cat visual cortex synapse with the cell bodies of both pyramidal and nonpyramidal cells, as well as proximal dendrites.

5. Functional Considerations

The fact that the axon terminals of chandelier cells form axo-axonal synapses which are symmetric in form led Somogyi (1977, 1979) and Fairén and Valverde (1980) to suggest that they are inhibitory neurons. Evidence in favor of this suggestion has been presented by Peters *et al.* (1982) who have shown that axon terminals believed to belong to chandelier cells contain GAD, the enzyme involved in the synthesis of the neurotransmitter GABA, which is a likely inhibitory neurotransmitter in cerebral cortex (see Ribak, 1978; Sillito, 1975). Using an antiserum specific to GAD and visualizing the binding sites by an HRP reaction product (Ribak *et al.*, 1976), Peters *et al.* (1982) have shown GAD-positive axon terminals to be associated with vertically oriented axon initial segments in rat visual cortex (Figs. 12 and 14). These axon initial segments pass through layer II/III and in some cases can be traced back to their origins from pyramidal cell bodies, and in anti-GAD-reacted material in which an optimal reaction occurs, all of the axon terminals synapsing with pyramidal cell axon initial segments are GAD positive. Some of the GAD-positive axon terminals forming symmetric synapses with the axon initial segments have rather irregular shapes, are often in groups, and may be more than 10 μm distant from the cell body (Figs. 12 and 14). All of these features are shown by chandelier cell axon terminals and favor the interpretation that the chandelier cell axon terminals are GAD positive. Other GAD-positive axon terminals synapsing with pyramidal cell axon initial segments are probably derived from smooth or sparsely spinous stellate cells, for in rat visual cortex the axon terminals of such cells can form symmetric synapses with the axon hillocks and proximal axon initial segments of pyramidal cells (Peters and Fairén, 1978), but the terminals of these nonpyramidal cells occur individually. It is pertinent to mention that in anti-GAD-stained preparations of rat visual cortex, individual GAD-positive axon terminals can also form symmetric synapses with the axon initial segments of layer V pyramidal cells, but groups of GAD-positive axon terminals similar to those associated with the axon initial segments of supragranular pyramidal cells are not encountered.

→

Figure 13. Electron micrograph showing a length of axon initial segment (is) with associated profiles of a gold-labeled chandelier cell axon (At). The axon initial segment then enters a nest of unlabeled and irregularly shaped axon terminals (At₁–At₄) containing pleomorphic vesicles. The synaptic junction formed by terminal, At₁ is sectioned obliquely (arrow), and terminal At₂ synapses with a spine (S) of the axon initial segment. Rat visual cortex. Bar equals 1 μm.

Figure 14. Electron micrograph of visual cortex treated with GAD antiserum. A short length of axon initial segment (is) is surrounded by GAD-labeled axon terminals (At), one of which is forming a symmetric junction (arrow). In serial sections, the axon initial segment could be seen to curve to the left to become associated with the second group of GAD-positive axon terminals (At₁) beneath. Two of these terminals are synapsing with a spine (S) of the axon initial segment. Compare this image with that shown in Fig. 13. Bar equals 1 μm.

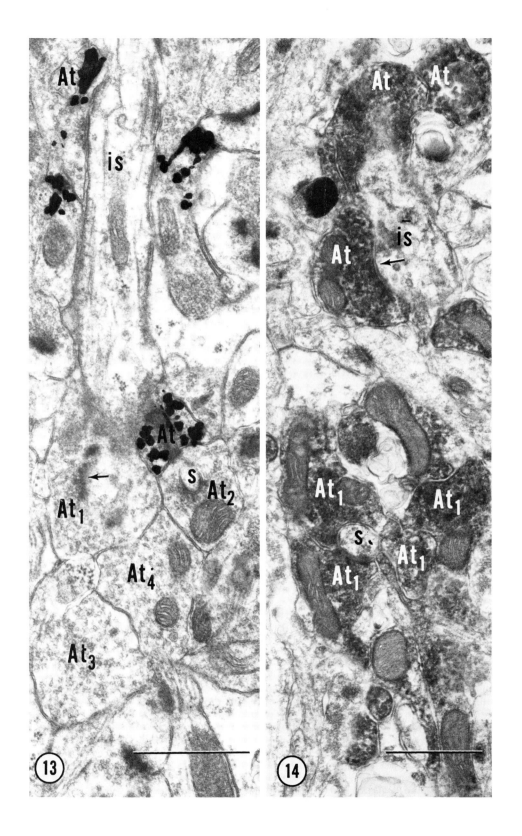

This observation is consistent with the fact that no chandelier cell axon terminals have yet been impregnated in deeper layers of this cortex.

In rat visual cortex, GAD-positive axon terminals not only synapse with the axon hillock and axon initial segments of pyramidal cells but also with the cell body and the shafts of the dendrites (Ribak, 1978). On the basis of our present knowledge, it seems likely that all of the symmetric axodendritic and axosomatic synapses, as well as those on the axon hillock and the proximal portion of the axon initial segment are formed by the smooth and sparsely spinous stellate cells (see Peters and Fairén, 1978; Peters and Proskauer, 1980b; Parnavelas et al., 1977). Thus, both these smooth and sparsely spinous stellate cells and the chandelier cells seem to form inhibitory synapses with the pyramidal neurons. In cat and monkey cortex, on the other hand, the situation is more complicated, for in these cortices it is almost certain that basket cells also form symmetric synapses with the cell bodies of pyramidal neurons (see Peters and Regidor, 1981, for a discussion). Whether the double bouquet cells, which also form symmetric synapses in monkey and cat visual cortex (Somogyi and Cowey, 1981), make additional synapses with the cell bodies, dendritic shafts, and spines of pyramidal neurons is not yet clear, but if they do, and if all symmetric synapses are inhibitory, then the pyramidal cells of cat and monkey cerebral cortex may be subject to inhibition derived from at least four nonpyramidal cell types.

What is the role of the chandelier cells which occur in the cerebral cortices of the wide range of mammals extending from the hedgehog to the monkey? They seem to be involved, preferentially, in the inhibition of pyramidal neurons and since a chandelier cell forms many axonal candles, each presumably synapsing with the axon initial segment of a different pyramidal cell, every chandelier cell should be able to inhibit numerous pyramidal cells. In most cortices, the chandelier cells seem to primarily exert their effects on pyramidal cells in the supragranular layers, but even there, not every pyramidal cell receives chandelier cell axon terminals and some pyramidal cells appear to receive terminals from more than one chandelier cell.

Which particular pyramidal cells are inhibited by chandelier cells is not completely known, but at least some of the pyramidal cells in rat visual cortex are ones with callosally projecting axons, as shown by Somogyi et al. (1979). The observations of Peters et al. (1982) also support the concept that the chandelier cells may be inhibiting callosally projecting pyramidal neurons. These authors have shown that the majority of Golgi-impregnated chandelier cells in rat visual cortex are located at the border of area 17 with 18a, while there are fewer impregnated chandelier cells at the area 17/18 border and least in area 17, a distribution similar to that of callosally projecting neurons (Schober et al., 1976; M. Miller, personal communication). Interestingly though, lateral area 17 and adjacent area 18a receive a very dense callosal projection, while fewer callosal terminals are present in area 18 (or 18b as it is sometimes termed), and almost none in medial area 17 (e.g., Lund and Lund, 1970; Cipolloni and Peters, 1979; Cusick and Lund, 1981). Thus, the distribution of callosal afferents and projecting cells coincides with the distribution of Golgi-impregnated chandelier cells. If the chandelier cells and the supragranular pyramidal cells receive callosal afferents, then they would both be monosynaptically excited by these afferents, and this excitation would be followed by inhibition of the pyramidal cells by the chandelier cells. Hence, the role of the chandelier cells might be to prevent repetitive activity across the corpus callosum.

If may also be significant that the visual midline of the rat is represented at the borders of area 17 with area 18a (Adams and Forrester, 1968; Montero *et al.*, 1973). Chandelier cells are also most concentrated at the area 17/18 border in cat visual cortex, as shown by Fairén and Valverde (1980), so that here again their concentration coincides with the distribution of callosally projecting neurons. However, before it can be accepted that the role of chandelier cells is to inhibit groups of pyramidal cells with specific inputs or projections, such as ones involved in the callosal connections between the two hemispheres, more information must be obtained. In particular, it is necessary to obtain data about the sources of the axon terminals which impinge on the chandelier cells, for although the sites of termination of the chandelier cell axons are becoming well known, nothing is known about the inputs to these neurons.

ACKNOWLEDGMENTS. I wish to thank Drs. M. L. Feldman and E. G. Jones for carefully reading the manuscript and making helpful comments to improve this account. The skilled assistance of Charmian C. Proskauer and Dan Kara is also acknowledged. Support for this work was provided by Grant NS07016 from the National Institute of Neurological and Communicative Disorders and Stroke of the United States Public Health Service.

6. References

Adams, A. D., and Forrester, J. M., 1968, The projection of the rat's visual field on the cerebral cortex. *Q. J. Exp. Physiol.* **53**:327–336.

Cipolloni, P. B., and Peters, A., 1979, The bilaminar and banded distribution of the callosal terminals in the posterior neocortex of the rat, *Brain Res.* **176**:33–47.

Cusick, C. G., and Lund, R. D., 1981, The distribution of the callosal projection to the occipital visual cortex in rats and mice, *Brain Res.* **241**:239–259.

Fairén, A., and Valverde, F., 1980, A specialized type of neuron in the visual cortex of cat: A Golgi and electron microscope study of chandelier cells, *J. Comp. Neurol.* **194**:761–779.

Fairén, A., Peters, A., and Saldanha, J., 1977, A new procedure for examining Golgi impregnated neurons by light and electron microscopy, *J. Neurocytol.* **6**:311–337.

Jones, E. G., 1975, Varieties and distribution of non-pyramidal cells in the somatic sensory cortex of the squirrel monkey, *J. Comp. Neurol.* **160**:205–268.

Lund, J. S., and Lund, R. D., 1970, The termination of callosal fibers in the paravisual cortex of the rat, *Brain Res.* **17**:25–45.

Lund, J. S., Henry, G. H., MacQueen, C. L., and Harvey, A. R., 1979, Anatomical organization of the primary visual cortex (area 17) of the cat: A comparison with area 17 of the macaque monkey, *J. Comp. Neurol.* **184**:599–618.

Lund, J. S., Hendrickson, A. E., Ogren, M. P., and Tobin, E. A., 1981, Anatomical organization of primate visual cortex area VII, *J. Comp. Neurol.* **202**:19–45.

Montero, V. M., Rojas, A., and Torrealba, F., 1973, Retinotopic organization of striate and peristriate visual cortex in the albino rat, *Brain Res.* **53**:197–201.

Norita, M., and Kawamura, K., 1981, Non-pyramidal neurons in the medial bank (Clare–Bishop area) of the middle syprasylvian sulcus: A Golgi study in the cat, *J. Hirnforsch.* **22**:9–28.

Palay, S. L., Sotelo, C., Peters, A., and Orkand, P. M., 1968, The axon hillock and the initial segment, *J. Cell Biol.* **38**:193–201.

Parnavelas, J. G., Sullivan K, Lieberman, A. R., and Webster, K. E., 1977, Neurons and their synaptic organization in the visual cortex of the rat: Electron microscopy of Golgi preparations, *Cell Tissue Res.* **183**:499–517.

Peters, A., 1981, The Golgi–electron microscope technique, in: *Current Trends in Morphological Techniques*, Vol. 2 (J. Johnson, ed.), pp. 187–212, CRC Press, Cleveland.

Peters, A., and Fairén, A., 1978, Smooth and sparsely-spined stellate cells in the visual cortex of the rat: A study using a combined Golgi–electron microscope technique, *J. Comp. Neurol.* **181**:129–172.

Peters, A., and Kimerer, L. M., 1981, Bipolar neurons in rat visual cortex: A combined Golgi–electron microscope study, *J. Neurocytol.* **10**:921–946.

Peters, A., and Proskauer, C. C., 1980a, Smooth or sparsely-spined cells with myelinated axons in rat visual cortex, *Neuroscience* **5**:2079–2092.

Peters, A., and Proskauer, C. C., 1980b, Synaptic relationships between a multipolar stellate cell and a pyramidal neuron in the rat visual cortex: A combined Golgi–electron microscope study, *J. Neurocytol.* **9**:163–183.

Peters, A., and Regidor, J., 1981, A reassessment of the forms of non-pyramidal neurons in area 17 of cat visual cortex, *J. Comp. Neurol.* **203**:685–716.

Peters, A., Proskauer, C. C., and Kaiserman-Abramof, I. R., 1968, The small pyramidal neuron of the rat cerebral cortex: The axon hillock and initial segment, *J. Cell Biol.* **39**:604–619.

Peters, A., Proskauer, C. C., and Ribak, C. E., 1982, Chandelier cells in rat visual cortex, *J. Comp. Neurol.* **206**:397–416.

Ribak, C. E., 1978, Aspinous and sparsely-spinous stellate neurons in the visual cortex of rats contain glutamic acid decarboxylase, *J. Neurocytol.* **7**:461–478.

Ribak, C. E., Vaughn, J. E., Saito, K., Barber, R., and Roberts, E., 1976, Immunocytochemical localization of glutamate decarboxylase in rat substantia nigra, *Brain Res.* **116**:287–298.

Schober, W., Luth, H.-J., and Gruschka, H., 1976, Die Herkunft afferenter Axone im striaten Kortex der Albinoratte: Eine Studie mit Meerrettich-Peroxidase, *Z. Mikrosk. Anat. Forsch.* **90**:399–415.

Sillito, A. M., 1975, The effectiveness of bicuculline as an antagonist of GABA and visually evoked inhibition in the cat's striate cortex, *J. Physiol. (London)* **250**:287–304.

Sloper, J. J., and Powell, T. P. S., 1979, A study of the axon initial segment and proximal axon of neurons in the primate motor and somatic sensory cortices, *Philos. Trans. R. Soc. London Ser. B* **285**:173–197.

Somogyi, P., 1977, A specific axo-axonal neuron in the visual cortex of the rat, *Brain Res.* **136**:345–350.

Somogyi, P., 1979, An interneuron making synapses specifically on the axon initial segment (AIS) of pyramidal cells in the cerebral cortex, *J. Physiol. (London)* **296**:18–19.

Somogyi, P., and Cowey, A., 1981, Combined Golgi and electron microscopic study on the synapses formed by double bouquet cells in the visual cortex of the cat and monkey, *J. Comp. Neurol.* **195**:547–566.

Somogyi, P., Hodgson, A. J., and Smith, A. D., 1979, An approach to tracing neuron networks in the cerebral cortex and basal ganglia: Combination of Golgi staining, retrograde transport of horseradish peroxidase and anterograde degeneration of synaptic boutons in the same material, *Neuroscience* **4**:1805–1852.

Somogyi, P., Freund, T. F., and Cowey, A., 1982, The axo-axonic interneuron in the cerebral cortex of the rat, cat and monkey, *Neuroscience* **7**:2577–2607.

Szentágothai, J., 1975, The "module-concept" in cerebral cortex architecture, *Brain Res.* **95**:475–496.

Szentágothai, J., and Arbib, M., 1974, Conceptual models of neural organization, *Neurosci. Res. Program Bull.* **12**:307–510.

Tömböl, T., 1978, Comparative data on the Golgi architecture of interneurons of different cortical areas in cat and rabbit, in: *Architectonics of the Cerebral Cortex* (M. A. B. Brazier and H. Petsche, eds.), pp. 59–76, Raven Press, New York.

Valverde, F., and Lopez-Mascaraque, L., 1981, Neocortical endeavor: Basic neuronal organization in the cortex of hedgehog, in: *Glial and Neuronal Cell Biology*, Part A (S. Fedoroff, ed.), pp. 281–290, Liss, New York.

Vogt, B. A. and Peters, A., 1981, Form and distribution of neurons in rat cingulate cortex: Areas 32, 24 and 29, *J. Comp. Neurol.* **195**:603–625.

11

Bipolar Cells

ALAN PETERS

A typical bipolar cell has a vertically elongate and narrow dendritic tree formed by two principal dendrites, one ascending from the upper pole of the ovoid or spindle-shaped body and the other one descending from the lower pole. The axonal plexus is also vertically elongate and commonly the axon takes origin from one of the primary dendrites.

1. Light Microscopy

1.1. Rat Cortex

To date the most extensively examined population of bipolar cells is that contained within rat cerebral cortex. In Golgi preparations (Feldman and Peters, 1978; Peters and Kimerer, 1981; Vogt and Peters, 1981), impregnated examples of these neurons are encountered throughout layers II to V. In rat visual cortex, the cell bodies are most frequent in layer II/III and in layer IV (Fig. 1), while in cingulate cortex they are mainly found in layers III and V (Fig. 2), and in both areas the perikarya of bipolar cells have relatively uniform dimensions, so that they vary only between 9 and 12 μm for the minor axis and 16 and 25 μm for the major axis. Thus, the cell bodies of the bipolar cells are among the smallest of the neurons in these cortical areas.

Most commonly, each end of the elongate cell body gives rise to a single primary dendrite, although sometimes two parallel dendrites may emerge from one pole of the cell body (Fig. 1, cells a and d; Fig. 2, cell b). In addition, some

ALAN PETERS • Department of Anatomy, Boston University School of Medicine, Boston, Massachusetts 02118.

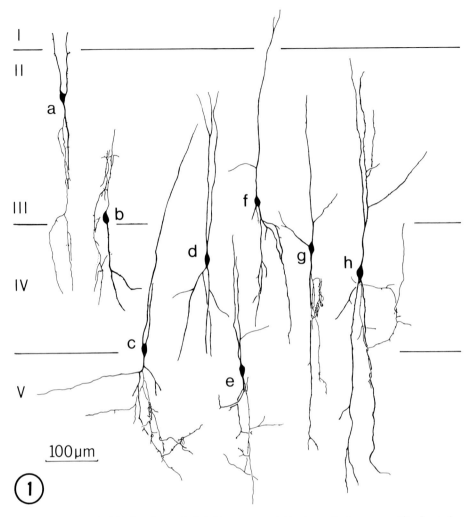

Figure 1. Camera lucida drawings of Golgi-impregnated bipolar cells from area 17 of rat visual cortex. The boundaries between the cellular layers are indicated by horizontal lines and the numbers of the layers are given on the left. From Peters and Kimerer (1981).

bipolar cells have a single and quite thin dendrite emerging from one side of the cell body, but these laterally projecting dendrites are generally shorter than the ones emerging from the poles of the cell body (Fig. 1, cell g). Indeed, the vertically oriented dendrites can pass for considerable distances through the depth of the cortex. Some of the bipolar cells, and especially those with cell bodies in layer IV or in layer V of rat visual cortex, can have ascending dendrites which reach almost to the outside of layer I, and descending dendrites which pass into lower layer V or into layer VI (Fig. 1, cells c, g, and h). Not all of the bipolar cells in the visual cortex stretch over such long distances, however, for some of the ones in layer II/III may have descending dendrites which remain in this layer (Fig. 1, cell a) or reach layer IV (Fig. 1, cells b and f). Thus, the

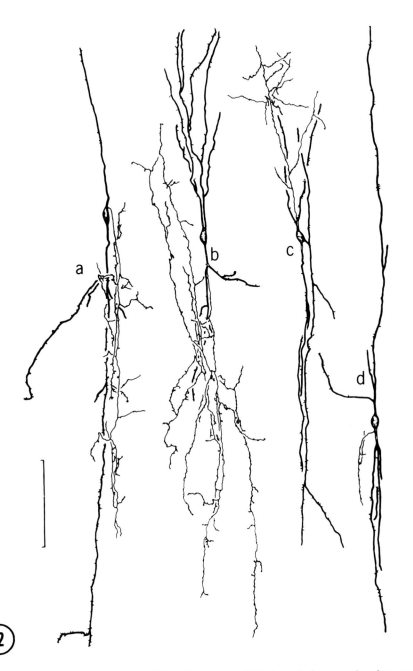

Figure 2. Camera lucida drawings of Golgi-impregnated bipolar cells from rat cingulate cortex. Cell a has its cell body in layer III of area 24b, and cell b in layer III of area 24a. Cell c is from layer V of area 24b, and cell d from layer V of area 29c. Calibration line equals 100 μm. Redrawn from Vogt and Peters (1981).

overall lengths of bipolar cells are variable, but as a group they are the most vertically extensive of the nonpyramidal cells in rat cortex, and their lengths are matched only by the pyramidal cells.

The other important feature of the bipolar cells is their narrow dendritic trees. This results from the fact that the two or three primary dendrites extending from the poles of the cell body are vertically oriented, and the secondary and tertiary branches arising from these dendrites also usually follow a vertical, or only slightly oblique course. Where the first branching of the primary dendrites takes place is variable. Sometimes, an ascending or descending primary dendrite can extend for long distances before forming secondary branches, in which case the dendrite usually forms a terminal tuft, whereas in other examples the first branching may occur close to the cell body. Also, the branching of the descending and ascending dendrites is rarely symmetrical (Figs. 1 and 2), and the asymmetry may be accentuated by two other factors. One is the location of the cell body within the depth of the cortex. Thus, bipolar cells with cell bodies in the lower half of the cortex tend to have short descending and longer ascending dendritic systems (Fig. 1, cells c and d; Fig. 2, cell d), while for neurons with their cell bodies in layer II/III the opposite is often true (Fig. 2, cells a and b). The other factor affecting the symmetry is the lateral spread of the dendrites, and frequently the descending system has a greater lateral spread than the ascending one. Nevertheless, the overall lateral spread of the dendritic tree is rarely more than about 100 μm.

Finally, although many of the bipolar cells in rat cortex have smooth-surfaced dendrites, it is not uncommon for a few, relatively short, spines to be present. Indeed, in rat visual cortex, smooth and sparsely spined varieties of bipolar cells are present in about equal number.

Although these vertically elongate neurons have been referred to as *bipolar cells* in the preceding paragraphs, in their account of the neurons in rat visual cortex Werner *et al.* (1979) refer to these same neurons as *double bouquet cells*. This name is used by them in recognition of the existence of the two dendritic tufts which emanate from these cells, and use of the term *double bouquet* will be discussed in more detail later in this chapter.

In both visual (Feldman and Peters, 1978; Peters and Kimerer, 1981) and cingulate (Vogt and Peters, 1981) cortices of the rat, the axons of the bipolar cells are commonly seen to arise from one of the vertically oriented dendrites and much less frequently from the perikaryon (Figs. 1–3). In the majority of cases, the descending primary dendrite gives rise to the axon, and it often emerges from 10 to 30 μm distant from the cell body. In all cases, however, the axon assumes a vertical trajectory initially and if it emerges from a dendrite it may bend to assume this trajectory, after which it can be either descending or ascending. Then, having passed for some distance, the axon branches form collaterals. These may arise at oblique angles and pass laterally, but most of the branches of the axonal plexus have an essentially vertical orientation, and like the dendritic tree, the axonal plexus tends to be quite narrow. The vertical extent of the plexuses vary though, for some neurons have the branches of the plexus extending in only one direction away from the cell body and this can be either ascending or descending, while other bipolar cells have axonal plexuses with

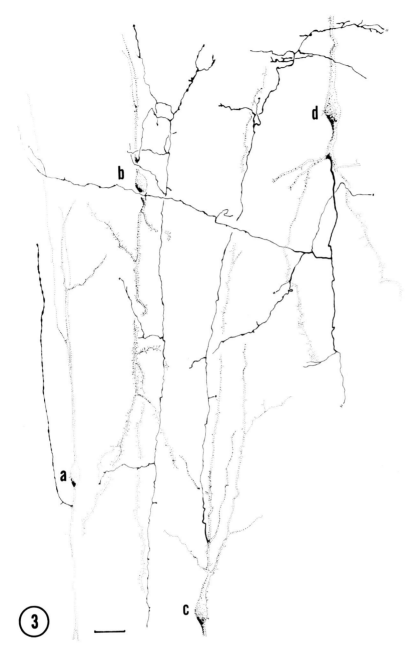

Figure 3. Camera lucida drawings of the axonal distributions of four bipolar cells in rat visual cortex. The neurons are a lower layer II/III spine-free cell (a), a midlayer II/III sparsely spinous cell (b), and two layer IV sparsely spinous bipolar cells (c and d). Calibration line equals 25 μm. From Feldman and Peters (1978).

both descending and ascending branches, whose vertical extent is almost as great as that of the dendrites (Figs. 1–3).

In most examples, the axons of the bipolar cells in rat cortex have relatively simple branching patterns and the axons are not richly endowed with swellings. In a few instances, however, examples of quite intricate vertical interweaving of axonal branches have been encountered (Fig. 1, cells c and g; Fig. 2, cells a and b). At these complexes, the axons can have many swellings, or boutons, and it has been observed that apical dendrites of pyramidal cells may pass through these complexes (Peters and Kimerer, 1981).

1.2. Other Cortices

The features of bipolar cells in rat cortex have been emphasized because information about the form, and existence of bipolar cells in the cortices of other species is relatively sparse.

From the account of Peters and Regidor (1981), it is clear that bipolar cells are present in cat visual cortex, and in their Golgi preparations these authors find such neurons to be preferentially located in layer IV, with a few in layer V. As in rat, these bipolar cells have quite small cell bodies, with average dimensions of 18 μm for the vertical axis and 10 μm for their widths. Also, major dendritic trunks arise from each pole of the spindle-shaped body (Fig. 4), but the branches of the ascending and descending dendrites tend to have a rather more oblique orientation than in the rat, and one or two of the dendritic branches may pass laterally, outside the otherwise narrow dendritic domain. In addition, a branch from the ascending dendrite may sometimes change direction and turn back, so that it descends toward the cell body (Fig. 4, cell b). Again, there is some variability on the overall lengths of the bipolar cells. The longest ones have dendrites extending from layer II to layer V, while the shortest ones only traverse two cellular layers, and while some bipolar cells in the cat have smooth dendrites, others possess a few spines.

As in the rat, the bipolar cells in cat visual cortex commonly have their axons originating from one of the dendritic trunks. Most frequently, it is the descending one, but none of the bipolar cells encountered by Peters and Regidor (1981) have well-impregnated axons. However, some information about the axonal distribution may be gleaned from one of the illustrations of Ramón y Cajal (1911). In his book, Ramón y Cajal has an illustration of neurons in the stellate cell layer, layer IV, of cat visual cortex and in that illustration, which is reproduced here (Fig. 5), are two neurons which he calls *fusiform cells* (cells B and C). These neurons are clearly bipolar in form, for they have spindle-shaped cell bodies, and the thin major dendrites that extend from the poles of the cell body give rise to vertically oriented, long and narrow, dendritic trees. The axons of these neurons (labeled a) are shown to arise from the descending dendrite, and as the axons descend, they give off a few collaterals before bifurcating and forming branches which curve upwards, in an arc, as recurrents (also see Chapter 6).

In the rabbit, the existence of bipolar cells in the auditory cortex has recently been demonstrated in a Golgi study by McCullen and Glaser (1982), who show bipolar cells to be present in layers II/III and IV. These neurons have fusiform

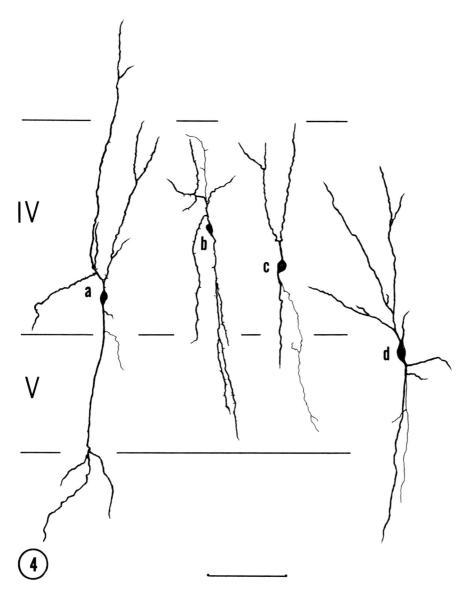

Figure 4. Camera lucida drawings of Golgi-impregnated bipolar cells from area 17 of cat visual cortex. Calibration line equals 100 µm. Redrawn from Peters and Regidor (1981).

somata and vertically oriented dendrites that emerge from the upper and lower poles of the cell body. The sizes of the cell bodies of bipolar neurons in layers II and upper III are given as 9 and 20 µm for their minor and major axes, while those in layers IV and lower III appear to range in size from 8 × 16 up to 12 × 24 µm. The dendritic systems of the neurons with cell bodies in layers IV and lower III are long, for they frequently extend across three or more cellular laminae, while the more superficially located cells in layer II and upper III have dendrites that only descend as far as the bottom of layer III. Interest-

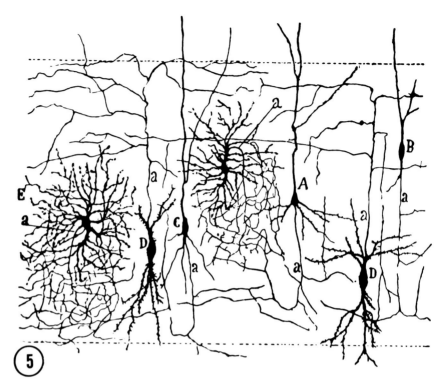

Figure 5. A reproduction of Fig. 387 from Ramón y Cajal (1911), showing various Golgi-impregnated cells in the stellate cell layer of the visual cortex of a 28-day-old cat. Cells B and C are described as small fusiform cells with descending axons, labeled a. Cells labeled D are large fusiform cells, cell A is a small pyramidal neuron, and cell E is a spider or neurogliaform cell.

ingly, these authors state that some of the bipolar cells have "eccentric" dendrites, characterized by a complete reversal of direction of one of the dendrites, somewhat similar to that shown by Peters and Regidor (1981) in cat visual cortex (see Fig. 4, cell a). As in the cat and rat, the bipolar cells in rabbit auditory cortex are either smooth or sparsely spinous and the axons typically emerge from one of the primary dendrites to form vertically oriented collaterals.

Additional information about bipolar cells in rabbit cortex comes from the account of Globus and Scheibel (1967) who studied neurons in the visual cortex. In their group of class II neurons, Globus and Scheibel (1967) show fusiform neurons which they describe as being bipolar in form (see their Fig. 6). The dendrites of these neurons bear few spines and can extend from layer I to layer VI, while the axons are described as being confined to the dendritic tree in their distribution. Shkol'nik-Yarros (1971) also shows examples of bipolar cells in rabbit visual cortex, as well as in dog visual cortex, and interestingly, like Ramón y Cajal (1911), she refers to them as *fusiform neurons.*

There is little information about the bipolar cells in the cortices of primates, but there is evidence that bipolar cells are present. An example of a Golgi-impregnated bipolar cell from macaque visual cortex is shown in Fig. 6. This particular neuron shows the same features as the bipolar cells in other animals.

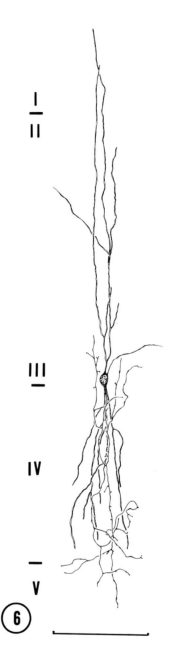

Figure 6. A Golgi-impregnated bipolar cell from area 17 of the visual cortex of a 1-year-old macaque monkey. The cell body is at the border between layers II and IV, and the narrow dendritic tree stretches from layer I to lower layer IV. The axon arises from a descending dendrite and forms a narrow plexus in which the branches are mostly vertical in their orientation. Calibration line equals 100 μm.

The cell body is at the level of the border between layers III and IV and is quite small, having dimensions of only 10 × 16 μm, and the narrow dendritic tree is formed by one ascending and two descending primary dendrites, which extend from layer I to lower layer IV. Also, the axon arises from one of the descending dendrites and forms a plexus that is essentially vertical in orientation and narrow. As for the human, Ramón y Cajal (1911) shows a variety of neurons that are clearly bipolar in form in some of his illustrations of human cerebral cortex (see

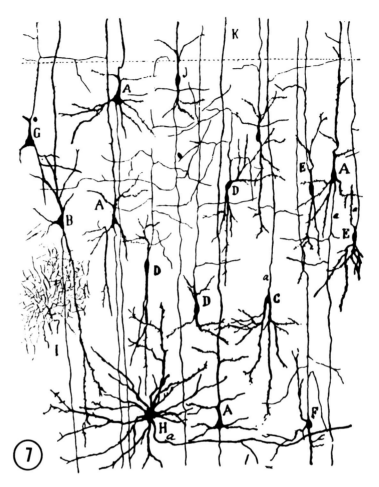

Figure 7. A reproduction of Fig. 373 from Ramón y Cajal (1911), showing Golgi-impregnated neurons in the parietal cortex of a 1-month-old human infant. The neurons are in upper layer V, and cells D and E are clearly examples of bipolar cells with ascending axons.

his Figs. 373, 375, and 395). As shown in Fig. 7, which is a reproduction of Fig. 373 from Ramón y Cajal (1911), these neurons, such as cells D and E, are vertically elongate, have long and narrow dendritic trees, and the axons emerge from one of the primary dendrites. Very little is shown of the axons of these cells, but the axons always pass in a vertical direction, either ascending or descending, and give off a few lateral branches.

1.3. Conclusions

There is evidence, then, for the presence of bipolar neurons in the cerebral cortices of rat, rabbit, cat, dog, monkey, and human, and in each case these neurons have rather small ovoid or spindle-shaped cell bodies from which arise two or three primary dendrites that typically produce a narrow and elongate dendritic field. The axons of such neurons frequently arise from one of the primary dendrites and form a plexus that is also narrow in its spread and essentially vertical in orientation, but not, apparently, extremely profuse.

One question that arises is whether these bipolar cells are different from the neurons that others have referred to as *double bouquet cells*. The term originates from Ramón y Cajal (1911) who described a variety of neurons as "cellules à double bouquet dendritique" in the auditory and other cortices. Examining the drawings of such cells by Ramón y Cajal (1911), for example in his Figs. 345, 347, 384, 393, it is apparent that the neurons described as "cellules à double bouquet dendritique" usually have a number of dendrites arising from the upper and lower poles of the cell body, and although the dendrites may be long, they always seem to have a wider spread than those of the neurons described here as being bipolar. Hence, most of the double bouquet cells are bitufted in form (Feldman and Peters, 1978). Moreover, the double bouquet cells generally have axons that produce long fascicular plexuses, which are either descending or both ascending and descending. Indeed, as described by Szentágothai (1973), their axons resemble a horse tail, and good examples of the axons of such cells are also illustrated by Jones (1975), who refers to them as *type 3 cells*. Thus, bipolar cells and double bouquet cells have different features and need to be distinguished from each other (for additional discussion, see Chapter 6).

In this context, reference might be made to a recent article by Somogyi and Cowey (1981). In their recent Golgi–EM study of some neurons in cat and monkey visual cortex, Somogyi and Cowey (1981) show that the double bouquet cells whose axons produce vertically oriented fascicles of collaterals have axon terminals which form symmetric synapses. On the other hand, a different type of neuron, which they also include in the double bouquet category, has an axon forming symmetric synapses. This latter type of neuron is in layer IV of monkey visual cortex. It has rather spiny dendrites, and forms a long and narrow dendritic field that is 20 to 50 μm wide. The axon originates from the lower pole of the perikaryon and takes a descending course while giving off a few collaterals. In its form, this type of neuron resembles what is here described as a bipolar cell, and interestingly, in common with the bipolar cells of rat visual cortex (Peters and Kimerer, 1981) its axon forms asymmetric synapses.

2. Electron Microscopy

2.1. Cell Body and Dendrites

The fine structure of bipolar cells in rat visual cortex has been examined by Peters and Kimerer (1981). They employed the technique of Fairén *et al.* (1977), so that Golgi-impregnated bipolar cells were gold-toned before being embedded in plastic for electron microscopy. This technique allows the neurons to be first examined in the light microscope to determine their overall morphology, after which the neurons can be thin-sectioned and their fine structure determined, for the presence of gold particles within the cytoplasm allows profiles of the various portions of the neurons to be identified in the electron microscope (Figs. 8–15).

As shown by light microscopy, the cell bodies of many bipolar cells are quite small and this is particularly true of bipolar cells in layer II/III. Thus, when the sections are taken through their cell bodies, the rather irregular nucleus almost fills the cell body, leaving only a thin rim of cytoplasm between the nuclear envelope and the plasma membrane of the perikaryon (Figs. 8 and 9). Moreover, the nucleus is commonly invaginated by a deep cleft which is often oriented parallel to the long axis of the cell body, and the cleft may be so deep that the profile of the nucleus appears in two parts separated by a narrow strip of cytoplasm. At the ends of the elongate cell body, where the ascending and descending primary dendrites emerge (Figs. 8 and 9), the cell body tapers to form cones of cytoplasm, and it is in these regions, where the cytoplasm becomes more abundant, that the Golgi apparatus and granular endoplasmic reticulum are most evident. Even then, the endoplasmic reticulum may consist of little more than a few isolated cisternae and stacks of two or three cisternae.

In contrast to these features shown by the smaller bipolar cells, the larger ones have more abundant cytoplasm at the poles of the cell body (Fig. 10). Larger bipolar cells are frequently, but not exclusively, encountered in layers IV and V, and in the cytoplasm at the poles of their cell bodies may be numerous cisternae of granular endoplasmic reticulum stacked in arrays that are oriented parallel to the surface of the cell body. This arrangement of the cisternae of granular endoplasmic reticulum is quite striking and the cisternae have many free polyribosomes lying both between and around them.

Regardless of their size, the cell bodies of bipolar cells in rat visual cortex receive only few axosomatic synapses (Figs. 8–10). Thus, in any one section through a cell body, it is rare to encounter more than three to five axosomatic synapses. These are of both the symmetric and the asymmetric varieties and usually the symmetric synapses are formed by larger axon terminals than the asymmetric ones. Also, the symmetric synapses are most common, so that in a survey of 100 axosomatic synapses on bipolar cells, Peters and Kimerer (1981) find about three symmetric synapses for every asymmetric synapse encountered.

As the perikarya of bipolar cells taper at their upper and lower poles to give rise to the ascending and descending primary dendrites, there is a gradual reduction in the number of ribosomes and cisternae of granular endoplasmic reticulum in the cytoplasm, and a gathering together of the microtubules as they funnel into the bases of the dendrites. As they enter the dendrites, the microtubules become arranged parallel to each other and they quite soon dominate the dendritic cytoplasm, for it contains little more than microtubules with mitochondria and tubular cisternae lying between them (Fig. 11). Some groups of ribosomes and short cisternae of granular endoplasmic reticulum may be en-

$\longrightarrow$

Figure 8. Electron micrograph of the cell body of a layer V bipolar cell from rat visual cortex. This Golgi-impregnated and gold-toned cell is shown as cell e in Fig. 1. The nucleus (N) almost fills the cell body and has a deep cleft. At the upper pole of the perikaryon, the cytoplasm contains a few cisternae of granular endoplasmic reticulum (ER) and portions of the Golgi apparatus (G). Only one axosomatic synapse (arrow) is apparent. Calibration line equals 5 μm.

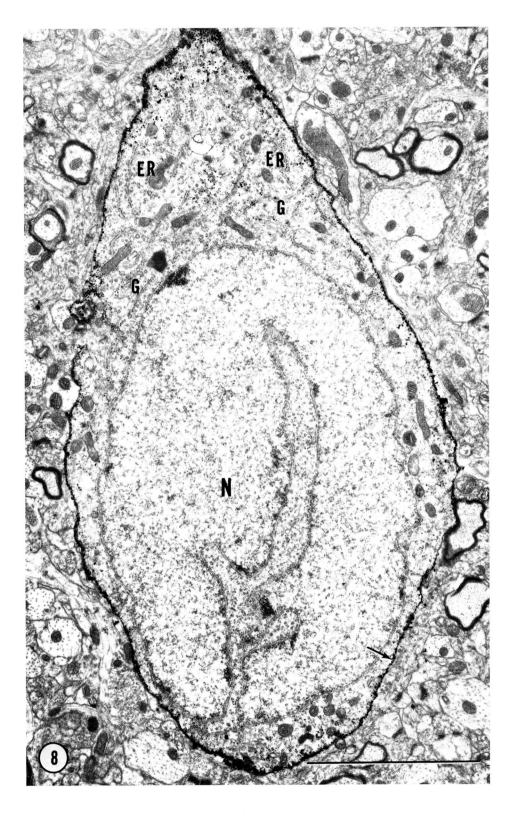

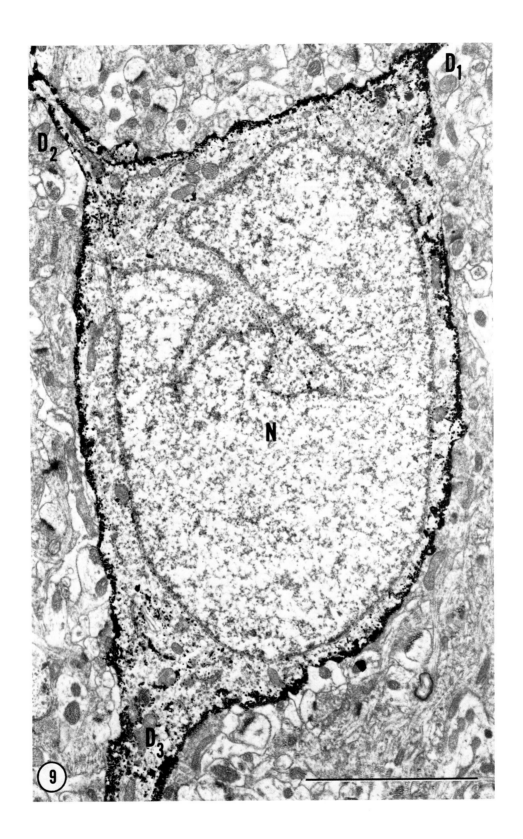

countered in the cytoplasm at the periphery of dendrites, however, but such groups become less common with increasing distance from the cell body as the dendrites taper and become thinner.

Because they have few if any spines, the dendrites of bipolar cells in rat visual cortex have rather smooth and regular contours, and like the cell body, they receive axon terminals forming both asymmetric and symmetric synapses (Fig. 11). In general, the symmetric synapses are most frequent along the surfaces of the proximal portions of the dendrites, with asymmetric synapses predominating more distally, where they occur both on the surface of the dendritic shaft and on any spines that may be present.

2.2. Axons

As shown by light microscopy, the axons of bipolar cells most commonly extend from one of the primary dendrites. The axons can be either myelinated or unmyelinated, and when the axon is myelinated, the Golgi impregnation stops where the axon enters its myelin sheath (Fig. 12). Consequently, the impregnated portion of a myelinated axon is rarely than 20 to 30 μm long. In all cases, however, the initial segments of the bipolar cell axons, like the initial segments of all neurons in the cerebral cortex, are characterized by a dense undercoating of the axolemma and the fasciculation of microtubules within its cytoplasm. If the axon is myelinated, these cytoplasmic characteristics of the initial segment stop where the axon enters its myelin sheath. In unmyelinated axons, the characteristics also persist for a distance of about 25 μm before being lost (Peters and Kimerer, 1981), after which the axon becomes thinner. Except where it swells to form terminals, the more distal lengths of the axon contain little more than isolated microtubules, a few tubular cisternae, and occasional mitochondria.

It should also be noted that in contrast to the axon initial segments of some pyramidal cells, no axo-axonic synapses have been seen on initial segments of bipolar cells.

When the axonal boutons, or terminals, of bipolar cells are examined in Golgi-impregnated and gold-toned preparations, they are found to form asymmetric synapses (Figs. 13–15). The neuronal elements most commonly postsynaptic to the boutons are dendritic spines (Figs. 14 and 15). Some bipolar cell axon terminals synapse with other neuronal elements, however, and Peters and Kimerer (1981) encountered examples in which shafts of apical dendrites of pyramidal cells, dendrites of nonpyramidal cells (Fig. 13), and even the cell bodies of nonpyramidal cells are postsynaptic to bipolar cell axons.

To determine the origins of the dendritic spines with which the bipolar cell axon terminals synapse is a problem, but since most of the spines in the cerebral cortex arise from the pyramidal cells, it is most likely that these are the neurons

---

$\leftarrow$

Figure 9. Electron micrograph of the cell body of a layer IV bipolar cell from rat visual cortex. The Golgi-impregnated and gold-toned cell is shown as cell g in Fig. 1, in which the ascending (D$_1$) and descending (D$_3$) dendrites as well as the laterally extending one (D$_2$) are evident. The nucleus (N) almost fills the cell body so that it is surrounded by only a thin rim of perikaryal cytoplasm. Calibration line equals 5 μm.

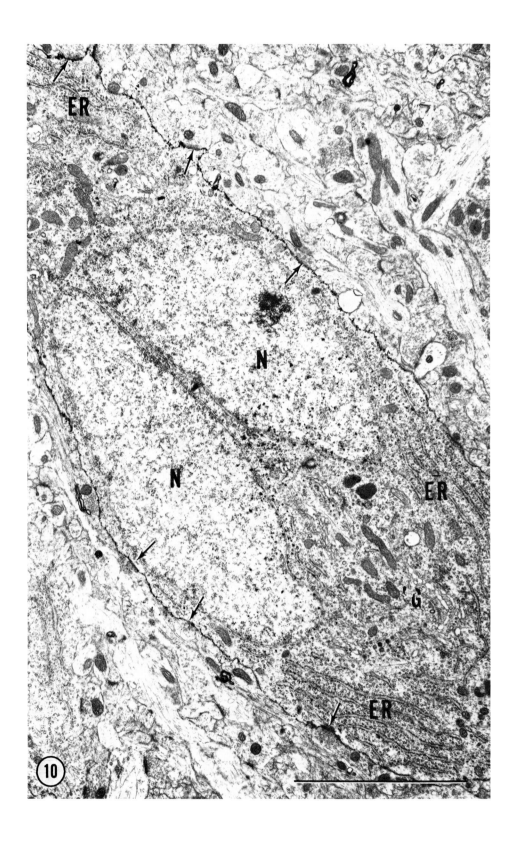

with which the majority of bipolar cell terminals synapse. There is no doubt that at least some of the spines originate from apical dendrites of pyramidal cells for this has been shown by Peters and Kimerer (1981). They examined a Golgi preparation in which the impregnated axon of a bipolar cell ran parallel to the apical dendrite of an impregnated layer III pyramidal neuron in rat visual cortex, and after gold-toning, study of this preparation in the electron microscope revealed two synapses between the labeled spines of the apical dendrite and terminals of the bipolar cell axon. That the axon terminals of bipolar cells might frequently synapse with apical dendrites is suggested by observations that bipolar cell axons are often seen to pass parallel to apical dendrites, and apical dendrites have been seen to pass through the vertical plexuses that are sometimes formed by bipolar cell axons (Peters and Kimerer, 1981).

As stated earlier, Somogyi and Cowey (1981) have also examined a type of neuron in layer IV of monkey visual cortex which is probably a bipolar cell. The axon of this neuron also formed asymmetric synapses, and Somogyi and Cowey (1981) state that of nine terminals they were able to find in the electron microscope, seven of them synapsed with dendritic shafts and two with spines. This distribution is different from that of the synapses formed by the axon terminals of bipolar cells in rat visual cortex, but whether it is significant can only be ascertained by further studies.

3. Peptides

There seems to be little doubt that in rat cortex, bipolar cells are one of the types of neuron which Lorén *et al.* (1979) and Sims *et al.* (1980) have shown to combine with antisera to vasoactive intestinal polypeptide (VIP). Both of these groups of authors comment that the cell bodies of the VIP-positive neurons occur throughout layers II to V, although the greatest number of them are present in layer II/III and are characterized by ovoid cell bodies from which vertically oriented, long processes extend (Fig. 16). The fact that some of the VIP-positive neurons in rat cortex are bipolar cells is also emphasized by Emson and Hunt (1981) who show the comparison between the forms of these neurons and the bipolar cells described by Feldman and Peters (1978). Furthermore, as observed by Emson and Hunt (1981), VIP-positive boutons are concentrated in layers I–IV, and many of them form vertical strings (Fig. 16), which correlates well with the features of the axonal plexuses of bipolar cells impregnated in Golgi preparations (Figs. 1 and 2). Morrison *et al.* (1981) and Parnavelas *et al.* (1981) have also observed that VIP-positive neurons in cerebral cortex are most numerous in layers II and III. They state that the cell bodies of some of these

Figure 10. Electron micrograph of the cell body of a layer III bipolar cell in rat visual cortex. The neuron is Golgi-impregnated and gold-toned, and is shown as cell b in Fig. 1. This is a large bipolar cell. The nucleus (N) appears as two profiles separated by a thin strip of cytoplasm. At the poles of the cell body, the granular endoplasmic reticulum (ER) is composed of cisternae stacked parallel to the cell surface, and these surround a cytoplasm containing the Golgi apparatus (G) and mitochondria. Axosomatic synapses are indicated by arrows. Calibration line equals 5 μm.

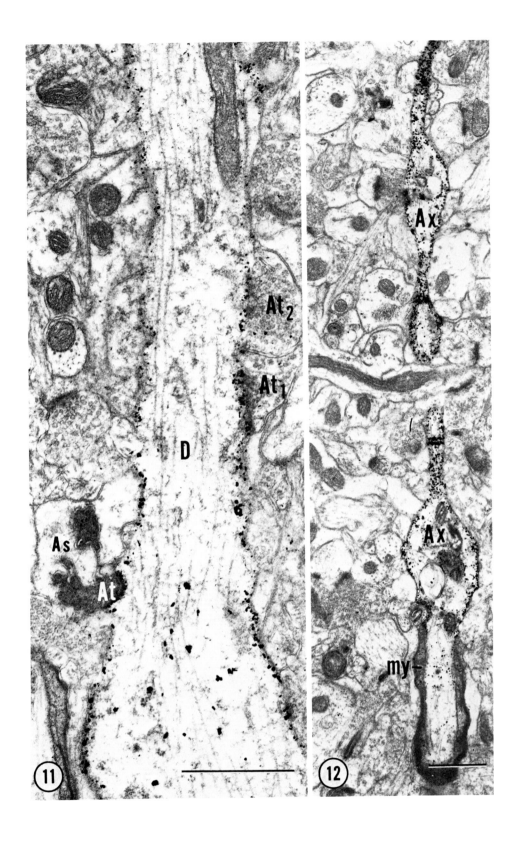

neurons are ovoid, measuring 8–10 μm across and 15 μm in length, and give rise to long dendrites which are vertically oriented, branch infrequently, and extend for long distances.

Emson *et al.* (1979) have examined the development of VIP-positive neurons to rat cortex and find that they can be first demonstrated at postnatal day 7, when the neurons occur in groups within the deeper layers of the neocortex. By postnatal day 14, the VIP-positive neurons have apparently reached their final positions in the cortex and some are evident as fusiform neurons in layers II to IV. Between days 14 to 28, the numbers of VIP-positive terminals increase substantially, but at the same time there is a drop in the cell body content of VIP in these neurons, making them less easily demonstrable by immunochemistry. Interestingly, the increase in the number of VIP-positive terminals during the period from days 14 to 28 correlates well with a dramatic increase in the amount of VIP that can be determined in the cortex by radioimmunoassay. Emson and Hunt (1981) suggest that this increase reflects the development of the adult form of the axonal terminals of the VIP-positive cells.

VIP-positive bipolar cells are also present in cat visual cortex (Fig. 17), although their concentration is less than in rat cortex. Also, as would be expected from Golgi preparations (Fig. 4), the bipolar cells in cat cortex lack the straight and vertically oriented dendrites that make rat bipolar cells so striking in appearance.

At present, the role of VIP in the cerebral cortex is unknown, but it is pertinent to mention that application of VIP to cortical neurons produces a strong excitation (Phillis *et al.,* 1978; Dodd *et al.,* 1979).

Antisera to cholecystokinin (CCK) also combine with bipolar cells in rat cortex (Innis *et al.,* 1979; Emson and Hunt, 1981), and Peters *et al.* (1983) have shown that among the CCK-positive cells in rat cerebral cortex, the bipolar cells are the most frequently labeled cells and are the most strongly reactive (Fig. 18). Peters *et al.* (1983) have emphasized the strong similarity between the form of the bipolar cells impregnated by the Golgi technique and the appearance of bipolar cells after treatment of the cortex with CCK antiserum, and observe that when the axons of the CCK-positive cells are evident, they often arise from one of the primary dendrites, and usually the descending one. Upon examination of CCK-positive bipolar cells in the electron microscope, Peters *et al.* (1983) have shown the HRP reaction product to form a granular deposit, which occurs

---

←

Figure 11. Electron micrograph of a gold-toned dendrite (D) from a bipolar cell in rat visual cortex. The dendrite is synapsing with a degenerating geniculocortical axon terminal (At) partially surrounded by astrocytic processes (As). A lesion was placed in the lateral geniculate nucleus of this animal 3 days before the brain was fixed. The dendrite also forms synapses with two normal axon terminals. One of them (At₁) is forming an asymmetric synapse, and the other (At₂) a symmetric synapse. Calibration line equals 1 μm.

Figure 12. Electron micrograph of the axon initial segment (Ax) of the Golgi-impregnated and gold-toned bipolar cell shown as cell f in Fig. 1. In the light microscope, the axon could only be followed for a short distance. The reason is that where the axon enters its myelin sheath (my), the impregnation, as indicated by the distribution of gold particles, comes to an end. Calibration line equals 1 μm.

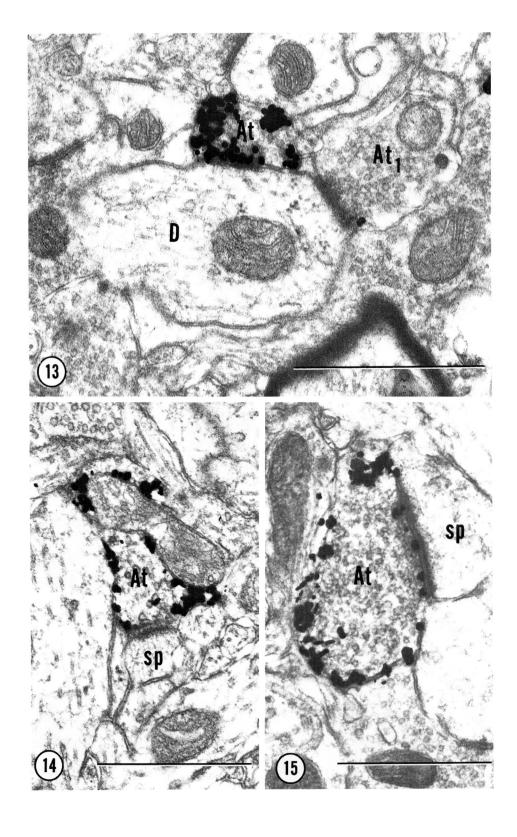

throughout the cytoplasm and nucleoplasm and is not associated with any particular type of organelle.

Like VIP, CCK applied iontophoretically to the cerebral cortex excites neurons (Rehfeld, 1980; Phillis and Kirkpatrick, 1980), and this action of these two peptides may correlate with the observation that the axon terminals from bipolar cells form asymmetric synapses (Peters and Kimerer, 1981), for such synapses are generally supposed to be excitatory in function. However, it is not known if these peptides are the primary neurotransmitters of the bipolar cells. According to Emson and Hunt (1981), the number of CCK-positive neurons is substantially greater than that of VIP-positive neurons, and on this basis they suggest that the two sets of bipolar neurons belong to different populations. Whether this is true has not been established.

4. The Role of Bipolar Cells in the Cortex

Since no physiological recordings have been made from bipolar cells, their functional role in the cortex is not known, but some suggestions can be made. If it is accepted that the axons of bipolar cells form asymmetric synapses in which dendritic spines are the predominant postsynaptic element, then it is likely that the bipolar cells have an excitatory effect on pyramidal neurons.

Because of their long dendritic fields, bipolar cells extend through appreciable depths of the cerebral cortex. The longest ones, those with cell bodies in layers IV and V, often stretch from layer I to layer V, while the bipolar cells with cell bodies in layer II/III are often shorter and their descending dendrites may reach no further than layer IV or lower III. Nevertheless, most of the bipolar cells have some portion of their dendritic trees passing through layers IV and lower III where the greatest numbers of thalamic afferents terminate, and there is evidence that bipolar cells do receive these afferents. Thus, Peters and Kimerer (1981) have shown a bipolar cell with its cell body in upper layer IV of rat visual cortex to receive geniculocortical axon terminals which form asymmetric synapses with one of its dendrites (see Fig. 11). In addition, White (1978) has shown a bipolar cell in mouse SmI cortex to receive thalamocortical afferents. This particular bipolar cell is interesting, because it receives thalamic terminals on both its cell body and dendrites, and of the cortical neurons examined by White (1978) the bipolar cell receives the greatest number of thalamocortical axon terminals per unit length of dendrite. Thus, as shown in Fig. 19, thalamocortical afferents can be expected to monosynaptically excite bipolar cells and pyramidal cells (e.g., White, 1978; Peters *et al.*, 1979). The fact that

---

Figures 13–15. Electron micrographs showing the gold-labeled axon terminals (At) of bipolar cells forming asymmetric synapses in rat visual cortex. In Fig. 13 the axon terminal is synapsing with the dendrite (D) of a nonpyramidal cell, which is also forming a second asymmetric synapse with an unlabeled axon terminal (At$_1$). In Figs. 14 and 15 the bipolar cell axon terminals are synapsing with dendritic spines (sp). Calibration lines equal 1 μm.

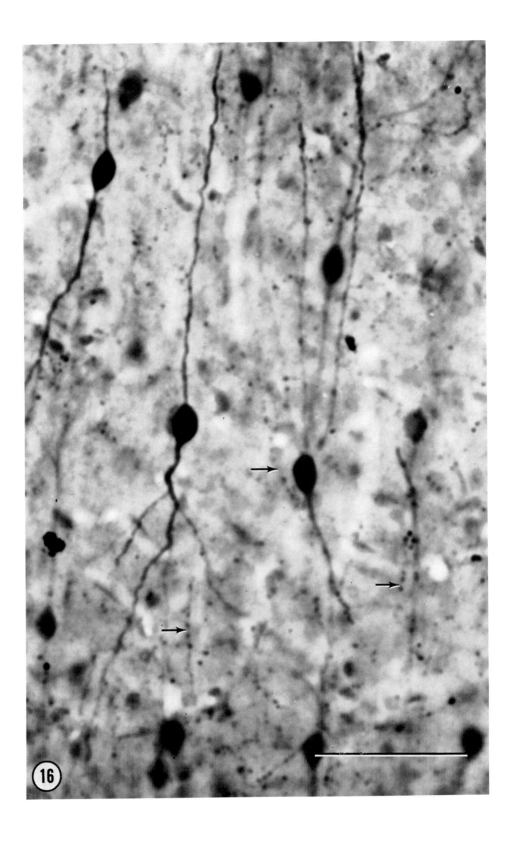

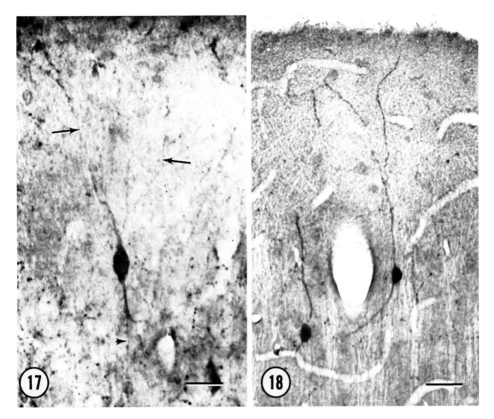

Figure 17. A VIP-positive bipolar cell in layer II of cat visual cortex. Section stained by the immunoperoxidase technique. The ascending dendrites (arrows) of the neuron reach the pial surface, and the axon (arrowhead) arises from the descending dendrite. Preparation by Dr. James D. Connor. Calibration line equals 25 μm.

Figure 18. Two CCK-immunoreactive bipolar cells in layer II of area 18a of rat cerebral cortex. Section stained by the immunoperoxidase technique. Calibration line equals 25 μm.

bipolar cells form asymmetric synapses with pyramidal neurons would lead to the further excitation of the pyramidal cells.

The sources of the other axon terminals forming asymmetric synapses with the cell bodies and dendrites of bipolar cells are not yet known. Most of the axon terminals forming asymmetric synapses in the cortex are probably derived from pyramidal neurons, and therefore it may be reasonable to suggest that the axons of the pyramidal neurons themselves synapse with bipolar cells. If this is so, then there may be an excitatory convergence, via the bipolar cells, onto the pyramidal neurons, which might synchronize their activity. In this respect, it is

←

Figure 16. VIP-immunoreactive bipolar cells in layer II/III of rat occipital cortex. Section stained by the immunoperoxidase technique. The bipolar cells are strongly reactive and show their ascending and descending dendrites. Note the vertical strings of axonal boutons (arrows) formed by the axons of the bipolar cells. Preparation by Dr. James D. Connor. Calibration line equals 25 μm.

interesting to note that Bullier and Henry (1979) have assessed the ordinal, or serial positions of different types of neurons after stimulation of the optic radiations in the cat. They have shown that while some neurons receive monosynaptic inputs, others have a convergence of both monosynaptic and other inputs. Yet for other neurons, ones not receiving direct thalamic input, the lowest order of excitatory input is disynaptic.

What of the symmetric synapses upon bipolar cells? In rat visual cortex, at least, most of the axon terminals which form symmetric synapses with the cell bodies and dendrites of neurons appear to be derived from the smooth or sparsely spinous multipolar and bitufted cells (Peters and Fairén, 1978; Peters

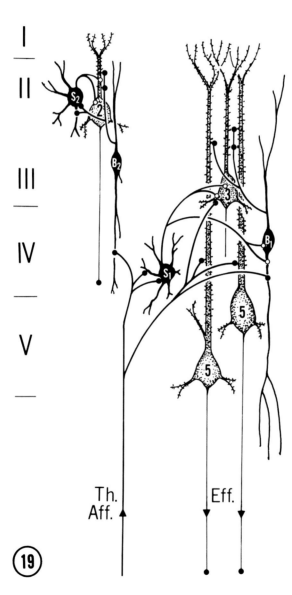

Figure 19. Diagram to show some of the synaptic relationships between bipolar cells (B_1 and B_2), smooth or sparsely spinous nonpyramidal cells (S_1 and S_2), and pyramidal cells (2, 3, and 5) in rat visual cortex. Potentially, the thalamic afferents (Th. Aff) can synapse with all postsynaptic surfaces capable of forming asymmetric synapses in layers IV and lower III, and they form asymmetric synapses (filled circles), as do the axons of the bipolar cells. The smooth and sparsely spinous cells, on the other hand, form symmetric and inhibitory synapses (open circles). Reproduced from Peters and Kimerer (1981).

and Proskauer, 1980; also see Chapter 13). Further, as shown by Ribak (1978), some axon terminals which form symmetric synapses in this cortex label with an antibody to GAD. Consequently, it can be concluded that they use GABA as their neurotransmitter and have an inhibitory function. Thus, these neurons would be expected to inhibit the bipolar cells, but they would also inhibit pyramidal neurons, for Peters and Fairén (1978) have shown axon terminals of the smooth or sparsely spinous stellate cells to synapse with the cell bodies and dendritic shafts of pyramidal neurons.

Some of these synaptic relationships of bipolar neurons are illustrated in Fig. 19, in which the bias is directed toward the bipolar cells exciting the pyramidal neurons. Whether this bias is correct is not presently known. On the basis of the forms of the bipolar cells and the character of their axonal plexuses, it would seem that the bipolar cells might be designed to reinforce the excitation that at least layer VI, layer V, and layer III pyramidal cells receive from the thalamocortical afferents (Peters *et al.*, 1979; White and Hersch, 1981; Hersch and White, 1981). In addition, because the axons of bipolar cells form long, vertically oriented, and narrow plexuses, they may reinforce the excitation of pyramidal neurons, synchronizing the activity of vertical arrays of pyramidal cells. This would be consistent with the fact that the axons of bipolar cells are frequently observed to pass parallel to apical dendrites which are arranged in clusters, which at least contain the apical dendrites of layer V and III pyramids (Peters and Walsh, 1972; Fleischhauer *et al.*, 1972; Feldman and Peters, 1974). The relationship between bipolar cells and clusters of apical dendrites is not yet known, but given that the center-to-center spacing of the clusters is between 40 and 60 μm, only a small number of clusters would be encompassed by the axon of any one bipolar cell.

ACKNOWLEDGMENT. This work was supported by Research Grant NS 07016 from the National Institutes of Health.

5. References

Builler, J., and Henry, G. H., 1979, Ordinal position of neurons in cat striate cortex, *J. Neurophysiol.* **42**:251–263.

Dodd, J., Kelly, J. S., and Said, S. I., 1979, Excitation of CA1 neurones of the rat hippocampus by the octacosapeptide, vasoactive intestinal polypeptide (VIP), [Proceedings] *Br. J. Pharmacol.* **66**:125P.

Emson, P. C., and Hunt, S. P., 1981, Anatomical chemistry of the cerebral cortex, in: *The Organization of the Cerebral Cortex* (F. O. Schmitt, F. G. Worden, G. Adelman, and S. G. Dennis, eds.), pp. 325–346, MIT Press, Cambridge, Mass.

Emson, P. C., Gilbert, R. F. R., Lorén, I., Fahrenkrug, J., Sundler, F., and Schaffalizky de Muckadell, O. B., 1979, Development of vasoactive intestinal polypeptide (VIP) containing neurones in rat brain, *Brain Res.* **177**:437–444.

Fairén, A., Peters, A., and Saldanha, J., 1977, A new procedure for examining Golgi impregnated neurons by light and electron microscopy, *J. Neurocytol.* **6**:311–337.

Feldman, M. L., and Peters, A., 1974, A study of barrels and pyramidal dendritic clusters in the cerebral cortex, *Brain Res.* **77**:55–76.

Feldman, M. L., and Peters, A., 1978, The forms of non-pyramidal neurons in the visual cortex of the rat, *J. Comp. Neurol.* **179**:761–794.

Fleischhauer, K., Petsche, H., and Wittowski, W., 1972, Vertical bundles of dendrites in the neocortex, *Z. Anat. Entwicklungsgesch.* **136:**213–223.

Globus, A., and Scheibel, A. B., 1967, Pattern and field in cortical structures: The rabbit, *J. Comp. Neurol.* **131:**155–172.

Hersch, S. M., and White, E. L., 1981, Thalamocortical synapses involving identified neurons in mouse primary somatosensory cortex: A terminal degeneration and Golgi/EM study, *J. Comp. Neurol.* **195:**253–263.

Innis, R. B., Correa, F. M. A., Uhl, G. R., Schneider, B., and Snyder, S., 1979, Cholecystokinin octapeptide-like immunoreactivity: Histochemical localization in rat brain, *Proc. Natl. Acad. Sci. USA* **76:**521–525.

Jones, E. G., 1975, Varieties and distribution of non-pyramidal cells in somatic sensory cortex of the squirrel monkey, *J. Comp. Neurol.* **160:**205–268.

Lorén, I., Emson, P. C., Fahrenkrug, J., Bjorklund, A., Alumets, J., Håkanson, R. P., and Sundler, F., 1979, Distribution of vasoactive intestinal polypeptide in the rat and mouse brain, *Neuroscience* **4:**1953–1976.

McMullen, M. T., and Glaser, E. M., 1982, Morphology and laminar distribution of non-pyramidal neurons in the auditory cortex of the rabbit, *J. Comp. Neurol.* **208:**85–106.

Morrison, J. H., Magistretti, P. J., Benoit R., and Bloom, F. E., 1981, The immunohistochemical characterization of somatostatin (SS) and vasoactive intestinal polypeptide (VIP) neurons within the cerebral cortex, *Soc. Neurosci. Abstr.* **7:**99.

Parnavelas, J. G., McDonald, J. K., Lin. C.-S., and Brecha, N. C., 1981, Localization of vasoactive intestinal polypeptide-like immunoreactivity in identified neurons in the visual cortex of the developing and mature rat, *Soc. Neurosci. Abstr.* **7:**98.

Peters, A., and Faírén, A., 1978, Smooth and sparsely spined stellate cells in the visual cortex of the rat: A study using a combined Golgi–electron microscope technique, *J. Comp. Neurol.* **181:**129–172.

Peters, A., and Kimerer, L. M., 1981, Bipolar neurons in rat visual cortex: A combined Golgi–electron microscope study, *J. Neurocytol.* **10:**921–946.

Peters, A., and Proskauer, C. C., 1980, Synaptic relationships between a multipolar stellate cell and a pyramidal neuron in rat visual cortex: A combined Golgi–electron microscope study, *J. Neurocytol.* **9:**163–183.

Peters, A., and Regidor, J., 1981, A reassessment of the forms of nonpyramidal neurons in area 17 of cat visual cortex, *J. Comp. Neurol.* **203:**685–716.

Peters, A., and Walsh, J. M., 1972, A study of the organization of apical dendrites in the somatic sensory cortex of the rat, *J. Comp. Neurol.* **144:**253–268.

Peters, A., Proskauer, C. C., Feldman, M. L., and Kimerer, L., 1979, The projection of the lateral geniculate nucleus to area 17 of the rat cerebral cortex. V. Degenerating axon terminals synapsing with Golgi impregnated neurons, *J. Neurocytol.* **8:**331–357.

Peters, A., Miller, M., and Kimerer, L. M., 1983, Cholecytokinin-like immunoreactive neurons in rat cerebral cortex, *Neuroscience* **8:**431–448.

Phillis, J. N., and Kirkpatrick, J. R., 1980, The actions of motilin, luteinizing hormone releasing hormone, cholecystokinin, somatostatin, vasoactive intestinal polypeptide and other peptides on rat cerebral cortical neurons, *Can. J. Physiol. Pharmacol.* **58:**612–623.

Phillis, J. N., Kirkpatrick, J. R., and Said, S. I., 1978, Vasoactive intestinal polypeptide excitation of central neurons, *Can. J. Physiol. Pharmacol.* **57:**337–340.

Ramón y Cajal, S., 1911, *Histologie du Système Nerveux de l'Homme et des Vertébrés* (translated by L. Azoulay), Vol. II, Maloine, Paris.

Rehfeld, J. F., 1980, Cholecystokinin, *Trends Neurosci.* **3:**65–67.

Ribak, C. E., 1978, Aspinous and sparsely-spinous stellate neurons in the visual cortex of rats contain glutamic acid decarboxylase, *J. Neurocytol.* **7:**461–478.

Shkol'nik-Yarros, E. G., 1971, *Neurons and Interneuronal Connections of the Central Visual System*, Plenum Press, New York.

Sims, K. B., Hoffman, D. L., Said, S. I., and Zimmerman, E. A., 1980, Vasoactive intestinal polypeptide (VIP) in mouse and rat brain: An immunocytological study, *Brain Res.* **186:**165–183.

Somogyi, P., and Cowey, A., 1981, Combined Golgi and electron microscopic study on the synapses formed by double bouquet cells in the visual cortex of the cat and monkey, *J. Comp. Neurol.* **195:**547–566.

Szentágothai, J., 1973, Synaptology of the visual cortex, in: *Handbook of Sensory Physiology,* Vol. VII/3, *Central Processing of Information,* Part B, *Visual Centers of the Brain* (R. Jung, ed.), pp. 269–324, Springer, Berlin.

Vogt, B. A., and Peters, A., 1981, Form and distribution of neurons in rat cingulate cortex: Areas 32, 24 and 29, *J. Comp. Neurol.* **195:**603–625.

Werner, L., Hedlich, A. Winkelmann, E., and Brauer, K., 1979, Versuch einer Identifizierung von Nervenzellen des visuellen Kortex der Ratte nach Nissl- und Golgi–Kopsch-Darstellung, *J. Hirnforsch.* **20:**121–139.

White, E. L., 1978, Identified neurons in mouse SmI cortex which are post-synaptic to thalamocortical axon terminals: A combined Golgi–electron microscopic and degeneration study, *J. Comp. Neurol.* **181:**627–662.

White, E. L., and Hersch, S. M., 1981, Thalamocortical synapses of pyramidal cells which project from SmI to MsI cortex in the mouse, *J. Comp. Neurol.* **198:**167–181.

12

Neurogliaform or Spiderweb Cells

EDWARD G. JONES

1. Background

Ramón y Cajal (1909–1911) described small neurons resembling neuroglial cells in both the striatum and the cerebral cortex (Fig. 1) (see also Fig. 1 of Chapter 8). Usually Ramón y Cajal termed these *cellules neurogliforme*. He notes that in the cerebral cortex, he had first observed them in the human visual area in 1899. His most extensive description of the cells comes in his general account of layer II of the cortex, though he notes that they are found in all layers and are especially common in the deeper layers. In layer II he refers to them as "cellules naine ou neurogliforme" and he illustrates them by reference to preparations of the human motor cortex (his Fig. 345) and of the cat visual cortex (his Fig. 347). Elsewhere he describes them in human visual and auditory cortex and in cat auditory cortex as well.

According to Ramón y Cajal the neurogliaform cell is very small, even "minuscule" (1922) with a "feeble" cell body and a large number of fine, radiating dendrites that are short, varicose, and rarely branched. The short length and lack of lateral branches on the dendrites, coupled with the difficulty of identifying an axon, was what in Ramón y Cajal's eyes caused these neurons to resemble neuroglial cells. The axon, when seen, is extremely thin, and never deeply im-

EDWARD G. JONES • James L. O'Leary Division of Experimental Neurology and Neurological Surgery and McDonnell Center for Studies of Higher Brain Function, Washington University School of Medicine, Saint Louis, Missouri 63110.

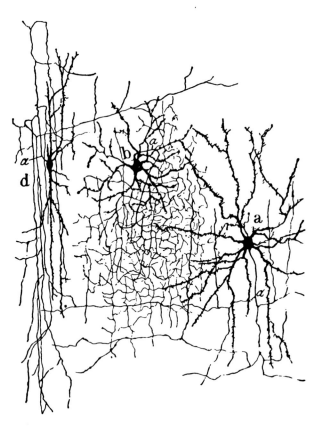

Figure 1. Drawing by Ramón y Cajal (1911) showing three forms of short-axon neurons from the visual cortex of a cat. Cell b is called a "dwarf cell" in the legend, one of Ramón y Cajal's synonyms for a neurogliaform or spiderweb cell.

pregnated. Shortly after its origin, it breaks up into a very dense, highly ramified arborization composed of delicate, beaded intertwined branches. Later, in his description of the visual cortex, he emphasizes the fact that the axonal arborization tends to remain within the territory of the dendrites. The cells, he says, are less common in the dog and cat than in man but in those species are remarkable for their larger size and extreme richness of their axonal arborizations.

As Ramón y Cajal's account of the cerebral cortex proceeds, he commences using the term *cellule araneiforme* or spiderweb cell as a synonym for *neurogliforme*, sometimes referring to a drawing of a cell by one name in the text and by the other in the figure legend (e.g., Fig. 387). By the time he wrote his account of the cat visual cortex (1922), he had generally come to refer to the cells as *araneiforme, aracniforme,* or *spinnenförmige,* all terms with the connotation of a spiderweb and emphasizing the axonal arborization as the distinguishing feature of the cell.

It seems doubtful that spiderweb or neurogliaform cells were clearly identified for more than half a century following Ramón y Cajal's last account. Neither term is mentioned by Lorente de Nó (1922), in his description of what he took to be the mouse auditory cortex but which we now know to be somatosensory cortex. Certain small cells shown in his drawings of layer IV have the dendritic patterns of spiderweb cells, and axonal ramifications that intertwine in what he called a "glomerular" or "basket" manner among the terminal ramifications of thalamic afferents. In both this and his later work (1949), he emphasized the extremely local nature of the effect that such cells should exert. The axonal ramifications drawn on some cells by O'Leary (1941) and O'Leary and Bishop (1938) in the visual cortex of the cat and rabbit are too incomplete for a positive identification, and even in more recent times it is doubtful that many workers have been successful in fully impregnating the axon and, therefore, in recognizing spiderweb cells.

2. Recent Studies

2.1. Distribution

Probably the first author to draw attention to spiderweb cells in recent times was Valverde (1971, 1978) who refers to them as *clewed cells,** the name, again, emphasizing the distinctive axonal plexus. Valverde's first description of such cells was from the visual cortex of the monkey. He found the cells to be especially characteristic of layer IVc and, from the extent of their axonal plexus, considered that each should embrace some 300–500 somata of the small spiny cells that also dominate layer IV. Both clewed and spiny cells he regarded as major recipients of the terminations of thalamic afferents. The composite arrangement of thalamic afferent terminations, clewed cell axons, and contained layer IV somata, he termed a *glomerulus*.

Spiderweb cells were also identified in the somatosensory and motor cortex of monkeys by Jones (1975) who referred to them as *type 5 cells*. They were especially concentrated in layer IV of the sensory area but could be observed in layer III of the motor area and in layer II of both areas. Jones confirmed Valverde's account of the extent of the axonal plexus showing an almost invariable diameter in all dimensions of 300–400 μm. Peters and Regidor (1981) later reported the presence of neurogliaform or spiderweb cells in all layers of area 17 of the cat visual cortex, noting that they are the smallest nonpyramidal cells in the cortex. Fairén and Valverde (1980) and Feldman and Peters (1978) have remarked on the apparent absence of these cells from the visual cortex of rodents. Tömböl (1978) has observed them in all layers of monkey visual cortex but has found them especially concentrated in layers I, II, IV, and V. See Chapter 6 for other accounts.

2.2. Description

The identification of a cell as a spiderweb cell depends always on the ability to stain the distinctive axonal plexus (Figs. 2, 3). When only the dendrites are stained, the cell, though obviously small, could easily be mistaken for any one of a number of other nonpyramidal cell types.

---

* *Clew,* a very old English word, means a ball of thread or yarn.

The soma is spherical and rarely more than 10–12 μm in diameter. Seven to ten thin dendrites radiate out symmetrically from the soma; some branch once or twice, many do not. Single and branched dendrites are of approximately equal length and extend for 50–75 μm, rarely more. Together, they form a very symmetrical, spherical dendritic field. Within this, it is common for some of the dendrites to curve back toward the soma. The dendrites are thin (1–2 μm), occasionally beaded, though not overtly so, and virtually never bear dendritic spines. Even those occasional spines seen intermittently on most aspiny, non-pyramidal neurons appear to be lacking.

The axon is extremely thin (0.5–1 μm) and can arise from any part of the soma or from the base of the dendrite. Almost immediately it branches and rebranches so frequently and the branches become so entangled that it is difficult to follow all the branches in continuity. Though there is a tendency for the

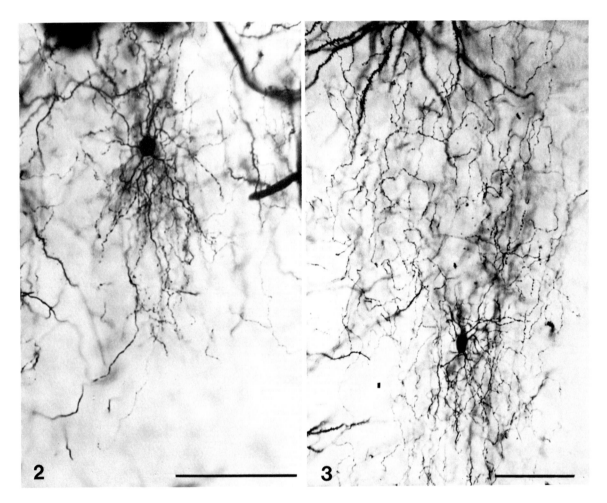

Figures 2 and 3. Photomicrographs of spiderweb or type 5 cells, from material illustrated in Jones (1975). Golgi–Kopsch preparations, from layer IV of the somatosensory cortex of squirrel monkeys. Parts of the complicated axonal plexus are out of the plane of focus or in the two adjacent sections. Bars represent 100 μm.

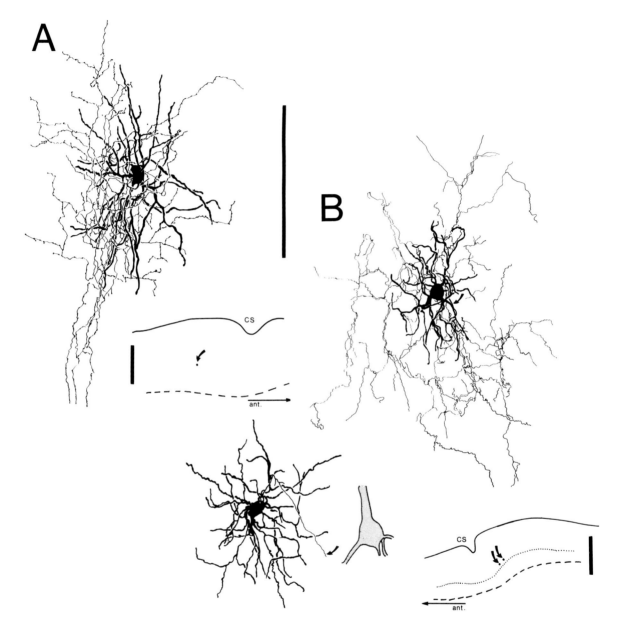

Figure 4. Camera lucida drawings of spiderweb cells from layer IV of the squirrel monkey somatosensory cortex. From material illustrated in Jones (1975). Only the parts of the axon found in one section are drawn; the axonal plexus formed by each cell usually extends through three or four 100-μm-thick sections. Lower cell in (B) has axon omitted to show dendritic field. Bars represent 100 μm and 1 mm (inset).

branches of the axon to be beaded, the diameter of each bead is not much greater than that of the axon, so the appearance is one of sinuosity rather than of a heavy boutonal investment. Such an axon is presumably unmyelinated. The axon branches suffer very little reduction in diameter so that the plexus has a homogeneous appearance. Characteristically, small "holes" appear in the plexus, representing the positions occupied by the unstained somata of other cells (Fig. 4).

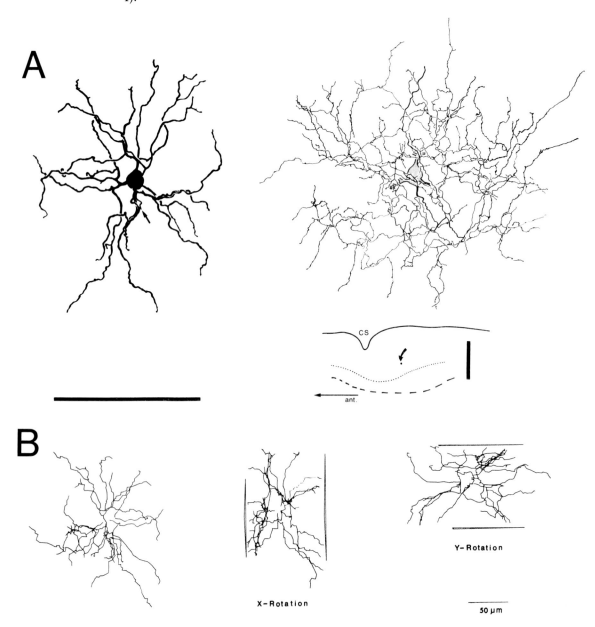

Figure 5. Camera lucida drawing (A) and computer reconstruction (B) of a spiderweb cell to show small extent and symmetry of dendritic field. In (A), dendrites and axon are drawn separately. In (B), lines represent surfaces of section. Bars represent 100 μm (A) and 50 μm (B). From Jones (1975).

Though the greater part of the axonal plexus is confined to the general vicinity of the dendritic field, in the monkey at least, it can extend for considerable distances beyond that. Figure 2 shows a spiderweb cell from the monkey somatosensory cortex with a dendritic field approximately 175 μm in diameter and an axonal field approximately 350 μm in diameter. Figures 4 and 5 show cells with even smaller dendritic fields.

To date there has been no direct identification of the spiderweb cell at the electron microscopic level. A cell from layer I of the visual cortex of an immature cat shown by LeVay (1973) to have an axon that gives rise to symmetric synapses is the only possible example. The smallest nonpyramidal cells of layer IV, from the accounts of Powell and his colleagues (Sloper *et al.,* 1979; Winfield *et al.,* 1980), have a rather low density of cytoplasmic organelles and receive relatively few axosomatic synapses, by contrast with larger nonpyramidal cells. At the electron microscopic level, layer IV contains a relatively dense plexus of fine, unmyelinated axons that are mildly beaded, contain flattened synaptic vesicles, and give off repeated en passant, symmetrical synapses (Jones and Powell, 1970). Axons of this type would be expected for the spiderweb cell, from its light microscopic appearances, but this also remains to be verified.

2.3. Are They GABAergic?

A substantial proportion (approximately 40%; Fig. 6) of the small-cell somata in layer IV of the monkey and rat cerebral cortex concentrate [^{3}H]-GABA and stain immunocytochemically for GAD (Ribak, 1979; Hendry and Jones, 1981; Hendry *et al.,* 1983; Houser *et al.,* 1983). It is rarely possible to stain the dendrites of such cells much beyond their proximal parts, though it can be confirmed that they are nonspiny. Sometimes dendrites that recurve toward the soma, like those of spiderweb cells, can be discerned but it would be premature to state that the spiderweb cells are proven GABAergic interneurons. Similarly, at the fine structural level, long segments of thin, beaded, unmyelinated GAD-positive axons can be seen making multiple en passant synapses on GAD-positive and GAD-negative neurons in layer IV (Hendry *et al.,* 1983), but as pointed out above, these axons have not been established as belonging to spiderweb cells.

3. Functions

No cells resembling spiderweb cells have been labeled by intracellular dye injections to date and it seems doubtful that many such small cells have been encountered electrophysiologically. Certainly none have been positively identified. In the absence of any physiological information and with no positively confirmed data regarding the synaptic relationships of the spiderweb cells, it is not possible to make more than extremely tentative suggestions as to their functions.

The highly branched and tightly intertwined axon of the spiderweb cell gives the cell some resemblance to the Golgi neuron of the cerebellum and to other known inhibitory interneurons elsewhere. If it can be tentatively thought

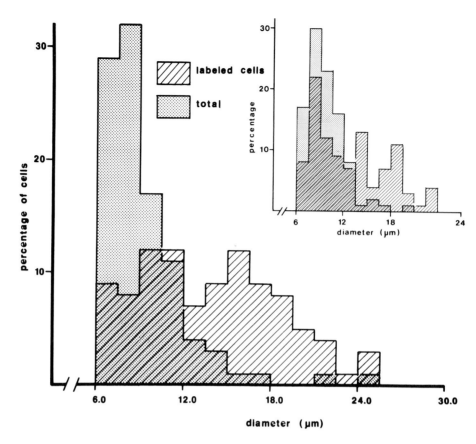

Figure 6. Histograms showing the percentages of [³H]-GABA-accumulating neurons in layer IV of area 3b relative to the total cell population of layer IV. Cells categorized according to somal diameter. Note that in small size range, at least 30% are GABA-accumulating and, therefore, probably GABAergic. Similar results are obtained with counts of immunocytochemically labeled GABA neurons. Main figure, frozen section autoradiographs; inset, plastic section autoradiographs. From Hendry and Jones (1981).

of as an inhibitory interneuron, and if all of the slight dilations on its highly branched axon are synaptic terminals, then the spiderweb cell would be in a position to exert a powerful inhibitory effect on a large number of neurons in a local area. Concentrated as it is in layer IV, where it probably receives thalamic axon terminations (Valverde, 1971), and possibly making synapses mainly on the small spiny neurons of that layer, the spiderweb cell, as an inhibitory interneuron, could play an important role in setting up surround inhibition. Supposing its action were similar to that of a Golgi cell in the cerebellum, the spiderweb cell could serve to inhibit the spiny and other layer IV cells less powerfully excited at the perimeter of a zone of focal thalamic input. In this way it could serve to maintain the focal nature of the input, much as a Golgi cell is thought to focus mossy fiber inputs to granule cells in the cerebellum. Such focusing would seem to be one essential prerequisite for setting up the columnarity of information flow through other cortical layers (Fig. 7). Such a theory (Jones, 1981) is entirely speculative and requires much additional work before it can be said to be confirmed or disproven.

4. References

Fairén, A., and Valverde, F., 1980, A specialized type of neuron in the visual cortex of cat: A Golgi and electron microscope study of chandelier cells, *J. Comp. Neurol.* **194:**761–780.

Feldman, M., and Peters, A., 1978, The forms of non-pyramidal neurons in the visual cortex of the rat, *J. Comp. Neurol.* **179:**761–794.

Hendry, S. H. C., and Jones, E. G., 1981, Sizes and distributions of intrinsic neurons incorporating tritiated GABA in monkey sensory-motor cortex, *J. Neurosci.* **1:**390–408.

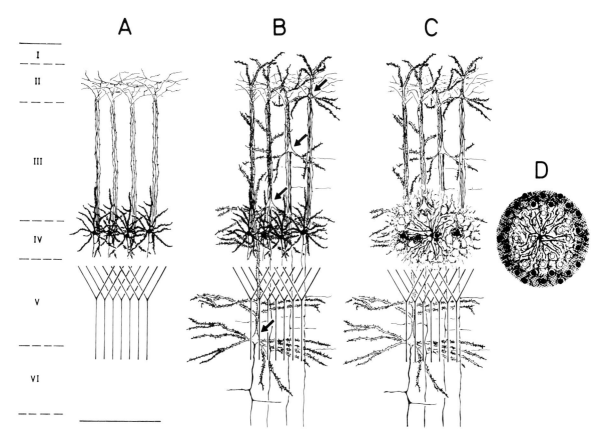

Figure 7. Schematic figure from Jones (1981) illustrating hypothetical mode of action of spiderweb cells, assuming they are inhibitory. Focal bundle of thalamocortical axons (A) terminates on a small group of spiny cells of layer IV, whose vertical axons synapse on pyramidal cells of all layers (arrows, B) converting focus into a column. Focus and column are maintained (C, D) by putatively inhibitory spiderweb cells which inhibit spiny cells less strongly excited at perimeter of thalamic input zone. Synaptic relationships shown do not exclude thalamocortical synapses on other cell types in cortex.

Hendry, S. H. C., Houser, C. R., Jones, E. G., and Vaughn, J. E., 1982, Synaptic organization of immunocytochemically identified GABAergic neurons in the monkey sensory-motor cortex, *J. Neurocytol.* **12:**639–660.

Houser, C. R., Hendry, S. H. C., Jones, E. G., and Vaughn, J. E., 1982, Morphological diversity of GABA neurons demonstrated immunocytochemically in monkey sensory-motor cortex, *J. Neurocytol.* **12:**617–638.

Jones, E. G., 1975, Varieties and distribution of non-pyramidal cells in the somatic sensory cortex of the squirrel monkey, *J. Comp. Neurol.* **160:**205–268.

Jones, E. G., 1981, Anatomy of cerebral cortex: Columnar input–output relations, in: *The Cerebral Cortex* (F. O. Schmitt, F. G. Worden, G. Adelman, and S. G. Dennis, eds.), pp. 199–235, MIT Press, Cambridge, Mass.

Jones, E. G., and Powell, T. P. S., 1970, Electron microscopy of the somatic sensory cortex of the cat. III. The fine structure of layers IV–VI, *Philos. Trans. R. Soc. London Ser. B* **257:**23–28.

Le Vay, S., 1973, Synaptic patterns in the visual cortex of the cat and monkey: Electron microscopy of Golgi preparations, *J. Comp. Neurol.* **150:**53–86.

Lorente de Nó, R., 1922, La corteza cerebral del ratón (Primera cortribucion-La corteza acústica), *Trab. Lab. Invest. Biol. Madrid* **20:**41–78.

Lorente de Nó, R., 1949, Cerebral cortex: Architecture, intracortical connections, motor projections, in: *Physiology of the Nervous System* (J. F. Fulton, ed.), 3rd ed., pp. 288–313, Oxford University Press, London.

O'Leary, J. L., 1941, Structure of the area striata of the cat, *J. Comp. Neurol.* **75:**131–164.

O'Leary, J. L., and Bishop, G. H., 1938, The optically excitable cortex of the rabbit, *J. Comp. Neurol.* **68:**423–478.

Peters, A., and Regidor, J., 1981, A reassessment of the forms of nonpyramidal neurons in area 17 of the cat visual cortex, *J. Comp. Neurol.* **203:**685–716.

Ramón y Cajal, S., 1909–1911, *Histologie du Système Nerveux de l'Homme et des Vertébrés* (translated by L. Azoulay), Vol. II, Maloine, Paris.

Ramón y Cajal, S., 1922, Studien über die Sehrinde der Katze *J. Psychol. Neurol.* **29:**161–181.

Ribak, C. E., 1978, Aspinous and sparsely-spinous stellate neurons in the visual cortex of rats contain glutamic acid decarboxylase, *J. Neurocytol.* **7:**461–478.

Sloper, J. J., Hiorns, R. W., and Powell, T. P. S., 1979, A quantitative and qualitative electron microscopic study of the neurons in the primate motor and somatic sensory cortices, *Philos. Trans. R. Soc. London Ser. B* **285:**141–171.

Tömböl, T., 1978, Some Golgi data on visual cortex of the rhesus monkey, *Acta Morphol. Acad. Sci. Hung.* **26:**115–138.

Valverde, F., 1971, Short axon neuronal subsystems in the visual cortex of the monkey, *Int. J. Neurosci.* **1:**181–197.

Valverde, F., 1978, The organization of area 18 in the monkey, *Anat. Embryol.* **154:**305–334.

Winfield, D. A., Gatter, K. C., and Powell, T. P. S., 1980, An electron microscopic study of the types and proportions of neurons in the cortex of the motor and visual areas of the cat and rat, *Brain* **103:**245–258.

13

Smooth and Sparsely Spinous Nonpyramidal Cells Forming Local Axonal Plexuses

ALAN PETERS and RICHARD L. SAINT MARIE

1. Introduction

In the cerebral cortex there exists a population of nonpyramidal cells with locally ramifying axonal plexuses which partially or completely overlap their dendritic trees. These neurons have smooth or sparsely spinous dendrites and, in addition to the local plexus, the axons of many of these neurons have branches which extend into cortical layers either above or below the one containing the cell body. In some cases, it has been shown that these branches give rise to a second plexus. So far as is known, the axons of these neurons do not leave the cerebral cortex and so these cells are variously referred to as short-axon, local-circuit, or Golgi type II neurons. Further, their axons do not form easily characterized terminal arborizations, as do the axons of chandelier cells (Chapter 10) and basket cells (Chapter 8).

   The group of neurons with smooth or sparsely spinous dendrites and locally distributed axonal collaterals lacking distinctive terminal arborizations have not yet been systematically classified, although Valverde (1976) and Fairén and Val-

ALAN PETERS and RICHARD L. SAINT MARIE • Department of Anatomy, Boston University School of Medicine, Boston, Massachusetts 02118.

419

verde (1979) have developed a classification scheme for those present in mouse visual cortex. One major difficulty in classifying these neurons across species is that only isolated examples of them have been described by the various authors who have studied Golgi preparations of different cortices. Yet another is that even those neurons which have been described may have possessed only partially impregnated axons. This is especially true in cases in which the axons of these neurons are myelinated in the mature cortex (see Peters and Proskauer, 1980b). To overcome this latter difficulty, many investigators have examined immature or even fetal brains in order to reveal the axonal morphology before myelination becomes completed. Extrapolation from incompletely developed brains, however, requires some caution, since such material often does not adequately reflect the form of the axons in the adult.

Apart from the Golgi methods, the only other useful method for revealing the axonal plexuses of cortical neurons with intracortically distributed branches is that of injecting individual neurons either with a fluorescent dye (e.g., Kelly and Van Essen, 1974) or with HRP (e.g., Gilbert and Weisel, 1979, 1981; Lin *et al.*, 1979). Dye-filling techniques have the distinct advantage of rendering the entire neuron visible (see Figs. 3 and 4) and frequently reveal a richness of axonal arborization rarely seen in Golgi-impregnated preparations. This procedure is not without its drawbacks, however, for it is time-consuming, technically difficult, and, of necessity, reveals only a few neurons per preparation. Also the procedure may preferentially select the larger and more abundant neuronal types. Undoubtedly such injection procedures will eventually contribute significantly to understanding intracortical circuitry and the form of the axonal plexuses of neurons, but to date the results of few such studies have been published. Consequently, any classification and categorization of neurons on the basis of their axonal and dendritic distribution patterns must largely proceed from the existing descriptions of Golgi-impregnated neurons. Bearing this in mind, the following is an attempt to classify the most commonly reported types of multipolar and bitufted neurons with smooth or sparsely spinous dendrites and local axonal plexuses lacking distinctive axonal terminals.

2. Neurogliaform Cells

The neurogliaform or clewed cell is one of the most frequently described local-circuit neurons in the cortex. These cells are small, multipolar neurons with short, sinuous dendrites which are smooth and, very often, beaded. The axons of these neurons have numerous, prominent varicosities and arborize profusely around the cell body, intertwined among the dendrites. Because of the profusion of axonal branches, Valverde (1971) has likened these axons to a ball of thread and, by analogy, refers to the neurons as *clewed cells*. Such cells have been encountered in all areas of cortex examined so far with the Golgi techniques and they are described in more detail in Chapters 6 and 12.

Other neurons with similar axons but with longer, radiating, smooth dendrites also exist and these have been described in layer IV of monkey extrastriate cortex by Lund *et al.* (1981), who refer to them as *type b* and *type c neurons*. Like the smaller neurogliaform cells, the axons of these larger neurons also form a

421

SMOOTH AND
SPARSELY
SPINOUS
NONPYRAMIDAL
CELLS

dense, intertwined local plexus and exhibit many prominent varicosities. Similar neurons with long dendrites and a dense axonal plexus have also been described by McMullen and Glaser (1982, their Fig. 6) in rabbit auditory cortex.

3. Neurons with Axons Forming Arcades

The next most commonly reported cell with a local axonal plexus is a medium-sized multipolar neuron with smooth radiating dendrites and an axon that arises directly from the cell body or from one of the proximal dendrites. Usually the axon ascends up to, or just beyond, the limits of the superficial dendritic tree and then breaks up into a shower of recurving collaterals. These collaterals form arcades that descend into the dendritic tree, somewhat in a manner reminiscent of the branches of a weeping willow tree. Some of the descending collaterals may pass well beyond the range of the deepest dendrites (Fig. 1, cell a; Fig. 2).

Neurons with arcade axons correspond to the class III neurons described by Valverde (1976) in mouse visual cortex, and such a cell from this same cortex is illustrated in Fairén and Valverde (1979). Neurons with similar axons have also been described in the visual cortex of the rat (Fig. 19 in Feldman and Peters, 1978; Fig. 1 in Peters and Proskauer, 1980a), rabbit (Fig. 14.1 in O'Leary and Bishop, 1938; Fig. 19.3 in Shkol'nik-Yarros, 1971), cat (Fig. 9 in O'Leary, 1941), and monkey (Fig. 29 in Lund, 1973) as well as in the rat cingulate cortex (Figs. 9c, 11b in Vogt and Peters, 1981), mouse somatosensory cortex (Fig. 1 in Woolsey *et al.,* 1975; Woolsey, 1978; Fig. 73 in Lorente de Nó, 1938), and cat suprasylvian gyrus (Fig. 2b in Norita and Kawamura, 1981). In monkey somatosensory cortex, Jones (1975) refers to such neurons as *type 2 cells.*

These neurons appear most frequently in layers II through IV of the cortex, although they have also been described in the infragranular layers (O'Leary, 1941; Feldman and Peters, 1978). Such a neuron has been depicted by Tömböl (1978) in layer V of cat striate cortex (her Fig. 1e) and it is interesting that although the neuron she illustrates has a classic arcade axon, the cell itself is a sparsely spinous bitufted cell.

In most of the Golgi-impregnated examples of these neurons, the axons have a relatively limited distribution. But one cell of this type illustrated by Fairén and Valverde (1979, their Fig. 1b) has a very profuse local plexus resembling that of the HRP-filled neuron from cat visual cortex shown here in Fig. 3. This may be the result of a better visualization of the axon, but alternatively there may exist varieties of these neurons, some with a more limited and less profuse axonal plexus than others. Continuing this discussion of the extent of the axonal plexus, it is interesting to note that although many of the axons in this group are largely confined to the vicinity of the cell body, some of the descending processes can be quite long (Fig. 2). Also, the initial portion of the axonal plexus of these neurons can closely resemble that formed by double bouquet cells. This point is made by Jones (1975), who refers to the typical double bouquet cells as *type 3 neurons.* He points out that both type 3 and type 2 neurons have arcade axons, the major difference being that the main axonal branches of the double bouquet cells become thicker as they pass away from the cell body and enter the

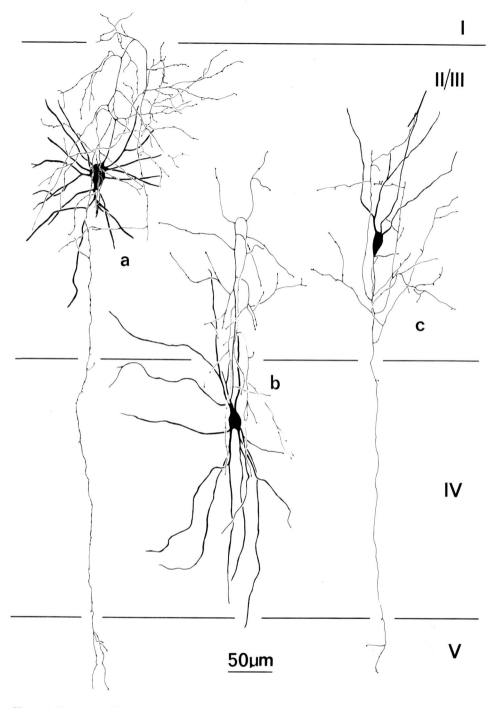

Figure 1. Camera lucida drawings of Golgi-impregnated local plexus neurons from rat visual cortex. Cell a has an axon forming arcades, and a descending axonal branch that extends in layer V. In cell b the axon ascends and then loops back toward the cell body. Cell c has a descending axon that forms a local plexus around the cell body before continuing into layer V. Redrawn from Peters and Fairén (1978).

423

**SMOOTH AND
SPARSELY
SPINOUS
NONPYRAMIDAL
CELLS**

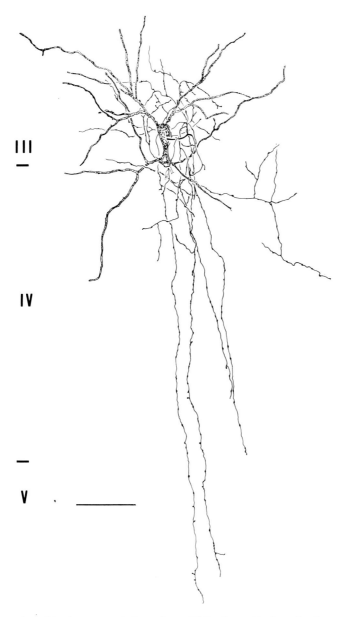

III

IV

V

Figure 2. A smooth multipolar neuron in lower layer II/III of area 18 of rat visual cortex. The axon arises from the left side of the cell body and forms a local plexus of arcades in the vicinity of the cell body. In addition a number of vertically descending branches reach layer V. Golgi–Kopsch preparation. Bar equals 50 μm.

radial bundles of axons and dendrites that characterize the double bouquet cell. Yet another neuron whose axon can appear to form arcades when viewed from certain directions is the basket cell (see Peters and Regidor, 1981, their Fig. 5).

Although most neurons with arcade axons described in the literature have axons ascending only to, or just beyond, the superficial limits of the dendritic

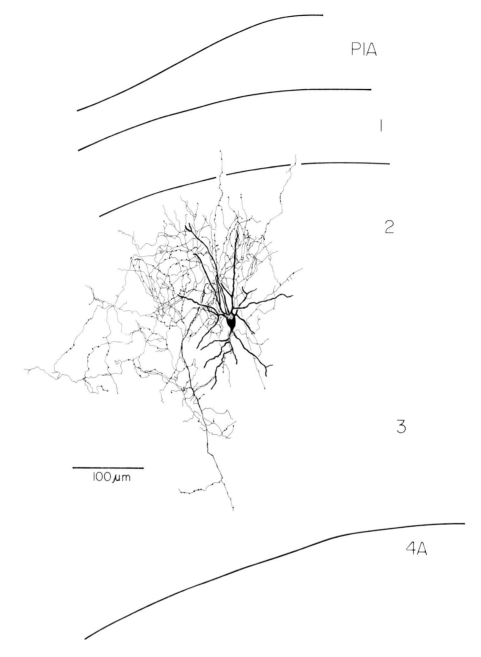

PIA

I

2

3

100 μm

4A

Figure 3. An HRP-injected neuron from layer II of area 17 of cat visual cortex. The axon of this smooth multipolar neuron arises from the upper surface of the cell body and produces a profuse local plexus overlapping the superficial dendritic tree. The main axonal stem then continues to descend below the level of the cell body. Preparation and drawing by Dr. Kevan Martin. Physiologically, this is a Y-driven neuron with a complex receptive field and is disynaptically excited by the thalamic input.

tree before curving back again, there are examples in which the axon ascends for some distance before recurving. An example of such a neuron is shown in Fig. 1, cell b. This neuron has its cell body in layer IV and its axon ascends into the middle of layer II/III before recurving. The axon of the neuron shown in Fig. 4 behaves similarly. This large, smooth multipolar neuron is from the somatic sensorimotor cortex of the rat and was injected with HRP by Dr. John Donoghue. The neuron has its cell body in layer V and the extremely long dendrites radiate out for a distance of some 250 μm. The axon emerges from the upper surface of the cell body and soon bifurcates, giving off one branch which forms a local plexus to one side of the cell body and another that ascends. This ascending branch gives off a series of horizontal collaterals in layer IV and, as it approaches layer III, curves back and descends, finally giving off collaterals in layer IV which contribute to the local plexus. Except for the distance traveled by the axon

425

SMOOTH AND
SPARSELY
SPINOUS
NONPYRAMIDAL
CELLS

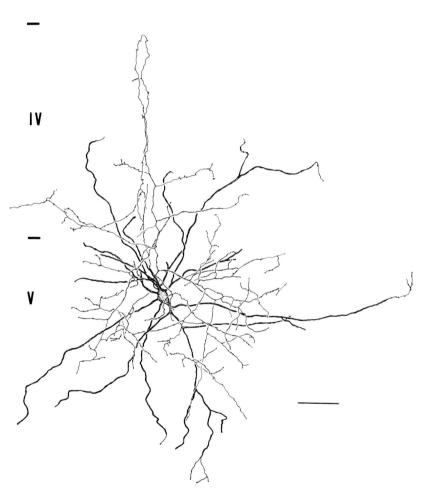

Figure 4. Drawing of an HRP-injected smooth multipolar cell with its cell body in layer V of rat somatic sensory motor cortex. The axon emerges from the upper surface of the cell body. One branch forms a plexus to the right of the cell body while another ascends giving off horizontal branches before curving back again to reach the level of the cell body and contributing to the local plexus. Preparation by Dr. John P. Donoghue. Bar equals 50 μm.

before it curves back, both of these neurons resemble those forming arcades more locally. Interestingly, a neuron with a similar axon has also been described by Lund *et al.* (1979) in layer IV of cat visual cortex (see their Fig. 6, cell B).

4. Neurons with Superficial Axonal Plexuses

Neurons of this type are equivalent to the class I neurons described by Valverde (1976) in mouse visual cortex. The axon ascends from the cell body to form a dense local plexus which has most of its bifurcations and collaterals

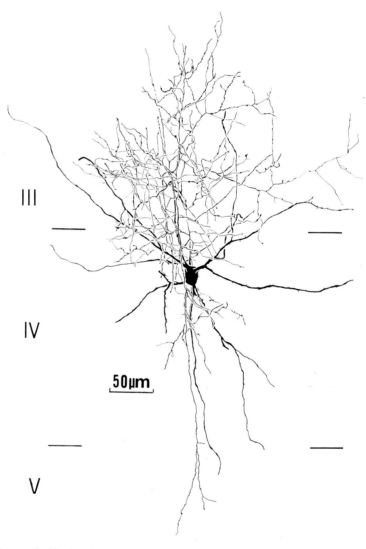

Figure 5. Camera lucida drawing of Golgi-impregnated sparsely spinous neuron from layer IV in rat visual cortex. The axon forms a profuse plexus superficial to the cell body. From Peters and Fairén (1978).

427

SMOOTH AND
SPARSELY
SPINOUS
NONPYRAMIDAL
CELLS

situated above the level of the cell body (Figs. 5 and 6). Some of the collaterals may descend beyond the longest descending dendrites, but most of the axonal plexus is contained within a cylindrical or ovoid territory which extends above and partially overlaps that of the ascending dendrites. There is, however, a wide variation in the vertical extent of the axonal plexus. Sometimes, as shown in Fig. 6, the axonal plexus is widespread laterally and does not extend far in the vertical direction. In other examples, however, as with the neuron shown in Fig. 7 from rat cingulate cortex (Vogt and Peters, 1981), the branches of the axonal plexus may extend for long distances in both their vertical and lateral extent, and so spread well beyond the limits of the dendritic tree.

Neurons with such superficially located axonal plexuses are medium to large, multipolar or bitufted neurons, having smooth or sparsely spinous dendrites. These cells have been reported in layer II through VI and, in addition to mouse visual cortex (Valverde, 1976), they have been described in rat (Figs. 5 and 6), rabbit (Fig. 14 in O'Leary and Bishop, 1938), and cat visual cortex (Fig. 5B in Lund et al., 1979). They are also found in monkey striate (Fig. 30, cell z, and Fig. 36 in Lund, 1973), and extrastriate cortex, in which Lund et al., (1981) refer to them as *type f stellate cells,* as well as in monkey somatosensory cortex, for some of the cells described by Jones (1975) as type 1 and type 2 cells have axons with this type of distribution. There is also evidence for their existence in human visual cortex (Fig. 62.9 in Shkol'nik-Yarros, 1971), and Ramón y Cajal (1911) shows examples of such neurons in both human frontal (his Fig. 337, cells C and D) and motor cortex (his Fig. 345, cell G).

5. Neurons with Long Ascending Axons

This group includes a range of neuronal types whose axons form a dense local plexus and then give rise to a branch, sometimes the main axonal stem, which ascends above the level of the cell body to form a second plexus.

A neuron of this type is shown in Fig. 8 (cell A) which is taken from the account given by Lund et al. (1979) of the neurons in the visual cortex of the cat. This particular neuron has its cell body in layer 4B. It has a local axonal arborization in layer 4B and a second one within layer 3. The local plexus produced by the collaterals of the axon are largely horizontal in their orientation and similar neurons are described by Lorente de Nó (1938) in mouse somato-sensory cortex (his Fig. 73) and by O'Leary and Bishop (1938) in rabbit visual cortex (their Fig. 13, cell 3). In each of these examples the cell bodies of the neurons are situated in layers IV through VI and the ascending axon gives off several collaterals before extending into layer II/III to form the dense terminal tuft.

A second distinct population of cortical neurons with a local dense plexus formed by an ascending axon is described by Valverde (1976) in mouse visual cortex. Valverde (1976) refers to these cells as *class II neurons.* The dendrites of these neurons are smooth or moderately spined, and Fairén and Valverde (1979) state that in some examples from mature animals the dendrites are so well endowed with spines that the neurons might almost be regarded as spiny in form. In mouse visual cortex the axons of these neurons emerge from the upper

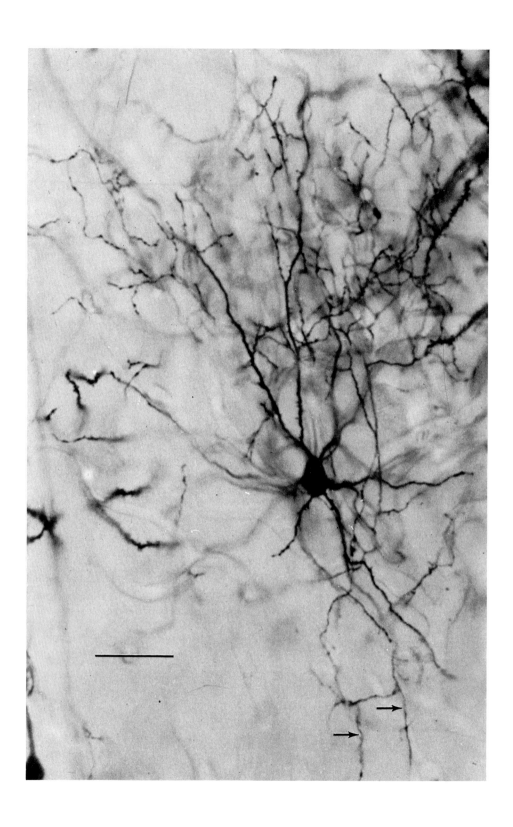

429

SMOOTH AND
SPARSELY
SPINOUS
NONPYRAMIDAL
CELLS

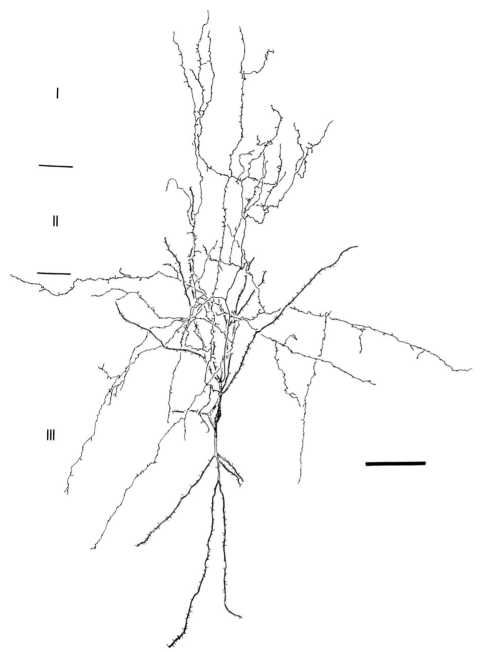

I

II

III

Figure 7. A sparsely spinous bitufted neuron from layer III of area 32 of rat cingulate cortex. The axon forms a local plexus before ascending into layer I. Drawing by Dr. B. A. Vogt. Rapid Golgi impregnation. Bar equals 50 μm.

←

Figure 6. A sparsely spinous multipolar neuron from layer II/III of area 17 of rat visual cortex. The axon emerges from the right side of the cell body. One branch ascends to form a local plexus situated above the cell body in a territory overlapping that of the superficial dendrites. Another branch of the axon gives rise to descending collaterals (arrows). Golgi–Kopsch preparation. Bar equals 50 μm.

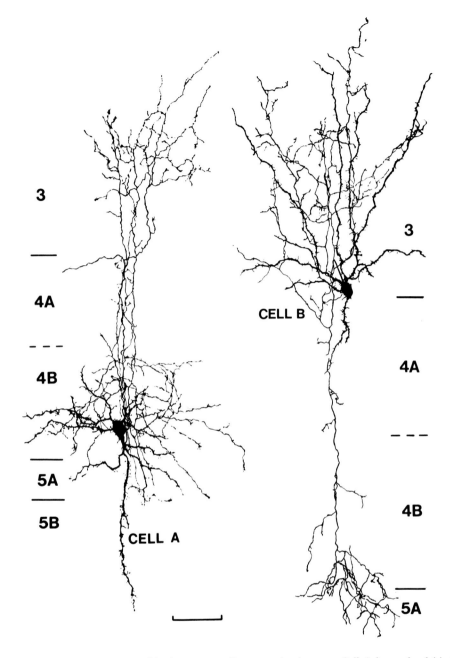

Figure 8. Two immature multipolar neurons from cat visual cortex. Cell A has a dendritic field largely confined to laminae 4B and 5A. Its axon has a double arborization, one around the dendritic field and a second in layer 3. Cell B has its dendritic field and one axonal arborization within layer 3. A second arborization is formed by a descending axon trunk in lower 4B and 5A. Kittens aged 5 weeks. Rapid Golgi impregnations. Bar equals 50 μm. From Lund *et al.* (1979).

surface of the cell body. After ascending for some distance the axon gives rise to a dense plexus of recurving axon collaterals which descend into the dendritic field to form the local plexus. The main axon then continues to ascend vertically until it reaches layer I, where it gives rise to a second series of collaterals which project horizontally through layer I. When the cell bodies of these neurons are in the deeper layers of the cortex, namely layers IV and VI, the two plexuses formed by the axon are separated and quite distinct, being connected only by the ascending axonal stem. On the other hand, when the neurons have their cell bodies in supragranular layers, the two plexuses are so close that they may overlap. Nevertheless, these neurons can be distinguished from those forming arcade or superficial axonal plexuses by the long horizontal collaterals which pass through layer I. Neurons similar to Valverde's (1976) class II neurons have been described, for example, in mouse somatosensory cortex (Fig. 73 in Lorente de Nó, 1938), rabbit visual cortex (Fig. 9 in O'Leary and Bishop, 1938), and cat visual cortex (Fig. 9 in O'Leary, 1941). Valverde (1976) makes the observation that neurons of this type with cell bodies located in layers IV through VI may correspond to a cell type described by Martinotti (1889) and later referred to by Ramón y Cajal (1911) as *Martinotti cells* (see Chapter 6).

6. Neurons with Long Descending Axons

Neurons of this group have axons which form a local plexus and, in addition, form a second plexus below the level of the cell body. These are smooth or sparsely spinous neurons and, in some respects, they are the reciprocal of those neurons with long ascending axons just described.

An example of a neuron with both a local plexus and a descending axon is shown in Fig. 8. Cell B in this illustration is in layer 3 of cat visual cortex (Lund *et al.,* 1979) and has an axon which arises from the upper surface of the cell body and soon bifurcates. One branch ascends to form a plexus which largely overlaps the territory of the superficial dendrites in its distribution. The other branch descends, giving off a few collaterals before reaching the border between layers 4B and 5A, where it forms a second plexus. As is evident, cells B and A in this same illustration are nearly reciprocals of each other.

Although cell B in Fig. 8 has a descending portion to its axon, the local plexus is similar in appearance to that produced by neurons which have only a superficial axonal plexus (see Fig. 5). Some of these latter neurons also have descending branches, although these branches have not been traced to a second plexus. Similarly, some of the examples of neurons with axons forming arcades have descending branches. For example, cell a in Fig. 1 has a descending branch which passes into layer V. In contrast, the smooth multipolar neuron from layer II of cat visual cortex shown in Fig. 10 has an axon which forms some recurving collaterals in the territory of the ascending dendrites and a branch which curves down and descends to give rise to a loose plexus of horizontal branches below the level of the descending dendrites. In this particular example, the local and deeper plexuses are hardly separated, so that there are some parallels between

431

SMOOTH AND
SPARSELY
SPINOUS
NONPYRAMIDAL
CELLS

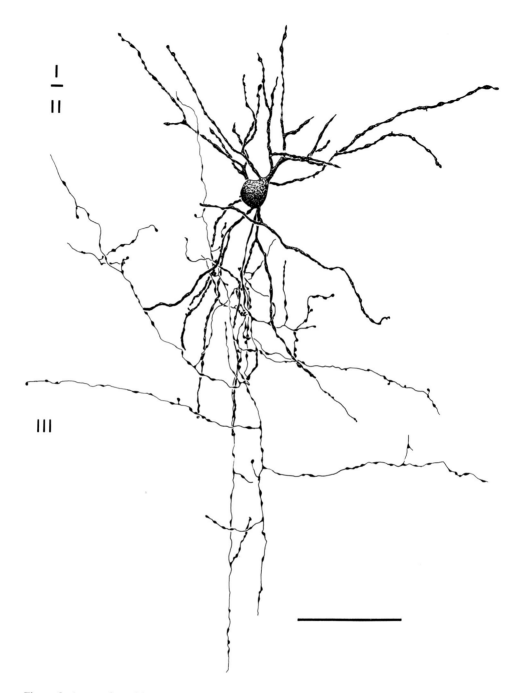

Figure 9. A smooth multipolar neuron with its cell body in layer II of monkey visual cortex. The axon extends from the lower surface of the soma and forms a local plexus with many recurrent branches just below the cell body. A descending branch of the axon forms horizontal collaterals. Rapid Golgi impregnation. Bar equals 50 μm.

433

SMOOTH AND
SPARSELY
SPINOUS
NONPYRAMIDAL
CELLS

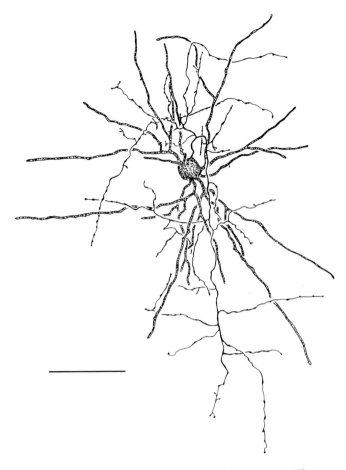

Figure 10. A smooth multipolar cell from layer II in area 17 of cat cortex. The axon emerges from the upper surface of the cell body and provides a local plexus as well as a descending branch with horizontal collaterals. Golgi–Kopsch impregnation. Bar equals 50 μm.

this arrangement and that of the plexuses formed by the class II neurons described by Valverde (1976) in the supergranular layers of mouse visual cortex (see preceding section).

Each of the neurons described above has the axon emerging from the upper surface of the cell body, but there is another group of neurons which have axons emerging from the lower surface of the cell body. Thus, cell c in Fig. 1, which is from rat visual cortex, has a descending axon which forms a local plexus of ascending branches and then continues to descend into layer V, and the neuron from monkey visual cortex shown in Fig. 9 has a similar descending axon. This latter neuron is in layer II and the local plexus is largely formed by horizontal and oblique collaterals which ramify below the level of the cell body. The main descending axon continues toward layer IV. Both of these neurons are similar to the class V neurons described by Valverde (1976) in layer II/III of mouse visual cortex, and similar neurons have been described by a number of authors. For example, O'Leary (1941, his Fig. 9.6) has described them in cat visual cortex as has Ramón y Cajal (1922, his Fig. 12), while Lund (1973, her Fig. 31, cells X and Z) shows examples in monkey visual cortex. Such neurons also appear to be present in the auditory cortex of the rabbit (Fig. 7c in McMullen and Glaser, 1982) and in the extrastriate cortex of the human (Fig. 67.1 in Shkol'nik-Yarros, 1971).

This concludes our summary of the most commonly reported smooth and sparsely spinous nonpyramidal neurons with locally distributed axons. Many other examples of such neurons abound in the literature but these could not be neatly categorized, either because too few examples are available or because their axons are insufficiently impregnated. This classification scheme is, therefore, only partial and suggestive and will, very likely, improve as new and more precise information on this important class of neurons becomes available.

7. A Consideration of the Morphology of Local Plexus Neurons

On the basis of Golgi studies, it seems that while local plexus neurons are probably the dominant form of smooth or sparsely spinous multipolar and bi-tufted cells with unmyelinated axons in the rodent cortex, in which they have rather stereotyped forms, in cats and primates such neurons become more diversified. At the same time, other nonpyramidal cells with more specialized forms of axonal plexuses make their appearance in these higher mammalian forms. Thus, the rodent cortex appears to have no well-defined counterpart of the basket cells and double bouquet cells. Yet despite the increase in variety of nonpyramidal cells, the electron microscopic analysis carried out by Winfield *et al.* (1980) suggests that the ratio between pyramidal and nonpyramidal cells is essentially similar in the cerebral cortex of the rat, cat, and monkey, as well as in the human (see Powell, 1981). Thus, Winfield *et al.* (1981) find that in the motor and visual cortices of each of these species, there are from 62 to 72% of pyramidal cells, 3 to 5% of large nonpyramidal cells, and 23 to 33% of small nonpyramidal cells.

In terms of function, the most relevant anatomical features of any neuron are its afferent and efferent connections; if such information were available about neurons, it would render most other morphological characteristics superfluous. Nevertheless, the connections of the neurons must ultimately depend on the distribution of their axons and dendrites within the cortex, since this distribution must determine the pre- and postsynaptic components with which any particular neuron can form synapses. If this fact is conceded, then the laminar position of any local plexus neuron and the distribution pattern of its axon must be of fundamental importance. Consequently, different distributions of axons and dendrites must be taken as indications that the various types of local plexus neurons have somewhat different roles in the internal circuitry of the cerebral cortex. Obviously, at present we have no idea what these differences might be, and to evaluate them will require bridging the gap between light and electron microscopy, so that correlations can be made between the morphology of the neuron and its synaptic connections. Several laboratories have embarked

435

SMOOTH AND
SPARSELY
SPINOUS
NONPYRAMIDAL
CELLS

on such studies using either Golgi–electron microscopic techniques (Section 7), or the examination of HRP-injected neurons, but the amount of data so far available about local plexus neurons allows suggestions to be made only about their general role in the internal circuitry of the cerebral cortex (Section 9).

8. Electron Microscopy

The fine structure of neurons definitively identified as smooth or sparsely spinous multipolar neurons with local axonal plexuses has been examined using combined Golgi–electron microscopic techniques. LeVay (1973) has examined such cells in monkey and cat, and Parnavelas *et al.* (1977), Peters and Fairén (1978), and Peters and Proskauer (1980a) have studied them in rat visual cortex. Of these reports, only those of Peters and Fairén (1978) and Peters and Proskauer (1980a) show the cytological details of the neurons, for they used a gold-toning procedure which partially replaces the silver chromate Golgi deposit with fine gold particles (Fairén *et al.,* 1977). In the studies by LeVay (1973) and Parnavelas *et al.* (1977), the Golgi precipitate was not removed and the cytoplasmic features of the neurons are largely masked. However, all of these studies agree that the axon terminals of the local plexus cells form symmetric synapses.

From the studies of Peters and Fairén (1978) and Peters and Proskauer (1980a), it is evident that local plexus neurons in rat visual cortex have perikarya with a cytoplasm darkened by the presence of well-developed cisternae of rough endoplasmic reticulum and many ribosomes (Fig. 11). The nuclei have rather irregular contours often in the form of deep folds. They also have prominent nucleoli and may contain intranuclear rods. The presence of nuclear rods cannot be used as a definitive means for identifying these neurons, however, for such rods have been encountered in the nuclei of a number of different types of neurons in rat cortex, including pyramidal cells. On the cell body, the axosomatic synapses are of two types, namely asymmetric and symmetric (Colonnier, 1968). Except for the spiny stellate cells of layer IV (LeVay, 1973), this feature seems to be common to all nonpyramidal cells so far examined by electron microscopy. Also, it is not uncommon for short bulbous spines to project from the cell body (see Peters, 1971; Feldman and Peters, 1978). In rat visual cortex, the dendrites of the smooth or sparsely spined multipolar cells arise rather abruptly from the cell body, so that they soon achieve a relatively uniform diameter and, as would be expected on the basis of light microscopy, the dendrites have relatively smooth contours. Like the perikarya, the dendrites also receive axon terminals forming both symmetric and asymmetric synapses although there is a tendency for symmetric synapses to be more frequent along the proximal portions of the dendrites and to become less common further away from the cell body, so that asymmetric synapses dominate the more distal portions of the dendrites.

In the electron microscope, the axons of the smooth or sparsely spinous multipolar cells are found to arise from rather small axon hillocks and to promptly assume the features of the axon initial segment, which is characterized by an undercoating of the axolemma and the presence of fascicles of microtubules in the axoplasm. Just at the site where the axon undergoes its first bifurcation, the

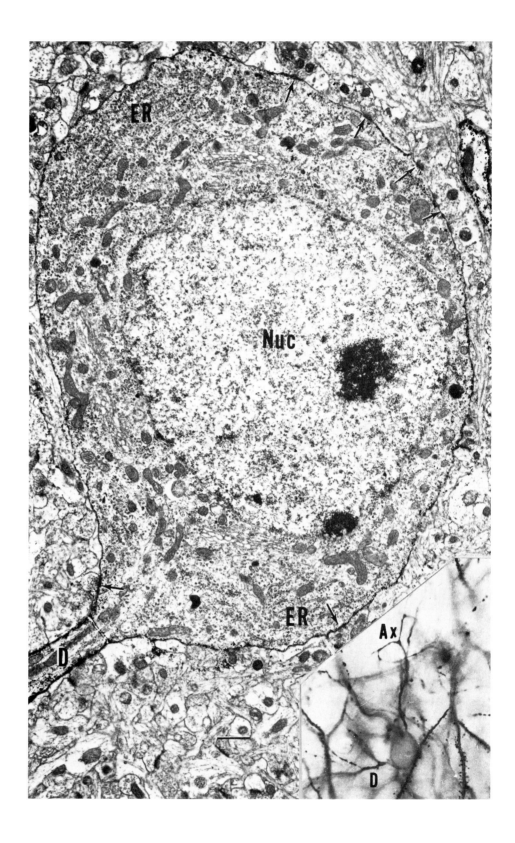

undercoating is lost and the fascicles of microtubules disappear. Consequently, the thin collateral branches of the axon contain little more than evenly spaced microtubules and vesicles in their cytoplasm. In common with other nonpyramidal cells so far examined in rat visual cortex, namely the bipolar cells (Peters and Kimerer, 1981) and chandelier cells (Peters *et al.*, 1982), the axon initial segments of the smooth or sparsely spinous multipolar cells receive few axon terminals forming axo-axonal synapses.

When the unmyelinated axons are traced, they are found to form boutons en passant and boutons terminaux, and, as mentioned above, these presynaptic boutons consistently form symmetric synapses (Figs. 11 and 12). At the synapses, the junctions have clefts about 200 Å wide and show a relatively even distribution of dense material attached to the cytoplasmic sides of the plasma membranes of both the axon terminal and the postsynaptic element. In addition, the synaptic complexes vary in length. Sometimes they occupy almost the entire interface between the synapsing membranes, whereas in other examples the complexes are short. The vesicles contained within these terminals are ellipsoidal or elongate in shape, as is characteristic of symmetric synapses in material fixed with aldehydes (see Colonnier, 1968; Peters *et al.*, 1976); although in gold-toned Golgi preparations, many of the synaptic vesicles may either be mutilated or hidden by the deposition of gold particles.

In their account of the local plexus neurons, Fairén and Valverde (1979) refer to these neurons as being "generalized," and this seems to be borne out by the observations of Peters and Fairén (1978) who show that their axon terminals synapse with a wide variety of postsynaptic elements. Thus, these intracortical neurons form symmetric synapses with the cell bodies and dendritic shafts of both pyramidal and nonpyramidal cells, as well as with axon initial segments (Figs. 12–14). Indeed, so far as the rat visual cortex is concerned, the tentative conclusion is that these neurons, along with similar neurons having myelinated axons (Peters and Proskauer, 1980b), are probably the source of most of the axonal boutons forming symmetric synapses. The exceptions are the axo-axonic synapses formed by the chandelier cells, which appear to synapse exclusively with the axon initial segments of some pyramidal cells (Somogyi, 1977; Fairén and Valverde, 1980; Peters *et al.*, 1982; also see Chapter 10).

That a smooth multipolar neuron with a local axon plexus can synapse with different portions of the surface of a single pyramidal cell has been shown by Peters and Proskauer (1980a), who examined a Golgi preparation containing both an impregnated local plexus neuron and an impregnated layer III pyramidal cell. On examination in the electron microscope it became apparent that the smooth multipolar cell formed symmetric synapses with the cell body, apical dendrite, and basal dendritic stem of the pyramidal cell. This particular smooth

437

SMOOTH AND
SPARSELY
SPINOUS
NONPYRAMIDAL
CELLS

←———————————————————————————————

Figure 11. A multipolar neuron from layer II/III of rat visual cortex. The inset at the bottom right is a light micrograph of the Golgi-impregnated and gold-toned neuron, showing the smooth dendrites and a portion of the axon (Ax) which forms arcades. The electron micrograph is taken through the middle of the soma of this neuron and extending from it is the dendrite (D) labeled in the inset. The nucleus (Nuc) has an irregular envelope and is surrounded by dark cytoplasm containing cisternae of rough endoplasmic reticulum (ER). Presynaptic axon terminals are indicated by arrows. This is the non-pyramidal neuron described in Peters and Proskauer (1980a). Bar on electron micrograph equals 1 μm.

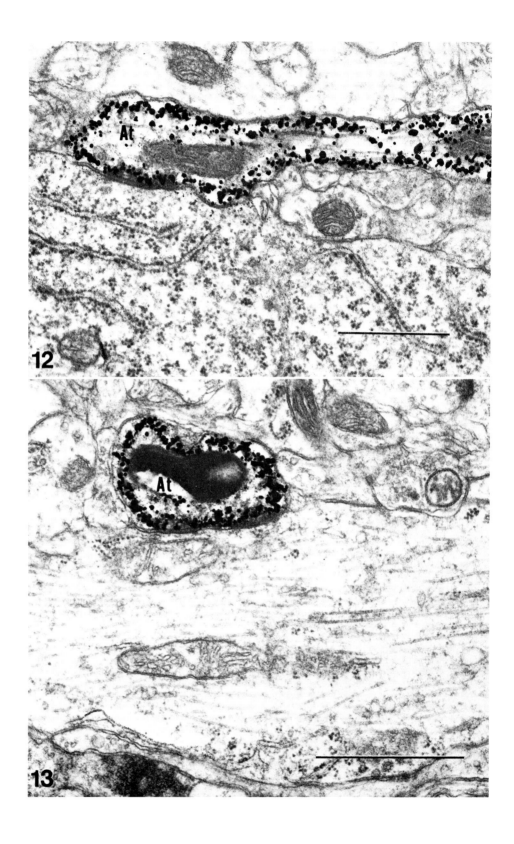

439

SMOOTH AND
SPARSELY
SPINOUS
NONPYRAMIDAL
CELLS

multipolar cell formed only a small proportion of the symmetric synapses on the pyramidal cell, however, indicating that a number of such neurons converge onto each pyramidal cell. As a point of interest, and to emphasize that this smooth multipolar cell, like others of its kind, shows no particular preference in choosing its postsynaptic partners, it should be mentioned that Fig. 12–14 show other axon terminals of this local plexus cell synapsing with the cell body (Fig. 12) and dendrite (Fig. 13) of a nonpyramidal cell, and with the axon hillock and axon initial segment of another pyramidal cell (Fig. 14). In addition, as shown by Peters and Proskauer (1980a), one of the axonal boutons of the neuron synapses with one of its own dendrites, to form an autapse.

How many synapses are formed by each local plexus neuron in rodent cortex is not known. However, by estimating the number of synapses by counting the boutonal swellings within impregnated axonal plexuses, Peters and Fairén (1978) determined that one of the neurons they examined had 75 synapses and another about 200.

Whether the local plexus neurons in cat and monkey also synapse on a variety of postsynaptic elements is not known. LeVay (1973) states that the axon terminals of these cells synapse with the shafts, and occasionally with the spines of spiny dendrites, but no further information is yet available. Nor is it known whether the terminals of local plexus cells with different types of axonal plexuses have similar or different distributions with respect to their postsynaptic targets. This needs to be determined in order to ascertain whether differences in the axonal plexuses reflect fundamental differences in the functions of various types of local plexus neurons in the cerebral cortex.

Again, it needs to be mentioned that many of the smooth or sparsely spinous multipolar neurons in rat visual cortex, and indeed in all cortices, have myeliniated axons. So far, nothing is known about the distribution patterns of these myelinated axons.

Undoubtedly, some of the neurons described in general accounts of the fine structure of nonpyramidal cells in the cortex are local plexus neurons. But in these accounts (e.g., Colonnier, 1968; Jones and Powell, 1970; Peters, 1971; Sloper, 1973; Tömböl, 1974; Braak, 1976; Winfield *et al.*, 1980), there is no direct correlation between the light microscopic appearance of the nonpyramidal cells and their fine structure. Thus, although they serve as useful general accounts demonstrating criteria by which nonpyramidal cells can be distinguished from pyramidal ones, they do not present information that can be considered specific to local plexus neurons.

9. Neurotransmitters

The fact that the axons of local plexus neurons form symmetric synapses suggests they have an inhibitory function. By examining the distribution of GAD

←———————————————————————————

Figures 12 and 13. Axon terminals of the multipolar neuron shown in Fig. 11. The terminals (At) are labeled by gold particles. In Fig. 12 an axon terminal is forming a symmetric synapse with the cell body of a nonpyramidal cell. In Fig. 13 the axon terminal is synapsing with the dendrite of a nonpyramidal cell. Bars equal 1 μm.

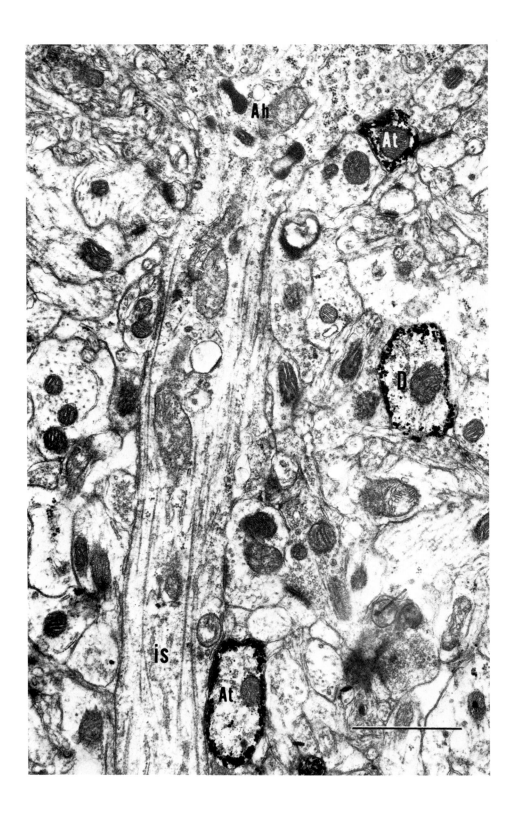

441

SMOOTH AND
SPARSELY
SPINOUS
NONPYRAMIDAL
CELLS

in rat visual cortex using an antiserum to GAD, Ribak (1978) finds that this enzyme is present in axon terminals which form symmetric synapses with the dendritic shafts and soma of both pyramidal and nonpyramidal cells, as well as with axon initial segments and some dendritic spines. This distribution of GAD-positive axon terminals essentially mirrors that of the axon terminals of the smooth and sparsely spinous multipolar neurons in this cortex (Peters and Fairén, 1978). Consequently, this finding provides strong evidence that these neurons are inhibitory, since GAD is the enzyme which synthesizes GABA, an amino acid which when topically applied suppresses the firing of cortical neurons (e.g., Krnjevic and Phillis, 1963; Krnjevic and Schwartz, 1967; Dichter, 1980). The question of the distribution of GAD in rat visual cortex will be discussed more fully in Volume 2.

Additional evidence for smooth multipolar cells in rat visual cortex being GABAergic comes form studies such as that of Somogyi *et al.,* (1981) who injected radioactive GABA into the cortex, and then examined semithin sections of Golgi-impregnated and gold-toned neurons to determine the types of neurons accumulating the [³H]-GABA. They find multipolar neurons with smooth dendrites to accumulate the isotope, and these neurons closely resemble some of the cells examined by Peters and Fairén (1978). Chronwall and Wolff (1980) also find that only nonpyramidal cells in rat visual cortex accumulate [³H]-GABA, and further demonstrate that neurons first accumulate [³H]-GABA at embryonic day 16. Until embryonic day 18, the prevelant positions for the [³H]-GABA-accumulating neurons are lamina I and below the cortical plate. As development continues, however, the [³H]-GABA-accumulating cells become spread throughout the layers of the cortex.

Which neurons accumulate [³H]-GABA in the monkey sensory motor cortex is less clear although it is evident that they are all nonpyrmidal cells. Hendry and Jones (1981) find the labeled cells to have two general forms; some are multipolar cells with large-diameter (15–20 μm) somata which probably correspond to the basket cells, and others with smaller (6–12 μm) somata, which may belong to several neuronal types. This result seems to reflect the increase in the number of different types of nonpyramidal cells in the monkey as compared with the rodent cerebral cortex and, in all likelihood, the local plexus neurons are included in the group of neurons with smaller somata.

10. The Role of Local Plexus Neurons

It seems, then, that smooth or sparsely spinous multipolar neurons with local axonal plexuses are present in the cerebral cortices of a wide range of species. They are the predominant type of nonpyramidal cell in rodent cortex,

←————————————————————————————

Figure 14. Two gold-labeled axon terminals (At) from the smooth multipolar cell shown in Fig. 11 are forming symmetric synapses, one with the axon hillock (Ah) and another with the axon initial segment (is) of a layer III pyramidal cell. Also contained in the field is a profile of a dendrite (D) of the multipolar cell. Bar equals 1 μm.

but in cat, monkey, and probably human cortex, there is a greater variety of nonpyramidal cells present. Despite this change, however, the ratio of pyramidal to nonpyramidal cells does not seem to alter greatly (Winfield *et al.,* 1980).

Even in the rodent there are classes of local plexus neurons with different forms of axonal plexuses and these classes can still be recognized in the cortices of the cat and monkey. Further, many of these neurons have been shown to have branches which form a second plexus some distance from the cell body, and in a different cortical layer. The axons of these neurons form symmetric synapses with the soma, dendritic shafts, and axon initial segments of both pyramidal and nonpyramidal cells, and since the local plexus cells appear to be GABAergic, they are probably inhibitory in function. That being so, then the local plexus neurons can be expected to form inhibitory synapses with the neuronal cell bodies and processes in their immediate vicinity, and in some cases, through ascending and descending processes, with neurons in other layers.

In both rat visual cortex (Peters *et al.,* 1979) and mouse primary somatosensory cortex (White, 1978; White and Rock, 1981; Hersch and White, 1981), thalamic afferents terminating in layers IV and lower III synapse with both smooth multipolar neurons and layer III and V pyramidal cells. Since the smooth multipolar cells synapse in turn with pyramidal cells, this could lead to thalamic excitation of the pyramidal cells followed, after a synaptic delay, by their inhibition. This is exactly the type of response recorded from cat visual cortex following stimulation of the geniculocortical afferents (see Watanabe *et al.,* 1966; Armstrong, 1968). Further, Winfield *et al.* (1981) have shown that about 60% of the axon terminals belonging to a supragranular pyramidal cell in the somatosensory cortex of the monkey formed asymmetric synapses on the shafts of smooth dendrites. If some of these smooth dendrites belong to local plexus neurons and other inhibitory cells, then as suggested by Winfield *et al.* (1981), activation of pyramidal cells themselves would lead to additional excitation of the local plexus cells. This could provide the basis for recurrent lateral inhibition (also see Powell, 1981) and for a means of sustaining the inhibition.

These are, at least, the beginnings of an interpretation of the role that local-circuit neurons might play in the cerebral cortex. However, studies of the distribution and connectivity of the axon terminals of the different classes of local-circuit neurons in rodent cortex still need to be carried out, while the connections of these neurons in the cortices of higher mammals are almost entirely unknown.

ACKNOWLEDGMENT. This work was supported by Research Grant NS07016 and Training Grant T32-NS07152 from the National Institutes of Health and Public Service.

11. References

Armstrong, C. M., 1968, The inhibitory pathway from the lateral geniculate body to the optic cortex in the cat, *Exp. Neurol.* **21**:427–439.
Braak, E., 1976, On the fine structure of the small heavily pigmented non-pyramidal cells in lamina II and upper lamina III of the human isocortex, *Cell Tissue Res.* **169**:233–245.

Chronwall, B., and Wolff, J. R., 1980, Prenatal and postnatal development of GABA-accumulating cells in the occipital neocortex of rat, *J. Comp. Neurol.* **190**:187–208.

Colonnier, M., 1968, Synaptic patterns on different cell types in the different laminae of the cat visual cortex: An electron microscope study, *Brain Res.* **9**:268–287.

Dichter, M. A., 1980, Physiological identificatiron of GABA as the inhibitory transmitter for mammalian cortical neurons in cell culture, *Brain Res.* **190**:111–121.

Fairén, A., and Valverde, F., 1979, Specific thalamo-cortical afferents and their presumptive targets in visual cortex: A Golgi study, in: *Development and Chemical Specificity of Neurons*, Vol. 51 (M. Cuneod, G. W. Kreutzberg, and F. E. Bloom, eds.), pp. 419–438, Elsevier, Amsterdam.

Fairén, A., and Valverde, F., 1980, A specialized type of neuron in the visual cortex of cat: A Golgi and electron microscope study of chandelier cells, *J. Comp. Neurol.* **194**:761–779.

Fairén, A., Peters, A., and Saldanha, J., 1977, A new procedure for examining Golgi impregnated neurons by light and electron microscopy, *J. Neurocytol.* **6**:311–337.

Feldman, M. L., and Peters, A., 1978, The forms of non-pyramidal neurons in the visual cortex of the rat, *J. Comp. Neurol.* **179**:761–794.

Gilbert, C. D., and Wiesel, T. N., 1979, Morphology and intracortical projections of functionally characterized neurones in the cat visual cortex, *Nature (London)* **280**:120–125.

Gilbert, C. D., and Wiesel, T. N., 1981, Laminar specialization and intracortical connections in cat primary visual cortex, in: *The Organization of the Cerebral Cortex* (F. O. Schmitt, F. G. Worden, G. Adelman, and S. G. Dennis, eds.), pp. 165–191, Press, Cambridge, Mass.

Hendry, S. H. C., and Jones, E. G., 1981, Sizes and distributions of intrinsic neurons incorporating tritiated GABA in monkey sensory-motor cortex, *J. Neurosci.* **1**: 390–408.

Hersch, S. M., and White, E. L., 1981, Thalamocortical synapses involving identified neurons in mouse primary somatosensory cortex: A terminal degeneration and Golgi/EM study, *J. Comp. Neurol.* **195**:253–263.

Jones, E. G., 1975, Varieties and distribution of non-pyramidal cells in the somatic sensory cortex of the squirrel monkey, *J. Comp. Neurol.* **160**:205–268.

Jones, E. G., and Powell, T. P. S., 1970, Electron microscopy of the somatic sensory cortex of the cat. 1. Cell types and synaptic organization, *Philos. Trans. R. Soc. London* **257**:1–11.

Kelly, J. P., and Van Essen, D. C., 1974, Cell structure and function in the visual cortex of the cat, *J. Physiol. (London)* **328**:515–547.

Krnjevic, K., and Phillis, J. W., 1963, Iontophoretic studies of neurons in the mammalian cerebral cortex, *J. Physiol. (London)* **165**:274–304.

Krnjevic, K., and Schwartz, S., 1967, The action of γ-aminobutyric acid on cortical neurones, *Exp. Brain Res.* **3**:320–336.

LeVay, S., 1973, Synaptic patterns in the visual cortex of the cat and monkey, *J. Comp. Neurol.* **150**:53–86,

Lin, C.-S., Friedlander, J., and Sherman, M., 1979, Morphology of physiologically identified neurons in the visual cortex of the cat, *Brain Res.* **172**:344–348.

Lorente de Nó, R., 1938, Cerebral cortex: Architecture, intracortical connections, motor projections, in: *Physiology of the Nervous System* (J. F. Fulton, ed.), 2nd ed., pp. 288–313, Oxford University Press, London.

Lund, J. S., 1973, Organization of neurons in the visual cortex, area 17, of the monkey *(Macaca mulatta)*, *J. Comp. Neurol.* **147**:455–496.

Lund, J. S., Henry, G. H., MacQueen, C. L., and Harvey, A. R., 1979, Anatomical organization of the primary visual cortex (area 17) of the cat: A comparison with area 17 of the macaque monkey, *J. Comp. Neurol.* **184**:599–618.

Lund, J. S., Hendrickson, A. E., Ogren, M. P., and Tobin, E. a., 1981, Anatomical organization of primate visual cortex area VII, *J. Comp. Neurol.* **202**:19–45.

McMullen, N. T., and Glaser, E. M., 1982, Morphology and laminar distribution of nonpyramidal neurons in the auditory cortex of the rabbit, *J. Comp. Neurol.* **208**:85–106.,

Martinotti, C., 1889, Contributo allo studio della corteccia cerebrale, ed all'origine centrale dei nervi, *Ann. Freniatria Sci. Affini* **1**:314–381.

Norita, M., and Kawamura, K., 1981, Non-pyramidal neurons in the medial bank (Clare–Bishop area) of the middle suprasylvian sulcus: A Golgi study in the cat, *J. Hirnforsch.* **22**:9–28.

O'Leary, J. L., 1941, Structure of the area striata of the cat, *J. Comp. Neurol.* **75**:131–164.

443

SMOOTH AND
SPARSELY
SPINOUS
NONPYRAMIDAL
CELLS

O'Leary, J. L., and Bishop, G. H., 1938, The optically excitable cortex of the rabbit, *J. Comp. Neurol.* **68**:423–478.

Parnavelas, J. G., Sullivan, K., Lieberman, A. R., and Webster, K. E., 1977, Neurons and their synaptic organization in the visual cortex of the rat: Electron microscopy of Golgi preparations, *Cell Tissue Res.* **183**:499–517.

Peters, A., 1971, Stellate cells of the rat parietal cortex, *J. Comp. Neurol.* **141**:345–374.

Peters, A., and Fairén, A., 1978, Smooth and sparsely spined stellate cells in the visual cortex of the rat: A study using a combined Golgi–electron microscope technique, *J. Comp. Neurol.* **181**:129–172.

Peters, A., and Kimerer, L. M., 1981, Bipolar neurons in rat visual cortex: A combined Golgi–electron microscope study, *J. Neurocytol.* **10**:921–946.

Peters, A., and Proskauer, C. C., 1980a, Synaptic relationships between a multipolar stellate cell and a pyramidal neuron in the rat visual cortex: A combined Golgi–electron microscope study, *J. Neurocytol.* **9**:163–183.

Peters, A., and Proskauer, C. C., 1980b, Smooth or sparsely spined cells with myelinated axons in rat visual cortex, *Neuroscience* **5**:2079–2092.

Peters, A. and Regidor, J., 1981, A reassessment of the forms of non-pyramidal neurons in area 17 of cat visual cortex, *J. Comp. Neurol.* **203**:685–716.

Peters, A., Palay, S. L., and Webster, deF. H., 1976, *The Fine Structure of the Nervous System: The Neurons and Supporting Cells*, Saunders, Philadelphia.

Peters, A., Proskauer, C. C., Feldman, M. L., and Kimerer, L., 1979, The projection of the lateral geniculate nucleus to area 17 of the rat cerebral cortex. V. Degenerating axon terminals synapsing with Golgi impregnated neurons, *J. Neurocytol.* **8**:331–357.

Peters, A., Proskauer, C. C., and Ribak, C. E., 1982, Chandelier cells in rat visual cortex, *J. Comp. Neurol.* **206**:397–416.

Powell, T. P. S., 1981, Certain aspects of the intrinsic organization of the cerebral cortex, in: *Brain Mechanisms and Perceptual Awareness* (O. Pompeiano and C. A. Marsan, eds.), pp. 1–19, Raven Press, New York.

Ramón y Cajal, S., 1911, *Histologie du Système Nerveux de l'Homme et des Vertébrés* (translated by L. Azoulay), Maloine, Paris.

Ramón y Cajal, S., 1922, Studien über die Sehrinde der Katze, *J. Psychol. Neurol.* **29**:161–181.

Ribak, C. E., 1978, Aspinous and sparsely-spinous stellate neurons in the visual cortex of rats contain glutamic acid decarboxylase, *J. Neurocytol.* **7**:461–478.

Shkol'nik-Yarros, E. G., 1971, *Neurons and Interneuronal Connections of the Central Visual System* (translated by B. Haigh), Plenum Press, New York.

Sloper, J. J., 1973, An electron microscopic study of the neurons of the primate motor and somatic sensory cortices, *J. Neurocytol.* . **2**:351–359.

Somogyi, P., 1977, A specific axo-axonal neuron in the visual cortex of the rat, *Brain Res.* **136**:345–350.

Somogyi, P., Freund, T. F., Halasz, N., and Kisvarday, Z. F., 1981, Selectivity of neuronal [^{3}H]-GABA accumulation in the visual cortex as revealed by Golgi staining of the labelled neurons, *Brain Res.* **225**:431–436.

Tömböl, T., 1974, An electron microscopic study of the neurons of the visual cortex, *J. Neurocytol.* **3**:525–531.

Tömböl, T., 1978, Comparative data on the Golgi architecture of interneurons of different cortical areas in cat and rabbit, in: *Architectonics of the Cerebral Cortex* (M. A. B. Brazier and H. Petsche, eds.), pp. 59–76, Raven Press, New York.

Valverde, F., 1971, Short axon neuronal subsystems in the visual cortex of the monkey, *Int. J. Neurosci.* **1**:181–187.

Valverde, F., 1976, Aspects of cortical organization related to the geometry of neurons with intra-cortical axons, *J. Neurocytol.* **5**:509–529.

Vogt, B. A., and Peters, A., 1981, Form and distribution of neurons in rat cingulate cortex: Areas 32, 24 and 29, *J. Comp. Neurol.* **195**:603–625.

Watanabe, S., Konishi, M., and Creutzfeldt, O., 1966, Postsynaptic potentials in the cat's visual cortex following electrical stimulation of afferent pathways, *Exp. Brain Res.* **1**:272–283.

White, E. L., 1978, Identified neurons in mouse SmI cortex which are postsynaptic to thalamocortical axon terminals: A combined Golgi–electron microscopic and degeneration study, *J. Comp. Neurol.* **181**:627–662.

White, E. L., and Rock, M. P., 1981, A comparison of thalamocortical and other synaptic inputs to dendrites of two non-spiny neurons in a single barrel of mouse SmI cortex, *J. Comp. Neurol.* **195:**265–277.

Winfield, D. A., Gatter, K. C., and Powell, T. P. S., 1980, An electron microscopic study of the types and proportions of neurons in the cortex of the motor and visual areas of the cat and rat, *Brain* **103:**245–258.

Winfield, D. A., Brook, R. N. L., Sloper, J. J., and Powell, T. P. S., 1981, A combined Golgi–electron microscopic study of the synapses made by the proximal axon and recurrent collaterals of a pyramidal cell in the somatic sensory cortex of the monkey, *Neuroscience* **6:**1217–1230.

Woolsey, T. A., 1978, Some anatomical bases of cortical somatotopic organization, *Brain Behav. Evol.* **15:**325–371.

Woolsey, T. A., Dierker, M. L., and Wann, D. F., 1975, Mouse SmI cortex: Qualitative and quantitative classification of Golgi-impregnated barrel neurons, *Proc. Natl. Acad. Sci. USA* **72:**2165–2169.

445

SMOOTH AND
SPARSELY
SPINOUS
NONPYRAMIDAL
CELLS

Neurons of Layer I

A Developmental Analysis

MIGUEL MARIN-PADILLA

1. Introduction

Only two types of intrinsic neurons are recognized in layer I of the mammalian cerebral cortex: a large type with long horizontal processes, unique to this layer and a variety of smaller, local-circuit, neurons which appear later in prenatal cortical ontogenesis. Although the neurons of layer I are not very abundant, they have been the subject of considerable controversy, some of which will be briefly analyzed and discussed below.

The morphology of these neurons can only be considered in the context of that of other components of layer I as well as with their overall structural organization. Their origin, development, and maturation must also be closely correlated with that of the other elements, both within and outside layer I, with which they establish synaptic connections. Furthermore, to understand the possible role of these neurons in the overall organization of the cerebral cortex it is necessary to comprehend clearly the origin and nature of the enigmatic superficial lamination of the mammalian cerebral cortex. Our present understanding of layer I has evolved from the works of classic (Ramón y Cajal, 1891, 1896, 1897, 1899, 1900, 1911; Retzius, 1891, 1893, 1894; Veratti, 1897; Ranke, 1909; Oppermann, 1929; Lorente de Nó, 1922, 1949; Tello, 1934, 1935) and recent investigators (Marin-Padilla, 1970, 1971, 1972, 1974, 1978; König et al., 1975,

MIGUEL MARIN-PADILLA • Department of Pathology, Dartmouth Medical School, Hanover, New Hampshire 03756.

1977; Raedler and Sievers, 1976; Raedler and Raedler, 1978; Raedler *et al.*, 1980; Rickmann *et al.*, 1977; Sousa-Pinto *et al.*, 1975; Tömböl, 1978; Shoukimas and Hinds, 1978; Takashima *et al.*, 1980; König and Marty, 1981; Lorroche, 1981; Larroche *et al.*, 1981; Larroche and Houcine, 1982; Marin-Padilla and Marin-Padilla, 1982; Rakic, 1982; Molliver, 1982; Morrison *et al.*, 1978).

Layer I (the marginal zone, the molecular layer, the plexiform lamina of Ramón y Cajal, the external or most superficial lamina of the cerebral cortex) has a simple plexiform organization characterized by an abundance of fibers and scarcity of neurons; a fact which has always puzzled investigators (Jones and Powell, 1970; Szentágothai, 1970, 1971, 1978). Layer I is composed of six essential elements: two types of neurons—Cajal–Retzius (CR) cells and the smaller neurons; three types of fibers—the specific afferents, the axonal terminals of Martinotti neurons, and terminals from afferent systems of lower cortical strata; and an extensive receptive surface formed by the apical dendritic bouquets of all pyramidal neurons of the cerebral cortex which represents the principal functional outlet of this lamina. These six basic elements and their structural organization within layer I are essentially similar in all mammalian species studied, including man, and in all regions of the cerebral cortex that have been analyzed.

Layer I has a very primitive cortical organization. As early as 1899, Ramón y Cajal pointed out this fact stating "The plexiform or molecular layer is one of the oldest cerebral formations in the phylogenetic series. It presents characteristics which are similar to those of the human cortex in all vertebrates, except the fishes." The phylogenetic antiquity of this superficial lamination has been corroborated in recent studies (Sas and Sanides, 1970; Marin-Padilla, 1971, 1978; Kirsche, 1974). Ontogenetically, layer I is also an old cortical structure. It is established very early in cortical neurogenesis and seems to remain essentially unchanged during the course of development (Marin-Padilla, 1971; Marin-Padilla and Marin-Padilla, 1982).

The simple structural organization of layer I and the fact that it has remained essentially unchanged in the course of both phylogenetic and ontogenetic evolution contrast paradoxically with some of the ideas and confusion expressed about it in the literature (Brun, 1965; Baron, 1976; Marin-Padilla and Marin-Padilla, 1982). A possible explanation for some of the controversy surrounding layer I might be the fact that it has always been considered to become incorporated in the mammalian neocortex late in neurogenesis. This generally held idea has recently been challenged by a new concept, which considers layer I to be different from and a much older entity in the mammalian neocortex than those layers which are derived from the cortical plate, namely layers VI, V, IV, III, and II, respectively (Marin-Padilla, 1971, 1978).

The first hypothesis concerning the origin of layer I was originally suggested by His (1904). He proposed that the earliest neurons accumulate between the intermediate zone and the neuronal-free marginal zone (layer I) of the telencephalic vesicle, establishing the cortical or pyramidal cell plate. According to this hypothesis, the appearance of the cortical plate marks the beginning of cortical development. Consequently, the marginal zone (layer I) would be deprived of neurons during its early developmental stages. This hypothesis promulgated by the Boulder Committee (1970) is still supported today (Rakic, 1972, 1974, 1975, 1982). It has been corroborated by autoradiographic studies (Sidman and Rakic, 1973; Smart and Smart, 1982; Smart and McSherry, 1982) including the original one of Angevine and Sidman (1961). However, the late arrival of neurons in the marginal zone (layer I) described in some of these studies (Smart and Smart, 1982) could represent the smaller neurons of this lamina which are known to arrive much later than the CR neurons (König and Marty, 1981). Perhaps, these studies were not extended early enough in cortical development to detect a population of neurons destined to populate the marginal zone prior to the appearance of the cortical plate.

The second hypothesis, proposed by Marin-Padilla (1971), pointed out that the early arrival of corticipetal fibers to the developing telencephalic vesicle establishes within it a superficial or external layer of white matter, composed of fibers and neurons which coincide anatomically with the so-called marginal zone. This primitive cortical organization was named the *primordial plexiform layer,* and the appearance and formation of this layer, which precede those of the cortical plate, mark the actual beginning of cortical neurogenesis. If this is so, then the marginal zone would not be deprived of neurons early in development. This hypothesis has also been corroborated by autoradiographic studies, which were carried out much earlier in cortical neurogenesis (König et al., 1977; Raedler and Raedler, 1978; Raedler et al., 1980; König and Marty, 1981). This hypothesis has also been corroborated by light (Marin-Padilla, 1978; Raedler and Raedler, 1978; Rickmann et al., 1977) and electron microscopic studies (König et al., 1975; Raedler and Raedler, 1978). Recently, it has been confirmed for the human cerebral cortex by both Golgi (Marin-Padilla and Marin-Padilla, 1982) and electron microscopic studies (Larroche, 1981; Larroche and Houcine, 1982).

The above brief outline discussing various aspects of layer I of the mammalian cerebral cortex should facilitate the morphologic analysis of its various components, of their interrelationships and overall organization.

2. Composition of Layer I

The structure of layer I of the mammalian cerebral cortex, including that of man, is simple, plexiform, and apparently quite stable in evolution. Its components can be separated into primary and secondary ones. The first group includes: the CR neurons, the specific afferent (primitive monoaminergic elements) fibers, the axonal terminals of the Martinotti neurons, and the apical dendritic bouquets of all pyramidal neurons of lower cortical strata. Together they constitute the basic structural and functional organization of this lamina. All of them are recognized throughout the entire course of cortical ontogenesis. Their distribution is universal throughout the entire surface of the brain, and their function is also considered to be generalized throughout the entire cerebral cortex. The secondary components of layer I include: the small neurons and terminal axons from the various afferent systems of lower cortical strata. Both are incorporated into layer I late in prenatal cortical ontogenesis. Their distribution is limited and therefore their functional role is also considered to be limited rather than generalized. The various components of layer I will be analyzed separately, i.e., neurons, axons, and dendrites entering from other layers.

2.1. Neurons of Layer I

There are two basic types of neurons in layer I: large neurons with long horizontal processes (horizontal neurons of Ramón y Cajal), and smaller neurons with short processes. Both types were originally described by Ramón y Cajal (1890, 1891, 1899, 1911) and considered to be specific to this layer. The presence of large neurons was soon confirmed in the human cerebral cortex by Retzius (1891, 1893, 1894) and that of small neurons in the mouse cerebral cortex by Lorente de Nó (1922). Subsequently, large and small neurons have been described in layer I in a variety of mammals including man (Veratti, 1897; Ranke, 1909; Oppermann, 1929; Novack and Purpura, 1961; Poliakov, 1961; Marty, 1962; Fox and Inman, 1966; Marin-Padilla, 1970, 1971, 1972, 1974, 1978; Sas and Sanides, 1970; Shkol'nik-Yarros, 1971; Sousa-Pinto *et al.,* 1975; Shoukimas and Hinds, 1978; Tömböl, 1978; Wolff, 1978; Takashima *et al.,* 1980; Braak, 1980; Larroche, 1981; Larroche and Houcine, 1982; Marin-Padilla and Marin-Padilla. 1982).

The CR Neurons

Despite other interpretations (Molliver and Van der Loos, 1970; König, 1978), the large horizontal neurons of layer I are usually still recognized today as the Cajal–Retzius neurons. One of the best reasons for selecting this name is the fact that Retzius, a co-discoverer, acknowledged in 1893 the discovery of these same neurons by Ramón y Cajal and proposed that they should be called *Die Cajalszellen.* These neurons are primary neuronal elements of layer I and are unique to this superficial lamina. Because of misconceptions concerning some of their structural and anatomical peculiarities, these neurons have been the subject of much controversy. Their variable morphologic appearance, the fact that they are more common in younger than in adult brains, and the fact that they may be absent from some cortical regions have been perhaps the major sources of controversy. The significant structural modifications undergone by these neurons in the course of prenatal cortical development have also contributed to the controversy, as their variations have often been interpreted as other neuronal types. Furthermore, staining problems have made the study of these neurons very difficult, often impossible, and have resulted in many incomplete descriptions of them. The silver precipitates which cover the surface of the cerebral cortex, in silver methods, often obscure the morphology of these neurons, giving rise to misconceptions about their structure and possible function.

The variable morphologic appearance of these CR neurons was recognized by Ramón y Cajal (1891, 1899, 1911), but he never suggested that these variations represented different neuronal types. In the human cerebral cortex, he described at least three different varieties of neurons: the marginal or pyriform, the horizontal or bipolar, and the triangular or irregular neuron (Fig. 1). These three distinct morphologic varieties which are characteristic of the human cortex have seldom been described in the cerebral cortex of experimental mammals, but the presence of these three varieties of neurons has been corroborated in a recent study of the human cerebral cortex (Marin-Padilla and Marin-Padilla, 1982). The variations are considered to represent adaptations of the CR cells to their particular location within layer I. Neurons located under the pial surface (marginal cells) tend to assume a pyriform appearance; those located in the middle of the lamina, entrapped among the numerous fibers, tend to assume a bipolar or horizontal appearance; and those located lower within layer I tend to assume a more irregular appearance (Figs. 2, 3).

It should be clearly understood that these morphologic variations affect or involve only the shape of the neuronal body and the origin of its main dendrites; and that all CR neurons are characterized by a distinct descending process which is transformed into a long horizontal axonal fiber at the lower half of layer I (Figs. 1–5). Therefore, a morphologic variation which only involves the shape of the neuronal body and the origin of its dendrites, but not its axonal process, is insufficient reason for considering the existence of different neuronal types among the CR neurons of the human cerebral cortex.

In the human brain, the most commonly described CR neuron is the marginal or pyriform neuron (Figs. 1–5) followed by the horizontal or bipolar one. However, the horizontal or bipolar neuron is the most commonly described type of CR neuron in experimental mammals. The more uncommon type of CR neuron is the irregular one located at the lower region of layer I. The scarcity and unusual lower position of these neurons within layer I suggests an abnormal displacement (Fig. 3).

The fact that the CR neurons are more common in the younger than in the adult brain has been the source of controversy and of lack of interest about them. Thus, there are studies in which they are either ignored or only mentioned briefly, while in others their existence is even questioned (His, 1904; Godina, 1951; Nañagas, 1923; Rabinowicz, 1964; Sholl, 1956; Colonnier, 1968; Armstrong-James and Johnson, 1970; Boulder Committee, 1970; Jones and Powell,

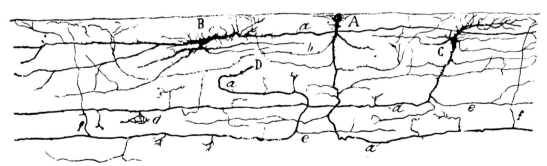

Figure 1. Ramón y Cajal's original drawing of the horizontal neurons of layer I of the human cerebral cortex. He described this figure as follows (translated from Spanish by the author): "Some horizontal neurons of the first lamina of the motor cerebral cortex (anterior central gyrus) from a month-old child. A, marginal or pyriform cell; B, bipolar cell; C, triangular cell; D, axon from a nonimpregnated neuron; e, initial thick collateral; d, terminal short and varicose branches; b, tangential long dendrites; c, short dendrites; a, axonic processes." From Ramón y Cajal's *Textura del Systema Nervioso del Hombre y de los Vertebrados*, Moya, Madrid (1904).

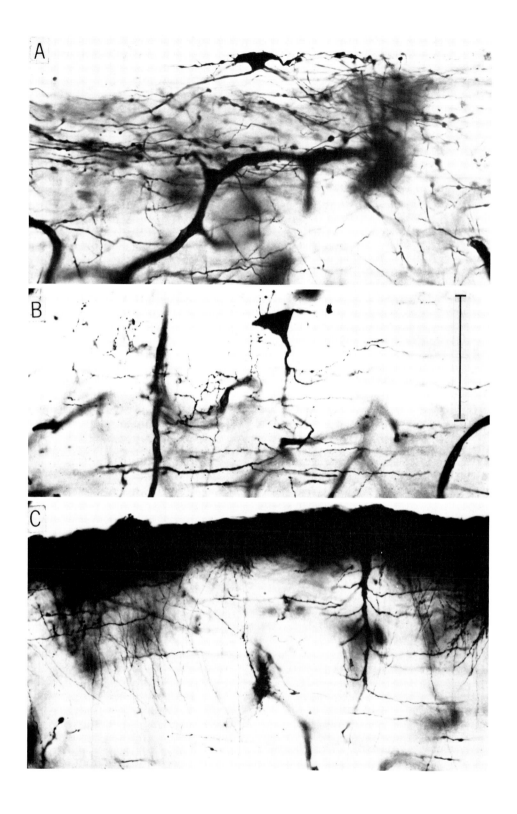

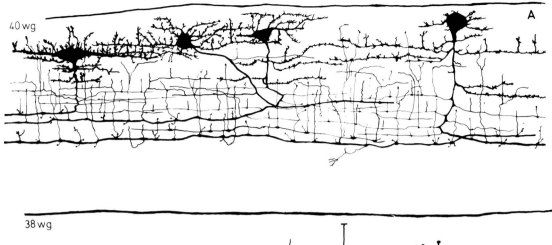

40 wg

A

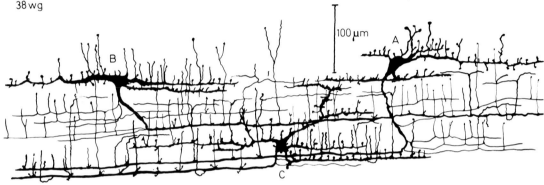

38 wg

100 μm

B

A

C

Figure 3. Composite figure of camera lucida drawings obtained from rapid Golgi preparations of the motor cortex of newborn infants (40 and 38 weeks of gestation, respectively) illustrating the overall structure of CR neurons, the variable shape of their bodies and main dendrites, and their variable location within layer I. The numerous long and short ascending processes (dendritic and axonal) which characterize these neurons and which are considered to be the essential components of the neuropil of this layer are also illustrated. Reproduced with permission from *Anat. Embryol.* **164:**161–206 (1982).

1970; Lund and Lund, 1970; Adinolfi, 1972; Rakic, 1982). Some investigators have suggested that although these neurons are common in embryonic brains, they progressively disappear in the adult, in which it is difficult to locate them (Conel, 1941, 1947, 1951; Purpura *et al.*, 1960; Åström, 1967; Duckett and Pearse, 1968; Bradford *et al.*, 1978). On the other hand, this phenomenon has recently been interpreted as resulting from the "dilution" that these neurons undergo in the course of brain growth (Marin-Padilla, 1971, 1972, 1978; Raedler

←

Figure 2. Rapid Golgi preparations of the motor cortex of a 2-month-old infant (A) and of two newborn infants (B, C) illlustrating the different morphologic appearances of CR neurons of layer I, which only involve the shape of the neuronal body and the origin of the main dendrites. All CR neurons are characterized by a single descending process which is transformed into a long horizontal axon at the lower half of the lamina. Camera lucida reproductions of the two neurons illustrated in (B) and (C) are shown in Fig. 3A. Scale: 100 μm. Reproduced with permission from *Anat. Embryol.* **164:**161–206 (1982).

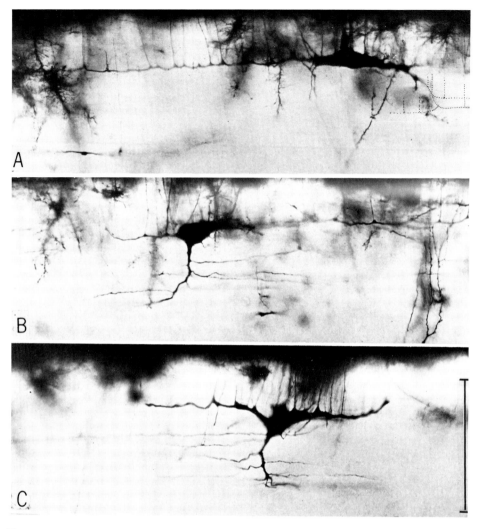

Figure 4. Rapid Golgi preparations of the motor cortex of a prematurely born infant (30 weeks of gestation) illustrating the variable morphology involving the body and main dendrites (A, horizontal; B, pyriform; C, triangular cells) of CR neurons. All of these neurons are characterized by a prominent descending process which is transformed into the horizontal axonal fiber of the neuron. Scale: 100 μm. Reproduced with permission from *Anat. Embryol.* **164**:161–206 (1982).

and Sievers, 1976; Raedler and Raedler, 1978; Rickmann *et al.*, 1977; Marin-Padilla and Marin-Padilla, 1982). Since the number of CR neurons is established very early in cortical development and remains unchanged, they must undergo a progressive dilution as the cerebral cortex grows.

Furthermore, CR neurons may be found only within strategic and possibly old regions of the cerebral cortex (Marin-Padilla and Marin-Padilla, 1982). They have been most often described in primary areas of the cerebral cortex, such as the motor (Ramón y Cajal, 1899; Retzius, 1893; Marin-Padilla, 1970; Marin-Padilla and Marin-Padilla, 1982), the visual (Ramón y Cajal, 1899; Purpura,

1975; Takashima *et al.*, 1980), and the acoustic regions (Ramón y Cajal, 1900). They may be absent from more recently evolved cortical regions such as the associative areas, and this could explain the apparent absence of CR neurons from large areas of the human cerebral cortex (Braak, 1980). But it should be clearly understood that while the body and main dendrites of CR neurons may be absent from some cortical regions, no area is deprived of their long horizontal (tangential) axons which extend over the entire surface of the cerebral cortex (Marin-Padilla and Marin-Padilla, 1982).

There have been other curious opinions expressed about the CR neurons for which there are not adequate or supportive data. The following opinions belong in this category: that they represent a special type of glia (von Koelliker, 1896), that they represent precursors of the giant pyramidal neurons (Duckett and Pearse, 1968), that they may be anaxonic (Gallego, 1972; Baron and Gallego, 1971; Baron, 1976), that they undergo progressive degenerative change and eventually disappear (Purpura *et al.*, 1960, 1964; Åström, 1967; Bradford *et al.*, 1978), and that they may not participate in neuroelectric activity (Novack and Purpura, 1961). All of these opinions only reflect the incompleteness of our knowledge about these neurons.

There have been few good descriptions of the structure of the CR superficial neurons from either man or experimental mammals. The most complete and accurate descriptions of CR neurons are those derived from Golgi studies of the cerebral cortex, and the classic descriptions of these neurons made by Ramón y Cajal and Retzius are undoubtedly the best ones available; they are as valid today as they were at the end of the last century (Fig. 1). Ramón y Cajal was the first to point out that one of the horizontal processes of these neurons represented its axon which could be followed for a long distance within layer I. He also pointed out that this axon acquired a myelin sheath very early in development and that it corresponded with the so-called tangential fibers of Retzius

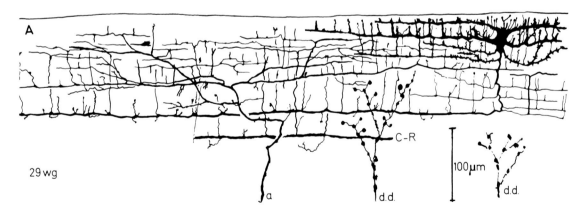

Figure 5. Composite figure of camera lucida drawings obtained from rapid Golgi preparations of the motor cortex of a premature infant (29 weeks of gestation) illustrating the location, structure, and distribution of a single CR neuron and of a single specific afferent fiber (a). While the horizontal axons of CR neurons occupy the lower half of layer I, the terminal branches of the specific afferent fibers tend to occupy its upper half. These two elements are found throughout the entire cerebral cortex even in areas deprived of neuronal bodies. Reproduced with permission from *Anat. Embryol.* **164**:161–206 (1982).

in layer I. He and Retzius also described developmental modifications in the structure of these neurons. Ramón y Cajal described a fetal and an adult type, while Retzius described in young human fetuses a candelabrum-like appearance for some of these neurons. All of these features as well as the developmental modifications of these neurons have recently been confirmed and corroborated in a Golgi study of the prenatal development of the CR neurons of the human cortex (Marin-Padilla and Marin-Padilla, 1982).

During prenatal cortical neurogenesis, the CR neurons assume at least three different morphological appearances which could be referred to as their neonatal, fetal, and embryonic morphologies, respectively. These structural variations involve only the shape of the neuronal body and its main dendrites since their horizontal axonal process remains essentially unchanged during cortical development.

The neonatal morphology of the CR neurons (29 to 40 weeks of gestation) is well known because it has been most often described. The neurons are characterized by a large and prominent body which could assume a variety of shapes depending on their location within layer I (Figs. 1–5). The bodies of these neurons can be pyriform or triangular, horizontal or bipolar, or irregular. Several main dendrites, which also contribute to the particular shape of the neuron, originate from the cell body. These dendrites are thick and irregular and are horizontally oriented. They are long and tortuous and are covered by numerous ascending branchlets and irregular short, spinelike processes (Figs. 1–5). The dendrites are oriented in an anteroposterior direction and often they can be visualized in their entirety in sagittal sections (Fig. 4). The morphology of some of these neurons in premature infants (29–30 weeks of gestation) resembles that of the so-called fetal type of Ramón y Cajal (Figs. 3, 4). It is possible that in addition to the large horizontally oriented dendrites, these neurons may also have other, and shorter dendrites oriented more randomly since some dendrites appear to be cut in the preparations (Figs. 2, 3). The dendrites of these neurons do not have the typical dendritic spines which characterize some other cortical neurons.

The most distinctive feature of the dendrites of CR neurons is their numerous short and long ascending branchlets. They are quite prominent in neurons of premature infants (Fig. 4) in which they appear to be most numerous. Ramón y Cajal believed that many of these ascending dendritic branchlets disappear progressively as the neurons assume their adult morphology, but the apparent reduction of the ascending branchlets observed during the maturation of CR neurons has recently been interpreted differently. Marin-Padilla and Marin-Padilla (1982) suggest that CR neurons undergo a progressive horizontal lengthening (horizontalization) of all of their processes during the course of cortical development, so that the distance between these ascending dendritic branchlets (as well as that of the ascending axonal terminals) increases progressively as development continues. Thus, in a given territory, the number of these ascending branchlets will seem to decrease progressively during cortical development, which could be misinterpreted as progressive disappearance of some of them.

All CR neurons, regardless of their shape or location, are characterized by a single descending process which becomes transformed into a thick and long horizontal axonal fiber within the lower half of layer I (Figs. 1–5). The horizontal (tangential) axons of CR neurons can be followed for a long distance as they extend over the surface of the cerebral cortex. They are recognized in all regions of the cerebral cortex, even in those lacking recognizable CR cell bodies. The horizontal axon of CR neurons acquires a myelin sheath before birth and together they form the prominent system of tangential fibers which is so characteristic of layer I of the mammalian cerebral cortex. The descending process of the CR neurons, as it extends from the neuronal body, gives off several thin and horizontal dendritic collaterals originally described by Ramón y Cajal (Fig. 1). Below, it gives off several thin and long horizontal axonal collaterals before it is transformed into the main horizontal axonal fiber (Figs. 1–5).

The main horizontal axonal process of the CR neuron, as well as the thin horizontal axonal collaterals, invariably give off numerous short and long ascending and fewer descending terminal fibrils throughout their entire length (Figs. 1, 3, 5). The numerous ascending terminals of the axons of CR neurons impart to layer I one of its most distinctive morphologic features (Figs. 1, 3, 5). They are recognized throughout the entire extent of the cerebral cortex as they come off the tangential fibers, and they are one of the most important components of the neuropil of this layer. They are believed to establish synaptic connections with the apical dendritic bouquets of all pyramidal neurons of the cerebral cortex regardless of location, size, or functional role of these neurons (see Fig. 13).

The fetal morphology of the CR neurons of the human cerebral cortex (15 to 28 weeks of gestation) is also quite characteristic (Figs. 6, 7). These neurons are smaller and more compact in appearance than those of the neonatal cortex. They have shorter dendrites with numerous ascending branchlets which are very close to one another and some of them resemble the "candelabrum-like" neurons described by Retzius (1891) in younger human fetuses. The cell bodies of these neurons are small and can assume various shapes (Figs. 6, 7). Their most distinctive feature is the numerous ascending branchlets which can originate from the neuronal body, the short dendrites, and the descending process and all bend upwards toward the pial surface (Figs. 6, 7). The branchlets are very close to each other and give the neurons a primitive and unexpanded appearance, but the compact and unexpanded appearance simply reflects a more primitive stage of the development than the ones in the neonatal animal. During the course of the subsequent cortical development, these CR neurons will expand progressively by elongating all of their processes horizontally.

All CR neurons analyzed during this developmental period are also characterized by a single descending process which is transformed into a main horizontal axonal fiber in the lower portion of layer I (Figs. 6, 7). The horizontal axonal processes of these neurons can be recognized through the entire extent of the cerebral cortex, and they give off many ascending terminal fibrils throughout their entire length (Fig. 7).

The embryonic morphology of the CR neurons of the human cerebral cortex (7 to 14 weeks of gestation) is less well understood because only a few examples of them have been described in the literature (Marin-Padilla and Marin-Padilla,

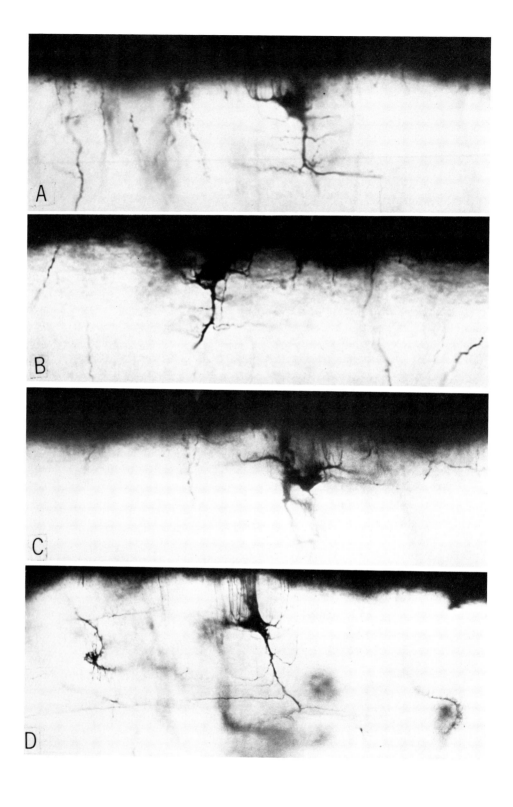

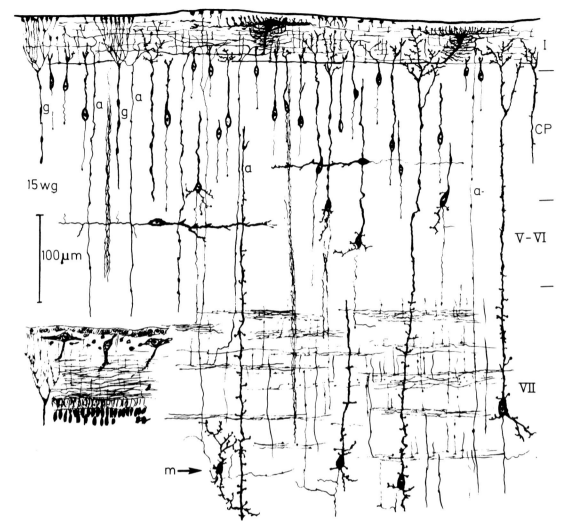

Figure 7. Composite figure of camera lucida drawings obtained from rapid Golgi preparations of the motor cortex of a premature infant (15 weeks of gestation) illustrating its overall structural organization. All pyramidal neurons of the cortical plate have apical dendritic bouquets within layer I. The CR neurons, at this developmental age, have a rather compact and unexpanded appearance with their ascending processes still quite close to one another, reflecting their primitive and unexpanded developmental stage. The deep pyramidal neurons of layer VII also have apical dendritic bouquets within layer I. At this age they appear partially embedded into the growing white matter. The CR cells seem to be quite numerous at this age (insert) because they are closer to one another in this expanding cerebral cortex. Reproduced permission from *Anat. Embryol.* **164:**161–206 (1982).

Figure 6. Rapid Golgi preparations of the motor cortex of a premature infant (22 weeks of gestation) illustrating the variable morphologic appearance of CR neurons including (A, B) pyriform, (C) horizontal, and (D) the candelabrum-like appearance described originally by Retzius. All of them are characterized by a single descending process, which is clearly illustrated in all neurons depicted. Reproduced by permission from *Anat. Embryol.* **164:**161–206 (1982).

1982; Larroche and Houcine, 1982). They are essentially bipolar or horizontal neurons with few ascending branchlets (Fig. 8). One of the horizontal processes of the neuron is its axon. The youngest human CR neuron described belongs to an 11-week-old embryo, and the morphology of these neurons prior to this time remains unknown.

The changing morphology of the CR neurons can be better understood if it is correlated with the development of layer I as a whole. In the course of prenatal cortical development, this superficial layer increases in size both vertically and horizontally. Layer I increases in thickness from less than 25 μm at the 11 weeks of gestation to more than 250 μm by the time of birth. This extraordinary vertical increase in size is accomplished without any change in its basic plexiform organization. The number of horizontal fibers simply increases progressively and they tend to be separated into an upper and a lower plexus. The number and particularly the vertical growth of the apical dendritic bouquets also increases progressively in the course of development, and consequently the embryonic bipolar CR neuron will be forced to grow vertically. This vertical growth could explain the prominent descending axonal process of the CR neurons of the human cerebral cortex. The extraordinary development of the descending axonal process of the human CR neurons has not been described in other mammalian species which have a thinner layer I. This vertical progressive

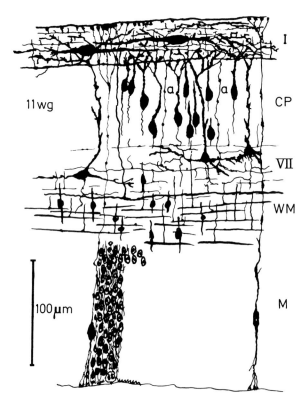

Figure 8. Composite figure of camera lucida drawings obtained from rapid Golgi preparations of the cerebral cortex of a premature infant (11 weeks of gestation) illustrating its overall structural organization. At this age, the CR neurons are horizontal cells with long processes one of which is the axon; all pyramidal neurons of the developing cortical plate have apical dendritic bouquets within layer I, as do the deep pyramidal neurons of layer VII. Also illustrated are the white matter (WM) and the matrix (M). Reproduced with permission from *Anat. Embryol.* **164:**161–206 (1982).

growth could also explain the numerous ascending and descending dendritic branchlets and axonal terminals which characterize these neurons. In addition, the surface of layer I also expands considerably as the cortex develops, and this expansion could explain the progressive horizontal lengthening (horizontalization) that all processes of CR neurons undergo.

NEURONS OF LAYER I

Our knowledge about the morphology of CR neurons of the cerebral cortex of experimental mammals also remains fragmentary and rather incomplete. There have been few descriptions of these neurons in the cerebral cortex of mouse, rat, rabbit, cat, dog, and sheep. Almost invariably the structure of these neurons is bipolar or horizontal. They are usually located toward the middle of the lamina. Their dendrites have ascending branchlets and one of its polar processes represents the axon. This axon does not descend, as it does in man, to the lower region of the layer, but it appears intermingled with the other fibrillar elements of layer I, without showing any preferential distribution. These axons also have many ascending terminal fibrils throughout their entire length. It should be emphasized that CR neurons of the nonhuman cerebral cortex do not reach the degree of development achieved by the human neurons. Instead, their morphology is comparable with that of the embryonic or fetal human CR neurons.

There have been few systematic Golgi studies of the prenatal development of the CR neurons in experimental animals (Marin-Padilla, 1972; Sousa-Pinto *et al.*, 1975). The embryonic CR neurons of cat cerebral cortex have horizontal dendrites and a descending axon which terminates in a lower layer (Fig. 9). In the course of cortical development, these neurons undergo a progressive horizontalization of their processes and by the time of birth they have acquired all their essential characteristics (Fig. 9). At this time, they are bipolar neurons with

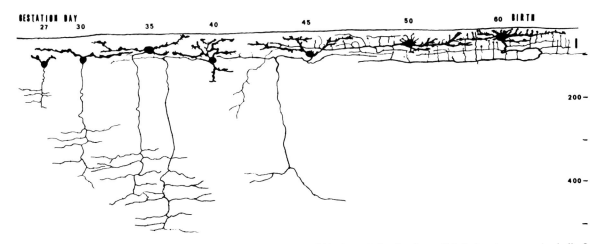

Figure 9. Composite figure of camera lucida drawings illustrating the entire prenatal development of the CR neurons of the cat cerebral cortex. The descending axonal processes possessed by these neurons early in their development disappear progressively as they assume a more horizontal shape within layer I. By the time of birth they have acquired all of their essential morphological characteristics. Scale: 100 μm. Reproduced with permission from *Z. Anat. Entwicklungsgesch.* **136:**125–142 (1972).

horizontal dendrites, with many ascending branchlets, and a long horizontal axon with many ascending terminal fibrils which can be followed for long distances within layer I (Fig. 9).

The ultrastructure of the CR neurons is quite characteristic (see Figs. 14, 15). It has been described in both man (Larroche, 1981; Larroche and Houcine, 1982) and rat (König *et al.*, 1975, 1977; König and Marty, 1981; Raedler and Sievers, 1976). These neurons are characterized by a prominent rough endoplasmic reticulum with its cisternae arranged in prominent parallel rows which extend into the bases of its main dendrites. Frequent axodendritic synapses of a primitive nature have been described on these primitive neurons (see Figs. 14, 15), and axosomatic synaptic contacts have also been described later in their development.

The CR neurons of the mammalian cerebral cortex are the first to appear in development and are among the first to achieve functional maturity (see Figs. 14, 15). The arrival of primitive corticipetal fibers to the undifferentiated telencephalic vesicle is considered to be the stimulus for the appearance and maturation of these neurons. The CR neurons are considered to be a link between these primitive, possibly monoaminergic, fibers and all the pyramidal neurons of the cerebral cortex.

The small neurons of layer I were also first described by Ramón y Cajal (1897) and confirmed by Lorente de Nó (1922). Their presence has been mentioned in a variety of other mammals including man (Ramón y Cajal, 1899, 1911; Meller *et al.*, 1968; Colonnier, 1968; Lund and Lund, 1970; Sousa-Pinto *et al.*, 1975;

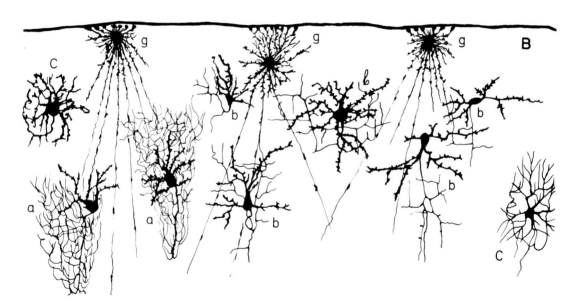

Figure 10. Composite figure of camera lucida drawings illustrating the variable appearance of the small neurons of layer I of the human motor cortex of newborn infants. Some small neurons are characterized by rich axonal arborizations (a) while others have very poor ones (b). Other small neurons resemble the "neurogliaform" cells of Ramón y Cajal (c). Also illustrated are some typical glial elements of layer I (g). Reproduced with permission from *Anat. Embryol.* **164:**161–206 (1982).

Baron, 1976; Marin-Padilla and Marin-Padilla, 1982). Undoubtedly, they are different from the CR neurons since their distribution within layer I is restricted. Our knowledge about them remains incomplete.

The small neurons of layer I are essentially stellate cells with short axonal and dendritic processes (Fig. 10). Their dendrites are short, irregular with a few spinelike structures and short collaterals. While the dendritic distribution of these neurons is nonspecific, their axonal arborization varies, but is more characteristic. It is possible to distinguish small neurons with rich axonal plexuses which extend into the upper region of layer II, from those with very poor axonal arborizations (Fig. 10). In addition, there are small neurons in layer I with undistinguishable axonal and dendritic processes. They correspond to the so-called "neurogli-aform" cells of Ramón y Cajal and could represent still immature and developing neurons (see Chapter 7).

The small neurons of layer I become progressively incorporated into this layer during the course of cortical development. They are first recognized around the 24th to 26th week of gestation in man, and at this time they are quite small and immature neurons. The territory of the distribution of their dendritic and axonal arborizations is not extensive even when they are fully mature neurons. Therefore, their functional role is also considered to be limited and restricted within layer I. A possible inhibitory functional role has recently been suggested for the small neurons of layer I (Hendry and Jones, 1981).

2.2. Fibers of Layer I

Layer I has, in addition to the horizontal axons of the CR neurons, three different types of fibers: the specific afferent fibers, the axonal terminals of Martinotti neurons, and terminal fibrils from the various afferent systems of lower cortical strata. The specific afferent fibers and the axonal terminals of Martinotti neurons are recognized throughout the entire course of prenatal cortical ontogenesis and are considered to be essential components of layer I. In contrast, the terminal fibrils of the various afferent systems derived from the lower cortical strata are progressively incorporated into layer I late in prenatal development. Their time of incorporation into layer I depends on the arrival time of the afferent system from which they originate. These terminal fibrils are considered to be nonprimary components of layer I and their distribution in it is limited.

The specific afferent fibers of layer I are the first elements to arrive at the undifferentiated telencephalic vesicle, and their arrival marks the beginning of cortical neurogenesis. They are considered to be the stimulus for the appearance and development of the CR neurons. The presence of these fibers in the telen-cephalic vesicle prior to the appearance of the cortical plate has been demonstrated in both human and experimental embryos (Marin-Padilla, 1971, 1978; König *et al.*, 1975; Raedler and Raedler, 1978; Rickmann *et al.*, 1977; Larroche, 1981; Marin-Padilla and Marin-Padilla, 1982).

The existence of specific ascending fibers which arise from the white matter and terminate in layer I has seldom been described in the literature. There were mentioned in some of Ramón y Cajal's early works (1899, 1900), as well as by

Lorente de Nó (1922) and Tello (1934, 1935); the latter pointed out the early arrival of these fibers within the developing cortex and showed they form two plexuses, one above and one below the cortical plate. The presence of these specific fibers have been corroborated in the cerebral cortex of normal and abnormal infants (Marin-Padilla, 1970, 1974), as well as normal and abnormal (Reeler) mice (Pinto-Lord and Caviness, 1979). Poliakov (1961, 1974) and Shkol'nik-Yarros (1971) have also mentioned the presence of ascending fibers which terminate in layer I, where they become long horizontal fibers.

Our understanding of the morphologic characteristics of these specific fibers has evolved from rapid Golgi studies of the cerebral cortices of mouse, cat, and human embryos (Figs. 11, 12). They are first recognized as they penetrate externally into the telencephalic vesicle and extend throughout its entire surface establishing in it an external white matter, named the *primordial plexiform layer*. The subsequent appearance of the cortical plate separates these fibers into two distinct plexuses, one above and the other below it.

In later developmental stages, they are seen ascending from the white matter crossing vertically in the developing cortical plate and terminating in layer I in a characteristic manner (Figs. 11, 12). As they penetrate into layer I, they bifurcate into two or more long horizontal collaterals which can be followed for a long distance. They are preferentially distributed through the upper half of layer I where they form a rich plexus of fibers (Figs. 11, 12). This plexus is clearly distinguishable from that formed by the axonal process of CR neurons in the lower half of this layer. It is composed of thinner, beaded, and more abundant fibers than that formed by the axonal processes of CR neurons (compare Fig. 12 with Figs. 3, 5). The horizontal collaterals of these fibers also give off numerous ascending and fewer descending terminals throughout their entire length not unlike those formed by the axonal processes of CR neurons (Fig. 12).

The number of these ascending specific afferent fibers undergo a considerable dilution as the brain grows and it may be difficult to locate them in the adult (Marin-Padilla, 1971; Rickmann *et al.*, 1977). The actual number of these ascending afferent fibers become established very early in cortical neurogenesis and remain unchanged throughout its course. As new fibers (thalamic, callosal, and cortico-cortical) become progressively incorporated into layer I in the course of cortical development, the number of ascending specific afferent fibers undergoes further dilution. They may be absent from those cortical regions which become incoporated later in development, such as the associative areas. However, it should be pointed out that the original plexus of thinner fibers formed by them in the upper half of layer I (human studies) can be recognized throughout the entire surface of the cerebral cortex. This plexus continues to grow horizontally in cortical development, although the number of original fibers which form it remain unchanged.

Figure 11. Rapid Golgi preparations of the motor cortex of a premature infant (29 weeks of gestation) illustrating the structure and distribution of several specific afferent fibers (A, B) and their relationships with the horizontal axons (arrows) of CR neurons and the terminal axonal fanlike branches of a Martinotti neuron (m) with its characteristic long, spinelike extensions. Scale: 100 μm. Reproduced with permission from *Anat. Embryol.* **164:**161–206 (1982).

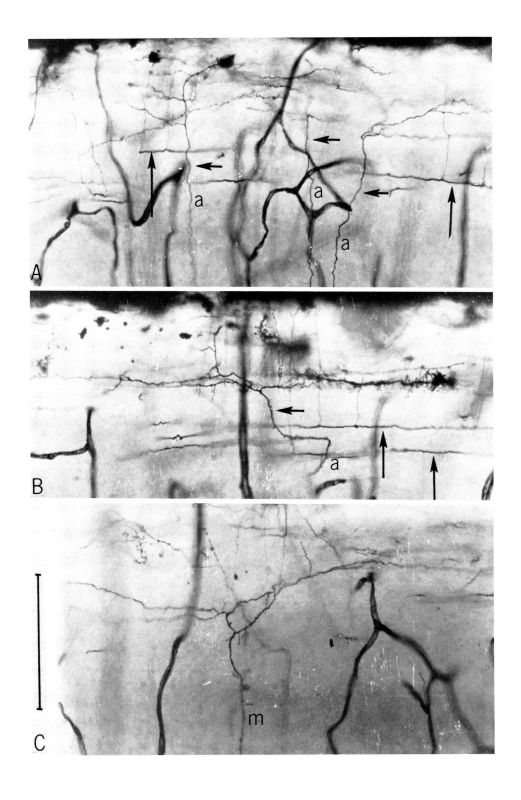

The main target of these specific fibers is considered to be the CR neurons which represent a link between them and all the pyramidal neurons of the cerebral cortex. Although the nature of these fibers remains unknown, all experimental studies support the idea that they may be monoaminergic in nature (Ungersted, 1971; Olson *et al.*, 1973; Schlumpf *et al.*, 1980; Morrison *et al.*, 1978; Molliver, 1982; Levitt and Rakic, 1982). These fibers are believed to originate from lower centers of the neuraxis. They are considered to play an important role, together with the CR neuron, in the overall organization of the cerebral cortex. Further studies are needed to elucidate their nature, origin, and possible functional role.

The axonal terminals of Martinotti neurons represent an important fibrillar component of layer I (Martinotti, 1890). These neurons have received little attention in the literature (Ramón y Cajal, 1911; Szentágothai, 1978; Marin-Padilla, 1970, 1971, 1972, 1974). Martinotti neurons are probably present at all cortical levels. Those of the deep plexiform lamina (layer VII or subplate zone) are among the first neurons to develop in cortical neurogenesis. Probably, Martinotti neurons appear progressively in an "inside-out" fashion together with the pyramidal neurons of similar cortical depth, establishing dual pyramidal–Martinotti sets at the various cortical levels. Therefore, the axonic terminals of Martinotti neurons become progressively incorporated into layer I in the course of cortical ontogenesis. The penetration of the axons of Martinotti neurons into layer I perhaps coincides with the formation of the apical dendritic bouquets of the pyramidal neurons of the same cortical depth.

The axons of Martinotti neurons terminate in layer I in a characteristic manner which is clearly distinguishable from the other fibrillar components of this layer. As the axons of these neurons approach layer I, they bifurcate into

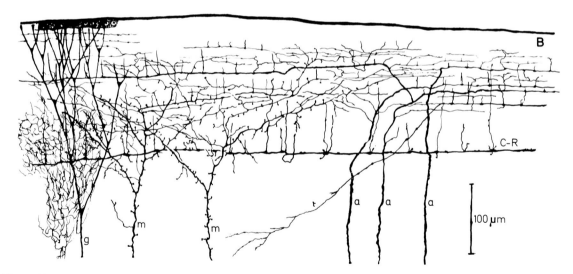

Figure 12. Composite figure of camera lucida drawings from rapid Golgi preparations of the motor cortex of newborn infants illustrating the distribution of three specific afferent fibers (a) and of two axonal terminals (m) from Martinotti neurons, and their relationships to the axon (C-R) of CR neurons within layer I. Reproduced with permission from *Anat. Embryol.* **164**:161–206 (1982).

several fanlike branches which penetrate layer I obliquely (Figs. 11, 12). These fanlike branches have a few, long spinelike processes which are quite characteristic (Figs. 11, 12). The extent of these branches within layer I is limited and might depend on the size or cortical depth of the cells of origin. The morphology of the axonal termination of Martinotti neurons resembles and mimics quite closely the arborization of the dendritic bouquets of the pyramidal neurons. This resemblance strongly suggests structural as well as functional interrelationships between Martinotti neurons and the dendritic bouquets of the pyramidal neurons of the same cortical depth. Based on their characteristic morphology, a possible inhibitory role has recently been suggested for the Martinotti neurons (Marin-Padilla and Marin-Padilla, 1982). That inhibition would be restricted and would take place between the axonal terminals of a given Martinotti neuron and the dendritic bouquets of pyramidal neurons of the same cortical depth.

Terminal fibrils from afferent systems of lower cortical strata represent another fibrillar component of layer I. In Golgi preparations, they are seen approaching layer I obliquely. They penetrate into it and branch only sparsely. They are progressively incorporated into layer I in the course of cortical development. The time of arrival of the different terminal fibrils depends on the time of arrival of the afferent systems from which they originate. Terminal fibrils from the deepest afferent systems arrive in layer I earlier than those from more superficial strata. During the course of cortical development, it is possible to trace some of them back to afferent systems composed of thicker fibers, which run more or less horizontally through deep (layers VI–V), intermediate (layers V–IV), and superficial (layers III–II) cortical strata.

It is possible that some of these terminal fibrils may be present in only specific regions of the cerebral cortex, such as the primary sensory and motor areas. Their distribution within layer I is limited and they do not extend throughout the entire surface of layer I as do the specific afferent fibers or the axonal processes of CR neurons. Since most of them arrive after the basic organization of this lamina has already been established, they are considered to be a nonprimary component. Although they enter layer I, the main target of the afferent systems from which these terminal fibrils originate is not this superficial lamina. Although terminal fibrils from nonspecific thalamic, specific thalamic, callosal, and cortico-cortical afferent systems could progressively reach layer I in the course of cortical ontogenesis, they will be unable to significantly modify either the basic structural organization or the postulated primitive functional role of this superficial lamina. Layer I is thus considered to be part of a primitive cortical organization which is older than the cortical plate.

2.3. Receptive Surfaces of Layer I

The apical dendritic bouquets of practically all pyramidal neurons of the cerebral cortex regardless of their size, functional roles, cortical location, or cortical depth become progressively incoporated into layer I in the course of cortical ontogenesis. Together, they constitute an extensive receptive surface and their parent cells represent the principal, if not the only, functional outlet of this superficial layer (Fig. 13). The apical dendritic bouquets of the different pyramidal neurons become progressively incorporated into layer I starting with the deep neurons of layer VII, and followed by those of layer VI, V, IV, III, and II, respectively. In reality, the first portion of a pyramidal neuron to develop is its terminal dendritic bouquet, which penetrates layer I early in its development (see Fig. 15). As the future pyramidal neurons progressively come in contact with layer I, during the "inside-out" formation of the cortical plate, they first grow their terminal dendritic bouquets and become anchored to this primitive layer. Thereby, the pyramidal neurons of the cerebral cortex retain their original connections with layer I and therefore remain "suspended" from it during the course of cortical ontogenesis.

The original dendritic bouquets of all pyramidal neurons continue to grow and expand as cortical ontogenesis continues. Their branches eventually occupy all the available space within layer I forming the well-known dendritic bouquets (Fig. 13), which tend to expand preferentially in the upper half of the lamina (Fig. 13) and become covered by typical dendritic spines. In Golgi preparations, multiple axospinous contacts are often observed between the ascending terminals of the axonal processes of the CR neurons and the spines of the dendritic bouquets (Fig. 13). Probably similar types of contacts might be established between the ascending terminals of the specific afferent fibers and the spines of the dendritic bouquets. All pyramidal neurons throughout the cerebral neocor-

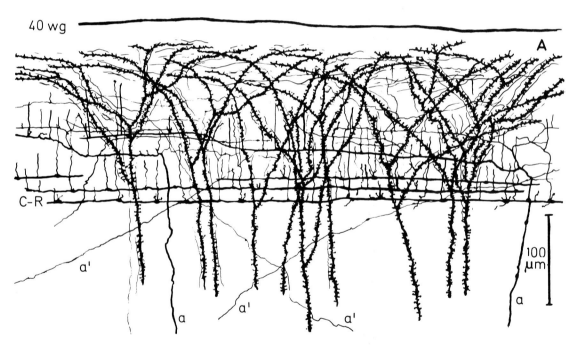

Figure 13. Composite figure of camera lucida drawings from rapid Golgi preparations of the motor cortex of newborn infants illustrating the preferential distribution of the apical dendritic bouquets of pyramidal neurons through the upper half of layer I. Also illustrated are the numerous ascending terminals from the horizontal axons of CR neurons and the horizontal collaterals of the specific afferent fibers (a) which seem to establish synaptic contacts with the spines of the dendritic bouquets of the pyramidal neurons. Also illustrated are several terminal fibrils (a′) from afferent systems of lower cortical strata. Reproduced with permission from *Anat. Embryol.* **164:**161–206 (1982).

tex, regardless of their eventual functional roles, receive the same kind of primitive information through their dendritic bouquets. It is the first information they receive and may be necessary for their subsequent growth and maturation.

3. Origin and Development of Layer I

To understand the interrelationships among the various components of layer I and their overall organization, it is first necessary to determine the origin of this layer and how it becomes established. The mammalian cerebral cortex, including that of man, undergoes two fundamental transformations early in its development, and these result in the establishment of layer I as a distinct cortical stratum.

The first transformation occurs after the arrival of the corticipetal fibers to the undifferentiated telencephalic vesicle, early in embryonic development (around the 12th day of gestation in the rat, the 20th in the cat, and the 50th in man). These primitive corticipetal fibers penetrate into the telencephalic vesicle and extend throughout its entire surface, establishing within it a distinct superficial or external white matter, which corresponds anatomically to the so-called marginal zone (Fig. 14). Perhaps stimulated by the arrival of these primitive fibers, neurons start to appear and to develop in this external white matter, establishing a primitive fibrillo-neuronal organization called the *primordial plexiform layer.* Although the duration of this primordial plexiform layer is relatively short, it is considered to be functionally active since primitive synaptic contacts have been demonstrated between its fibers and the neurons (Figs. 14 and 15).

The second transformation in mammalian cortical ontogenesis is the appearance of the cortical plate (pyramidal cell plate) which is considered to represent the actual mammalian neocortex (Fig. 15). It appears that the migrating neuroblasts which will form the cortical plate, guided by radial glial fibers, are progressively attracted toward the primordial plexiform layer and start to accumulate *within it.* Therefore, the appearance of the cortical plate divides the primordial plexiform layer into a superficial plexiform zone, layer I, and a deep plexiform layer VII (the subplate zone). The division of the primordial plexiform layer obviously results in the separation of its components (fibers and neurons) into two different groups (Fig. 15). The neurons retained in layer I become horizontal cells and are recognized as embryonic CR neurons. Early in their development, these embryonic CR neurons have a descending axonal process which terminates in layer VII. However, as cortical ontogenesis continues, these neurons undergo a progressive horizontalization of all of their processes and their axons become long horizontal (tangential) fibers within layer I, losing their original connections with layer VII (Fig. 9). The neurons retained in layer VII are transformed into pyramidallike neurons, with recurrent axonal collaterals to layer I, and Martinotti neurons which have ascending axons terminating in layer I. In this early cortical organization, the pyramidallike neurons represent the projection neurons, while the CR and Martinotti neurons represent the associative elements. The primitive corticipetal fibers are also divided by the appearance of the cortical plate, and form two distinct plexuses, one located just

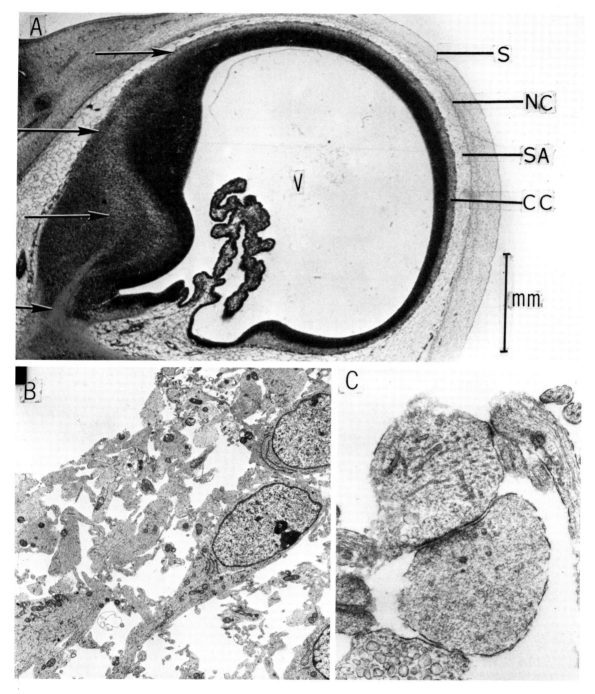

Figure 14. General view of the entire cerebral hemisphere of a 7-week-old human embryo illustrating the primordial plexiform layer stage which occurs in cortical ontogenesis, and precedes the appearance of the cortical plate (which in man occurs around the eighth week of gestation) by several days. Primitive horizontal neurons, recognized as embryonic CR neurons, have been described at this time in cortical development with the electron microscope. (B) Electron micrograph illustrating one of these embryonic CR neurons as well as numerous profiles of fibrillar elements which establish primitive synapses with the dendrites of these neurons as shown in (C). (B) and (C) reproduced with permission from *Anat. Embryol.* **162**:301–312 (1981).

above and the other one just below it. This early cortical organization is also characterized by the formation of synapses only above and below the newly formed cortical plate, so that the first synapses are present only in layers I and VII, respectively. The presence of synapses only in layers I and VII, at this time in cortical ontogenesis, presupposes that they are functionally active, while the primitive and growing cortical plate is functionally inactive early in its development.

It appears that all future pyramidal neurons of the cortical plate are progressively attracted to layer I, so that they can make synaptic connections with it. Therefore, any set of migrating neuroblasts must bypass all the preceding ones in order to establish direct contacts with layer I. Consequently, all newly arrived neurons will always occupy the most superficial zone of the cortical plate and will be in direct contact with layer I. These newly arrived neurons then grow apical dendritic bouquets which penetrate layer I (Fig. 15). Once these young pyramidal neurons have established synaptic connections with layer I, they are ready to be displaced by the arrival of the next set of migrating neuroblasts, but they do not lose their original connection with the superficial lamina. Thus, the first segments of pyramidal neurons to develop are their apical dendritic bouquets. The early formation of the terminal dendritic bouquets of pyramidal neurons has previously been recognized by several investigators (Berry and Rogers, 1965; Morest, 1970; Marin-Padilla, 1971, 1972; Peters and Feldman, 1973). Since it appears that these early connections do not disappear, but are retained throughout the course of cortical ontogenesis, all pyramidal neurons of the cerebral cortex become and remain anchored to layer I by their dendritic bouquets and are forced to grow in a unique manner.

The possible implication of this phenomenon is of considerable importance for understanding of the overall structural organization of the mammalian cerebral cortex. The universal need for all pyramidal neurons of the cerebral cortex to make and to retain connections with layer I will force them to grow in a unique manner. This universal need could also explain the so-called "inside-out" formation of the cortical plate. The pyramidal neurons must grow by the progressive upward elongation of their apical dendrites, increasing the distance between the neuronal body and the dendritic bouquet which is firmly anchored to layer I. Therefore, they must grow by the progressive lengthening of their apical dendrites. Consequently, the growth and maturation of pyramidal neurons can be expected to follow an "inside-out" progression. This unique type of growth implies that in addition to the usual terminal dendritic growth, pyramidal neurons are capable of adding new membrane to the midportion of their apical dendrite. The possible importance of this type of growth and its implication on the growth and maturation of the pyramidal neurons of the mammalian cerebral cortex should be further explored.

It should be pointed out that this unique type of growth could explain many of the peculiar features which characterize pyramidal neurons of the mammalian cerebral cortex, features which have previously not been satisfactorily explained. It could explain, first of all, the distinct morphology of these neurons since they could have no other. Also, it could explain: (1) the extraordinary structural uniformity of pyramidal neurons throughout phylogenetic evolution; (2) their universal radial orientation to the surface of the cerebral cortex and hence to layer I; and (3) their variety of sizes, which depend on the degree of apical

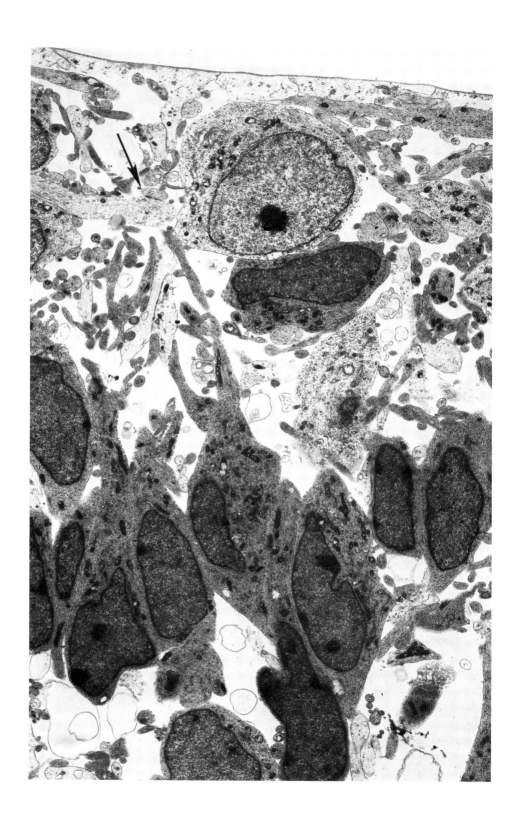

elongation, and hence of their developmental age, or the time of their original contacts with layer I. Perhaps, this unique type of growth could also explain the overall organization of the mammalian cerebral cortex with its numerous giant, large, medium, and small pyramidal neurons which are similar in distribution through the entire cortex. In conclusion, it can be stated that layer I must play a more important role in the overall organization of the cerebral cortex than has previously been suspected.

4. Structural–Functional Organization of Layer I

Based on the data gathered from this morphologic and developmental study, the structural–functional organization of layer I of the mammalian cerebral cortex is envisioned as follows.

First, the basic afferent system of layer I is represented by primitive corticipetal fibers which are the first elements to arrive during cortical ontogenesis. Experimental evidence supports the idea that these primitive fibers are monoaminergic in nature. Although their origin remains unknown, neurons from mesencephalic centers of the reticular formation (e.g., locus coeruleus) have been suggested as their possible source. These fibers penetrate into layer I and course horizontally through it. In the human cerebral cortex, they tend to occupy the upper half of layer I. Their principal target are the CR neurons, with which they seem to establish axodendritic synapses. They might also establish secondary connections with the apical dendritic bouquets of pyramidal neurons (Fig. 16, I).

Second, the basic neuronal element of layer I is the CR neuron. These neurons are the first neuronal elements to be recognized in cortical ontogenesis. They have various appearances, but the variation only involves the shapes of their cell bodies and the origins of the main dendrites, for all of them are characterized by a descending axonal process which becomes transformed into long horizontal (tangential) fibers which can be followed for a long distance within layer I. The long horizontal axonal processes of these neurons with their numerous ascending terminals are recognized throughout the entire cerebral cortex, even within regions lacking cell bodies of CR neurons. The main targets of these neurons are the apical dendritic bouquets of all pyramidal neurons of the cerebral cortex, and the numerous ascending terminals of the horizontal axonal processes of these CR cells are believed to establish synaptic contacts with the apical dendritic bouquets of all pyramidal neurons. The CR neurons are, therefore, considered to be a link between the early arriving monoaminergic

←

Figure 15. Electron micrograph of the structural organization of layer I of the cerebral cortex of a rat embryo (16 days of gestation) illustrating a CR neuron with horizontal dendrites and an axodendritic synaptic contact with one of the dendrites (arrow). The newly arrived neuroblasts (primitive pyramidal neurons) of the cortical plate have numerous apical dendritic bouquets growing into layer I. These primitive dendritic bouquets are clearly visible because they are darker than the numerous fibrillar profiles (specific afferent fibers) of layer I. Reproduced with permission from *Z. Anat. Entwicklungsgesch.* **148:**73–87 (1975).

fibers and the apical dendritic bouquets of all pyramidal neurons, and they transmit the same kind of primitive information to all pyramidal neurons regardless of their size, location, or eventual functional roles. This common and primitive information may be needed for the growth and maturation of all pyramidal neurons whether they be large or small or whether they be motor, sensory, visual, acoustic, or associative in nature (Fig. 16, II).

Third, the basic functional outlet of layer I is represented by the apical dendritic bouquets of all pyramidal neurons from the various cortical strata. Thus, during cortical development, the pyramidal neurons become progressively incoporated into layer I, and they become incorporated in an "inside-out" fashion, the deepest neurons being the first ones to become incorporated, followed sequentially by the most superficial ones. In addition, dual sets of pyramidal and Martinotti neurons are probably present at all levels of the cerebral cortex. All pyramidal neurons receive the same kind of primitive information from layer I, and they may be locally inhibited, at the level of the dendritic bouquets, by the axonal terminals of the accompanying Martinotti neurons of each of the different dual sets. This basic relationship probably occurs throughout the entire cerebral cortex (Fig. 16, III).

Fourth, the subsequent arrival of other afferent systems (nonspecific and specific thalamic fibers, callosal and cortico-cortical fibers) within the cerebral cortex will determine the particular specific function of its various regions and neuronal assemblages. Although terminal fibrils from all of these afferent sys-

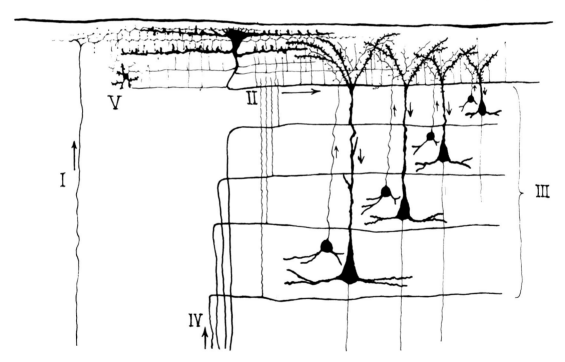

Figure 16. Schematic representation of the possible structural–functional organization of layer I of the mammalian cerebral cortex based on morphologic and developmental observations.

tems reach layer I, their functional role in this lamina is considered to be restricted and secondary (Fig. 16, IV).

Fifth, the small neurons of layer I become incorporated into it late in prenatal cortical ontogenesis. Their distribution within layer I is limited, and their functional role is considered to be restricted and possibly inhibitory (Fig. 16, V).

ACKNOWLEDGMENT. This work has been supported by Grant 09274 from the National Institute of Child Health and Human Development.

5. References

Adinolfi, A. M., 1972, Morphogenesis of synaptic function in layer I and II of the somatic sensory cortex, *Exp. Neurol.* **34:**372–382.

Angevine, J. B., and Sidman, R. L., 1961, Autoradiographic study of cell migration during histogenesis of cerebral cortex of the mouse, *Nature (London)* **192:**766–768.

Armstrong-James, M., and Johnson, R., 1970, Quantitative studies of postnatal changes in synapses in rat superficial motor cerebral cortex, *Z. Zellforsch. Mikrosk. Anat.* **110:**559–568.

Åström, K. E., 1967, On the early development of the isocortex in fetal sheep, in: *Progress in Brain Research*, Vol. 26 (C. G. Berhard and J. P. Shade, eds.), pp. 1–59, Elsevier, Amsterdam.

Baron, M., 1976, Organizacion funcional de la capa I de la corteza cerebral: Cellulas de Cajal [Doctoral thesis], *Ann. Ins. Farm. Esp.* **22:**23–240.

Baron, M., and Gallego, A., 1971, Cajal cells of the rabbit cerebral cortex, *Experientia* **27:**430–432.

Berry, M., and Rogers, A. W., 1965, The migration of neuroblasts in the developing cerebral cortex, *J. Anat.* **99:**691–709.

Boulder Committee, 1970, Embryonic vertebrate central nervous system: Revised terminology, *Anat. Rec.* **166:**257–262.

Braak, H., 1980, *Architectonics of the Human Telencephalic Cortex*, pp. 66, 77, Springer-Verlag, Berlin.

Bradford, R., Parnavelas, J. G., and Lieberman, A. R., 1978, Neurons in layer I of the developing occipital cortex of the rat, *J. Comp. Neurol.* **176:**121–132.

Brun, A., 1965, The subpial granular layer of the fetal cerebral cortex in man: Its ontogeny and significance of congenital cortical malformations, *Acta Pathol. Microbiol. Scand. Suppl.* **179:**1–98.

Colonnier, M., 1968, Synaptic patterns on different cell types in the different laminae of the cat visual cortex: An electron microscope study, *Brain Res.* **9:**268–287.

Conel, J. L., 1941, *The Postnatal Development of the Human Cerebral Cortex*, Vol. II, pp. 97–130, Harvard University Press, Cambridge, Mass.

Conel, J. L., 1947, *The Postnatal Development of the Human Cerebral Cortex*, Vol. III, pp. 132–148, Harvard University Press, Cambridge, Mass.

Conel, J. L., 1951, *The Postnatal Development of the Human Cerebral Cortex*, Vol. IV, pp. 158–177, Harvard University Press, Cambridge, Mass.

Duckett, S., and Pearse, A. G. E., 1968, The cells of Cajal–Retzius in the developing human brain, *J. Anat.* **102:**183–187.

Fox, M. W., and Inman, O., 1966, Persistence of the Retzius–Cajal cells in developing dog brain, *Brain Res.* **3:**192–194.

Gallego, A., 1972, Conexiones centrales entre neuronas: Cellulas moduladoras de las capas plexiformes, *Arch. Fac. Med. Madrid* **21:**69–116.

Godina, G., 1951, Istogenesi e differenziazione dei neuroni e digly elementi gliali della corteccia cerebrale, *Z. Zellforsch. Mikrosk. Anat.* **36:**401–435.

Hendry, S. H. C., and Jones, E. G., 1981, Sizes and distribution of intrinsic neurons incorporating tritiated GABA in monkey sensory-motor cortex, *J. Neurosci.* **1:**390–408.

His, W., 1904, *Die Entwicklung des menschlichen Gehirns wahrend der ersten Monate*, pp. 176–196, Hirzel, Leipzig.

Jones, E. G., and Powell, T. P. S., 1970, Electron microscopy of the somatic sensory cortex of the cat. II. The fine structure of layers I–II, *Philos. Trans. R. Soc. London Ser. B* **257:**13–21.

Kirsche, W., 1974, Zur vergleichenden Funktions bezogene Morphologie der Hirnrinde der Wirbeliere auf der Grundlage embryologische und neurohistologischer Untersuchunge, *Z. Mikrosk. Anat. Forsch.* **88:**21–51.

König, N., 1978, Retzius–Cajal or Cajal–Retzius cells?, *Neurosci. Lett.* **9:**361–363.

König, N., and Marty, R., 1981, Early neurogenesis and synaptogenesis in cerebral cortex, *Bibl. Anat.* **19:**152–162.

König, N., Roch, G., and Marty, R., 1975, The onset of synaptogenesis in rat temporal cortex, *Z. Anat. Entwicklungsgesch.* **148:**73–87.

König, N., Valat, J., Fulcrand, J., and Marty, R., 1977, The time of origin of Cajal–Retzius cells in the rat temporal cortex: An autoradiographic study, *Neurosci. Lett.* **4:**21–26.

Larroche, J.-C., 1981, The marginal layer in the neocortex of a 7-week-old human embryo, *Anat. Embryol.* **162:**301–312.

Larroche, J.-C., and Houcine, O., 1982, Le néo-cortex chez l'embryon et le fetus humain: Apport du microscope électronique et du Golgi, *Reprod. Nutr. Dev.* **22:**163–170.

Larroche, J.-C., Privat, A., and Jardin, L., 1981, Some fine structures of the human fetal brain, in: *Sam Levine International Symposium, Paris* (A. Minkowsky, ed.), pp. 350–358, Karger, Basal.

Levitt, P., and Rakic, P., 1982, The time of genesis, embryonic origin and differentiation of the brain stem monoaminergic neurons in the rhesus monkey, *Dev. Brain Res.* **4:**35–57.

Lorente de Nó, R., 1922, La corteza cerebral del ratón, *Trab. Lab. Invest. Biol. Madrid* **20:**41–78.

Lorente de Nó, R., 1949, Cerebral cortex: Architecture, intracortical connections, motor projections, in: *Physiology of the Nervous System* (J. F. Fulton, ed.), 3rd ed., pp. 288–313, Oxford University Press, London.

Lund, J. S., and Lund, R. D., 1970, The termination of callosal fibers in the paravisual cortex of the rat, *Brain Res.* **17:**25–45.

Marin-Padilla, M., 1970, Prenatal and early postnatal ontogenesis of the human motor cortex: A Golgi study. I. The sequential development of the cortical layers, *Brain Res.* **23:**167–183.

Marin-Padilla, M., 1971, Early prenatal ontogenesis of the cerebral cortex (neocortex) of the cat *(Felis domestica):* A Golgi study. I. The primordial neocortical organization, *Z. Anat. Entwicklungsgesch.* **134:**117–145.

Marin-Padilla, M., 1972, Prenatal ontogenetic history of the principal neurons of the neocortex of the cat *(Felis domestica):* A Golgi study. II. Developmental differences and their significance, *Z. Anat. Entwicklungsgesch.* **136:**125–142.

Martin-Padilla, M., 1974, Structural organization of the cerebral cortex (motor area) in human chromosomal aberrations. I. $D_1(13–15)$ trisomy, Patau syndrome, *Brain Res.* **66:**375–391.

Marin-Padilla, M., 1978, Dual origin of the mammalian neocortex and evolution of the cortical plate, *Anat. Embryol.* **152:**109–126.

Marin-Padilla, M., and Marin-Padilla, M. T., 1982, Origin, prenatal development and structural organization of layer I of the human cerebral (motor) cortex: A Golgi study, *Anat. Embryol.* **164:**161–206.

Martinotti, C., 1890, Beitrag zum Studium der Hirnrinde und dem Centralursprung der Nerven, *Int. Monatschr. Anat. Physiol.* **7:**69–90.

Marty, R., 1962, Development post-natal des responses sensorielles du cortex cerebrale chez le chat et le lapin, *Arch. Anat. Microsc. Morphol. Exp.* **51:**126–264.

Meller, K., Breipohl, W., and Glees, P., 1968, The cytology of the developing molecular layer of mouse motor cortex, *Z. Zellforsch. Mikrosk. Anat.* **96:**171–183.

Molliver, M. E., 1982, Monoamines in the development of the cortex, in: *Development and Modifiability of the Cerebral Cortex* (P. Rakic and P. S. Goldman-Rakic, eds.), pp. 492–507, MIT Press, Cambridge, Mass.

Molliver, M. E., and Van der Loos, H., 1970, The ontogenesis of cortical circuitry: The spatial distribution of synapses in somesthetic cortex of newborn dogs, *Adv. Anat. Embryol. Cell Biol.* **42:**7–53.

Morest, D. K., 1970, A study of neurogenesis in the forebrain of opossum pouch embryo, *Z. Anat. Entwicklungsgesch.* **130:**265–305.

Morrison, J. H., Grzanna, R., Molliver, M. E., and Coyle, J. T., 1978, The distribution and orientation of noradrenergic fibers in the neocortex of the rat: An immunofluorescence study, *J. Comp. Neurol.* **181:**17–40.

Nañagas, J. C., 1923, Anatomical studies on the motor cortex of macacus rhesus, *J. Comp. Neurol.* **35:**67–96.

Novack, C. R., and Purpura, D. P., 1961, Postnatal ontogenesis of neurons in cat neocortex, *J. Comp. Neurol.* **117**:291–307.

Olson, L., Boreus, L. O., and Seiger, A., 1973, Histochemical demonstration and mapping of 5-hydroxytryptamine and catecholamine containing neurons in the human fetal brain, *Z. Anat. Entwicklungsgesch.* **139**:259–282.

Oppermann, K., 1929, Cajalsche Horizontalzellen und Ganglienzellen des Marks, *Z. Neurol. Psychiat.* **120**:121–137.

Peters, A., and Feldman, M., 1973, The cortical plate and molecular layer of the late rat fetus, *Z. Anat. Entwicklungsgesch.* **141**:3–37.

Pinto-Lord, M. C., and Caviness, V. S., 1979, Determination of cell shape and orientation: A comparative Golgi study of cell–axon interrelationships in the developing neocortex of normal and Reeler mice, *J. Comp. Neurol.* **187**:49–70.

Poliakov, G. I., 1961, Some results of research into the development of the neuronal structure of the cortical ends of the analysers in man, *J. Comp. Neurol.* **117**:197–212.

Poliakov, G. I., 1974, Relations between some structural parameters of types and forms of neurons effecting different kinds of switches in the neocortex, *J. Hirnforsch.* **15**:249–268.

Purpura, D. P., 1975, Morphogenesis of visual cortex in the preterm infant, in: *Growth and Development of the Brain* (M. A. B. Brazier, ed.), pp. 33–49, Raven Press, New York.

Purpura, D. P., Carmichal, M. W., and Housepian, E. M., 1960, Physiological and anatomical studies of the development of superficial axodendritic synaptic pathways in neocortex, *Exp. Neurol.* **2**:324–347.

Purpura, D. P., Shofer, R. J., Housepian, E. M., and Noback, C. R., 1964, Comparative ontogenesis of structure–function relations in cerebral and cerebellar cortex, in: *Growth and Maturation of the Brain, Progress in Brain Research,* Vol. 4 (D. P. Purpura and J. P. Shadé, eds.), pp. 219–221, Elsevier, Amsterdam.

Rabinowicz, T. H., 1964, The cerebral cortex of the premature infant of the 8th month, in: *Growth and Maturation of the Brain, Progress in Brain Research,* Vol. 4 (D. P. Purpura and J. P. Shadé, eds.), pp. 39–92, Elsevier, Amsterdam.

Raedler, A., and Sievers, J., 1976, Light and electron microscopical studies on specific cells of the marginal zone in the developing rat cerebral cortex, *Anat. Embryol.* **149**:173–181.

Raedler, E., and Raedler, A., 1978, Autoradiographic study of early neurogenesis in rat neocortex, *Anat. Embryol.* **154**:267–284.

Raedler, E., Raedler, A., and Feldhaus, S., 1980, Dynamic aspects of neocortical histogenesis in the rat, *Anat. Embryol.* **158**:253–269.

Rakic, P., 1972, Mode of cell migration of the superficial layers of the fetal monkey neocortex, *J. Comp. Neurol.* **146**:61–84.

Rakic, P., 1974, Neurons in rhesus monkey visual cortex: Systematic relation between time of origin and eventual disposition, *Science* **183**:425–426.

Rakic, P., 1975, Timing of major ontogenetic events in the visual cortex of rhesus monkey, in: *Brain Mechanisms in Mental Retardation* (N. A. Buchwald, ed.), *UCLA Forum Med. Sci.* **18**:3–40.

Rakic, P., 1982, Early developmental events: Cell lineage, acquisition of neuronal position and areal and laminar development, in: *Developmental and Modifiability of Cerebral Cortex* (P. Rakic and P. S. Goldman-Rakic, eds.), pp. 439–451, MIT press, Cambridge, Mass.

Ramón y Cajal, S. R., 1890, Sobre la existencia de celulas nerviosas especiales de la primera capa de las circunvoluciones cerebrales, *Gaceta Med. Catalana* **1890**:225–228.

Ramón y Cajal, S., 1891, Sur la structure de l'écorce cérébrale de quelques mammifères, *Cellule* **7**:125–176.

Ramón y Cajal, S., 1896, Le bleue de methyléne dans les centres nerveux, *Rev. Trimest. Microsc.* **1**:21–82.

Ramón y Cajal, S., 1897, Las cellulas de cilindro-eje corto de la capa molecular del cerebro, *Rev. Trimest. Microsc.* **2**:104–127.

Ramón y Cajal, S., 1899, Comparative study of the sensory areas of the human cortex, in: *Clark University, 1889–1899, Decennial Celebration* (W. E. Story and L. N. Wilson, eds.), pp. 311–382, Norwood Press, Norwood, Mass.

Ramón y Cajal, S., 1900, Estudios sobre la corteza cerebral humana. III. Estructura de la corteza acústica, *Rev. Trimest. Microsc.* **5**:129–183.

Ramón y Cajal, S., 1911, *Histologie du Système Nerveux de l'Homme et des Vertébrés* (translated by L. Azoulay), Vol. II, pp. 519–646, Maloine, Paris.

Ranke, O., 1909, Kenntnis der normalen und pathologischen Hirnrindenbildung, *Beitr. Pathol. Anat. Allg. Pathol.* **47:**51–125.

Retzius, G., 1891, Über den Bau der Olerflächenschicht der Grosshirnrinde beim Menschen und bei Säugetieren, *Verh. Biol. Ver.* **3:**90–103.

Retzius, G., 1893, Die Cajalschen Zellen der Grosshirnrinde beim Menschen und bei Säugetieren, *Biol. Untersuch.* **4:**1–9.

Retzius, G., 1894, Weitere Beiträge zur Kenntnis der Cajalschen Zellen der Grosshirnrinde des Menschen, *Biol. Untersuch.* **6:**29–34.

Rickmann, M., Chronwall, B. M., and Wolff, J. R., 1977, On the development of nonpyramidal neurons and axons outside the cortical plate: The early marginal zone as a pallial anlage, *Anat. Embryol.* **151:**285–307.

Sas, E., and Sanides, F., 1970, A comparative Golgi study of the Cajal foetal cells, *Z. Mikrosk. Anat. Forsch.* **82:**385–396.

Schlumpf, M., Shoemaker, W. J., and Bloom, F. E., 1980, Innervation of embryonic rat cerebral cortex by catecholamine-containing fibers, *J. Comp. Neurol.* **192:**361–376.

Shkol'nik-Yarros, E., 1971, *Neurons and Interneuronal Connections of the Central Visual System*, pp. 22–31, Plenum Press, New York.

Sholl, D. A., 1956, *Organization of the Cerebral Cortex*, pp. 15–30, Methuen, London.

Shoukimas, G. M., and Hinds, J. W., 1978, The development of the cerebral cortex in the embryonic mouse: An electron microscopic serial section analysis, *J. Comp. Neurol.* **179:**795–830.

Sidman, R. L., and Rakic, P., 1973, Neuronal migration with special reference to developing human brain, *Brain Res.* **62:**1–35.

Smart, I. H. M., and Smart, M., 1982, Growth patterns in the lateral wall of the mouse telencephalon. I. Autoradiographic studies of the histogenesis of the isocortex and adjacent areas, *J. Anat.* **134:**273–298.

Smart, I. H. M., and McSherry, G. M., 1982, Growth patterns in the lateral wall of the mouse telencephalon. II. Histological changes during and subsequent to the period of isocortical neuron production, *J. Anat.* **134:**415–442.

Sousa-Pinto, A., Paula-Barbosa, M., and Carmo Matos, M., 1975, A Golgi and electron microscopical study of nerve cells in layer I of the cat auditory cortex, *Brain Res.* **95:**443–458.

Szentágothai, J., 1970, Les circuits neuronaux de l'écorce cérébrale, *Bull. Acad. R. Med. Belg.* **10:**475–492.

Szentágothai, J., 1971, Some geometric aspects of the neocortical neuropil, *Acta Biol. Acad. Sci. Hung.* **22:**107–124.

Szentágothai, J., 1978, The neuron network of the cerebral cortex: A functional interpretation. Ferrier Lecture, *Proc. R. Soc. London Ser. B* **201:**219–248.

Takashima, S., Chan, F., Becker, L. E., and Armstrong, D. L., 1980, Morphology of the developing visual cortex of the human infant: A quantitative and qualitative Golgi study, *J. Neuropathol. Exp. Neurol.* **39:**487–501.

Tello, J. F., 1934, Les différenciationes neurofibrillaires dans le prosencéphale de la souris de 4 a 15 millimetres, *Trab. Lab. Invest. Biol. Madrid* **29:**339–395.

Tello, J. F., 1935, Evolution des formations neurofibrillairs dans l'écorce cérébrale du foetus de souris blanche depuis les 15 mm. fusgu ara la naissance, *Trab. Lab. Invest. Biol. Madrid* **63:**139–171.

Tömböl, T., 1978, Comparative data of the Golgi architecture of interneurons of different cortical areas in cat and rabbit, in: *Architectonics of the Cerebral Cortex* (M. A. B. Brazier and H. Petsche, eds.), pp. 59–76, Raven Press, New York.

Ungersted, U., 1971, Sterotaxic mapping of the monoaminergic pathways in the rat brain, *Acta Physiol. Scand. Suppl.* **367:**1–48.

Veratti, E., 1897, Ueber einige Structurengentumlichkeiten der Hirnrinde bei deu Säugethieren, *Anat. Anz.* **13:**377–389.

von Koelliker, A., 1896, *Handbuch der Gewebelehre des Menschen*, pp. 644–650, Engelmann, Leipzig.

Wolff, J. R., 1978, Ontogenetic aspects of cortical architecture, lamination, in: *Architectonics of the Cerebral Cortex* (M. A. B. Brazier and H. Petsche, eds.), pp. 159–173, Raven Press, New York.

15

Layer VI Cells

TERÉZ TÖMBÖL

1. Introduction

The laminar parcellation of the cerebral cortex was first introduced by Meynert (1870) who distinguished five layers in the human cerebral cortex, with the exception of the visual area in which he described eight layers. In the following decades the understanding of this lamination was greatly advanced by Golgi analyses of the cortex, and Ramón y Cajal (1911) distinguished eight layers in most cortices and nine layers in the visual cortex. The deepest laminae he termed *layers VI–VII* and/or *VIII–IX,* although these are now referred to as *layer VI,* sublaminae VIa and VIb, on the basis of other cytoarchitectonic studies (Brodmann, 1909; Vogt and Vogt, 1919; von Economo and Koskinas, 1925; Woolsey, 1958; Otsuka and Hassler, 1962; Hassler and Muhs-Clement, 1964; Fleischhauer *et al.,* 1980).

Layer VI is present in all cortical fields, but its thickness is variable, with more or less conspicuous sublaminae VIa and VIb. According to Golgi studies, the cells are of different types (Ramón y Cajal, 1911; O'Leary and Bishop, 1938; O'Leary, 1941; Lorente de Nó, 1949). The classes of neurons that can be distinguished in both Golgi and cytoarchitectonic preparations have resulted in the use of the terms *polymorph* or *multiform* to describe the neurons in this layer.

The structure of layer VI clearly reflects its dual origin (Marin-Padilla, 1978): it consists of an outer columnar zone (sublamina VIa) and an inner zone of horizontal cells (sublamina VIb) (Raedler and Raedler, 1978; Wolff, 1978).

TERÉZ TÖMBÖL • First Department of Anatomy, Histology, and Embryology, Semmelweis University Medical School, Budapest 1450, Hungary.

479

2. General View of Layer VI

The thickness of the cortex and, with it, that of layer VI vary according to species. Thus, the motor cortex is three times thicker in the human brain than in the mouse brain and similar differences can be observed in the thickness of layer VI (Powell, 1981). Further, in the cortex the density of the cells varies from layer to layer and data obtained from measurements in the rat brain show that layer VI is one of the layers with highest cell density (Fleischhauer and Vossel, 1979).

Cytoarchitectonic maps of the cat (Otsuka and Hassler, 1962; Hassler and Muhs-Clement, 1964), rabbit (Fleischhauer *et al.,* 1980), and rat (Vogt and Peters, 1981) neocortex confirm that both sublaminae of layer VI occur throughout the cortex and that they are especially marked in the visual area (Otsuka and Hassler, 1962). In the koniocortex, however, lamina VI is less clearly subdivided than in the homotypical cortex (Jones and Burton, 1974, 1976). In the cat visual cortex (Otsuka and Hassler, 1962), layer VI consists of multiform cells constituting sublamina VIa, and of fusiform cells constituting sublamina VIb and in most locations sublamina VIb fuses gradually with the underlying white matter of the hemisphere. The cells are arranged into columns by radial fiber bundles. In the

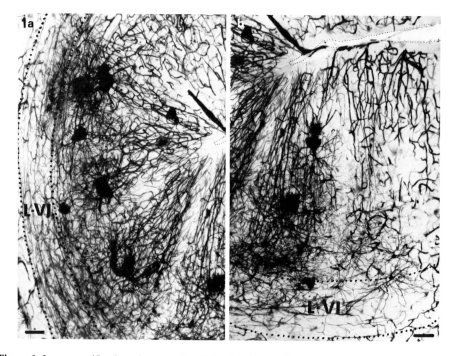

Figure 1. Low-magnification photographs of the visual cortical area of a cat at the depth (a) and on the side (b) of the sulcus splenialis. The thickness of layer VI changes in the two parts of the region. Bars equal 100 μm. (c,d) Schematic drawings showing the changes in thickness of the cortex with its curvature. (c) The convex and (d) the concave and the rather straight areas. The change of layer VI can be seen. The form of columnar slabs also varies with the curvature. The shapes of pyramidal neurons in layer VI also accommodate the change in their available space.

depths of sulci, layer VI is thinnest; the two sublaminae can hardly be distinguished and the columnar arrangement cannot be seen.

In his study on the architectonics of the human cortex, Braak (1980) showed that the multiform layer is dominated by modified pyramidal cells containing varying amounts of pigment (see Chapter 3). It appears often as a bipartite layer, which splits into a narrow, densely pigmented, upper part (VIa) and a broad, moderately pigmented lower one (VIb), although the amount of pigmentation of layer VI varies with the cortical area. The Golgi technique also reveals cortical lamination (Figs. 1a,b). The thickness of the cortex is strongly influenced by the number of gyri present in the cortex and this leads to fundamental changes in the lamination. At the tops of the gyri, where the convexity of the cortex is

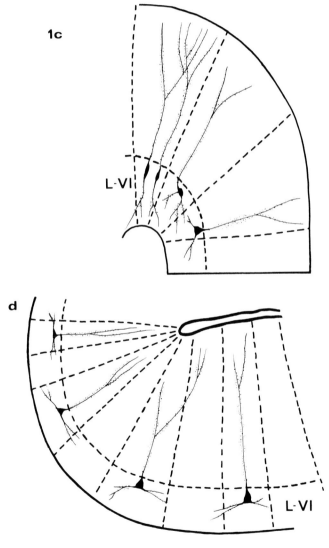

Figure 1. *(continued)*

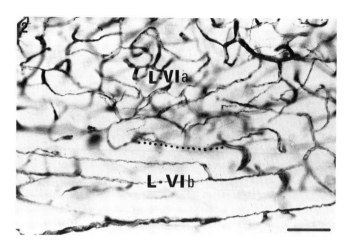

Figure 2. Angioarchitecture of layer VI. Golgi-impregnated vessels are seen. Bar equals 100 μm.

greatest, the outer layers are narrowest and the inner layers widest, while in the concavities—at the depths of the sulci—the outer layers become wider and the inner ones narrower (Figs. 1c,d). For this reason, the lamination and the thickness of the cortex can only be considered as typical in places where the curvature is least. The folding of the cortex also determines the shape of the neurons and very probably it also affects the shapes of functional cortical slabs (Figs. 1c,d).

The angioarchitecture of the cortex also shows some laminar differences. Wolff (1978) in his study claims that cortical angioarchitecture displays at least three sets of vascular modules. The phylogenetically oldest and largest modules mainly supply lamina VI. Golgi impregnation is also useful for the demonstration of the angioarchitecture of the cortex and striking differences in the sublaminae of layer VI can be revealed (Fig. 2). In sublamina VIb, horizontal vessels are connected to each other with short branches, while in sublamina VIa the angioarchitectonic pattern is irregular.

The development of the cortex also confirms the distinction between the two sublaminae of layer VI. According to the interpretation of Marin-Padilla (1978), the mammalian cerebral cortex has a dual origin (see Chapter 14). In his view, the different cell types of the cortex are generated both from the primordial plexiform layer and from the cortical plate, for the migrating cells which will form the cortical plate separate the primordial plexiform layer into a superficial and a deep plexiform lamina. The latter becomes sublamina VIb. Sublamina VIa, however, develops from the cortical plate. Indeed, the characteristics of the cell types of the two sublaminae suggest that they have different origins because in sublamina VIb the neuronal processes have a dominantly horizontal orientation (Raedler and Raedler, 1978; Wolff, 1978). The maturation process of interneurons in layer VI is similar to that in the outer layers (Marin-Padilla, 1975; Rakic, 1975, 1981; Tömböl, 1980), i.e., the maturation of interneurons follows, with a few days' lag, that of pyramidal cells (Fig. 3).

3. The Golgi Architecture of Layer VI

The first Golgi studies (Golgi, 1886; Meynert, 1870; Martinotti, 1890; Schaffer, 1897; Ramón y Cajal, 1911) provided basic data on the neuronal elements of the CNS, and in the second era of the Golgi method (O'Leary and Bishop, 1938; O'Leary, 1941; Lorente de Nó, 1949) some morphological structures were given tentative functional correlations. Further detailed analysis of the Golgi architecture of the CNS has been carried out during the third revival of the Golgi method in the past two decades, emphasizing the continuing value of the method (Shkolnik-Yarros, 1960; Szentágothai, 1969, 1975, 1978a,b; Peters and Walsh, 1972; Tömböl, 1972, 1978a,b; Szentágothai and Arbib, 1974; Jones, 1975b; Feldman and Peters, 1978; Lund *et al.*, 1979, 1981; Peters and Regidor,

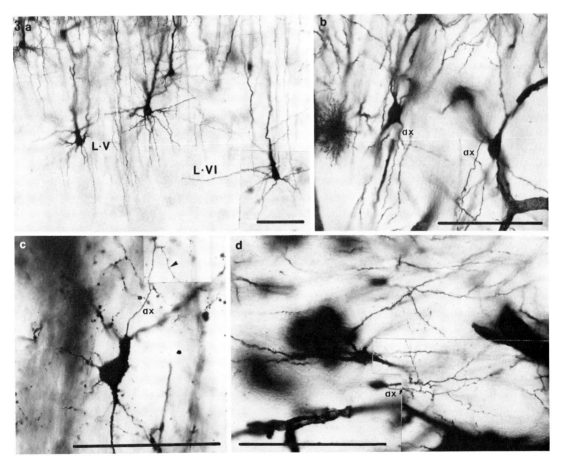

Figure 3. (a,c) One-day-old kitten brain. Pyramidal neurons (a) and LCNs (c) demonstrate the difference between the two types of neurons during the process of maturation. (b,d) Pyramidal neurons (b) and LCNs (d) at day 9. ax, axon; arrowhead in (c) points to an axonal collateral. Bars equal 100 μm.

1981). The recent application of the Golgi method at the EM level had added further to its value (Peters and Fairén, 1978; Somogyi *et al.*, 1981, Peters *et al.*, 1982).

The present Golgi analysis is an account of the use of the Golgi technique in examining neurons in layer VI of the cortex. For this purpose, serial sections of adult cat brains were impregnated by the perfusion Golgi–Kopsch method.

Neuron Types of Layer VI

Ramön y Cajal (1911) divided cortical neurons into two basic groups: neurons with long or short axons. To the first group belong the projection neurons of the cortex which establish projection, commissural, and/or association connections. The short-axon neurons are called *interneurons* (Lenhossék, 1895) but following Rakic's proposal (1975) they will be referred to as *local-circuit neurons*. These neurons belong to the short-axon group, whose axons arborize locally. Their axons never leave the gray metter.

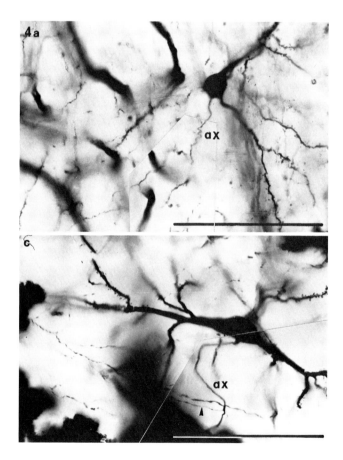

Figure 4. Pyramidal neurons of different types: (a) small pyramidal and (b) medium-size pyramidal neurons in sublamina VIa; (c) triangular pyramidal neuron in sublamina VIb; (d) small pyramidallike neuron in sublamina VIa. Bars equal 100 μm.

The Projection Neurons of Layer VI

1. In sublamina VIa, pyramidal and pyramidallike neurons of different sizes comprise the projection neurons. Ramón y Cajal (1911) distinguished three types of long-axon cells in his layers VI and VII: medium-size pyramidal neurons, the apical dendrites of which ascend to the plexiform layer and whose axons emit four to six axonal collaterals; triangular neurons with three dendrites of equal length (they have no apical dendrites); fusiform neurons with vertically oriented dendrites, one of which ascends to the plexiform layer and the other descends toward the white matter, while their axons give off two or three collaterals.

Further Golgi descriptions added several new types to the group of long-axon cells. The pyramidallike, medium-size neuron is one of them (Jones, 1975b; Feldman and Peters, 1978, Tömböl, 1978a).

In sublamina VIa, the shapes of the medium-size *pyramidal neurons* are strongly influenced by the curvature of the cortex (Figs. 1c,d). The typical shapes of the neurons can be observed in those areas where the curvature of the cortex is at a minimum (Fig. 4a). In contrast, in those areas where the convexity of the cortex is significant, the pyramidal neurons appear elongated, or *vertically fusiform,* while

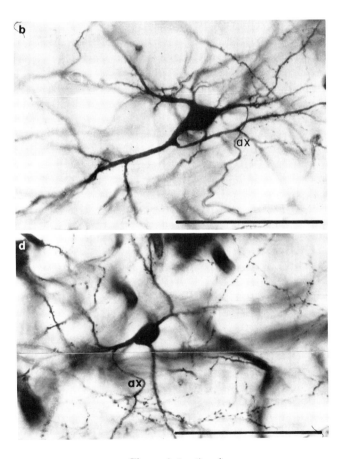

Figure 4. *(continued)*

at the bottoms of sulci the widths of the cells increase, so that the somata of pyramidal neurons become rather flat, or *triangular* (Figs. 1c,d). The vertically oriented fusiform projection neurons described by Ramón y Cajal are identical with the pyramidal neurons found in the thick layer VI of the convex cortical areas. Their ascending dendrites are apical dendrites, while the descending dendrites are identical with basal dendrites. The dendrites are spinous, like those of other pyramidal neurons. (See Chapter 5.)

The medium-size pyramidal neurons—packed tightly on top of each other in a column—develop horizontally elongated cell bodies instead of pyramide shaped ones. Their apical dendrites originate from the sides of the cell bodies to follow a curved course, avoiding the soma of the neurons situated more superficially in the column. These are the so-called "altered" pyramidal or pyramidallike neurons (Figs. 5a,b) of sublamina (VIa (Jones, 1975a; Tömböl, 1978b).

In the middle of the layer there are medium-size pyramidal neurons, the apical dendrites of which are only as thick as their basal ones and, entering layer V, they arborize. The apical dendrites branch, however, and only reach layers IV and III. These neuron types are identical with the triangular neurons (Figs. 4b,c) described by Ramón y Cajal and with those referred to as pyramidal neurons of layer VI, the apical dendrites of which do not reach the outer layers. Their basal dendrites follow a horizontal trajectory. In the group of medium-size projection neurons there are cell types with *multipolar* shapes (Fig. 5c). Their spiny dendrites ascend only to the level of layer V and their axons follow a curved course, while giving off several collaterals.

Small pyramidal and *ovoid neurons* (Fig. 4d) can also be observed in sublamina VIa (O'Leary, 1941). Their apical dendrites are thin and extend to layers III–IV. The basal dendrites do not branch profusely and the dendrites are moderately covered by spines. Their axons enter the white matter after giving rise to a few horizontal collaterals.

The projection neurons in sublamina VIa have spinous dendrites and the apical dendrites of the pyramidal neurons have the most dense covering of spines. The axons of pyramidal neurons of other cortical layers always take a straight course; by contrast, the projection neurons in sublamina VIa have curved axons with collaterals that are generally thick and extend horizontally in both directions. The length of these collaterals is 500–1000 μm. Some side branches arise at sharp angles from the collaterals and are also oriented horizontally. Apart from their proximal parts the axon collaterals are varicose, and the sizes of the varicosities decrease along the distal portions of the collaterals. Some spinelike processes also appear on the side branches of the axonal collaterals.

2. *The polymorph lamina, sublamina VIb,* has been so-named because its cells have various shapes and sizes. Ramón y Cajal distinguished two kinds of projection neurons in this lamina: fusiform neurons with vertical dendritic trees, and triangular pyramidal cells. In addition, horizontally oriented neurons have been described by other authors (Tömböl *et al.*, 1975a,b; Tömböl, 1978a,b; Peters and Regidor, 1981). These neurons are fusiform, but they are not identical with the vertically fusiform neurons of Ramón y Cajal.

In lamina VIb four types of projection neurons of different orientation and shape can be found. There are the *medium-size pyramidal neurons* of lamina VIb,

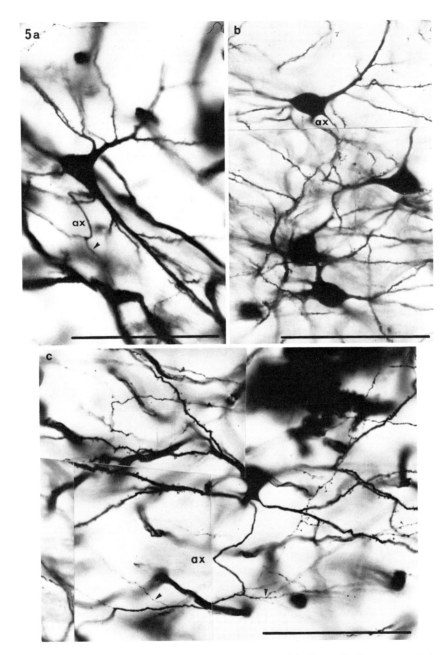

Figure 5. Pyramidal (a), pyramidallike (b) neurons, and a multipolar projection neuron (c) in sublamina VIa. Arrowheads point to axonal collaterals. Bars equal 100 μm.

which have *fusiform shapes* at the convexity of gyri and *triangular shapes* with tangentially elongated cell bodies in the depth of sulci. All these neurons have compact spinous apical and basal dendrites (Fig. 6a). Their apical dendrites ascend to layer IV, and their axons enter the white matter after giving off a few collaterals.

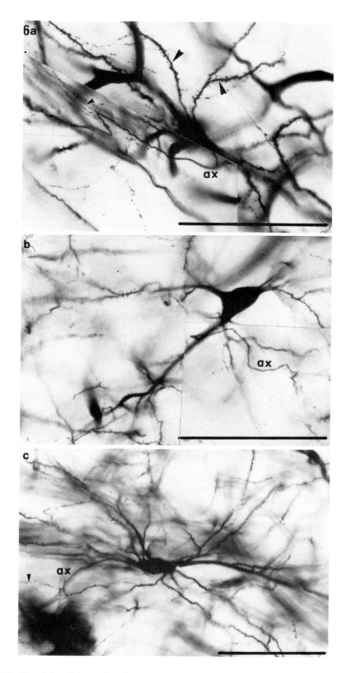

Figure 6. (a) The basal dendrites of a triangular pyramidal neuron. Arrowheads point to dendritic spines. (b) Tangential pyramidal neuron with ascending basal dendrite. (c) Medium-size ovoid multipolar neuron. These neurons are located in sublamina VIb. Arrowheads in (c) point to axonal collaterals. Bars equal 100 μm.

Tangential, or *horizontally pyramidal* neurons form an important group of projection neurons. Their somata have a pyramidal shape, are medium-size or small, and are found mostly in the middle of sublamina VIb. They have a variety of forms. In one group one of the basal dendrites of the neuron ascends into layer IV, while the apical dendrites follows a tangential course in the lamina (Figs. 6b,8a). All the dendrites are densely covered with spines. However, some of the tangential pyramidal neurons preserve their original pyramidal form. The basal dendrites ramify regularly and take an oblique course in the lamina, while the apical dendrites pass horizontally for varying distances (Figs. 7a,b). Some of the apical dendrites arborize after 150–200 μm although others extend for between 500–1000 μm (Fig. 7c). The axons of the tangential pyramidal neurons give off one or two collaterals and enter the white matter.

The *small pyramidallike neurons* belong to the third group of projection cells in sublamina VIb (Fig. 8b). These neurons can be found near the white matter. Their apical dendrites ascend to layer V, where they ramify, and the basal dendrites are arranged horizontally. The dendrites are spinous. The axons of these cells follow a long tangential course at the border of the white matter and before entering the white matter they give off some short varicose side branches.

In sublamina VIb *medium-size neurons with ovoid cell bodies* are occasionally impregnated (Fig. 6c). These cells have numerous (about 10–15) dendrites which ramify two or three times, to form a very rich dendritic tree. The dendrites are moderately spinous and the axon enters the white matter.

The most characteristic projection neurons of sublamina VIb are the *tangential fusiform neurons* (Fig. 9), of which there are both small and medium-size varieties. The horizontal fusiform neurons have two fundamental characteristics: a fusiform cell body with two obvious poles, and bilateral, narrow tangentially extended dendrites.

The cell body of each mediun size fusiform neuron is 30 × 10 μm in diameter, and the small varieties of this type of neuron are more elongated than fusiform. The dendrites originate from the two poles of the fusiform and elongated neurons, and most neurons have only one dendrite extending from each pole. Peters and Regidor (1981) have called them *deep bipolar neurons.* The long horizontal dendrites arborize once or twice, developing a very narrow dendritic tree, and each one extends for about 700–800 μm. The lengths of the two main, long dendrites are different; sometimes one is twice as long as the other. The dendritic trees of the small fusiform neurons are wider, because their dendrites have a richer ramification. The axons of the tangential fusiform neurons give off collaterals and enter the white matter, in which a few collaterals arise. These collaterals return to the cortical gray matter. The axonal collaterals of horizontal fusiform neurons give off small spinelike side branches.

The apical dendrites of the projection neurons which have pyramidal and pyramidallike shapes in sublamina VIb do not reach the plexiform layer, but enter layer IV. In this layer they may contact the terminal arborizations of specific afferents. The tangential pyramidal and fusiform (bipolar) neurons can collect input from distant regions, and they may contact the axonal collaterals, the afferent fibers, and the local axonal arborizations in the layer.

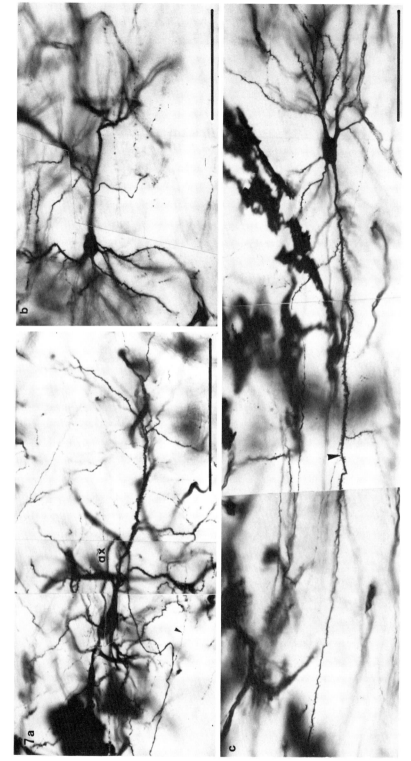

Figure 7. Tangential pyramidal neurons in sublamina VIb. Arrowhead in (a) points to an axonal collateral; arrowhead in (c) shows the long apical dendrite of the neuron. Bars equal 100 μm.

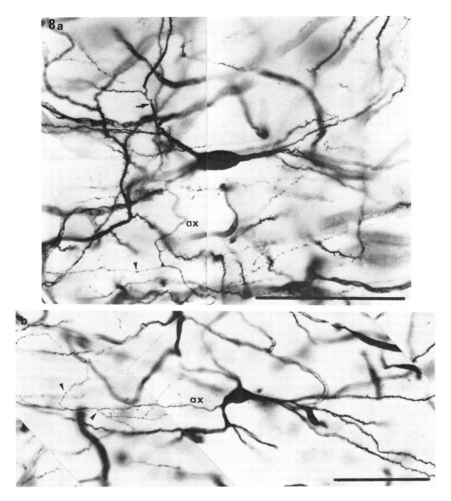

Figure 8. Tangential pyramidal neuron (a) with a short apical dendrite. The ascending basal dendrite is seen (arrow). (b) Small pyramidallike, ovoid neuron at the border between white matter and cortex. Arrowheads point to axonal collaterals. Bars equal 100 μm.

Local-Circuit Neurons (Interneurons) in Layer VI

Ramón y Cajal (1911) analyzed the local-circuit neurons (LCN) in the outer and inner parts of layer VI. He distinguished cells having ascending axons, neurogliaform neurons, and LCNs whose axons arborize in layer VI. He also described large stellate neurons in the outer part of the layer as well as neurons (Martinotti cells) with long ascending axons. On the other hand, O'Leary (1941) divided the short-axon cells into two groups: neurons with axons that arborize locally, usually within the confines of the layers to which the cell body belongs, and other neurons that ramify extensively within several layers. The cell bodies of the neurons having local axonal arborizations are often small and they have few dendrites. The cells of the other group have larger cell bodies and longer

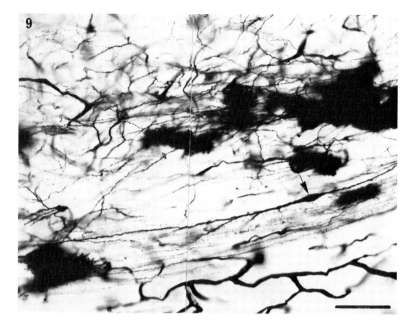

Figure 9. Fusiform bipolar projection neuron in sublamina VIb. Arrow points to the cell body. Bar equals 100 μm.

dendrites. O'Leary demonstrated five types of short-axon neurons in layer VI. One is a small basket neuron (see Chapter 8). Another has horizontal axonal arborizations, while a third type develops a roughly vertical axonal arborization which also ramifies in layer VI. The other two types have ascending axons, and one of then corresponds to the Martinotti cell. Recently, other types of cells have been identified in layer VI (Tömböl, 1978a,b; Peters and Regidor, 1981).

1. *In sublamina VIa,* LCNs of various shape, size, and orientation can be found.

a. One characteristic group of LCNs is composed of pyramidal cells with *medium-size* and *small cell bodies* (Figs. 10a–c). The medium-size pyramidal cell has ordinary apical and basal dendrites which are densely spinous. The apical dendrite ascends to the outermost layer. Several smooth, thick side branches arise from the axon which follows a horizontal course, giving off other varicose branches before it finally divides into two horizontal branches. The terminal arborization of the axon has not been observed so far. However, the axonal arborization pattern of another group of medium size pyramidal neurons is completely different from this, for the axon arises from the base of the cell body, descends for a distance of about 100 μm, and ramifies several times into fine varicose branches. In sublamina VIa small pyramidal neurons with short axons occur. The apical dendrites of the small pyramidal neurons ascend as far as layer IV and they are densely spinous. The remification of the basal dendrites is poor. The axon arborizes after it has passed for only a short distance, and develops a local terminal net.

b. The second group of short-axon cells consists of *pyramidal neurons* with nearly *tangential apical dendrites*. One form is the medium-size pyramidal neuron, which has spinous dendrites. The apical dendrites of these neurons are oriented horizontally, and their basal dendrites are arranged in different directions in layer VI. The axons of these cells ascend up to the outer layers and give off side branches in different layers. Very probably these neurons are the Martinotti cells (Fig. 11a). The other type of tangential pyramidal neuron is small and has smooth dendrites with swellings along their lengths. The axon arises from one of the primary basal dendrites and follows an ascending course to pass into layer IV, where it arborizes (Figs. 11b,c).

c. The *basket neurons of medium size* (Fig. 12) constitute a third group of short-axon cells. From the rounded cell bodies of basket neurons, 8 to 10 thick primary dendrites originate and extend in all directions. They ramify to produce smooth dendrites with conspicuous swellings. The axon of a basket cell arises usually from the cell body, ascends in the parent layer, and within a short distance it produces several thick, horizontal collaterals. These horizontal side branches give off several preterminals which emerge át right angles, and the final section of the axonal trunk arborizes into fine branches that are also oriented in the horizontal plane. Small basket neurons also occur in sublamina VIa (Fig. 13).

d. *Small neurons with round cell bodies*, relatively rich dendritic trees, and different axonal arborizations characterize the neurons in the fourth group of LCNs. The dendritic trees are spherical. Three special subtypes of these neurons can be distinguished: neurogliaform cells, small round cells, and medium round cells. The presence of neurogliaform neurons in layer VI was demonstrated by Ramón y Cajal (1911). The dendritic trees of *neurogliaform* neurons (Fig. 14c) are fairly dense, and are smooth, with irregular swellings (see Chapter 12). The impregnation of the axon is random and it is frequently difficult to recognize it among the relatively thin dendrites. The varicose axon branches to produce an extremely thick and fine axonal network, and there is considerable overlap between the dendritic tree and the axonal arborization. Both extend for about 250–350 μm in all directions.

Small round cells with sparsely spinous dendrites (Fig. 15b) have characteristic axonal arborizations. The number of their dendrites is less than that of the neurogliaform neurons. Thus, five to seven primary dendrites originate from the cell body, and they have a rather straight course with only a few branches. Spines can be observed on their surface only sporadically. The axon of this cell type ascends for a short distance, during which it gives off numerous side branches that extend from both sides, but usually asymmetrically. The axonal branches take a straight course in an oblique direction in the layer and form additional ramifications. The side branches are varicose, and the axonal plexus usually extends well beyond the territory occupied by the dendrites. The axonal plexus is so characteristic that it can even be recognized in kittens on the ninth postnatal day (Fig. 15a). The third subtype of *round cells* is *medium-size*. These cells have five to seven smooth dendrites, with numerous swellings along their lengths. The axons of these neurons originate from the upper surface of the soma and after a short distance they arborize to develop a fairly confined axonal net, which is composed of thin, but strongly varicose, branches (Fig. 14d). This type also has a variety with dendrites that are sparsely spinous (Fig. 10d).

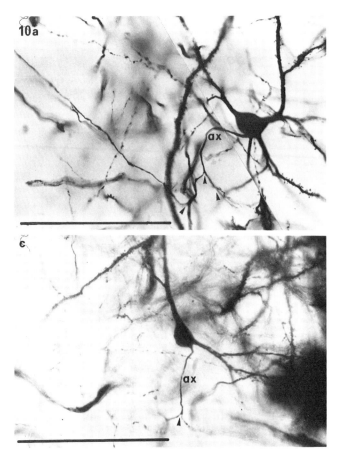

Figure 10. Medium-size pyramidal (a), pyramidallike (b), and small pyramidal (c) LCNs in sublamina VIa. The dendrites are densely spinous. Arrowheads point to the branching of the axons. (d)

e. *Ovoid neurons* of different size, with bipolar, tangentially expanded dendrites can be found in lamina VIa. Three to five dendrites arise from the poles of the ovoid cell body; the dendrites are short and produce tufted arborizations. The secondary dendrites are spiny (Fig. 16) or sparsely spinous (Figs. 14a,b). The neurons in this group show many variations, both in size and in dendritic features. Their axons ascend and ramify into fine, varicose branches. In this group are some vertically oriented, medium-size ovoid bipolar neurons (Fig. 17), with vertically oriented dendritic trees. The axon arises from one pole of the cell and after a short ascent it arborizes in an essentially horizontal plane.

f. The sixth type of LCN in lamina VIa is the *large fusiform neuron* (Fig. 18). The long axis of the neuron is tangentially oriented. The size of the cell body is 30 × 12 μm. The characteristically horizontal dendritic trees arise from two to four major trunks, which branch several times as they extend as far as 300–500 μm from the cell body. The secondary and tertiary dendrites are sparsely spi-

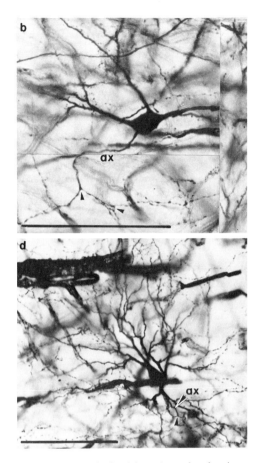

Multipolar, medium-size LCN with smooth dendrites. Arrowhead points to the first branching of the axon. Bars equal 100 μm.

nous. The major trunks originate at, or near, the two poles of the cell body, and although the branchings of dendrites occur at acute angles, the dendritic trees are contained within sublamina VIa. The axons arise from one of the polar dendritic trunks and begin to ramify only a short distance from their origin. The varicose side branches also extend horizontally.

2. *The LCNs in sublamina VIb* are of different types, and four main groups can be distinguished. In this sublamina the tangentially oriented and extended short-axon neurons are dominant.

a. The largest LCNs both in terms of the sizes of their cell bodies and the extensions of their dendritic trees are the *fusiform short-axon cells* or bipolar neurons (Fig. 19a). The dimensions of the cell bodies of the fusiform LCNs are about 30 × 12 μm. Their primary dendritic trunks arise from the two poles of the neuron; they are rather thick and extend for about 60–80 μm before they

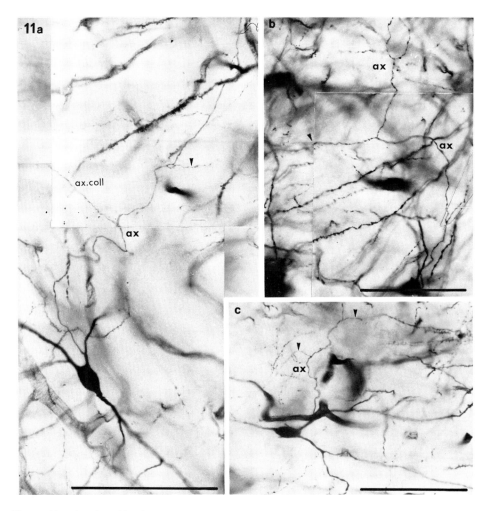

Figure 11. LCNs in sublamina VIa. (a) Martinotti cell with an axon ascending to the outer layers. Axonal collaterals (ax. coll., arrowhead) are given off in layer V. (b,c) Small neurons, pyramidallike, with axons ascending up to layer IV. Arrowheads point to axonal collaterals. Bars equal 100 μm.

bifurcate. Their overall length is 800–1000 μm, and the surfaces of the dendrites are densely covered with spines. The axon usually arises from one of the primary dendritic trunks, or directly from the cell body, and after a distance of about 100 μm it ramifies to form horizontally oriented branches which are varicose and have spinelike side extensions.

b. The second group is made up of *tangentially oriented smooth dendritic pyramidal neurons* (Fig. 20c). The axons arborize over a large field and encompass the width of layer VI. The basal and the apical dendrites branch several times, developing a fairly rich dendritic tree. There are swellings along the smooth dendrites. The axon arises from the cell body and ascends for a short distance before ramifying to form a long and wide axonal plexus located mainly to the

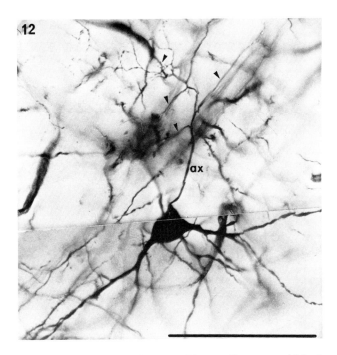

Figure 12. Large basket neuron in sublamina VIa with ascending axon, which gives off horizontal side branches (arrowheads) and forms a terminal plexus. Bar equals 100 μm.

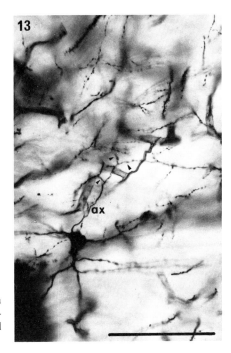

Figure 13. Small basket neuron with ascending axon in sublamina VIa. Arrowheads point to the horizontal side branches and descending preterminal branches. Bar equals 100 μm.

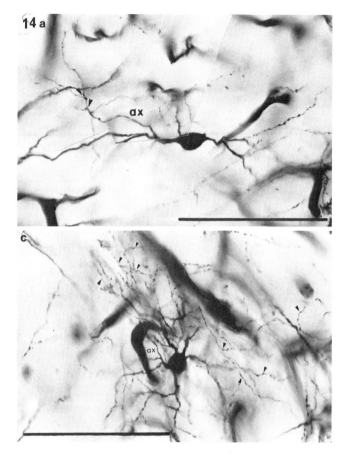

Figure 14. LCNs in sublamina VIa. (a,b) Small ovoid bipolar neurons with sparsely spinous dendritic tufts. Arrowheads point to the branching of the axon. (c) Neurogliaform neuron. The axon arises from one of the dendritic trunks. Arrowheads point to the varicose axonal branches. (d) Round cell

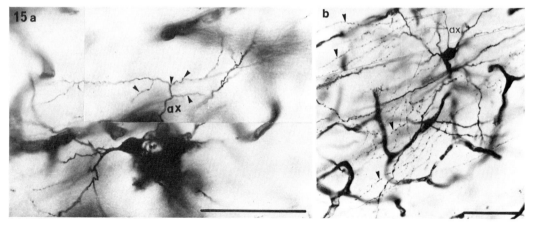

Figure 15. Small round cells with sparsely spinous dendrites in sublamina VIa. Their axons ascend and arborize; arrowheads point to the various axonal branches. (a) Small round cell from a 9-day-old kitten cortex and (b) from an adult cat brain. Bars equal 100 μm.

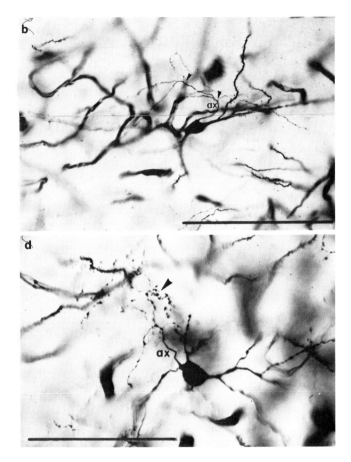

with smooth dendrites. The fairly large varicosities (arrowhead) along the branches of the axon are seen. Bars equal 100 μm.

side of the apical dendrite, but horizontally it extends 800–1000 μm beyond the dendritic tree.

c. The third group of cells in lamina VIb are *medium-size, bipolar neurons* with smooth or spinous dendrites that are tangentially oriented, and are near the border of the white and gray matter (Fig. 21). These ovoid bipolar neurons have densely spinous dendrites with asymmetric dendritic trees. One of their polar dendrites extends as far as 600–800 μm, giving off only a few side branches. The dendrites on the other side of the cell are much shorter. The axons of these neurons arborize parallel to, and adjacent with, the cortical border at the white matter. The dendritic trees of the medium-size bipolar neurons with smooth dendrites are symmetric with regard to both dendritic length, which is about 250 μm, and their pattern of branching. The surfaces of the dendrites are uneven, and swellings are found along their lengths. Axons arise from one of the primary dendritic trunks and become thicker along their course, as they give off varicose and branching side branches. The axonal arborization is only on

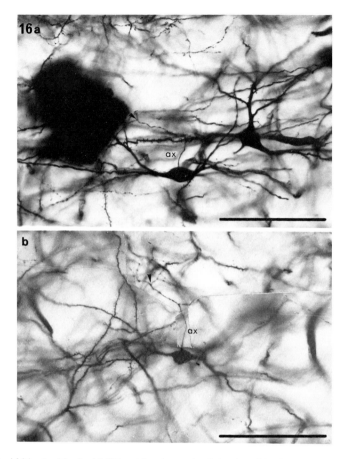

Figure 16. Ovoid bipolar bitufted LCNs with spinous dendrites in sublamina VIa. The axons ascend and arborize (arrowheads). Bars equal 100 μm.

one side of the neuron, and the axon extends far beyond the dendritic tree (Fig. 22).

   d. The fourth group of LCNs is composed of *small neurons with ovoid cell bodies,* with either spinous or smooth dendrites, and *small neurons with round cell bodies* and smooth dendrites. The small ovoid neurons with spinous dendrites are bipolar and are situated horizontally (Figs. 20a,b). At the poles of the ovoid cell body a few dendritic trunks originate and arborize at wide angles. The secondary dendrites are spinous. The axon bifurcates a short distance after its origin; the axonal branches are varicose and extend horizontally. Small ovoid neurons with smooth dendrites have dendrites on one pole of the cell body; at the other pole the axon arises, and this develops a fine varicose axonal net near the white matter (Fig. 19b). The small round cell is localized at the border of white matter and cortex (Fig. 20d). It has a roughly spherical dendritic tree, consisting of several sparsely branching dendrites which have numerous varicosities along their course. The axon arises from the cell body and arborizes to

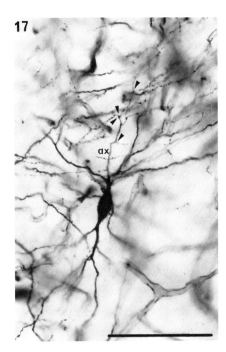

Figure 17. Vertically arranged ovoid LCN in sublamina VIa. The dendrites originate at the poles and are smooth. The axon arises from the ascending dendritic trunk and ramifies (arrowheads) into numerous fine branches. Bar equals 100 μm.

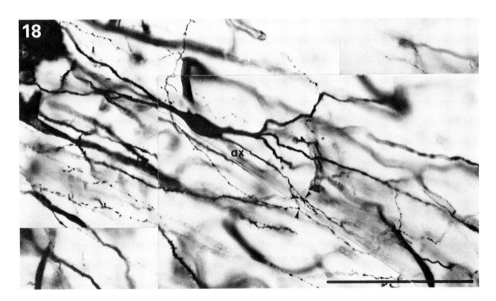

Figure 18. Large fusiform LCN with tangential extending dendrites in sublamina VIa. The axon arises from the cell body and after a short course it arborizes (arrowheads). Bar equals 100 μm.

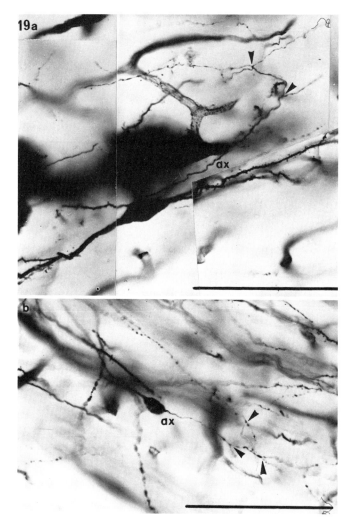

Figure 19. LCNs in sublamina VIb. (a) Large, tangential fusiform neuron with thick dendritic trunks originating at the poles of the cell body. The dendrites are thick and ramify poorly, and are densely spinous. The axon branches (arrowheads) to form varicose branches. (b) Small ovoid neuron with smooth dendrites and a varicose axon which branches (arrowheads) several times. Bars equal 100 μm.

produce fine varicose axonal branches that extend in all directions at the border of white matter and cortex.

The detailed analysis just given suggests that LCNs can be classified into six groups in sublamina VIa and four groups in sublamina VIb. Most of the inter-neuronal types present in the cat can also be observed in other species (Fig. 23). Such distinctions between cell types may seem at first sight to be rather theo-retical, but without doubt, the differences in the extension, orientation, pattern and size of the axonal and dendritic arborizations (Peters and Regidor, 1981), as well as spine density, varicosities, and swellings, must be important in determining the functions of the neurons. The location of the neurons in the sublaminae also seems to be of importance. Some types of LCNs occur only in sublamina VIa, i.e., basket neurons, short-axon pyramidal neurons, etc., while others occur only in sublamina VIb, i.e., tangentially located pyramidal neurons.

4. The Connections of Neurons of Layer VI

4.1. Efferent Connections

Layer VI became a focus of interest when the feedback connections from the cortex to thalamic relay nuclei established by the neurons of layer VI were confirmed. After the first experiments (Gilbert and Kelly, 1975; Gilbert, 1977)

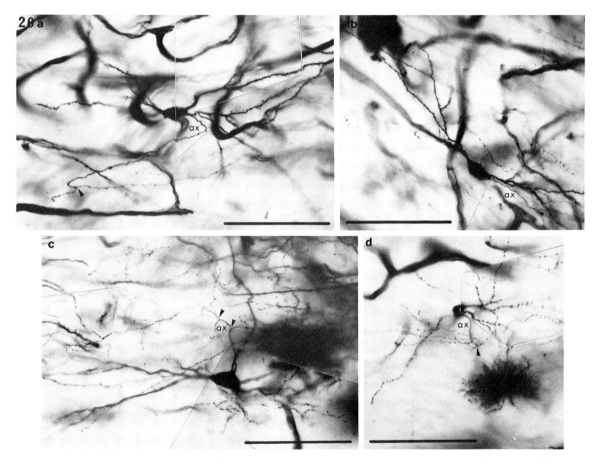

Figure 20. LCNs in sublamina VIb. Small ovoid, bipolar bitufted neurons with spinous dendrites can be seen in (a) and (b). The axon arises from one of the dendritic trunks. Arrowheads point to the ramification of the axon. (c) Tangential pyramidal neuron with smooth dendrites. The axon ascends, bifurcates, and ramifies (arrowheads). (d) Small round cell near the border of white matter. The axon arborizes (arrowhead) into fine varicose branches. Bars equal 100 μm.

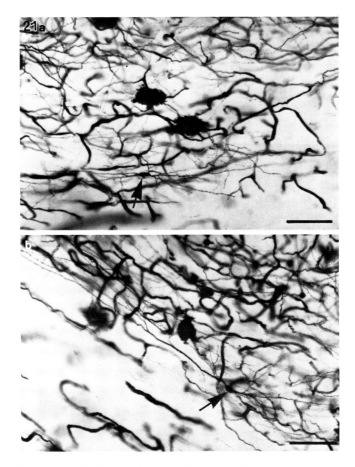

Figure 21. Medium-size ovoid bipolar LCNs at the border of white matter. Arrows point to the cell bodies. (a) Smooth dendritic bipolar cell; (b) ovoid bipolar cell with spinous dendrites. Bars equal 100 μm.

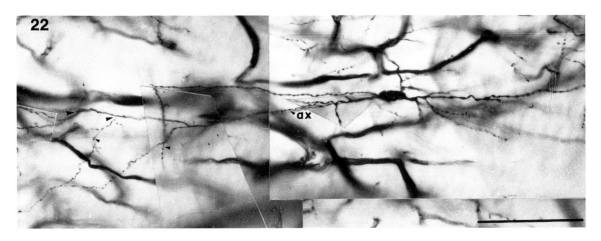

Figure 22. Medium-size ovoid, bipolar LCN with smooth dendritic tufts. The axon arises from one of the dendritic trunks and gives off side branches (arrowheads) which are varicose. Bar equals 100 μm.

a number of other studies were published concerning different cortical areas (Trojanowski and Jacobson, 1975, 1976; Schober *et al.*, 1976; Jones and Wise, 1977; Wong-Reilly, 1977; Somogyi *et al.*, 1978; Madarász *et al.*, 1979; Kelly and Wong, 1981; Lund *et al.*, 1981; Schober, 1981; Swadlow and Weyand, 1981). By injection of HRP, neurons participating in this feedback were identified (Tömböl *et al.*, 1976). It was shown that the pyramidal and pyramidallike and ovoid (multipolar) neurons in sublamina VIa send axons to the relay nuclei of the thalamus. In some cases the fusiform neurons in sublamina VIb were also labeled, probably due to the use of large HRP injections. These neurons may have connections with the nonspecific nuclei of the thalamus (Fig. 24). The efferent connections of layer VI neurons with the thalamic nuclei have not yet been demonstrated in all cortical areas, and it has to be emphasized that these connections may differ between species (Kawamura and Diamond, 1978).

4.2. The Connections of Layer VI Neurons with Cortical Afferents (Specific and Nonspecific)

The existence of a feedback from layer VI to the thalamic relay nuclei suggests that these neurons probably have direct contact with specific fibers arising from the thalamus. Direct contact may be established with the apical dendritic shafts or with apical dendritic tufts in layer IV. The ovoid (multipolar), tangential, pyramidal, and fusiform neurons lacking ascending dendrites have no connections with specific afferents in layer IV. Lorente de Nó (1949) suggested that all layers, including layer VI, contain cells that make synaptic contact with specific afferents from the thalamus. In our Golgi preparations the horizontal branches of specific afferents and their terminals were impregnated, so that their close contact with dendrites of neurons in layer VI could be demonstrated (Tömböl, 1976, 1978a,b). The termination of specific afferents in layer VI was demonstrated by EM degeneration and autoradiographic experiments (Killackey and Ebner, 1973; Sloper, 1973; Peters and Feldman, 1976; Ferster and LeVay, 1978; Lund *et al.*, 1979; Donoghue and Ebner, 1981; Michael, 1981; Schober, 1981; Vogt *et al.*, 1981), which have shown the termination of specific afferents in the outer part of sublamina VIa. According to the EM studies, the number of terminals is low, and they establish axospinous (axodendritic) synapses (Peters *et al.*, 1979). In Golgi-impregnated preparations the entering fiber bundles can rarely be impregnated, and this is particularly true of their side branches at the border of layers VI and V. The arborization of specific afferents is regular; they give off short terminal side branches and have a final terminal arbor which extends in a tangential direction. These terminals are similar to those found in layer IV. Very often close approximation between the terminals and spiny dendrites of projection neurons can be observed (Figs. 25a,b). Other cortical afferents [nonspecific thalamic (Lorente de Nó, 1949; Macchi and Bentivoglio, 1979) and commissural fibers (Sloper, 1973; Jones and Wise, 1977; Kelly and Wong, 1981; Vogt *et al.*, 1981)] can also terminate in layer VI. The association fibers pass through the layer without forming terminals in it (Kawamura and Otani, 1970). Very few neurons whose axons belong to either association or commissural fibers have been found in layer VI in studies employing the HRP method (Ka-

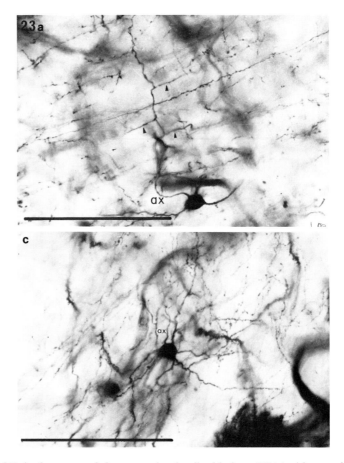

Figure 23. LCNs in the cortex of rhesus monkey localized in layer VI (a) with ascending axon; (b) round and (d) ovoid small LCNs with local axonal arborization; (c) neurogliaform neuron. Bars equal 100 μm.

wamura and Diamond, 1978; Hornung and Garey, 1981; Kelly and Wong, 1981; McKenna *et al.*, 1981; Tiggs *et al.*, 1981). Kelly and Wong (1981) suggest that these projection cells are not identical with the corticothalamic neurons.

In Golgi preparations long ascending vertical afferent fibers which emit several horizontal collaterals in layer VI can be observed. These short side branches are 100–150 μm long, and are fine and varicose. These vertical afferents are very probably either commissural or association fibers. The direction of the horizontal side branches is identical with the course of dendrites present in layer VI (Fig. 26a).

4.3. The Connections of Layer VI Neurons with Axons of Local Origin

1. Layer VI contains many horizontal axonal collaterals. The numerous horizontal axonal collaterals of layer V pyramidal neurons are in this layer, most

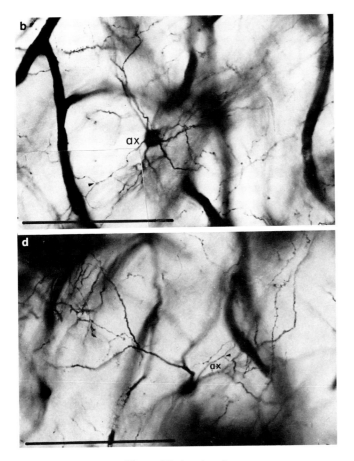

Figure 23. *(continued)*

of them in its outer and middle part (Valverde, 1978). The projection neurons of layer VI also produce several collaterals which have horizontal courses. The axonal collaterals of layer V pyramids give off several short, spinelike processes, while the axonal collaterals of layer VI neurons are varicose. The length of the collaterals is up to 800–1000 μm and they may contact different dendrites. The tangentially localized pyramidal neurons, both projection neurons and LCNs, as well as the bipolar neurons in sublamina VIb, are suitably oriented for contacting horizontal axonal collaterals. In lamina VIb some projection neurons give off their last collaterals while they are in the white matter, but these collaterals turn back into lamina VIb and take a horizontal course (Fig. 26c). The axons arising from pyramidal neurons of outer layers do not give off collaterals in layer VI. In their studies of the collaterals of pyramidal neurons in motor cortex, Landry *et al.* (1980) established that recurrent excitation and inhibition may occur by means of axonal collaterals. The recurrent excitation is produced monosynaptically, while the recurrent inhibition is produced disynaptically in large pyramidal-tract (PT) cells by collaterals of slow PT neurons. The direct

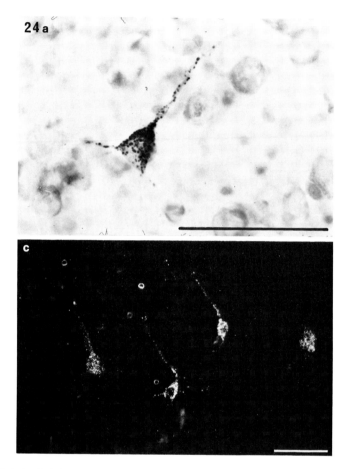

Figure 24. Labeled cells in layer VI in visual cortex (a,b), in somatosensory cortex (c), and in cingulate cortex (d) after HRP injection into the corresponding subcortical areas (i.e., into lateral geniculate body, ventrobasal nucleus, and nucleus anterior ventralis thalami). Pictures were taken by Hajdu, Somogyi, and Madarász in collaboration with the author. Bars equal 100 μm.

excitation has to be produced on the basal dendrites of slow PT cells, while the inhibition has to involve local-circuit neurons together with PT collaterals and slow PT neurons. One can assume that in layer VI the large number of collaterals may have a fundamental significance in controlling the function of the neurons, especially those in sublamina VIb.

2. The axonal terminals of certain LCNs (basket and chandelier neurons) invade layer VI, especially lamina VIa. The terminals of chandelier neurons play an extraordinary role by contacting the axons of projection neurons of layer VI. Golgi–EM studies have proven that the termination of the so-called candle-stick terminals is on the axons of pyramidal neurons (Somogyi *et al.*, 1982) and that the terminals have GABAergic characteristics (Peters *et al.*, 1982) (Figs. 25c,d

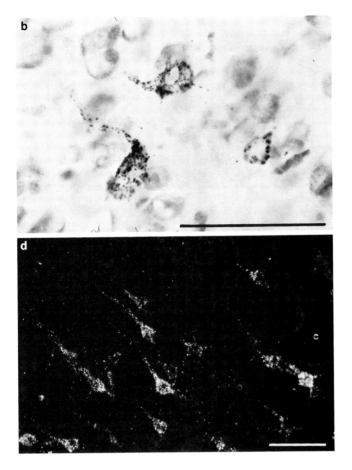

Figure 24. *(continued)*

and Chapter 10). The axonal branches and terminals of some of the "nonpyr-amidal" neurons located in layers II and III also reach layer VI (Somogyi *et al.*, 1981). Their GABAergic terminals are inhibitory (see Volume 2).

3. The axons of LCNs of layer VI have a significant role in the intrinsic synaptic organization of layer VI. There are basically two types of LCN axonal patterns: (1) an abundant axonal ramification in a circumscribed region and (2) a less abundant but long horizontally extended axonal plexus. Gatter and Powell (1978) studied the intrinsic connections in the motor cortex and suggested that short intrinsic cortical axons appear to be distributed predominantly horizontally within their laminae of origin. In addition, there are intrinsic connections ex-tending over 0.5–1.0 mm. The different distances over which the intrinsic fiber

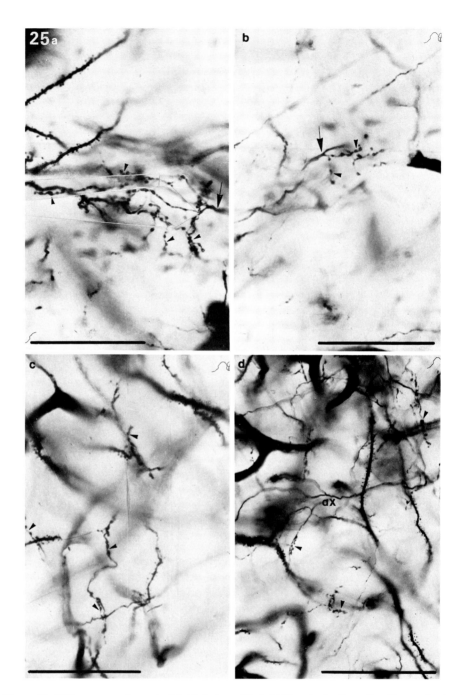

Figure 25. Different axonal terminal fields in layer VI. (a,b) Terminals of specific afferents in visual cortex of cat. Arrows point to the thick fibers and arrowheads show the terminals. (c,d) Axon and candlestick terminals of chandelier neuron (arrowheads). Bars equal 50 μm.

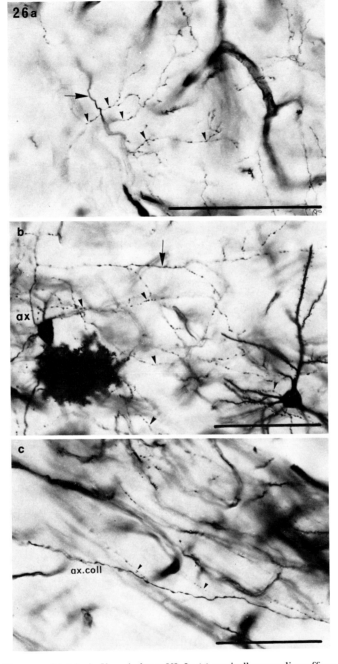

Figure 26. Afferent and intrinsic fibers in layer VI. In (a) vertically ascending afferent fiber (arrow) and its nearly horizontal side branches (arrowheads) can be seen. In (b) the connection between basket (on the left) and a pyramidal neuron (on the right) is demonstrated. The axon of the basket neuron ascends and gives off side branches (arrow) which produce further branches, preterminals, and terminals (arrowheads). In (c) an axonal collateral is seen returning from the white matter to layer VI, giving off very thin side branches (arrowheads). Bars equal 100 μm.

systems extend reflect the fact that they have various functional zones within layer VI. The LCNs of layer VI exert partly inhibitory and partly excitatory effects. The basket neurons which are known to be inhibitory interneurons (see Chapter 8) are present only in sublamina VIa, but one can predict that among LCNs found there, some of the others are also inhibitory (Fig. 26b).

5. Conclusion

Golgi impregnations allow some insight into the organization of the central nervous system. The connections that exist within a given structure can be analyzed only after the different cell types have been identified. The Golgi method by itself does not yield sufficient information about function, but the detailed analysis of the neurons of a region, together with the results obtained by other methods, enable some cautious functional conclusions to be drawn.

In several areas of the cortex the cells of layer VI definitely demonstrate a vertical arrangement (Hassler and Muhs-Clement, 1964); the Golgi architecture, however, reveals that horizontal connections also exist. The axonal collaterals of neurons located in the outer layers, and the axonal collaterals of layer VI projection neurons, and also the axonal arborizations of some LCNs, suggest a horizontal organization. In spite of these facts the neuronal elements of layer VI may indirectly contribute to the columnar organization. The long horizontal expansions of axons may contribute to the organization of large cortical slabs and indirectly they may play a role in the functional organization of small cortical columns.

The connections between the subcortical structures and layer VI became evident by use of the HRP method (Gilbert and Kelly, 1975; Schober *et al.*, 1976; Jones and Wise, 1977; Kawamura and Diamond, 1978; Somogyi *et al.*, 1978; Madarász *et al.*, 1979; Swadlow and Weyand, 1981). The sizes of the injections and the number of labeled cells show a direct correlation. A fairly high percentage of projection neurons (Kelly and Wong, 1981) in sublamina VIa establish contacts with the cells in the specific relay nuclei of the thalamus. The projection neurons of layer VI also contact nonspecific nuclei of the thalamus (Kawamura and Diamond, 1978; Macchi and Bentivoglio, 1979) and this connection may be effected by the neurons of sublamina VIb. The pyramidal neurons of layer VI have direct contacts with specific afferents, producing a monosynaptic feedback in layer VI (Hersch and White, 1981). In addition, ovoid neurons receive direct specific afferents in layer VI (Peters and Feldman, 1976; Donoghue and Ebner, 1981; Vogt *et al.*, 1981). The specific function of projection neurons of sublamina VIa probably has some relation with the specific pigmentation of these cells (Braak, 1980). The tangential fusiform and pyramidal neurons in sublamina VIb, which may contact the nonspecific thalamic centers, get most of their input from the axonal collateral systems. The feedback from these neurons to the nonspecific thalamic cells must be at least also influenced by other nonspecific fibers. The presence of different types of projection neurons, distinguished in Golgi preparations, has been confirmed by the analysis of the connections of

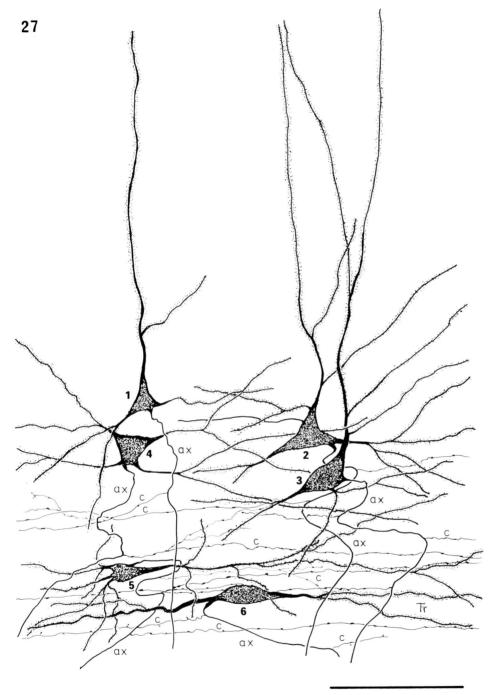

Figure 27. Schematic drawing of projection neurons of layer VI in the cortical area where the curvature is reduced to a minimum. 1 = Small pyramidal neuron; 2 = medium-size pyramidal neuron; 3 = pyramidallike neuron; 4 = multipolar neuron; 5 = tangential pyramidal neuron; 6 = fusiform neuron. c = axonal collateral. Bar equals 100 μm.

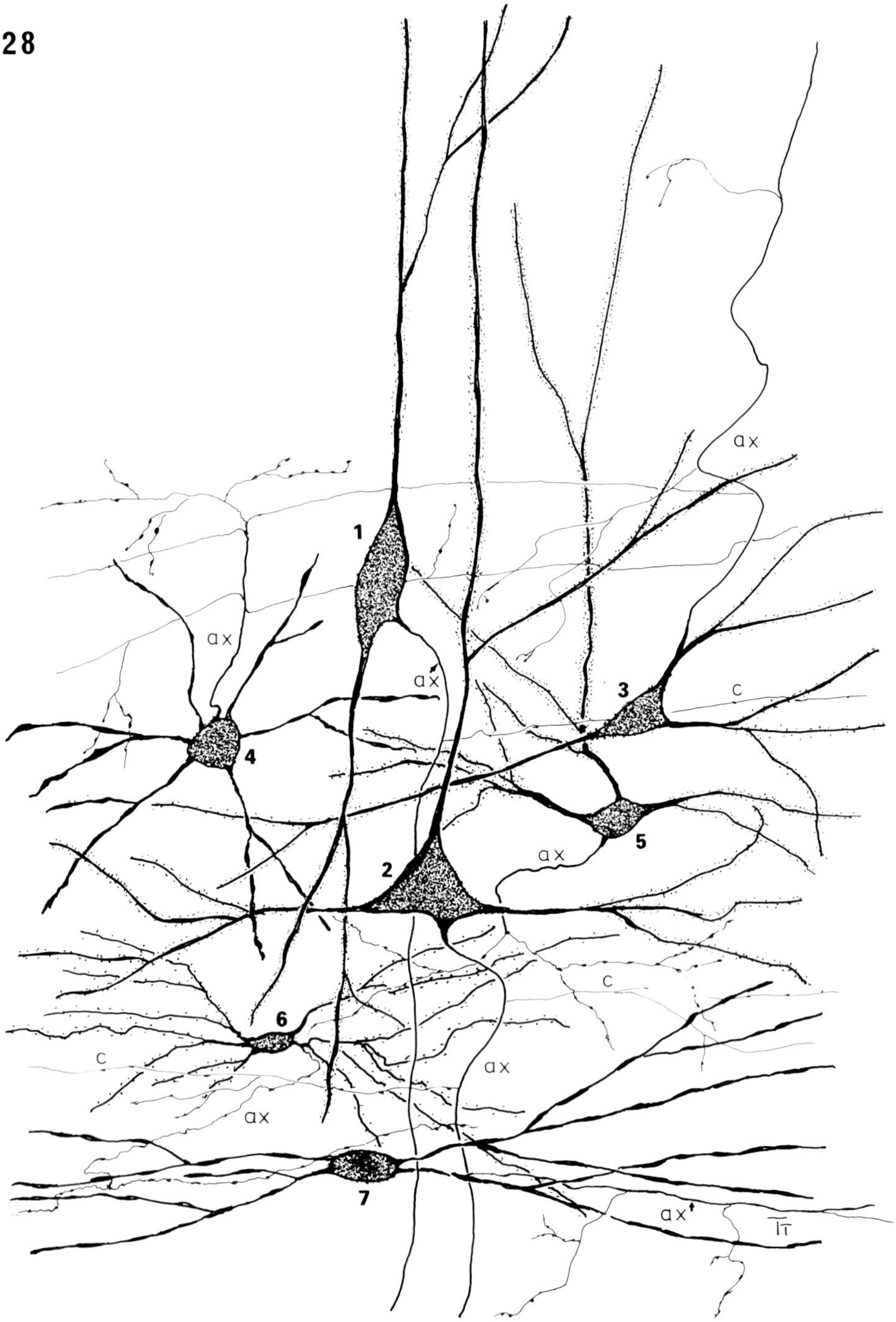

Figure 28. Schematic drawing of projection (1,2) and local-circuit (3–7) neurons of layer VI in a cortical region where the convex curvature is increased to a maximum. 1 = Vertically arranged pyramidal neuron; 2 = medium-size pyramidal neuron; 3 = Martinotti neuron; 4 = basket neuron; 5 = small pyramidal LCN; 6 = small ovoid, bipolar, spinous LCN; 7 = medium-size ovoid bipolar LCN. c = Axonal collateral. Bar equals 100 μm.

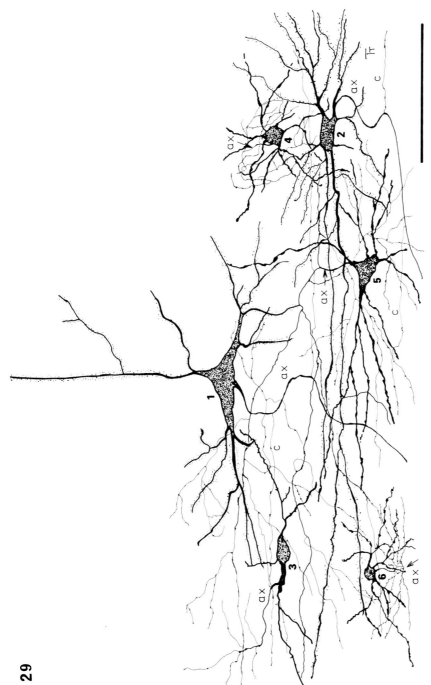

Figure 29. Schematic drawing of projection (1,2) and local-circuit (3–6) neurons of layer VI in a cortical region where the concave curvature is increased to a maximum. 1 = Triangular pyramidal neuron; 2 = tangential pyramidal projection neuron with long apical dendrite; 3 = small ovoid LCN with sparsely spinous dendrites; 4 = neurogliaform neuron; 5 = tangential pyramidal LCN with smooth dendrites; 6 = small round LCN with smooth dendrites. c = Axonal collateral. Bar equals 100 μm.

29

layer VI neurons. The pyramidal, pyramidallike, and also the ovoid (multipolar) projection neurons belong to the same group, because they have connections with specific thalamic nuclei. Another group of projection neurons in sublamina VIb are the bipolar tangential neurons, which are likely to have connections with nonspecific thalamic nuclei. A third group of projection neurons in sublamina VIb contribute to the commissural connections. The projection pyramidal neurons, and their different varieties formed by the convolutions of the cortex, evidently demonstrate a vertical organization within cortical slabs, while the tangential bipolar (fusiform) projection neurons and the tangential pyramidal neurons in sublamina VIb represent other groups with horizontal dendritic extensions (Figs. 27–29). The LCNs can also be divided into several (10) subgroups. The interpretation of this classification is difficult if it is based only on the Golgi method. Some of these neurons clearly participate in the columnar organization, while others are parts of the tangential neuronal network. Between the two main groups are the Martinotti cells with their horizontally extended apical dendrites and vertically ascending axons. The detailed analysis of lamina VI of different cortical areas in cat cerebral cortex suggests some general principles of structure. The principle established earlier (Creutzfeldt, 1978; Powell, 1981), that there are no fundamental differences between the different cortical areas, is also confirmed by the study of the Golgi architecture of layer VI. Moreover, the intrinsic connections of the neurons form links between layer VI and the cortical columnar system. Finally, the function of layer VI in different cortical areas is influenced by the specific afferents which arrive within the cortical areas.

6. References

Braak, H., 1980, Architectonics of the human telencephalic cortex, in: *Studies of Brain Function*, Vol. 4 (H. B. Barlow, E. Florey, O. J. Grüsser, and H. Van der Loos, eds.), Springer-Verlag, Berlin.

Brodmann, K., 1909, Vergleichende Lokalisationslehre der Grosshirnrinde, in: *Ihnen Prinzipien dargestellt auf Grund des Zellenbaues* (J. A. Barth, ed.), Leipzig.

Creutzfeldt, O. D., 1978, The neocortical link: Thoughts on the generality of structure and function of the neocortex, in: *Architectonics of the Cerebral Cortex* (M. A. B. Brazier and H. Petsche, eds.), pp. 357–383. Raven Press, New York.

Donoghue, J. P., and Ebner, F. F., 1981, The laminar distribution and ultrastructure of fibers projecting from three thalamic nuclei to the somatic sensory-motor cortex of the opossum, *J. Comp. Neurol.* **198:**389–420.

Feldman, M. L., and Peters, A., 1978, The forms of non-pyramidal neurons in the visual cortex of the rat, *J. Comp. Neurol.* **179:**761–794.

Ferster, D., and LeVay, S., 1978, The axonal arborizations of lateral geniculate neurons in the striate cortex of the cat, *J. Comp. Neurol.* **182:**923–944.

Fleischhauer, K., and Vossel, A., 1979, Cell densities in the various layers of the rabbit's striate area, *Anat. Embryol.* **156:**269–281.

Fleischhauer, K., Zilles, K., and Schleicher, A., 1980, A revised cytoarchitectonic map of the neocortex of the rabbit (*Oryctolagus cuniculus*), *Anat. Embryol.* **161:**121–143.

Gatter, K. C., and Powell, T. P. S., 1978, The intrinsic connections of the cortex of area 4 of the monkey, *Brain* **101:**513–541.

Gilbert, C. D., 1977, Laminar differences in receptive field properties of cells in cat primary visual cortex, *J. Physiol. (London)* **269:**391–421.

Gilbert, C. D., and Kelly, J. P., 1975, The projections of cells in different layers of the cat's visual cortex, *J. Comp. Neurol.* **163:**81–106.

Golgi, C., 1886, Sulla fina anatomia degli organi centrali del sistema nervoso, Pavia.

Hassler, R., and Muhs-Clement, K., 1964, Architektonischer Aufbau des sensomotorischen und parietalen Cortex der Katze, *J. Hirnforsch.* **6**:377–420.

Hersch, S. M., and White, E. L., 1981, Quantification of synapses formed with apical dendrites of Golgi-impregnated pyramidal cells: Variability in thalamocortical inputs, but consistency in the ratios of asymmetrical to symmetrical synapses, *Neuroscience* **6**:1043–1051.

Hornung, J. P., and Garey, L. J., 1981, Ultrastructure of visual callosal neurons in cat identified by retrograde axonal transport of horseradish peroxidase, *J. Neurocytol.* **10**:297–314.

Jones, E. G., 1975a, Lamination and differential distribution of thalamic afferents within the sensory-motor cortex of the squirrel monkey, *J. Comp. Neurol.* **160**:167–204.

Jones E. G., 1975b, Varieties and distribution of non-pyramidal cells in the somatic sensory cortex of the squirrel monkey, *J. Comp. Neurol.* **160**:205–268.

Jones, E. G., and Burton, H., 1974, Cytoarchitecture and somatic sensory connectivity of thalamic nuclei other than ventrobasal complex in the cat, *J. Comp. Neurol.* **154**:395–432.

Jones, E. G., and Burton, H., 1976, Areal differences in the laminar distribution of thalamic afferents in cortical fields of the insular, parietal and temporal regions of primates, *J. Comp. Neurol.* **168**:197–248.

Jones, E. G., and Wise, S. P., 1977, Size, laminar and columnar distribution of efferent cells in the sensory-motor cortex of monkeys, *J. Comp. Neurol.* **175**:391–438.

Kawamura, S., and Diamond, I. T., 1978, The laminar origin of descending projections from the cortex to the thalamus in *Tupaia glis, Brain Res.* **153**:333–339.

Kawamura, K., and Otani, K., 1970, Corticocortical fiber connections in the rat cerebrum: The frontal region, *J. Comp. Neurol.* **139**:423–448.

Kelly, J. P., and Wong, D., 1981, Laminar connections of the cat's auditory cortex, *Brain Res.* **212**:1–15.

Killackey, H. P., and Ebner, F. F., 1973, Convergent projections of three separate thalamic nuclei onto a single cortical area, *Science* **179**:283–285.

Landry, P., Labelle, A., and Deschênes, M., 1980, Intracortical distribution of axonal collaterals of pyramidal tract cells in the cat motor cortex, *Brain Res.* **191**:327–336.

Lenhossék, M. V., 1895, *Der feinere Bau des Nervensystem* (Fischer, ed.), Berlin.

Lorente de Nó, R., 1949, Cerebral cortex: Architecture, intracortical connections, motor projections, in: *Physiology of the Nervous System* (J. F. Fulton, ed.), 3rd ed., pp. 288–330, Oxford University Press, London.

Lund, J. S., Henry, G. H., MacQueen, C. L., and Harvey, A. R., 1979, Anatomical organization of the primary visual cortex (area 17) of the cat: A comparison with area 17 of the macaque monkey, *J. Comp. Neurol.* **184**:599–618.

Lund, J. S., Hendrickson, A. E., Ogren, M. P., and Tobin, E. A., 1981, Anatomical organization of primate visual cortex area VII, *J. Comp. Neurol.* **202**:19–45.

Macchi, G., and Bentivoglio, M., 1979, The use of axonal transport in the neuroanatomical study of the subcortical projections to the neocortex, *Arch. Ital. Anat. Embriol.* **84**(Suppl.):35–83.

McKenna, T. M., Whitsel, B. L., Dreyer, D. A., and Metz, C. B., 1981, Organization of cat anterior parietal cortex: Relations among cytoarchitecture, single neuron functional properties, and interhemispheric connectivity, *J. Neurophysiol.* **45**:667–697.

Madarász, M., Tömböl, T., Hajdu, F., and Somogyi, G., 1979, A combined horseradish peroxidase and Golgi study on the afferent connections of the ventrobasal complex of the thalamus in the cat, *Cell Tissue Res.* **199**:529–538.

Marin-Padilla, M., 1975, LCNs in the neocortex, in: *Local Circuit Neurons* (P. Rakic, ed.), pp. 91–98, MIT Press, Cambridge, Mass.

Marin-Padilla, M., 1978, Dual origin of the mammalian neocortex and evolution of the cortical plate, *Anat. Embryol.* **152**:109–126.

Martinotti, S., 1890, Beitrag zum Studium der Hirnrinde und der ventralen Ursprung der Nerven, *Int. Monatschr. Anat. Physiol.* **8.**

Meynert, T., 1870, Von Gehirne der Saugethiere, in: *Handbuch der Lehre von den Geweben des Menschen und der Thiere*, Vol. 2 (Stricker, ed.), pp. 694–808.

Michael, C. R., 1981, Columnar organization of color cells in monkey's striate cortex, *J. Neurophysiol.* **46**:587–604.

O'Leary, J. L., 1941, Structure of the area striata of the cat, *J. Comp. Neurol.* **75**:131–164.

O'Leary, J. L., and Bishop, G. H., 1938, The optically excitable cortex of the rabbit, *J. Comp. Neurol.* **68:**423–477.

Otsuka, R., and Hassler, R., 1962, Über Aufbau und Gliederung der corticalen Sehsphäre bei der Katze, *Arch. Psychiatr. Nervenkr.* **203:**213–234.

Peters, A., and Fairén, A., 1978, Smooth and sparsely-spined stellate cells in the visual cortex of the rat: A study using a combined Golgi–electron microscope technique, *J. Comp. Neurol.* **181:**129–172.

Peters, A., and Feldman, M., 1976, The projection of the lateral geniculate nucleus to the area 17 of the rat cerebral cortex, *J. Neurocytol.* **5:**85–107.

Peters, A., and Regidor, J., 1981, A reassessment of the forms of nonpyramidal neurons in area 17 of cat visual cortex, *J. Comp. Neurol.* **203:**685–716.

Peters, A., and Walsh, T. M., 1972, A study of the organization of apical dendrites in the somatic sensory cortex of the rat, *J. Comp. Neurol.* **144:**253–268.

Peters, A., Proskauer, C C., Feldman, M. L., and Kimerer, L., 1979, The projection of the lateral geniculate nucleus to area 17 of the rat cerebral cortex, V. Degenerating axon terminals synapsing with Golgi impregnated neurons, *J. Neurocytol.* **8:**331–357.

Peters, A., Proskauer, C. C., and Ribak, C. E., 1982, Chandelier cells in rat visual cortex, *J. Comp. Neurol.* **206:**397–416.

Powell, T. P. S., 1981, Certain aspects of the intrinsic organisation of the cerebral cortex, in: *Brain Mechanisms and Perceptual Awareness* (O. Pompeiano and C. Ajmone Marsan, eds.), pp. 1–19, Raven Press, New York.

Raedler, E. and Raedler, A., 1978, Autoradiographic study of early neurogenesis in rat neocortex, *Anat. Embryol.* **154:**267–284.

Rakic, P., 1975, Definition of the term, "local circuit neuron," and the concept of local neuronal circuits, in: *Local Circuit Neurons, Neurosci. Res. Program Bull.* **13:**299–309.

Rakic, P., 1981, Developmental events leading to laminar and areal organization of the neocortex, in: *The Organization of the Cerebral Cotex* (F. O. Schmitt, ed.), pp. 7–28, MIT Press, Cambridge, Mass.

Ramón y Cajal, S., 1911, *Histologie du Système Nerveux de l'Homme et des Vertébrés*, Vol. II, Maloine, Paris.

Schaffer, K., 1897, Zur feineren Structur der Stirnrinde und über die funktionelle Bedeutung der Nervenzellenforsatze, *Arch. Mikrosk. Anat. Entwicklungsmech.* **XLVIII.**

Schober, W., 1981, Efferente und afferente Verbindungen des Nucleus lateralis posterior thalami ("Pulvinar") der Albinoratte, *Z. Mikrosk. Anat. Forsch.* **95:**827–844.

Schober, W., Lüth, H. J., and Gruschka, H., 1976, Die Herkunft afferenter Axone im striären Cortex der Albinoratte: Eine Studie mit Meerrettich-Peroxidase, *Z. Mikrosk. Anat. Forsch.* **90:**399–415.

Shkol'nik-Yarros, E. G., 1960, Neurons of visual cortex in man, *Arch. Anat. Histol. Embryol.* **32:**24–38.

Sloper, J. J., 1973, An electron microscope study of the termination of afferent connections to the primate motor cortex, *J. Neurocytol.* **2:**361–368.

Somogyi, G., Hajdu, F., Tömböl, T., and Madarász, M., 1978, Limbic projections to the cat thalamus: A horseradish peroxidase study, *Acta Anat.* **102:**68–73.

Somogyi, P., Cowey, A., Halász, N., and Freund, T. F., 1981, Vertical organization of neurones accumulating ^{3}H-GABA in visual cortex of rhesus monkey, *Nature (London)* **294:**761–763.

Somogyi, P., Freund, T. F., and Cowey, A., 1982, The axo-axonic interneuron in the cerebral cortex of the rat, cat, and monkey, *Neuroscience* **7:**2577–2608.

Swadlow, H. A., and Weyand, T. G., 1981, Efferent systems of the rabbit visual cortex: Laminar distribution of the cells of origin, axonal conduction velocities, and identification of axonal branches, *J. Comp. Neurol.* **203:**799–822.

Szentágothai, J., 1969, Architecture of the cerebral cortex, in: *Basic Mechanisms of the Epilepsies* (H. H. Jasper, A. A. Ward, and A. Pope, eds), pp. 13–28, Little, Brown, Boston.

Szentágothai, J., 1975, The 'module-concept' in cerebral cortex architecture, *Brain Res.* **95:**475–496.

Szentágothai, J., 1978a, The neuron network of the cerebral cortex: A functional interpretation. Ferrier Lecture, *Proc. R. Soc. London Ser. B.* **201:**219–248.

Szentágothai, J., 1978b, Specificity versus (quasi-) randomness in cortical connectivity, in: *Architectonics of the Cerebral Cortex* (M. A. B. Brazier and H. Petsche, eds.), pp. 77–97, Raven Press, New York.

Szentágothai, J., and Arbib, M. A., 1974, Conceptual models of neural organization, *Neurosci. Res. Program Bull.* **12:**307–510.

Tigges, J., Tigges, M., Anschel, S., Cross, N. A., Letbetter, W. D., and McBride, R. L., 1981, Areal and laminar distribution of neurons interconnecting the central visual cortical areas 17, 18, 19 and MT in squirrel monkey *(Saimiri), J. Comp. Neurol.* **202**:539–560.

Tömböl, T., 1972, A Golgi analysis of the sensory-motor cortex in the rabbit, in: *Synchronization of EEG Activity in Epilepsies* (H. Petsche and M. A. B. Brazier, eds.), pp. 25–36, Springer, Berlin.

Tömböl, T., 1976, Golgi analysis of the internal layers (V–VI) of the cat visual cortex, in: *Afferent and Intrinsic Organization of Laminated Structures in the Brain* (O. Creutzfeldt, ed.), pp. 292–295, Springer-Verlag, Berlin.

Tömböl, T., 1978a, Comparative data on the Golgi architecture of interneurons of different cortical areas in cat and rabbit, in: *Architectonics of the Cerebral Cortex* (M. A. B. Brazier and H. Petsche, eds.), pp 59–76, Raven Press, New York.

Tömböl, T., 1978b, Some Golgi data on visual cortex of the rhesus monkey, *Acta Morphol. Acad. Sci. Hung.* **26**:115–138.

Tömböl, T., 1980, Some data on postnatal maturation of the cerebral cortex in cat, *Acta Biol. Acad. Sci. Hung.* **31**:341–365.

Tömböl, T., Hajdu, F., and Somogyi, G., 1975a, Identification of the Golgi picture of the layer VI cortico-geniculate projection neurons, *Exp. Brain Res.* **24**:107–110.

Tömböl, T., Hajdu, F., and Somogyi, G., 1975b, Medium range intracortical connections established by non-pyramidal neurons, *Verh. Anat. Ges.* **69**:527–530.

Tömböl, T., Madarász, M., Hajdu, F., and Somogyi, G., 1976, Some data on the Golgi architecture of visual areas and suprasylvian gyrus in the cat, *Verh. Anat. Ges.* **70**:271–275.

Trojanowski, J. Q., and Jacobson, S., 1975, A combined horseradish peroxidase–autoradiographic investigation of reciprocal connections between superior temporal gyrus and pulvinar in squirrel monkey, *Brain Res.* **85**:347–353.

Trojanowski, J. Q., and Jacobson, S., 1976, Areal and laminar distribution of some pulvinar cortical efferents in rhesus monkey, *J. Comp. Neurol.* **169**:371–392.

Valverde, F., 1978, The organization of area 18 in the monkey: A Golgi study, *Anat. Embryol.* **154**:305–334.

Vogt, B. A., and Peters, A., 1981, Form and distribution of neurons in rat cingulate cortex: Areas 32, 24, and 29, *J. Comp. Neurol.* **195**:603–625.

Vogt, B. A., Rosene, D. L., and Peters, A., 1981, Synaptic termination of thalamic and callosal afferents in cingulate cortex of the rat, *J. Comp. Neurol.* **201**:265–283.

Vogt, C., and Vogt, O., 1919, Allgemeinere Ergebnisse unserer Hirnforschung, *J. Psychol. Neurol.* **25**:279–462.

von Economo, C., and Koskinas, G. N., 1925, *Die Cytoarchitektonik der Hirnrinde des erwächsenen Menschen*, Springer, Berlin.

Wolff, J. R., 1978, Ontogenetic aspects of cortical architecture: Lamination, in: *Architectonics of the Cerebral Cortex* (M. A. B. Brazier and H. Petsche, eds.), pp. 159–173, Raven Press, New York.

Wong-Riley, M., 1977, Connections between the pulvinar nucleus and the peristriate cortex in the squirrel monkey as revealed by peroxidase histochemistry and autoradiography, *Brain Res.* **134**:225–236.

Woolsey, C. N., 1958, Organization of somatic sensory and motor areas of the cerebral cortex, in: *Biological and Biochemical Basis of Behavior* (H. Harlow and C. N. Woolsey, eds.), pp. 63–81, University of Wisconsin Press, Madison.

16

Laminar Distribution of Cortical Efferent Cells

EDWARD G. JONES

1. Introduction

Lamination is one of the hallmarks of the cerebral cortex. Despite the early recognition of this characteristic feature of cortical histology, however, there is still little understanding of the fundamental organizing principle that governs it. Does each lamina represent an aggregation of cells with like input connections? With like output connections? With both? Or is there some other unifying factor, such as a particular set of local-circuit neurons, that serves to bring together disparate cell types as a histological and perhaps functional entity? Though at the present time we have no definite answers to many of these questions, we are in a position to say that in large part each lamina represents the aggregation of somata of pyramidal cells that send their axons to a common target outside the cortical area in which they lie. The rest of the chapter is, therefore, devoted to describing the different types of connectional relationships exhibited by pyramidal cells in different layers.

The pyramidal cells are the output cells of the cerebral cortex (Chapter 5). There appears to be only a single well-documented case of nonpyramidal cells sending axons outside the cortical area in which they lie. (This relates to a particular class of large spiny cells, seemingly found only in layer IVb of the

EDWARD G. JONES • James L. O'Leary Division of Experimental Neurology and Neurological Surgery and McDonnell Center for Studies of Higher Brain Function, Washington University School of Medicine, Saint Louis, Missouri 63110.

primate visual cortex and referred to below.) Conversely, there appear to be few authenticated cases of pyramidal cells with axons that are confined to the cortical area in which they lie. Because of their long axons, pyramidal cells are more accessible to experimental manipulation than intrinsic neurons and over the years they have been studied by the methods of retrograde degeneration, antidromic stimulation, and retrograde axoplasmic transport. The more recent studies that made use of retrograde axoplasmic transport have given us a fairly clear idea of the laminar disposition of the parent cell somata of virtually every cortical efferent system in a variety of mammals and in many cortical areas.

2. Early Anatomical Studies

2.1. Early Studies of Cellular Degeneration

Many early experimental studies that attempted to define the cells of origin of cortical efferent pathways by retrograde cellular degeneration were unsuccessful. After sectioning various fiber systems, such as the corticospinal tract and the corpus callosum, it was widely reported that the cells of the cerebral cortex underwent little or no retrograde reaction. The belief thus grew up that the cells were in some way preserved from retrograde atrophy by their possession of substantial numbers of intracortical, collateral axon branches (Ramón y Cajal, 1928).

Despite this, however, a number of reports continued to appear suggesting not only that a retrograde reaction might indeed be identified in the cerebral cortical cells, but also that this could be used to localize the cell bodies of origin of certain efferent pathways. Among these reports were those of Campbell (1905) who discovered an 87.5% decrease in the number of Betz cells in the motor cortex of individuals suffering from amyotrophic lateral sclerosis. He also reported several cases in which he observed severe chromatolysis of Betz cells in appropriate parts of the motor representation following long-standing amputation of a limb (Fig. 1). A few years later, Holmes and Page May (1909) and Nissl (1908) found atrophy only of deep layers of the cortex (especially the large cells in layer V) in man and animals after destructive lesions of the spinal cord but atrophy of all layers after lesions of the subcortical white matter. Bielschowsky (1916) considered that he had confirmed the infragranular origin of the subcortical projections by the absence of corticofugal degeneration in the internal capsule following encephalitic destruction of only the superficial layers of the cortex in man. Findings such as this, coupled with indications of selective atrophy of the supragranular layers in long-standing cases of insanity, led Campbell (1905), Bolton (1910), and others to suggest that the infragranular layers were efferent or motor and the supragranular "associative."

Among later experimental studies, Pines and Maiman (1939) noted retrograde degeneration of large pyramidal cells in the deeper part of layer III and in layers V and VI of the dog cortex following section of the corpus callosum. These findings have been duplicated for layer III, many years later, in the cat and monkey by Shoumura (1974) and Glickstein and Whitteridge (1976).

523

**LAMINAR
DISTRIBUTION
OF CORTICAL
EFFERENT
CELLS**

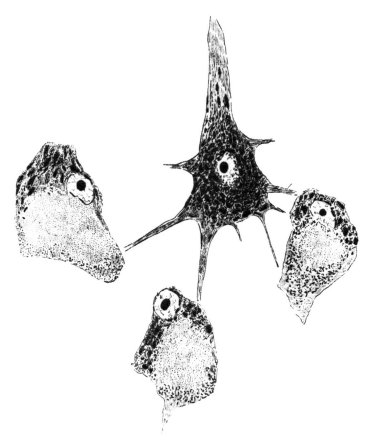

Figure 1. Campbell's camera lucida drawings of three giant cells in the medial part of the human cortex undergoing chromatolysis as the result of amputation of contralateral lower limb some years previously, with a normal cell from the same area for comparison. From Campbell (1905).

2.2. Studies with the Golgi Technique

Golgi studies have not been particularly useful in elucidating the differential projections of pyramidal neurons in separate cortical layers, for the obvious reason that, even if well impregnated, the axons can rarely be traced over long distances. Ramón y Cajal (1909–1911, 1922) was especially cautious about the efferent targets of the cells that he impregnated. With the possible exception of certain small pyramidal cells of layer IV in the cat visual cortex, that had strongly recurrent axons, he seems to have regarded pyramidal cells of all layers as having axons that entered the white matter. But, otherwise, he limited himself to the remark that callosal axons appeared to arise from small and medium-size cells and as collaterals of projection and association axons emanating from large pyramidal cells. He noted (1922) that some collaterals given off in the white matter could return to the area of origin.

Lorente de Nó (1922, 1949) noted the origins of callosal and corticorcortical axons from layer III pyramids and from short pyramidal cells at the border of layers V and VI in the mouse. He also mentioned that some of the irregularly shaped cells of layer VI gave rise to callosal and to short association fibers to neighboring fields and suggested that large layer V pyramids sent axons to subcortical sites with many collaterals in the basal ganglia. O'Leary and Bishop (1938) and O'Leary (1941) though noting that probably all pyramidal cells had axons that left the cortex, did not indicate their targets.

3. Electrophysiological Studies

Up until quite recent times, the methods of electrophysiology, in general, lacked sufficient resolution to detect the differential laminar origins of particular sets of cortical efferent axons. Even now the technique of intracortical micro-stimulation (Asanuma and Rosén, 1972) does not lend itself particulary well to this type of analysis because of the difficulty of determining whether the cell soma or some more distant part of a neuron is being activated and whether the effect is direct or transsynaptic (Jankowska *et al.*, 1975).

The electrophysiological method that lends itself best to the laminar analysis of the cells of origin of corticofugal axons, though not without interpretational problems, involves detecting the antidromic invasion of the parent soma by an action potential set up by electrical stimulation of the target site of the axon or of the axon itself. This type of work has a long history in regard to the cells of origin of the corticospinal tract (see Phillips and Porter, 1977, for a review) but until recently the method had been less widely used to seek the cells of origin of other output connections. In the case of the corticospinal tract, early studies (e.g., Towe *et al.*, 1963) had interpreted the antidromic field potentials and cellular responses in the cat motor cortex as indicating a localization of the somata of large, rapidly conducting neurons in layer V and the somata of small, slowly conducting neurons in layer III. More recent physiological and anatomical work has disproved this, showing the localization of the parent cells of both sets of axons in layer V (Asanuma and Rosén, 1972; Coulter *et al.*, 1976; Humphrey and Corrie, 1978)(Fig. 2).

Other studies that made use of the method of antidromic activation, coupled with careful histological reconstruction of recording sites, served to localize the cells of origin of corticomedullary axons to layer V of the cat sensory motor cortex (Gordon and Miller, 1969); those of the corpus callosum to layer III of the cat somatic sensory and cat and rabbit visual cortex (Miller, 1975; Toyama *et al.*, 1974; Swadlow and Weyand, 1981); those of corticotectal axons to layer V and of corticogeniculate axons to layer VI of the cat and rabbit visual cortex (Toyama *et al.*, 1974; Gilbert, 1977; Harvey, 1978, 1980; Palmer and Rosenquist, 1974; Swadlow and Weyand, 1981); and those of corticorubal axons to layer V of the cat and monkey motor cortex (Humphrey and Rietz, 1976; Humphrey and Corrie, 1978). For the purposes of localizing the cell bodies of origin of a particular set of efferent axons, however, the method has been largely superseded by the anatomical, retrograde tracing methods to be discussed in Section 4.1.

525

**LAMINAR
DISTRIBUTION
OF CORTICAL
EFFERENT
CELLS**

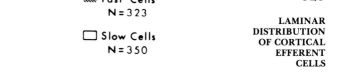

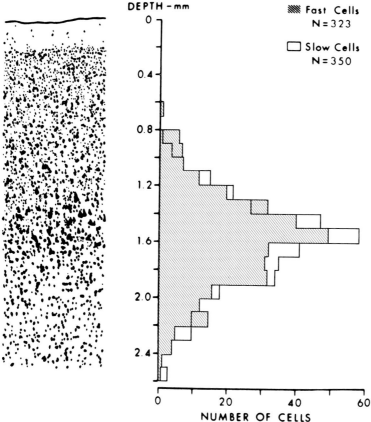

Figure 2. Laminar distribution of somata of pyramidal tract neurons in the wrist extensor area of the monkey motor cortex, as detected by antidromic invasion of the somata following electrical stimulation of the bulbar pyramid. From Humphrey and Corrie (1978).

One of the advantages of the antidromic method over the anatomical, retrograde labeling method is that it permits the discharge properties, receptive fields, and other features of a projecting neuron's behavior to be specified. In the cat visual cortex, for example, corticotectal neurons have receptive field properties that distinguish them from other "complex cells" (in particular, the lack of summation with stimulus length along the receptive field axis) (Palmer and Rosenquist, 1974). The corticotectal cells are binocularly activated and show selectivity for the direction of a moving stimulus. The latter property is also possessed by cells in the superficial layers of the superior colliculus but is lost by those cells if the visual cortex is ablated in the cat or rabbit (Wickelgren and Sterling, 1969; Berman and Cynader, 1975; Mize and Murphy, 1976; Graham *et al.*, 1982), though not in the monkey (Schiller *et al.*, 1974) or ground squirrel (Michael, 1972).

Layer V cells projecting from area 18 of the cat visual cortex to the visual area of the pontine nuclei also possess well-defined receptive field properties that distinguish them from other area 18 cells but are very similar to those of the pontine visual cells themselves (Gibson *et al.*, 1978a,b).

Corticorubral neurons in the motor cortex of the monkey when identified antidromically have been found to resemble red nucleus neurons more closely than they do pyramidal tract neurons (Fromm *et al.*, 1981). (Fig. 3). The background activity of corticorubral neurons is lower; corticorubral neurons tend to increase their discharge at or after the onset of a voluntary movement, rather than before; the two cell types show different responses to steady-state forces, joint position, and to passive changes in limb position. The axons of corticorubral neurons in the monkey motor cortex have conduction velocities estimated at about 15 m/sec as compared with 50–55 m/sec for fast pyramidal tract neurons and 8–12 m/sec for slow (Humphrey and Corrie, 1978; Fromm *et al.*, 1981). This implies that corticorubral neurons are smaller than most pyramidal tract neurons, an observation confirmed by anatomical tracing methods (Jones and Wise, 1977). Careful reconstruction of recording sites in the motor cortex is in accord with the anatomical results in indicating that the somata of these small, corticorubral neurons lie above those of the pyramidal tract neurons in the upper part of layer V (Humphrey and Rietz, 1976; Humphrey and Corrie, 1978). Approximately 10% of the motor cortex neurons projecting to the red nucleus, however, have antidromic latencies approaching those of pyramidal tract neurons and, moreover, can be antidromically activated by stimulation of the pyramidal tract as well as of the red nucleus, implying collateral branching to both sites (Humphrey and Corrie, 1978; Fromm *et al.*, 1981). There is some anatomical confirmation of this, though all such branched axons seem to terminate in the magnocellular red nucleus (Catsman-Berrevoets *et al.*, 1979). The somata of origin of branched axons seem to lie in the the deeper part of layer V and have discharge properties intermediate between those of corticorubral neurons and pyramidal tract neurons (Fromm *et al.*, 1981).

The preceding examples have been of cortical efferent neurons whose properties resemble those of neurons at their target sites and which differ from those of other neurons in the cortical area in which the lie. In one instance at least, however, the receptive field properties of a set of output neurons are quite varied and represent virtually the full range of receptive field types found in their area of origin. As recorded in the splenium of the cat corpus callosum, the receptive fields of the callosal axons can reflect all the receptive field types found in the visual cortex in which they arise and terminate (Berlucchi *et al.*, 1967; Hubel and Wiesel, 1967; Harvey, 1980). Similarly, corticogeniculate neurons identified antidromically in layer VI of the cat striate area include both simple and complex types and show a rather wide range of conduction velocities (Gilbert, 1977; Harvey, 1978).

Several studies of the cat visual cortex have concentrated on the types of receptive fields possessed by output neurons projecting to different sites, and also on determining which of these may receive monosynaptic thalamic connections. As already mentioned, both callosal and corticogeniculate neurons can have receptive field properties that result in them being classified as simple and complex cells and both types have been reported to receive monosynaptic thalamic connections (Gilbert, 1977; Bullier and Henry, 1979; Harvey, 1980; Ferster

527

**LAMINAR
DISTRIBUTION
OF CORTICAL
EFFERENT
CELLS**

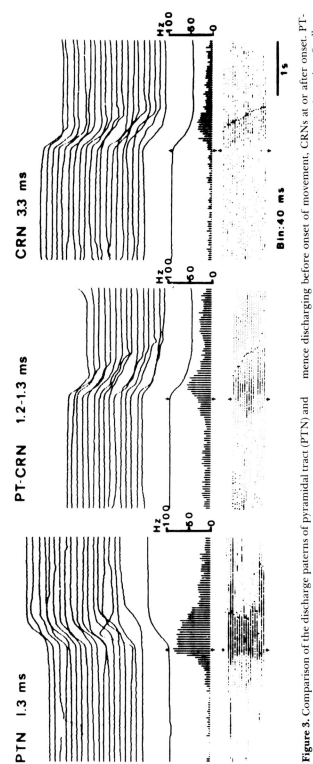

Figure 3. Comparison of the discharge paterns of pyramidal tract (PTN) and corticorubral (CRN) neurons and neurons with axons branching to both sites (PT-CRN) in the motor cortex of monkey performing a pronation–supination movement of the forearm. Movement indicated by upper trace. PTNs commence discharging before onset of movement, CRNs at or after onset. PT-CRNs have intermediate discharge patterns. Antidromic latencies of cells to stimulation of axon indicated at top. From Fromm *et al.* (1981).

and Lindstrom, 1983). Corticotectal neurons appear to form a special class of complex cells (Palmer and Rosenquist, 1974; Gilbert, 1977; Harvey, 1980), and corticopontine neurons a further class of complex cells (Gibson *et al.*, 1978a).

4. Retrograde Tracing Studies

4.1. Localization of Cell Somata

The introduction of anatomical techniques by means of which the cells of origin of any long tract could be readily labeled by retrograde axoplasmic transport led to a large number of studies on the laminar origins of cortical efferent systems. In a rather short time, knowledge of efferent lamination advanced more than it had in the preceding half-century.

The first studies seem to have been those of Holländer (1974) on the cells of origin of corticotectal fibers in the cat, of Jacobson and Trojanowski (1974) and Wong-Riley (1974) on the cells of origin of the corpus callosum in rats, cats, and monkeys, and of Maciewicz (1974) on cells with corticocortical projections in the visual areas of the cat. These were immediately followed by a number of studies that localized the cells of origin of a particular efferent pathway (Berrevoets and Kuypers, 1975; Jacobson and Trojanowski, 1975; Jones *et al.*, 1975; Magalhães-Castro *et al.*, 1975; Robson and Hall, 1975; Romagnano and Maciewicz, 1975; Spatz, 1975; Winfield *et al.*, 1975; Coutler *et al.*, 1976; Weisberg and Rustioni, 1976; Wise and Jones, 1976; Humphrey and Rietz, 1976; Gibson *et al.*, 1978a; Jones *et al.*, 1977, 1978; Wise and Jones, 1977a,b). Other studies surveyed the whole range of efferents arising from a particular area in a particular species (Gilbert and Kelly, 1975; Lund *et al.*, 1975a,b; Wise, 1975; Ravizza *et al.*, 1976; Jones and Wise, 1977; Wise and Jones, 1977a,b).

From these early studies, the following pattern of organization appeared to emerge. Subcortical projections all arise from infragranular neurons: those projecting to the thalamus arise from layer VI and to a lesser extent from layer V; those projecting to other subcortical sites such as spinal cord, tectum, medulla oblongata, pons, red nucleus, and striatum arise only from layer V; corticocortical and callosal projections arise predominantly from the supragranular layers with some species variation in that more significant numbers arise from infragranular layers in rodents than in primates (Figs. 4–8).

Further refinements of this basic pattern included evidence that the corticothalamic projection to the principal thalamic relay nucleus for a particular cortical area arises only from layer VI while that to the intralaminar or other "nonspecific" thalamic nuclei arises only from layer V (Gilbert and Kelly, 1975; Lund *et al.*, 1975; Catsman-Berrevoets and Kuypers, 1978). Within layer VI itself of the monkey visual cortex, superficially placed cells project to the parvo- and deeply situated cells to the magnocellular layers of the lateral geniculate nucleus (Lund *et al.*, 1975). In layer V the largest and most deeply situated cells project to the spinal cord (Fig. 6) while the most superficial and smallest project to the striatum. In between, tend to lie those projecting to other subcortical sites, though there is considerable overlap (Jones and Wise, 1977; Foster *et al.*, 1981) (Figs.

529

**LAMINAR
DISTRIBUTION
OF CORTICAL
EFFERENT
CELLS**

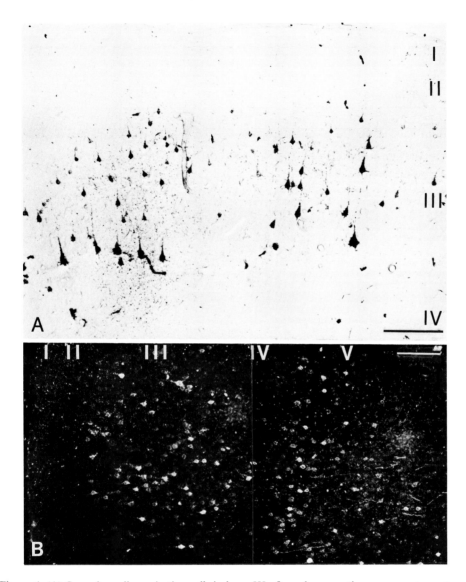

Figure 4. (A) Commissurally projecting cells in layer III of monkey somatic sensory cortex, retrogradely labeled by HRP injected into contralateral cortex. Uncounterstained; bar equals 200 μm. From Hendry and Jones (1983b). (B) Retrogradely labeled, commissurally projecting cells in all layers of rat somatic sensory cortex. Darkfield; surface of brain to left; bar equals 300 μm. From Wise and Jones (1976).

9–11). Similarly, although the cells of origin of some pathways tend to be much smaller (e.g., the corticorubral) than those of others (e.g., corticospinal), there is a good deal of overlap here too (Jones and Wise, 1977; Murray and Coulter, 1981) (Fig. 6). In the supragranular layers, at least of primates and cats, the larger, more deeply placed cells tend to project the furthest, i.e., across the corpus callosum or to distant ipsilateral cortical fields. The smaller, more superficially situated cells tend to project to ipsilateral fields situated nearby. However, there is, again, no rigid size or sublaminar separation of the parent cells of the different projections (Gilbert and Kelly, 1975; Jones and Wise, 1977; Tigges *et al.*, 1981; Lund *et al.*, 1981). Originally it appeared that only rodents possessed significant numbers of corticocortical or callosally projecting cells in the infragranular layers (Wise and Jones, 1976). Since then, however, large numbers of layer VI cells have been found to have ipsilateral corticocortical projections to adjacent (Rockland and Pandya, 1981; Tigges *et al.*, 1981) and distant (Friedman *et al.*, 1980) cortical fields in primates (Fig. 12). In some areas such as the motor cortex (Zant and Strick, 1978), additional large numbers of

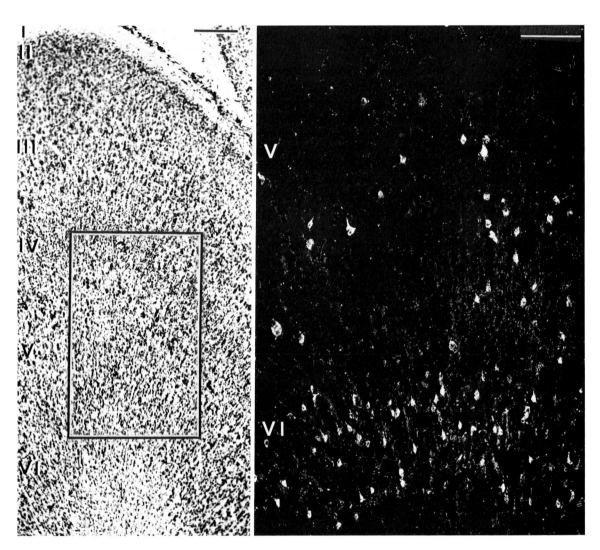

Figure 5. Retrogradely labeled corticothalamic cells (right) in layers V and VI of monkey somatic sensory cortex. Dark-field photomicrograph (B) is from boxed area of thionin-stained section shown in (A). Bars equal 250 μm (A) and 100 μm (B).

callosally projecting layer VI cells are also found whereas in the parietal cortex there is a significant population in layer V (Hedreen and Yin, 1981). There seems to be some areal variation in primates for no layer V and far fewer callosally projecting layer VI neurons are found in the somatic sensory areas (Jones *et al.*, 1979). Layer VI is also the origin of a rather substantial projection to the claustrum (LeVay and Sherk, 1981).

In cortical areas projecting to the amygdala, the cells of origin of the corticoamygdaloid projection lie in layers II and III (Mufson *et al.*, 1981). Corticostriatal cells, additional to those in layer V, have recently been described in these layers in the cat (Royce, 1982).

531

LAMINAR
DISTRIBUTION
OF CORTICAL
EFFERENT
CELLS

4.2. Patchy Distribution of Efferent Cell Somata

Early studies with retrograde tracers often emphasized the nonhomogeneous distribution of a particular set of efferent cells in the horizontal dimension (e.g., Jones *et al.*, 1975; Jacobson and Trojanowski, 1977a,b; Jones and Wise, 1977). For example, the cells of origin of corticospinal fibers in the monkey were demonstrated to form localized clusters of three or more cells with intervening unlabeled zones in the sensory motor cortex (Fig. 13), a feature that seemed to correlate with observations made using antidromic stimulation and single-unit recording (Humphrey and Corrie, 1978). Though in some instances the use of more sensitive retrograde labeling methods has shown that the dysjunctive nature of the cell somal distribution is far less clear-cut than previously supposed (e.g., Hedreen and Yin, 1981), in other instances there is an obvious patchiness of distribution. This is particularly true of the callosal projection. In some areas, not only are callosally projecting cells confined to one part (such as the representation of the vertical meridian of the visual field or that of more proximal body parts) but within that part there may be alternating patches of projecting and nonprojecting cells (Fig. 14). The foci of projecting cells are the same foci that receive the terminations of callosal axons coming from cells in contralateral cortex (Jones *et al.*, 1979; Cipolloni and Peters, 1979). In the cat auditory cortex, the callosally connected zones contain cells that show types of binaural responses different from those in the unconnected zones. Those in the connected zones exhibit summation of responses related to the two ears or ipsilateral dominance and suppression, while those in the unconnected zones exhibit monoaural contralateral responses or contralateral dominance and suppression (Imig and Brugge, 1978). In some areas of the monkey cortex, patches of callosally projecting cells may alternate, though with considerable overlap, with patches of cells in the same layers that project to ipsilateral cortical areas (Jones *et al.*, 1979; Goldman-Rakic and Schwartz, 1982). It is not known whether the patchy distribution of many cortically and subcortically projecting systems indicates that different sets of efferent cells belong to separate cortical columns or whether they can be differentially recruited under varying functional circumstances.

The rat somatic sensory cortex presents one of the clearest examples of a horizontal separation of cell classes with differential efferent connections. Here, callosally projecting cells are distributed only around and between the aggregations of layer IV granule cells that form the body map of the rat while the

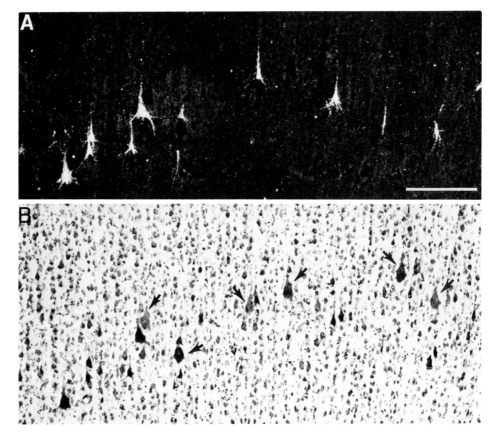

Figure 6. (A–D) Darkfield and brightfield photomicrographs from same fields of two different monkeys, showing retrogradely labeled corticospinal (A, B) and corticorubral (C, D) cells in motor cortex. Arrows indicate unlabeled giant cells in (B) and labeled cells in (C). Bars equal 200 μm. From Jones and Wise (1977).

majority of subcortically projecting cells lie deep to the granular aggregations (Wise, 1975; Wise and Jones, 1976; Wise *et al.*, 1979). (Fig. 15). The cortex of the patches is innervated by the thalamic ventrobasal complex but the thalamic input to the surrounding callosally connected zones is not yet clearly established (Wise and Jones, 1978).

4.3. Cell Types

All of the cells of origin of efferent projections emanating from layers II, III, V, or VI can be recognized as pyramidal in form (Fig. 8). Reports of other cell types retrogradely labeled after injections of tracer at a distance appear to

533

**LAMINAR
DISTRIBUTION OF
CORTICAL
EFFERENT
CELLS**

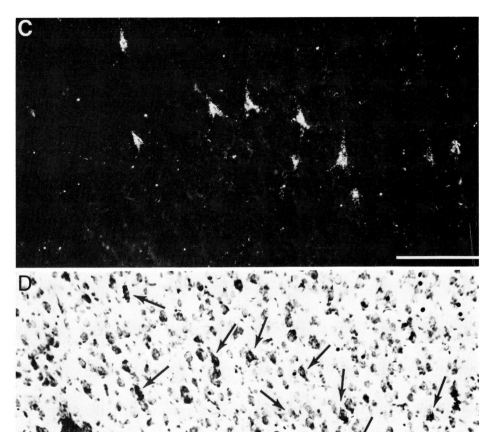

Figure 6. (*continued*)

derive mostly from labeling of the modified pyramids of layer VI (see Chapter 4) or from incomplete labeling of pyramidal cells in other layers.

Layer IV, however, though containing few or no efferent cells in most cortical areas, seems to furnish us with an example of a nonpyramidal source of efferent projections from the monkey striate cortex. Lund *et al.* (1975) discovered that a certain number of large multipolar cells of layer IVb could be retrogradely labeled following injections of HRP in the white matter of the hemisphere subjacent to the superior temporal gyrus. Shatz (1977) has reported a similar population of commissurally projecting nonpyramidal cells in the cat visual cortex. Such cells seem to be equivalent to the large spiny multipolar cells originally described in layer IV of the human and cat visual cortex by Ramón y Cajal (1909–1911, 1922).

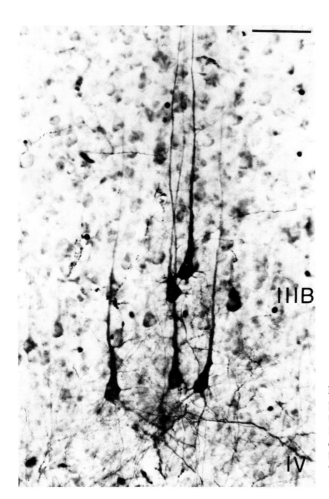

Figure 7. Retrogradely labeled pyramidal cells in layer IIIB of monkey somatic sensory cortex following injection of HRP in the corpus callosum. Reacted with cobalt-enhanced diaminobenzidine. Thionin counterstain; bar equals 100 μm.

As mentioned earlier, the sizes of the pyramidal somata that give rise to each set of efferent connections tend to fall into a particular range, though with some degree of variability, particularly in regard to the corticospinal projection. Lassek's (1941) observation that the number of giant pyramidal cells (Betz cells) in any animal cannot account for more than about 3% of the total population of pyramidal tract axons, seems amply confirmed from the wide range of sizes of the labeled somata. The differences in size, overall, of the cells of origin of the different pathways readily accounts for the wide range of conduction velocities of axons in the pyramidal tract through which many project (e.g., Evarts, 1965; Humphrey and Corrie, 1978). Certain corticofugal cells are absent from some cortical areas: corticorubral cells, for example, are not found outside the

Figure 8. Schematic diagram of laminar origins of efferent projections, based mainly on data from monkeys. Parentheses indicate a projection may not arise from the layer indicated in all species or all areas.

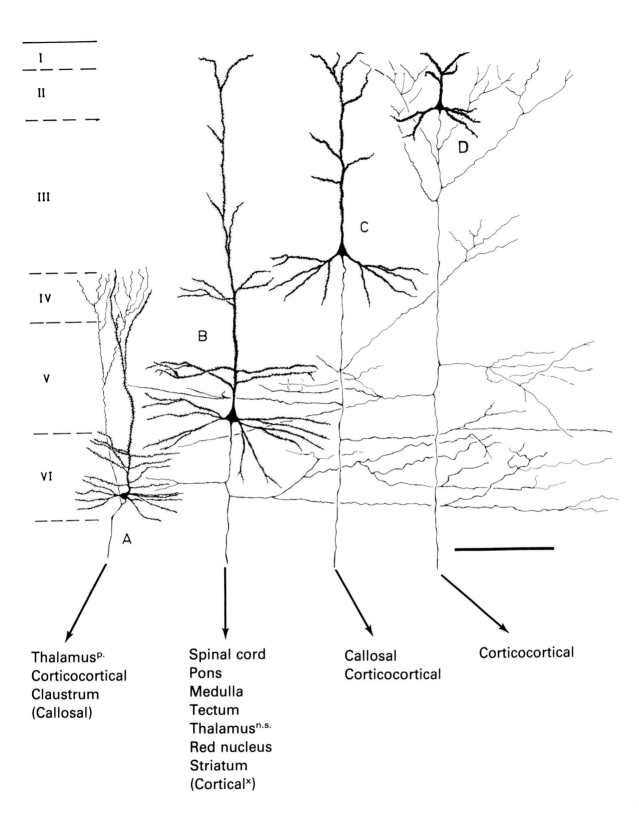

I

II

III

IV

V

VI

A

B

C

D

Thalamus[p.]
Corticocortical
Claustrum
(Callosal)

Spinal cord
Pons
Medulla
Tectum
Thalamus[n.s.]
Red nucleus
Striatum
(Cortical[x])

Callosal
Corticocortical

Corticocortical

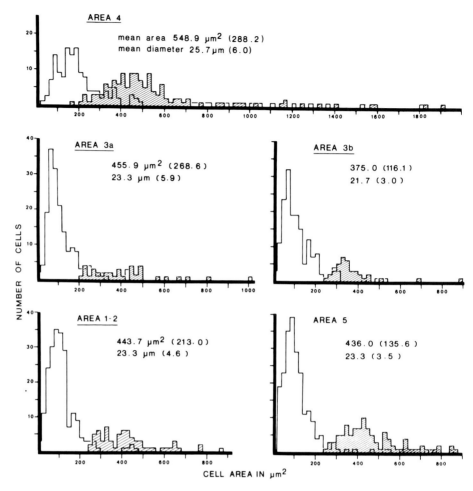

Figure 9. Areas and diameters of retrogradely labeled corticospinal cells (hatching) in several cytoarchitectonic fields of monkeys. Unhatched histograms indicate range of sizes of all cells of same layer. Standard deviations in parentheses. From Jones and Wise (1977).

motor or premotor cortex; some areas appear to lack corticotectal and some lack corticospinal cells. In other areas there are particularly large populations of corticotectal or corticospinal cells. Presumably variations in sizes, numbers, and distributions of the various kinds of pyramidal cells are significant elements in determining the cytoarchitectonic distinctiveness of a particular cortical field.

It is not yet clear whether the pyramidal cells of origin of a particular efferent system have a distinctive dendritic architecture that might make them recognizably different from those giving rise to another system. However, it is evident that pyramidal cells do differ in their dendritic branching patterns and in their populations of dendritic spines (Fig. 16). Local increases in dendritic branching or in spine populations on a pyramidal neuron can often be correlated with a layer of afferent fiber terminations though which the apical dendrite ascends or into which the basal dendrites descends (Fig. 16) (Lund and Boothe, 1975;

Hendry and Jones, 1983a,b). Others, however, do not and their dendrites traverse these layers without branching (Fig. 16). In an intracellular injection study, Deschênes *et al.* (1979) have reported that fast pyramidal tract neurons in the cat are less highly branched and their dendrites have fewer spines than slow pyramidal tract neurons, especially in layers I–III. Possibly in these differences among the corticofugal cells are clues to differences in their afferent connections, particularly to variations in afferent inputs that may drive them. There is evidence in the mouse somatic sensory cortex (White, 1979) that virtually all pyramidal cells with dendrites passing through layer IV receive thalamocortical synapses (Fig. 17). But corticothalamic cells receive the most and corticostriatal cells the least. Possibly there may be further variations of this type, even among corticofugal neurons projecting to the same region. Could, for example, corticorubral cells projecting to the magnocellular part of the red nucleus be innervated differently from those projecting to the parvocellular part and thus show differences in dendritic field architecture? Or slow and fast pyramidal tract neurons (Deschênes *et al.*, 1979); or motor cortex neurons altering their discharge in relation to slow controlled movements, but not to ballistic movements (Evarts and Fromm, 1977)?

It also seems possible that different classes of output neuron may have

537

**LAMINAR
DISTRIBUTION
OF CORTICAL
EFFERENT
CELLS**

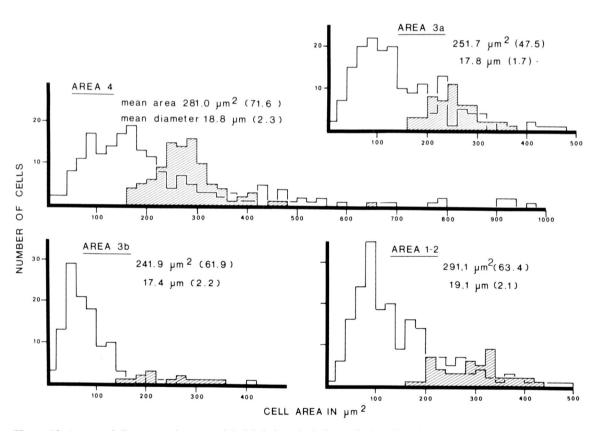

Figure 10. Areas and diameters of retrogradely labeled corticobulbar cells (hatching) in motor and somatic sensory areas of monkeys. From Jones and Wise (1977).

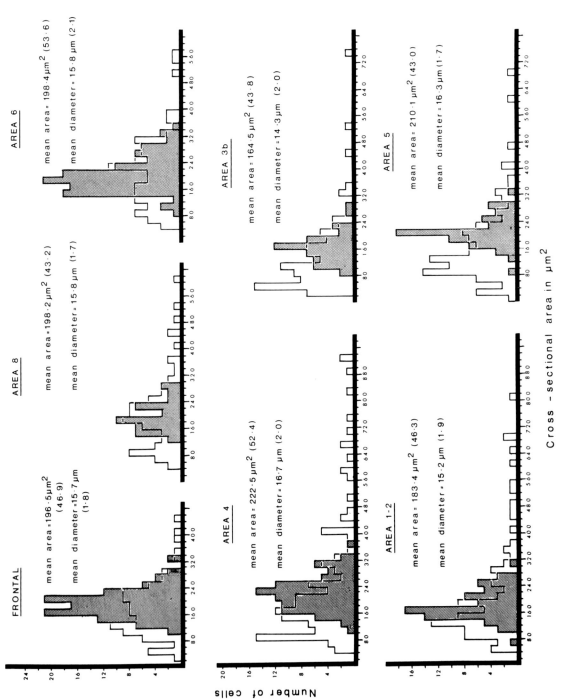

Figure 11. Areas and diameters of retrogradely labeled corticostriatal cells (hatching) from several cortical areas of monkeys. From Jones *et al.* (1977).

539

LAMINAR
DISTRIBUTION
OF CORTICAL
EFFERENT
CELLS

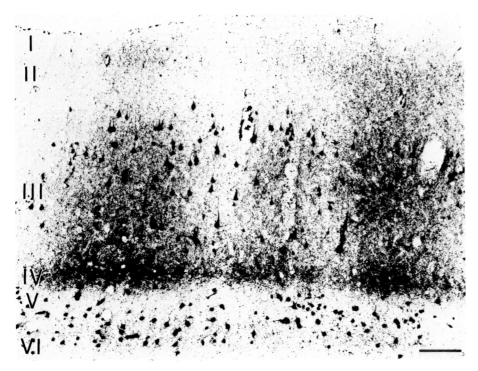

Figure 12. Retrograde labeling of corticocortical neurons and anterograde labeling of corticocortical axons in supra- and infragranular layers of monkey second somatic sensory area following injection of HRP in ipsilateral first somatic sensory area. Uncounterstained; bar equals 150 μm. From Friedman *et al.* (1981).

distinctive patterns of intracortical axon collaterals, perhaps causing them to influence selectively other classes of output cell. There are very few data available on the intracortical collaterals of pyramidal neurons. Probably in most Golgi studies they have not been fully impregnated. In their study of single injected cells in the cat visual cortex, Gilbert and Wiesel (1979) remark that some layer V cells, identified from receptive field mapping as "special complex cells," and therefore probably projecting to the superior colliculus, gave off less extensive collaterals as their axon traversed layer VI than others, identified as "standard complex cells," which had extensive layer VI collaterals. Possibly other differences of this kind will emerge with time and may provide support for some of the conjectures made throughout this section.

4.4. Collateral Projections

Given the fact that a sizeable percentage of the population of cells in a cortical layer (e.g., layer VI) can be retrogradely labeled from an injection of tracer in any one of its projection sites, and the number of sites to which such a layer projects, it seems not unreasonable to ask to what extent one projection is made up of collaterals of axons projecting to another site? Over the years, the question of collateralization of corticospinal axons to brain stem sites such as the red nucleus or pontine nuclei, has been the subject of repeated investigation by physiological techniques. There are many reports of antidromic invasion of single cortical neurons from stimulation sites in both the pyramidal tract and various other subcortical centers such as the striatum, thalamus, red nucleus, pontine nuclei, dorsal column nuclei, and medullary reticular formation (e.g., Endo *et al.*, 1973). Long before this, Ramón y Cajal (1909–1911) had noted in

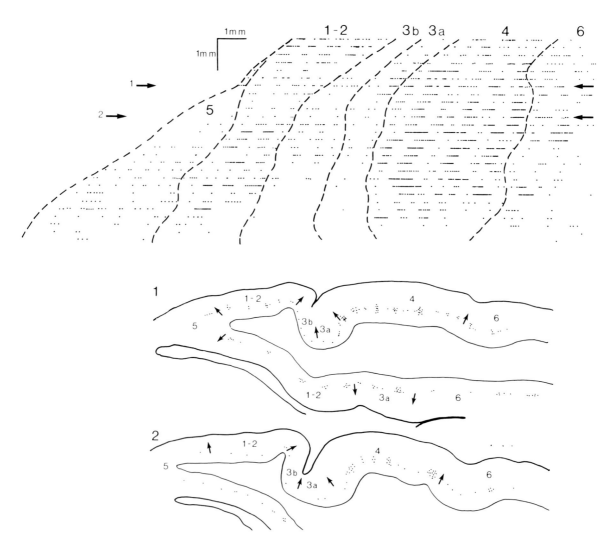

Figure 13. Unfolded map of monkey pre- and postcentral cortex, made from sagittal sections (1,2), showing patchy distribution of retrogradely labeled corticospinal neurons (dots). Broken lines indicate borders of architectonic fields. From Jones and Wise (1977).

541

LAMINAR
DISTRIBUTION
OF CORTICAL
EFFERENT
CELLS

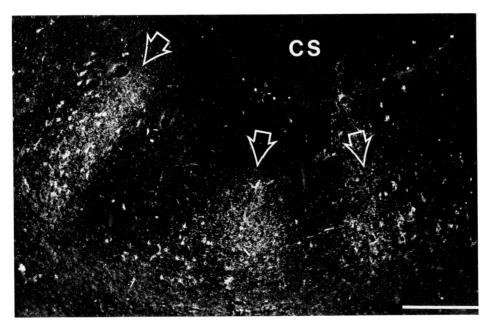

Figure 14. Retrograde labeling of callosal cells and anterograde labeling of callosal axons in columns in floor of central sulcus of a monkey following injection of HRP in contralateral cortex. Darkfield; bar equals 200 μm. From Jones *et al.* (1979).

his Golgi studies of the rodent brain that many corticofugal axons descending into the internal capsule gave off collaterals to the striatum or thalamus and that, further down the neuraxis, axons of the pyramidal tract gave off collaterals to the red nucleus, tectum, pons, and dorsal column nuclei. Virtually all of these connections have been reportedly confirmed by physiological studies at one time or another.

Perhaps the most thorough study of this type in recent times is that of Humphrey and Corrie (1978) in the arm area of the monkey motor cortex. In their sample of neurons responding antidromically to stimulation of the medullary pyramid, 75% projected to the spinal cord and 14% to the medulla oblongata. Though only 7.6% of the neurons appeared to send collaterals to the contralateral dorsal column nuclei, 72% of these arose from identified corticospinal axons. By contrast, in the cat Gordon and Miller (1969) could identify no collaterals of corticospinal neurons innervating the dorsal column nuclei. In the study of Humphrey and Corrie (1978), a relatively small percentage of the pyramidal tract axons gave collaterals to the red nucleus or medullary reticular formation. The number of collateral axons innervating the red nucleus was only one-quarter as large as the number of direct corticorubral axons. The higher proportion of nonbranched projections has been confirmed by Fromm *et al.* (1981) and Palmer *et al.* (1981). The collateral corticorubral projections arise from relatively rapidly conducting pyramidal tract axons and the direct projection from slowly conducting axons. Anatomical studies that earlier had reported

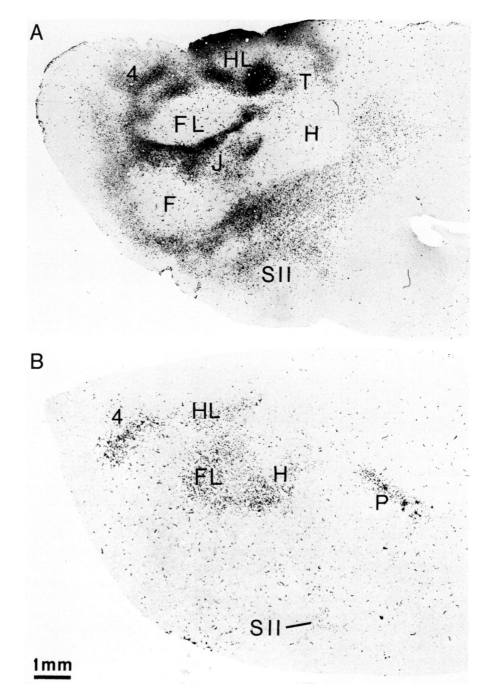

Figure 15. Sections passing through layers III (A) and V (B) of flattened rat brains showing patchy distribution of retrogradely labeled callosal (A) and corticospinal and corticotrigeminal neurons (B). Uncounterstained. (A) from Jones (1982); (B) from Wise *et al.* (1979). Face (F); lower jaw (J); head (H); truck (T); and forelimb (FL). Representations: 4, motor cortex; p, parietal cortex; SII, second somatic sensory area.

543

**LAMINAR
DISTRIBUTION
OF CORTICAL
EFFERENT
CELLS**

retrograde labeling of only small pyramidal cells in the upper part of layer V, above those of other cortical efferent cells, were presumably labeling only the cells of origin of the direct projection (Jones and Wise, 1977). Other antidromic studies have reported a small number of collaterals of pyramidal tract axons innervating the pontine nuclei of the cat (Gibson *et al.*, 1978b) and a relatively high proportion of corticotectal axons in the rabbit with collaterals to the lateral posterior thalamic nucleus (Swadlow and Weyand, 1981).

In another recent study of a small number of large, deep, layer V pyramidal neurons injected intracellularly in rats after antidromic activation from the cerebral peduncle, some of their filled axons entering the internal capsule were noted to give off collateral branches in the striatum (Donoghue and Kitai, 1981). These observations are difficult to correlate with retrograde labeling studies that showed most corticostriatal projections to arise from smaller pyramidal cells mainly in the more superficial parts of layer V (Jones *et al.*, 1975; Wise and Jones, 1977a; Jones and Wise, 1977).

In the cerebral cortex itself, Ramón y Cajal (1909–1911) had also reported collaterals of cortical efferent axons passing to other cortical areas both ipsilaterally and through the corpus callosum. The recent anatomical evidence that all subcortical projections arise from infragranular layers while most corticocortical projections arise from supragranular layers, makes it difficult to interpret these observations, though they were made in rodents in which, as stated above, the segregation of efferent cells is less clear-cut than in other species. Recently, Zarzecki *et al.* (1978) have shown by intracellular recording that the axons of some identified pyramidal tract neurons in the cat motor cortex can have collateral branches that enter the somatic sensory cortex. Swadlow and Weyand (1981) could not detect similar branching of efferent axons from the rabbit visual cortex, so the extent to which this represents a general rule is difficult to determine. Certain new anatomical observations suggest that such collateralization may be rather rare. For example, after injecting the fluorescent dye nuclear yellow in the prefrontal cortex of one side in monkeys and another dye (fast blue) in the contralateral parietal cortex, Schwartz and Goldman-Rakic (1982) found fewer than 5% of the cells in the uninjected prefrontal or parietal cortex "double-labeled" by the two dyes. Similar experiences have been reported by others investigating corticocortical and callosal connections of different cortical areas (Andersen *et al.*, 1982, and Fig. 18). Though the labeled ipsi- and contralaterally projecting cells can be closely intermingled in these experiments, most are labeled by one or the other retrogradely transported dye but very few by both.

Similar attempts have been made to retrogradely label subcortically projecting cells by dyes or other tracers injected at more than one subcortical site. Here, again, the results suggest that, contrary to the expectations raised by physiological experimentation, the extent of collateralization is rather modest. Catsman-Berrevoets *et al.* (1980) and Catsman-Berrevoets and Kuypers (1981) found no evidence for callosal or corticospinal collaterals emanating from corticothalamic cells in layer V of the rat sensory motor cortex. Catsman-Berrevoets *et al.* (1979) found only a limited number of double-labeled cells in the cat motor cortex after injections of the magnocellular red nucleus and spinal cord and none after injection of the parvocellular red nucleus and spinal cord. Rustioni

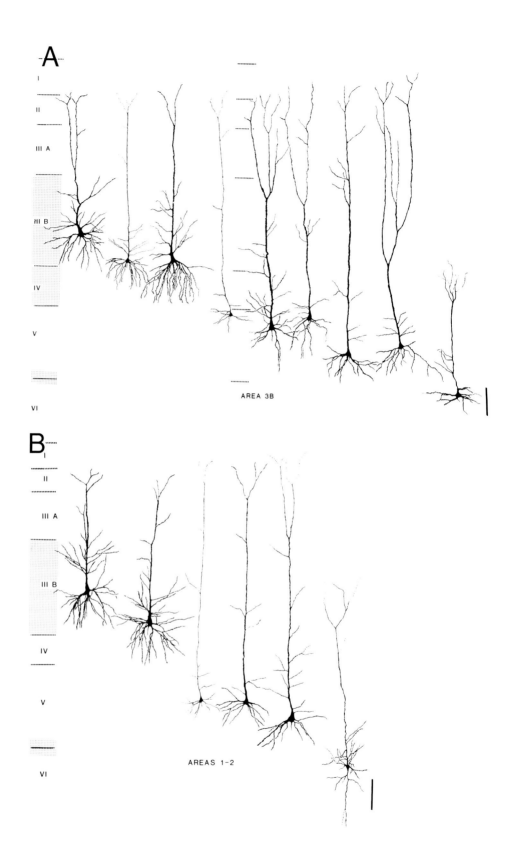

AREA 3B

AREAS 1-2

545

**LAMINAR
DISTRIBUTION
OF CORTICAL
EFFERENT
CELLS**

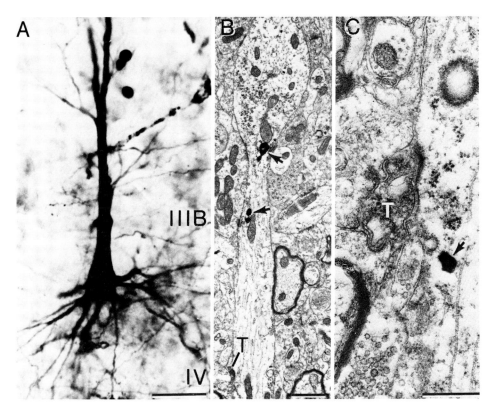

Figure 17. (A) Retrogradely labeled, callosally projecting, pyramidal cell with soma in layer IIIb and basal dendrites descending into layer IV of monkey somatic sensory cortex. (B, C) Serial electron micrographs showing a basal dendrite of a cell similar to (A) with a degenerating thalamocortical terminal (T) ending on it. Arrows indicate reaction product. Bars equal 50 μm (A), 5 μm (B), 1 μm (C). From Hendry and Jones (1983b).

and Hayes (1981) reported a comparably small number of double-labeled cells in the cat sensory motor cortex after injections of the dorsal column nuclei and spinal cord. Assuming that the presence of one retrogradely transported tracer in a cell does not in some way block effective labeling by a second, these anatomical results imply that the degree of subcortical collateralization of cortico-fugal fibers is also relatively limited.

5. Neurotransmitter

The corticofugal transmitter or transmitters still elude conclusive identification. Over the years there have been many suggestions (see review in Curtis

←——————————————————————————————

Figure 16. Varieties of pyramidal cells from layers IIIb, V, and VI of areas 3b (A) and 1–2 (B) of monkey somatic sensory cortex showing relationships of their dendritic branching patterns to layers of termination of thalamic afferents (stipple). Bars equal 100 μm. After Hendry and Jones (1983a).

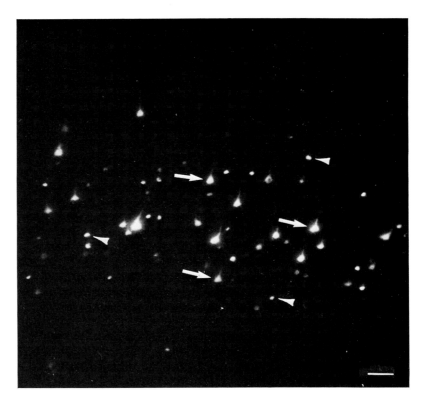

Figure 18. Fluroescence photomicrograph of retrogradely labeled cells in the supragranular layers of area 7a of a monkey following large injections of the dye fast blue into the contralateral area 7a and of the dye nuclear yellow into the ipsilateral prefrontal cortex (areas 8, 45, and 46). Arrows indicate examples of fast blue-labeled cells. Arrowheads indicate examples of nuclear yellow-labeled cells. No cells in this field were double-labeled. Bar equals 100 μm. Courtesy of Dr. C. Asanuma.

and Johnston, 1974) but none has yet been confirmed. GABA seems ruled out by its localization only in nonpyramidal neurons (Ribak, 1978; Houser *et al.*, 1983; Hendry *et al.*, 1983) and by the fact that the earliest cortical and subcortical responses to cortical stimulation are excitatory. The known brain-gut peptides also seem ruled out by their localization in nonpyramidal neurons (e.g., Emson and Hunt, 1981).

Of the putative corticofugal transmitters, circumstantial evidence points in favor of aspartate or glutamate. Each has an excitatory effect on neurons at sites to which the cortex projects, though this effect is, of course, shared by many neuronal systems (Curtis and Johnston, 1974). However, stimulation of the cortex leads to release of both amino acids from the spinal cord and other sites (Canzek *et al.*, 1981). Ablation of the cortex leads within a short time to a fall in L-glutamate levels and substantial reductions in the high-affinity uptake of glutamate and aspartate especially by synaptosomal fractions, in the dorsal lateral geniculate nucleus, superior colliculus, and striatum (e.g., Lund-Karlsen and Fonnum, 1978; Divac *et al.*, 1977; Reubi and Cuénod, 1979; McGeer *et al.*, 1977; Fonnum *et al.*, 1981). Finally, tritiated D-aspartate is taken up via a high-affinity uptake system by the axon terminals of corticothalamic, corticostriatal, and cor-

547

LAMINAR
DISTRIBUTION
OF CORTICAL
EFFERENT
CELLS

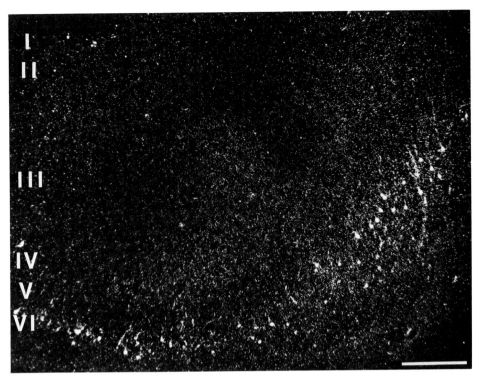

Figure 19. Retrograde labeling of corticothalamic neurons with [³H] D-aspartate in layer VI of monkey second somatic sensory cortex. Darkfield; bar equals 300 μm.

ticomedullary axons and retrogradely transported to their cell bodies of origin in the cerebral cortex (Streit, 1980; Baughman and Gilbert, 1980, 1981; Rustioni and Cuénod, 1982; Jones, 1982; Fig. 19). Being in the D form, it is not further metabolized and, thus, remains in the cell as a marker. It does not appear to accumulate by retrograde transport or by local uptake in the cell bodies of thalamocortical axons (Baughman and Gilbert, 1980, 1981). There are, however, hints that it may be transported retrogradely in corticocortical and callosal axons (Streit, 1980; Baughman and Gilbert, 1981).

These observations by no means confirm aspartate as a corticofugal transmitter and because aspartate and glutamate can substitute for one another in the same high-affinity uptake system, they do not permit a distinction to be made between the two. The selectivity of the effect, however, coupled with the knowledge of selective transport of their transmitter substances in other neuronal pathways (Streit and Cuénod, 1979; Streit *et al.*, 1979), suggests that it should be regarded seriously.

6. Summary

The pyramidal neurons are the output cells of the cerebral cortex and in most cortical areas no efferent axons arise from nonpyramidal neurons. It is not clear whether all pyramidal neurons have an axon that leaves the cortex though this seems likely.

Though the somata of subcortically projecting pyramidal neurons are mainly confined to the infragranular layers and these display specificity of laminar and even sublaminar location, those of corticocortically and callosally projecting pyramidal neurons are less clearly confined to the supragranular layers and display areal and species differences in distribution.

There is anatomical evidence that collateral branching of cortical efferent axons to innervate more than one site outside the cortical area of origin is not extensive and may affect only a small percentage of the neuronal population. Physiological experiments have tended to imply more extensive branching.

Different classes of corticofugal neuron projecting to the same site can often be identified physiologically. There are also significant differences in the dendritic branching patterns, dendritic spine populations, and possibly in intracortical axon collateralization, among pyramidal neurons. However, these morphological differences cannot, as yet, be corrected with the functional differences.

Many pyramidal neurons receive significant numbers of monosynaptic thalamic connections.

There is suggestive evidence that many or all corticofugal cells secrete glutamate or aspartate as their neurotransmitter.

ACKNOWLEDGMENT. Personal work reported herein was supported by Grant NS10526 from the National Institutes of Health, United States Public Health Service.

7. References

Andersen, R. A., Asanuma, C., and Cowan, W. M., 1982, Observations on the callosal and associational cortico-cortical connections of area 7a of the macaque monkey, *Soc. Neurosci. Abstr.* **8:**210.

Asanuma, H., and Rosén, I., 1972, Topographical organization of cortical efferent zones projecting to distal forelimb muscles in the monkey, *Exp. Brain Res.* **14:**243–256.

Baughman, R. W., and Gilbert, C. D., 1980, Aspartate and glutamate as possible neurotransmitters of cells in layer 6 of the visual cortex, *Nature (London)* **287:**848–849.

Baughman, R. W., and Gilbert, C. D., Aspartate and glutamate as possible neurotransmitters in the visual cortex, *J. Neurosci.* **1:**427–439.

Berlucchi, G., Gazzaniga, M. S., and Rizzolati, G., 1967, Microelectrode analysis of transfer of visual information by the corpus callosum, *Arch. Ital. Biol.* **105:**583–598.

Berman, N., and Cynader M., 1975, Receptive fields in cat superior colliculus after visual cortex lesions, *J. Physiol (London)* **245:**261–270.

Berrevoets, C. E., and Kuypers, H. G. J. M., 1975, Pericruciate cortical neurons projecting to brain stem reticular formation, dorsal column nuclei and spinal cord in the cat, *Neurosci. Lett.* **1:**257–262.

Bielschowsky, M., 1916, Über Hemiplegie bie intakter Pyramidalbahnen, *J. Psychol. Neurol.* **22:**225–287.

Bolton, J. S., 1910, A contribution to the localization of cerebral function, based on the clinicopathological study of mental disease, *Brain* **33:**26–147.

Bullier, J., and Henry, G. H., 1979, Laminar distribution of first order neurons and afferent terminals in cat striate cortex, *J. Neurophysiol.* **42:**1271–1281.

Campbell, A. W., 1905, *Histological Studies on the Localization of Cerebral Function,* Cambridge University Press, London.

Canzek, V., Wolfenberger, M., Amsler, U., and Cuénod M., 1981, In vivo release of glutamate and aspartate following optic nerve stimulation, *Nature (London)* **293:**572–573.

549

LAMINAR
DISTRIBUTION
OF CORTICAL
EFFERENT
CELLS

Catsman-Berrevoets, C. E., and Kuypers, H. G. J. M., 1978, Differential laminar distribution of corticothalamic neurons projecting to the VL and the center median: An HRP study in the cynomolgus monkey, *Brain Res.* **154**:359–365.

Catsman-Berrevoets, C. E., and Kuypers, H. G. J. M., 1981, A search for corticospinal collaterals to thalamus and mesencephalon by means of multiple retrograde fluorescent tracers in cat and rat, frontal projections to magnocellular and parvocellular red nucleus and superior colliculus in cynomolgus monkey: An HRP study, *Neurosci. Lett.* **12**:41–46.

Catsman-Berrevoets, C. E., Lemon, R. N., Verburgh, C. A., Bentivoglio, M., and Kuypers, H. G. J. M., 1980, Absence of callosal collaterals derived from rat corticospinal neurons: A study using fluorescent retrograde tracing and electrophysiological techniques, *Exp. Brain Res.* **39**:433–440.

Cipolloni, P. B., and Peters, A., 1979, The bilaminar and banded distribution of the callosal terminals in the posterior neocortex of the rat, *Brain Res.* **176**:33–48.

Coulter, J. D., Ewing, L., and Carter, C., 1976, Origin of primary sensorimotor cortical projections to lumbar spinal cord of cat and monkey, *Brain Res.* **103**:366–372.

Curtis, D. R., and Johnston, G. A. R., 1974, Amino acid transmitters in the mammalian central nervous system, *Ergeb, Physiol. Biol. Chem. Exp. Pharmakol.* **69**:97–188.

Deschênes, M., Labelle, A., and Landry, P., 1979, Morphological characterizations of slow and fast pyramidal tract cells in the cat, *Brain Res.* **178**:251–274.

Divac, I., Fonnum, F., and Storm-Mathisen, J., 1977, High affinity uptake of glutamate in terminals of corticostriatal axons, *Nature (London)* **266**:377–378.

Donoghue, J. P., and Kitai, S. T., 1981, A collateral pathway to the neo-striatum from corticofugal neurons of the rat sensory-motor cortex: An intracellular HRP study, *J. Comp. Neurol.* **201**:1–14.

Emson, P. C., and Hunt, S. P., 1981, Anatomical chemistry of the cerebral cortex, in: *The Organization of the Cerebral Cortex*, (F. O. Schmitt, F. G. Worden, G. Adelman, and S. G. Dennis, eds.), pp. 325–346, MIT Press, Cambridge, Mass.

Endo, K., Araki, T., and Yagi, N., 1973, The distribution and pattern of axon branching of pyramidal tract cells, *Brain Res.* **57**:484–491.

Evarts, E. V., 1965, Relation of discharge frequency to conduction velocity in pyramidal tract neurons, *J. Neurophysiol.* **28**:216–228.

Evarts, E. V., and Fromm, C., 1977, Sensory responses in motor cortex neurons during precise motor control, *Neurosci. Lett.* **5**:267–272.

Ferster, D., and Lindstrom, S., 1983, An intracellular analysis of geniculocortical connectivity in area 17 of the cat, *J. Physiol. (London)* (in press).

Fonnum, F., Storm-Mathisen, J., and Divac, I., 1981, Biochemical evidence for glutamate as neurotransmitter in corticostriatal and corticothalamic fibers in rat brain, *Neuroscience* **6**:863–874.

Foster, R. E., Donoghue, J. P., and Ebner, F. F., 1981, Laminar organization of efferent cells in the parietal cortex of the Virginia opossum, *Exp. Brain Res.* **43**:330–336.

Friedman, D. P., Jones, E. G., and Burton, H., 1980, Representation pattern in the second somatic sensory area of the monkey cerebral cortex, *J. Comp. Neurol* **192**:21–41.

Fromm, C., Evarts, E. V., Kröller, J., and Shinoda, Y., 1981, Activity of motor cortex and red nucleus neurons during voluntary movement, in: *Brain Mechanisms and Perceptual Awareness* (O. Pompeiano and C. Ajmone Marsan, eds.), pp. 269–294, Raven Press, New York.

Gibson, A., Baker, J., Mower, G., and Glickstein, M., 1978a, Corticopontine cells in area 18 of the cat, *J. Neurophysiol* **41**:484–495.

Gibson, A., Baker, J., Mower, G., Robinson, F., and Glickstein, M., 1978b, Bifurcation of the corticopontine pathway in the cat, *Soc. Neurosci. Abstr.* **4**:629.

Gilbert, C. D., 1977, Laminar differences in receptive field properties of cells in cat primary visual cortex, *J. Physiol. (London)* **268**:391–421.

Gilbert, C. D., and Kelly, J. P., 1975, The projections of cells in different layers of the cat's visual cortex, *J. Comp. Neurol.* **163**:81–105.

Gilbert, C. D., and Wiesel, T. N., 1979, Morphology and intracortical projections of functionally characterised neurons in the cat visual cortex, *Nature (London)* **280**:120–125.

Glickstein, M., and Whitteridge, D., 1976, Degeneration of layer III pyramidal cells in area 18 following destruction of callosal input, *Brain Res.* **104**:148–151.

Goldman-Rakic, P. S., and Schwartz, M. L., 1982, Interdigitation of contralateral and ipsilateral columnar projections to frontal association cortex in primates, *Science* **216**:755–757.

Gordon, G., and Miller, R., 1969, Identification of cortical cells projecting to the dorsal column nuclei of the cat, *Q. J. Exp. Physiol.* **54**:85–98.

Graham, J., Berman, N., and Murphy, E. H., 1982, Effects of visual cortical lesions on receptive-field properties of single units in superior colliculus of the rabbit, *J. Neurophysiol.* **47:**272–286.

Harvey, A. R., 1978, Characteristics of corticothalamic neurons in area 17 of the cat, *Neurosci. Lett.* **7:**177–181.

Harvey, A. R., 1980, The afferent connexions and laminar distribution of cells in area 18 of the cat, *J. Physiol. (London)* **302:**483–505.

Hedreen, J. C., and Yin, T. C. T., 1981, Homotopic and heterotopic callosal afferents of caudal inferior parietal lobule in *Macaca mulatta, J. Comp. Neurol.* **197:**605–622.

Hendry, S. H. C., and Jones, E. G., 1980, Electron microscopic demonstration of thalamic axon terminations on identified commissural neurons in monkey somatic sensory cortex, *Brain Res.* **196:**253–257.

Hendry, S. H. C., and Jones, E. G., 1983a, The organization of pyramidal and nonpyramidal cell dendrites in relation to thalamic afferent terminations in the monkey somatic sensory cortex, *J. Neurocytol.* **12:**278–298.

Hendry, S. H. C., and Jones, E. G., 1983b, Thalamic inputs to identified commissural neurons in the monkey somatic sensory cortex, *J. Neurocytol.* **12:**299–316.

Hendry, S. H. C., Houser, C. R., Jones, E. G., and Vaughn, J. E., 1983, Synaptic organization of immunocytochemically identified GABAergic neurons in the monkey sensory-motor cortex, *J. Neurocytol.* **12:**639–660.

Holländer, H., 1974, On the origin of the corticotectal projections in the cat, *Exp. Brain Res.* **21:**433–439.

Holmes, G., and Page May, W., 1909, On the exact origin of the pyramidal tract in man and other mammals, *Brain* **32:**1–43.

Houser, C. R., Hendry, S. H. C., Jones, E. G., and Vaughn, J. E., 1983, Morphological diversity of GABA neurons demonstrated immunocytochemically in monkey sensory-motor cortex, *J. Neurocytol.* **12:**617–638.

Hubel, D. H., and Wiesel, T. N., 1967, Cortical and callosal connections concerned with the vertical meridian of the visual fields in the cat, *J. Neurophysiol.* **30:**1561–1573.

Humphrey, D. R., and Corrie, W. S., 1978, Properties of pyramidal tract neuron system within a functionally defined subregion of primate motor cortex, *J. Neurophysiol.* **41:**216–243.

Humphrey, D. R., and Rietz, R. R., 1976, Cells of origin of corticorubral projections from the arm area of primate motor cortex and their synaptic actions in the red nucleus, *Brain Res.* **110:**162–169.

Imig, T. J., and Brugge, J. F., 1978, Sources and terminations of callosal axons related to binaural and frequency maps in primary auditory cortex of the cat, *J. Comp. Neurol.* **182:**637–660.

Jacobson, S., and Trojanowski, J. Q., 1974, The cells of origin of the corpus callosum in rat, cat, and rhesus monkey, *Brain Res.* **74:**149–155.

Jacobson, S., and Trojanowski, J. Q., 1975, Corticothalamic neurons and thalamocortical terminal fields: An investigation in rat using horseradish peroxidase and autoradiography, *Brain Res.* **85:**385–401.

Jacobson, S., and Trojanowski, J. Q., 1976a, Prefrontal granular cortex of the rhesus monkey. I. Intrahemispheric cortical afferents, *Brain Res.* **132:**209–234.

Jacobson, S., and Trojanowski, J. Q., 1976b, Prefrontal granular cortex of the rhesus monkey. II. Interhemispheric cortical afferents, *Brain Res.* **132:**235–246.

Jankowska, E., Padel, Y., and Tanaka, R., 1975, The mode of activation of pyramidal tract cells by intracortical stimuli, *J. Physiol. (London)* **249:**617–636.

Jones, E. G., 1982, The thalamus, in: *Chemical Neuroanatomy* (P. Emson, ed.), Raven Press, New York.

Jones, E. G., and Wise, S. P., 1977, Size, laminar and columnar distribution of efferent cells in the sensory-motor cortex of monkeys, *J. Comp. Neurol.* **175:**391–438.

Jones, E. G., Burton, H., and Porter, R., 1975, Commissural and cortico-cortical "columns" in the somatic sensory cortex of primates, *Science* **190:**572–574.

Jones, E. G., Coulter, J., Burton, H., and Porter, R., 1977, Cells of origin and terminal distribution of corticostriatal fibers arising in the sensory-motor cortex of monkeys, *J. Comp. Neruol.* **173:**53–80.

Jones, E. G., Coulter, J. D., and Hendry, S. H. C., 1978, Intracortical connectivity of architectonic fields in the somatic sensory, motor and parietal cortex of monkeys, *J. Comp. Neruol.* **181:**291–348.

Jones, E. G., Coulter, J. D., and Wise, S. P., 1979, Commissural columns in the sensory motor cortex of monkeys, *J, Comp. Neurol.* **188:**113–136.

Lassek, A. M., 1941, The pyramidal tract of the monkey, *J. Comp. Neurol.* **74:**192–202.

LeVay, S., and Sherk, H., 1981, The visual claustrum of the cat. I. Structure and connections, *J. Neurosci.* **1:**956–980.

551

LAMINAR
DISTRIBUTION
OF CORTICAL
EFFERENT
CELLS

Lorente de Nó, R., 1922, La corteza cerebral de ratón (Primera contribución-La corteza acústica), *Trab. Lab. Invest. Biol. Madrid* **20**:41–78.

Lorente de Nó, R., 1949, Cerebral cortex: Architecture, intracortical connections, motor projections, in: *Physiology of the Nervous System* (J. F. Fulton, ed.), 3rd ed., pp. 288–313, Oxford University Press, London.

Lund, J. S., and Boothe, R. G., 1975, Interlaminar connections and pyramidal neuron organisation in the visual cortex, area 17, of the macaque monkey, *J. Comp. Neurol.* **159**:305–334.

Lund, J. S., Lund, R. D., Hendrickson, A. E., Bunt, A. H., and Fuchs, A. F., 1975, The origin of efferent pathways from the primary visual cortex, area 17, of the macaque monkey as shown by retrograde transport of horseradish peroxidase. *J. Comp. Neurol.* **164**:287–304.

Lund, J. S., Hendrickson, A. E., Ogren, M. P., and Tobin, E. A., 1981, Anatomical organization of primate visual cortex area VII, *J. Comp. Neurol.* **202**:19–46.

Lund-Karlsen, R., and Fonnum, F., 1978, Evidence for glutamate as a neurotransmitter in the corticofugal fibres to the dorsal lateral geniculate body and the superior colliculus in rats, *Brain Res.* **151**:457–468.

McGeer, P. L., McGeer, E. G., Scherer, V., and Singh, K., 1977, A glutamatergic cortico-striatal path?, *Brain Res.* **128**:369–373.

Maciewicz, R. J., 1974, Afferents to the lateral suprasylvian gyrus of the cat traced with horseradish peroxidase, *Brain Res.* **78**:139–143.

Magalhães-Castro, H. H., Saraiva, P. E. S., and Magalhães-Castro, B., 1975, Identification of corticotectal cells of the visual cortex of cats by means of horseradish peroxidase, *Brain Res.* **83**:474–479.

Michael, C. R., 1972, Functional organization of cells in the superior colliculus of the ground squirrel, *J. Neurophysiol.* **35**:833–846.

Miller, R., 1975, Distribution and properties of commissural and other neurons in cat sensorimotor cortex, *J. Comp. Neurol.* **164**:361–374.

Mize, B. R., and Murphy, E. H., 1976, Alterations in receptive field properties of superior colliculus cells produced by visual cortex ablation in infant and adult cats, *J. Comp. Neurol.* **168**:393–424.

Mufson, E. J., Mesulam, M.-M., and Pandya, D. P., 1981, Insular interconnections with the amygdala in the rhesus monkey, *Neuroscience* **6**:1231–1248.

Murray, E. A., and Coulter, J. D., 1981, Organization of corticospinal neurons in the monkey, *J. Comp. Neurol.* **195**: 339–365.

Nissl, F., 1908, Experimental Ergebnisse zur Frage der Hirnrindenschichtung, *Monatsschr. Psychiat. Neurol.* **23**:186–188.

O'Leary, J. L., 1941, Structure of the area striata of the cat, *J. Comp. Neurol.* **75**:131–164.

O'Leary, J. L., and Bishop, G. H., 1938, The optically excitable cortex of the rabbit, *J. Comp. Neurol.* **68**:423–478.

Palmer, C., Schmidt, E. M., and McIntosh, J. S., 1981, Corticospinal and corticorubral projections from the supplementary motor area in the monkey, *Brain Res.* **209**:305–314.

Palmer, L. A., and Rosenquist, A. C., 1974, Visual receptive fields of single striate cortical units projecting to the superior colliculus in the cat, *Brain Res.* **67**:27–42.

Phillips, C. G., and Porter, R., 1977, *Corticospinal Neurons: Their Role in Movement*, Academic Press, New York.

Pines, L. J., and Maiman, R. M., 1939, Cells of origin of fibers of the corpus callosum: Experimental and pathological observations, *Arch. Neurol. Psychiatry* **42**:1076–1081.

Ramón y Cajal, S., 1909–1911, *Histologie du Système Nerveux de l'Homme et des Vertébrés* (translated by L. Azoulay), Maloine, Paris.

Ramón y Cajal, S., 1922, Studien über die Sehrinde der Katze, *J. Psychol. Neurol.* **29**:161–181.

Ramón y Cajal, S., 1928, *Degeneration and Regeneration of the Nervous System* (translated by R. M. May), Oxford University Press, London.

Ravizza, R. J., Straw, R. B., and Long, P. D., 1976, Laminar origin of efferent projections from auditory cortex in the golden Syrian hamster, *Brain Res.* **114**:497–500.

Reubi, J. C., and Cuénod, M., 1979, Glutamate release in vitro from corticostriatal terminals, *Brain Res.* **176**:185–188.

Ribak, C., 1978, Aspinous and sparsely-spinous stellate neurons in the visual cortex of rats contain glutamic acid decarboxylase, *J. Neurocytol.* **7**:461–478.

Robson, J. A., and Hall, W. C., 1975, Connections of layer VI in striate cortex of the grey squirrel (*Sciurus carolinensis*) *Brain Res.* **93**:133–139.

Rockland, K. S., and Pandya, D. N., 1981, Cortical connections of the occipital lobe in the rhesus monkey: Interconnections between areas 17, 18, 19 and the superior temporal sulcus, *Brain Res.* **212**:249–270.

Romagnano, M. A., and Maciewicz, R. J., 1975, Peroxidase labeling of motor cortex neurons projecting to ventrolateral nucleus in the cat, *Brain Res.* **83**:469–473.

Royce, G. J., 1982, Laminar origin of neurons which project upon the caudate nucleus: A horseradish peroxidase investigation in the cat, *J. Comp. Neurol.* **205**:8–29.

Rustioni, A., and Cuénod, M., 1982, Selective retrograde transport of D-aspartate in spinal interneurons and cortical neurons of rats, *Brain res.* **236**:143–155.

Rustioni, A., and Hayes, N. L., 1981, Corticospinal tract collaterals to the dorsal column nuclei of cats: An anatomical single and double retrograde tracer study, *Exp. Brain Res.* **43**:237–245.

Schiller, P. H., Stryker, M., Cynader, M., and Berman, N., 1974, Response characteristics of single cells in the monkey superior colliculus following ablation or cooling of visual cortex, *J. Neurophysiol.* **37**:181–194.

Schwartz, M. L., and Goldman-Rakic, P. S., 1982, Single cortical neurons have axon collaterals to ipsilateral and contralateral cortex in fetal and adult primates, *Nature (London)* **299**:154–156.

Shatz, C., 1977, Abnormal interhemispheric connections in the visual system of Boston Siamese cats: A physiological study, *J. Comp. Neurol.* **171**:229–246.

Shoumura, K., 1974, An attempt to relate the origin and distribution of commissural fibres to the presence of large and medium pyramids in layer III in the cat's visual cortex, *Brain Res.* **67**:13–25.

Spatz, W. B., 1975, An efferent connection of the solitary cells of Meynert: A study with horseradish peroxidase in the marmoset *Callithrix*, *Brain Res.* **92**:450–455.

Streit, P., 1980, Selective retrograde labeling indicating the transmitter of neuronal pathways, *J. Comp. Neurol.* **191**:429–464.

Streit, P., and Cuénod, M., 1979, Transmitter specificity and connectivity revealed by differential retrograde labeling of neural pathways, *Neurosci. Lett. Suppl.* **3**:340.

Streit, P., Knecht, E., and Cuénod, M., 1979, Transmitter-specific retrograde labeling in the striatonigral and raphe-nigral pathways, *Science* **205**:306–308.

Swadlow, H. A., and Weyand, T. G., 1981, Efferent system of the rabbit visual cortex: Laminar distribution of the cells of origin, axonal conduction velocities, and identification of axonal branches, *J. Comp. Neurol.* **203**:799–822.

Tigges, J., Tigges, M., Anschel, S., Cross, N. A., Ledbetter, W. D., and McBride, R. L., 1981, Areal and laminar distribution of neurons interconnecting the central visual cortical areas 17, 18, 19 and MT in squirrel monkey *(Saimiri)*, *J. Comp. Neurol.* **202**:539–560.

Towe, A. L., Patton, H. D., and Kennedy, T., 1963, Properties of the pyramidal system in the cat, *Exp. Neurol.* **8**:202–238.

Toyama, K., Matsunami, K., Ohno, T., and Tokashiki, S., 1974, An intracellular study of neuronal organization in the visual cortex, *Exp. Brain Res.* **21**:45–66.

Weisberg, J. A., and Rustioni, A., 1976, Cortical cells projecting to the dorsal column nuclei of cats: An anatomical study with the horseradish peroxidase technique, *J. Comp. Neurol.* **168**:425–437.

White, E. L., 1979, Thalamocortical synaptic relations: A review with emphasis on the projections of specific thalamic nuclei to the primary sensory areas of the neocortex, *Brain Res. Rev.* **180**:275–312.

Wickelgren, B. G., and Sterling, P., 1969, Influence of visual cortex on receptive fields of cat superior colliculus, *J. Neurophysiol.* **32**:16–23.

Winfield, D. A., Gatter, K. C., and Powell, T. P. S., 1975, Certain connections of the visual cortex of the monkey shown by the use of horseradish peroxidase, *Brain Res.* **92**:456–461.

Wise, S. P., 1975, The laminar organization of certain afferent and efferent fiber systems in the rat somatosensory cortex, *Brain Res.* **90**:139–142.

Wise, S. P., and Jones, E. G., 1976, The organization and postnatal development of the commissural projection of the rat somatic sensory cortex, *J. Comp. Neurol.* **163**:313–343.

Wise, S. P., and Jones, E. G., 1977a, Cells of origin and terminal distribution of descending projections of the rat somatic sensory cortex, *J. Comp. Neurol.* **175**:129–158.

Wise, S. P., and Jones, E. G., 1977b, Topographic and columnar distribution of the corticotectal projection from the rat somatic sensory cortex, *Brain Res.* **133**:223–235.

Wise, S. P., and Jones, E. G., 1978, Development studies of thalamocortical and commissural connections in the rat somatic sensory cortex, *J. Comp. Neurol.* **178**:187–208.

Wise, S. P., Murray, E. A., and Coulter, J. D., 1979, Somatotopic organization of corticospinal and corticotrigeminal neurons in the rat, *Neuroscience* **4**:65–78.

Wong-Reily, M. T. T., 1974, Demonstration of geniculo-cortical and callosal projection neurons in the squirrel monkey by means of retrograde axonal transport of horseradish peroxidase, *Brain Res.* **79:**267–272.

Zant, J. D., and Strick, P. L., 1978, The cells of origin of interhemispheric connections in the primate motor cortex, *Soc. Neurosci. Abstr.* **4:**308.

Zarzecki, P., Shinoda, Y., and Asanuma, H., 1978, Projections from area 3a to the motor cortex by neurons activated from group I muscle afferents, *Exp. Brain Res.* **33:**269–282.

Index